CATARACT SURGERY
AND ITS COMPLICATIONS

CATARACT SURGERY AND ITS COMPLICATIONS

NORMAN S. JAFFE, M.D., F.A.C.S., F.I.C.S.

Clinical Professor of Ophthalmology, Bascom Palmer Eye Institute,
University of Miami School of Medicine;
Chairman, Department of Ophthalmology, St. Francis Hospital,
Miami Beach, Florida

THIRD EDITION

with 1283 illustrations

The C. V. Mosby Company

ST. LOUIS • TORONTO • LONDON   1981

THIRD EDITION

The C. V. Mosby Company
11830 Westline Industrial Drive, St. Louis, Missouri 63141

Library of Congress Cataloging in Publication Data

Jaffe, Norman S   1924-
    Cataract surgery and its complications.

    Bibliography: p.
    Includes index.
    1. Cataract—Surgery.   2. Cataract—Surgery—
Complications and sequelae.   I. Title. [DNLM:
1. Cataract extraction.   2. Cataract extraction—
Adverse effects.   WW260 J23c]
RE451.J33 1980   617.7'42059   80-19355
ISBN 0-8016-2404-5

C/CB/B 9 8 7 6 5 4 3 2   01/B/013

Foreword

No other surgical specialty has been so dominated by a single operation as has ophthalmology by cataract extraction. It is estimated that more than 400,000 such procedures are performed annually in the United States, and many times that number are done throughout the world.

Cataract extraction is a simple, but extremely delicate, procedure. It is amazing that beginning residents may perform their first four or five cataract extractions without a flaw, and that thousands of such procedures may be performed in cataract camps, in about five minutes for each operation, with relatively good results. Yet I am sure that ophthalmologists who find it necessary to undergo the operation themselves seek the best cataract surgeon they know, for they realize that the success of each operation depends on the proper performance of every step of the procedure. The number of significant complications that can occur is astonishing.

The improvement in results and in the management of complications during the past 25 years has not been attributable so much to the increased mechanical skill of the physician as to the development of more efficient techniques and better safeguards such as sedation, the ability to lower intraocular pressure, antibiotics, and instrumentation, including the operating microscope.

• One might wonder how a single person could write a book about cataract surgery and its complications when a panel of experts can spend 8 hours a day for 5 days and still not cover the subject. Dr. Jaffe has done this by being selective in his emphasis of subject material. Yet he has extended his coverage widely, from the decision of when to operate and the psychologic preparation of the patient to the management of postoperative behavioral disturbances. Since each ophthalmic surgeon will have a favorite technique for cataract surgery, this area has been summarized on the basis of principles; yet, since all surgeons encounter major complications if they operate frequently enough, the physiologic basis for normalcy and the histopathologic alterations encountered as a result of the complications have been discussed in detail. The discussion here is almost encyclopedic, and very little could be added to this most scholarly and critical review of all surgical complications during or after a cataract extraction.

Probably the outstanding characteristic of this book is the author's ability to select critically the important contributions to the management of cataract problems. These are analyzed and evaluated on the basis of his vast experience as ophthalmic surgeon and consultant. Greatest attention is given to those areas that he has personally investigated, among them postoperative astigmatism, the management of impending and actual vitreous loss, late rupture of the face of the vitreous, postoperative endophthalmitis, hyperosmotic agents, and intraocular lens implantation.

Dr. Jaffe initiated the popularity of intraocular lenses in this country in 1967. It has been through his leadership that the surgical techniques and the materials for implantation have been constantly improved. Even more important has been his firm insistence that rational guidelines for lens implant surgery be maintained to ensure an orderly growth of this modality of cataract surgery. He has set an example for young ophthalmologists by energetically following the postoperative course of his patients. His statistical presentations have been voluminous. His colleagues have often heard him say, "We want facts, not opinion." Without question, the American Intra-Ocular Implant Society has been of immense service to the public, primarily through Dr. Jaffe's great energies and capabilities.

This book, since its first edition, has been the leading teaching text on cataract surgery of this generation, and it remains a credit to the author.

A. Edward Maumenee, M.D.

Preface

Old concepts change, and new ideas are plentiful in all fields of science and medicine. Cataract surgery and its complications are no exception. I have attempted to be highly selective in modifying older concepts and in including those changes that have gained wide acceptance and new modalities that promise to survive.

It will be apparent that this work is not intended to be an atlas of cataract surgery. Techniques in cataract surgery are presented as method guidelines on which the principles of this operation are based. The emphasis is clearly on complications. Whenever possible, I have made an attempt to correlate the pathogenesis, pathophysiology, and clinical picture of the seemingly endless number of complications that may confront the cataract surgeon. I hope this will provide a rational approach to their management.

Once again, as in the second edition, the innovator of a method has contributed a guest chapter. In addition to Dr. Charles D. Kelman's chapter on phacoemulsification is a chapter on keratophakia and keratomileusis, written by Dr. José I. Barraquer, the acknowledged pioneer of this technique.

It will undoubtedly be apparent to many readers that some subjects have received a greater emphasis than others. These represent areas of my special interest and widest experience. No single surgeon can speak authoritatively about every facet of surgical methods and complications. Nor can every aspect of the subject be covered. To avoid the high cost of an extremely large volume, certain topics such as anatomy, embryology, and the optic correction of aphakia have been omitted.

The major task of keeping abreast of the dynamic changes in cataract surgery is nearly indescribable. I am continually reminded that the responsibility of this and future editions is almost a full-time occupation. Whatever the effort, I have been more than adequately compensated by the gratitude expressed by both residents in ophthalmology and experienced practitioners. What more can one ask?

Norman S. Jaffe

Contents

CATARACT SURGERY
AND ITS COMPLICATIONS

PART ONE

CATARACT SURGERY AND SPECIAL TECHNIQUES

CHAPTER 1

The decision to operate

During the past 40 years, a much more liberal approach to the indication for cataract surgery has occurred among opthalmic surgeons, resulting in some criticism from those who maintain that this more liberal interpretation is not medically, socially, and economically justified. Nevertheless, a poll taken on this subject among ophthalmologists would likely show that opinions vary from never removing the cataract (no matter the state of maturity) as long as the opposite eye enables the patient to "get around" to removing the cataract if it "bothers" the patient (no matter what the state of the good eye).

Ophthalmic surgery has progressed far beyond the era of the old extracapsular extraction when it was almost mandatory to wait until vision was reduced virtually to light perception. The key factors favoring a bolder approach to surgery include the following:

1. Establishment of intracapsular lens extraction
2. Reduction of the incidence of unplanned extracapsular lens extractions
3. Reduction of operative loss of vitreous
4. Refinement of planned extracapsular cataract extraction
5. Introduction of phacoemulsification
6. Improvement in intraocular lenses and lens implant surgery
7. Improvement in cataract spectacles and contact lenses
8. Availability of anti-infectious and anti-inflammatory agents
9. Improvement in sutures and instrumentation
10. Improvement in results

These factors are discussed in other sections of the book. They have brought the patient a long way from the days when patients had to suffer through years of visual impairment before the cataract was "ripe" enough for surgery.

This whirl of technological advances has had an intoxicating effect on American ophthalmology. A dilemma faces every responsible ophthalmologist. The lay press, on the one hand, has heightened public expectation by making the most heroic surgical procedures appear conventional. Consumer groups, on the other hand, label new advances as bordering on human experimentation.

No rigid rules can be imposed on any surgeon or on every patient. Nevertheless, a painstakingly honest approach to the following question must be undertaken. Will the operation benefit the patient? The needs of the patient and not the ability to perform a technically perfect operation is the main consideration. Most elderly, inactive individuals can get along reasonably well with advanced nuclear sclerosis that reduces their visual acuity to 20/80 in the better eye, since they may retain adequate reading ability. However, a relatively small posterior subcapsular opacity may be very disabling even though distance visual acuity in the darkened examination room is 20/40 to 20/50. These patients read poorly and are practically helpless when crossing streets facing the sun. The increasing rigidity and miosis of the pupil with advancing age compound the difficulty. Many tragedies have resulted because cataract patients cannot meet the most imporant physical requirement for a license to operate a motor vehicle: adequate corrected distance visual acuity (usually 20/40 in the better eye).

There are many situations where a relatively small cataract in the axial position may make it impossible for the patient to earn a livelihood. Young patients whose pupils constrict briskly on attempted near vision are especially affected.

In planning cataract surgery on the second eye, one should be aware of any operative or postoperative complications in the first eye. These mishaps show an annoying tendency to repeat. One should be extremely conservative in considering surgery on the one-eyed patient. If the first eye was lost as a result of cataract surgery, surgery on the second eye should be delayed as long as possible. One may be slightly less conservative if the first eye was lost as a result of other nonoperative causes (trauma, infection, and so on).

These considerations are always tempered by the personal experience of the cataract surgeon. Surgeons confident in their surgical ability are likely to be influenced by this confidence in the approach to surgery. On the other hand, a surgical failure in a one-eyed patient is likely to have a sobering influence on the surgeon for the rest of that surgeon's professional life.

The surgeon should never lose sight of the fact that the aphakic eye with 20/20 corrected visual acuity often renders the patient more disabled than a phakic eye with 20/50 to 20/60 acuity. The limited field of vision with aphakic spectacles is an important problem in patients of all ages. If contact lens problems are anticipated because of extreme nervousness, hand tremor, arthritis, ocular allergy, and so on, the surgeon must approach surgery with greater caution. If an intraocular lens implantation is planned, the surgeon must appreciate the greater complexity of the procedure. Every surgeon wishes for the opportunity to reconsider the decision to operate for at least one patient.

There is a wide variance in opinion concerning the advisability of performing cataract surgery on both eyes during the same period of hospitalization. Bilateral cataract surgery on the same day is risky and warranted only in the rarest circumstance. Many surgeons have successfully removed cataracts from both eyes several days apart. The arguments in favor of this are as follows: one hospitalization, one convalescent period, avoidance of the problem of monocular aphakia, and convenience related to employment. These sur-

geons claim that the advantages outweigh the potential hazards: the risk of causing damage to both eyes by infection and injury, the risk of a late complication in the first eye such as expulsive hemorrhage, the risk of complications that tend to be bilateral such as cystoid macular edema, bilateral retinal detachments, corneal edema from vitreocorneal adherence, and the greater stress of two operations performed within a short period of time. Although I cannot document it, my impression is that the incidence of complications is higher. I prefer to postpone surgery on the second eye until I have assured myself that the first eye has fulfilled my expectations. Too often, I have learned something from the surgery on the first eye or from the months after the surgery that I have used with benefit on the second eye. However, I concede that circumstances may occur that favor a short interval between surgery on the two eyes. In spite of this personal preference, I am also aware that there is nearly an equally divided view on whether bilateral cataract surgery should be performed only days apart in each eye or whether a longer interval is more prudent.

There is also a wide diversity of opinion on the need for cataract extraction in the second eye of an elderly patient after successful cataract surgery on the first eye. Although I am aware that many ophthalmologists do not share my view, I am less conservative here. It is my opinion that if the patient had binocular visual function before the onset of cataracts, he will enjoy better visual function if both cataracts are removed. However, if the patient functions well for his needs and is minimally disturbed by the handicaps of monocular aphakia, I would not recommend surgery on the second eye. If the patient wears aphakic spectacles (with a balance lens before the phakic eye) and is suffering from the usual perceptual difficulties associated with monocular aphakia, I would recommend surgery on the second eye. If the patient has successfully managed a contact lens in the sole aphakic eye, cataract surgery on the second eye may not be necessary. The situation with intraocular lenses is discussed in Chapter 5.

PREOPERATIVE PHYSICAL EXAMINATION

Before planning cataract surgery, the surgeon must be made aware of the physical condition of the patient. This is best accomplished by requesting that the patient seek consultation with his personal physician. In many instances it is advisable to share the responsibility of the patient's hospitalization with his physician. This makes it convenient for the latter to supervise the patient's medical status.

Cataract surgery has progressed to the point that only a rare patient need be refused surgery because of physical disability. However, the surgeon must exercise good judgment when considering surgery on feeble, aged, and infirm individuals. Cataract surgery is usually unjustified on a patient with an overwhelming medical problem such as a terminal stage of malignancy. If an intelligent medical workup is obtained, most temporary contraindications may be eliminated.

If the patient is a diabetic, control should be adequate and the diabetic status monitored during the hospital stay. One should never neglect to inquire whether the patient is taking anticoagulation therapy. This therapy should be eliminated to allow the prothrombin level to return to normal before surgery. Severe anemia should be corrected, high blood pressure reduced, and all signs of congestive failure eliminated. Respiratory problems such as bronchitis and asthma should be controlled. The genitourinary tract should be investigated for infections and other problems. Prostatic hypertrophy is no contraindication to surgery because the patient will be permitted early ambulation. With the current popularity of administering hyperosmotic agents preoperatively, it is advisable to employ an agent with relatively little diuretic effect (glycerin) rather that one that might require an indwelling catheter (mannitol). Dental and otolaryngologic consultations should be obtained when indicated. The surgeon should also consider the patient's emotional status. A surgical procedure should not be undertaken on a depressed patient or one whose peptic ulcer is active or whose colitis is uncontrolled.

There is no better ally to the ophthalmic surgeon than the competent internist who has followed the patient for years and is familiar with his personal habits, his idiosyncrasies to drugs, his allergies, and his current medication regime. It is important to know whether systemic steroids or antibiotics may be used safely in case of postoperative complications or as a prelude to surgery

when indicated. I have a special medical clearance form to be filled out by the patient's personal physician. The physician may check a box affirmatively or negatively regarding a desire to observe the surgery and aid in the medical management of the patient while in the hospital. The physician also provides a list of the patient's medications to be used during hospitalization and is asked to sign the form. I confess that other than for medicolegal reasons I have rarely found this beneficial for the patient.

Many hospitals today require certain minimum laboratory tests on every admitted patient. Other tests may be performed as indicated by the results of physical examination or as recommended by the patient's internist.

A careful medical history is obtained, and a physical examination is performed on admission. This may be performed by house staff personnel, the patient's internist, or both.

PREOPERATIVE OCULAR EXAMINATION
Visual acuity

Visual acuity should be determined for both near and far distance. One should attempt to estimate the degree of visual impairment caused by the lens opacity. Occasionally a patient will have what appears to be a small opacity, but the vision may be reduced to low levels. However, using a direct ophthalmoscope or a Hruby lens, the examiner may observe badly distorted fundus details. This is seen in patients with nuclear sclerosis with a disorganized nucleus and with posterior subcapsular cataracts. If an indirect ophthalmoscope with its greater light intensity is used, this important finding may be missed completely, and the patient may be denied cataract surgery because the media appeared too clear to reduce vision severely. Retinoscopy is also useful in evaluating the media.

The surgeon should suspect the added factor of macular dysfunction if in the presence of nuclear sclerosis near vision is diminished more than far vision, since the opposite is the rule. Axial opacities cause greater impairment of near than of far vision, and they also cause greater disturbance in bright illumination than in dim light. In this regard, one does not properly estimate the patient's disability if the examination is performed in relative darkness. A simple technique is to flash a penlight into the patient's eye while he reads the vision chart. If the patient has difficulty making out the larger letters, he will have a serious visual handicap outdoors. As mentioned previously, 20/30 visual acuity may be reduced to finger counting in a patient with an axial cataract whose eye is illuminated by a light or in the sun.

These examples emphasize that the surgeon should not be influenced by a number for visual acuity. An acuity of 20/80 for one patient may represent a level of impairment entirely different from that of 20/80 for another patient.

Occasionally the patient will volunteer the statement that the eye under consideration for surgery was always a poor eye. If the cataract does not appear dense enough to reduce vision to the low level found, macular degeneration, optic nerve disease, or amblyopia may be present. There are two useful tests that can be applied. Place a variable-density or a light-polarizing filter (Polaroid) before the eye being tested. If the eye is amblyopic, little or no reduction in visual acuity will be found. If macular degeneration is present, a sharp reduction in acuity occurs. Additional information may be obtained by performing what amounts to a modified photostress test. If the patient's vision is markedly depressed after indirect ophthalmoscopy with use of at least 6 volts of illumination and if it requires an inordinately long time to recover, a maculopathy may be suspected. Amblyopia may be suspected if strabismus is present or if a past history of strabismus is reported. It may also be anticipated if the glasses worn by the patient show considerably more hypermetropic or astigmatic correction in the eye being considered for surgery.

For further testing for amblyopia, two additional techniques are available. If the lens opacity is not too dense and the macular reflex can be observed by the examiner, the fixation pattern can be tested with a visuscope. If the macula cannot be seen clearly, the afterimage transfer test may be used.[1] If the "transferred" afterimage runs vertically through the dot, fixation in the tested eye is centric. If it consistently falls either to the left or right of the dot, fixation is eccentric. Occasionally in cases of deep suppression a contralateral awareness of the afterimage will not be appreciated, and the second eye will not report an afterimage. In this case the test is of no value.

The Haidinger brush test may also provide information concerning the macula if the cataract is not too dense. Since many patients with normal maculas do not appreciate Haidinger's brushes, a negative response is difficult to interpret. However, a positive response is a very favorable sign.

Visual fields

With a cataract of little or moderate density, a careful and accurate visual field examination is possible. Less sophisticated methods must be used when cataracts reduce visual acuity to a range from 20/200 to light perception. The Amsler grid is useful in detecting a central scotoma or metamorphopsia except when vision is diminished to a very low level. Peripheral fields may be tested by the finger counting method or the technique of Kestenbaum.[2] Unless the cataract is very dense the patient should be able to count fingers held 1 foot from the eye at an angle of 45 degrees to the fixation target (examiner's nose or face). Tests used when acuity is reduced to hand movements or light perception are described subsequently.

Intraocular pressure

It is probably superfluous to emphasize the necessity to check the intraocular pressure of the eye, preferably by applantation, before cataract surgery. Glaucoma secondary to an intumescent lens, a phacolytic process, a subluxated lens, uveitis, a hemolytic process, or progressive narrowing of the angle of the anterior chamber will alter the technique of surgery.

Gonioscopy

If the intraocular pressure is elevated, the angle should be visualized. Chronic and subacute narrow-angle glaucoma can be effectively treated by removing the cataract and performing a sector or peripheral iridectomy. The ingenuity of the surgeon is tested when the pressure is above normal in the presence of an open angle or a traumatically recessed angle. This is discussed on p. 231.

Slit lamp examination

The health of the cornea should be estimated. The presence of an endothelial dystrophy of the Fuchs type influences the prognosis and also the choice of surgery (p. 338). There is no sure way of distinguishing cases of cornea guttata that remain unchanged indefinitely from those that are merely a prelude to a full-blown Fuchs' dystrophy.

The presence of keratitic precipitates or an active iridocyclitis may be detected. Posterior synechiae and their location should be noted. The presence of a tremulous iris points to subluxation or dislocation of the lens. The iris should be examined for rubeosis, which might indicate a central vein thrombosis concealed by the cataract. The type of cataract and the condition of the capsule can best be evaluated by slit lamp examination.

It is often possible to determine the health of the vitreous. Extensive liquefaction or cellular infiltration is often caused by a posterior uveitis.

Examination of the pupils

If the pupil reacts sluggishly to light on direct stimulation but briskly on indirect stimulation (Marcus Gunn pupil), the prognosis for restoration of central vision is extremely questionable.

The ability of the pupil to dilate adequately should be estimated before surgery. If the pupil demonstrates senile rigidity or fails to dilate adequately because of long-term miotic therapy, a sector iridectomy and marginal sphincterotomies, or both, should be considered. A soft cataract can easily be molded through a small pupil, but attempts to deliver an intumescent lens through an inadequate pupillary opening are fraught with danger of capsular rupture and loss of vitreous.

Fundus examination

Unless the cataract is almost mature, a reasonably adequate fundus examination is usually possible. Developmental anomalies such as coloboma, inflammatory changes, degenerative lesions, and other abnormalities should be noted so that a reasonable preoperative visual prognosis may be offered. The indirect ophthalmoscope with its intense illumination system is invaluable in this regard.

EVALUATION OF THE EYE WITH AN ADVANCED OR MATURE CATARACT

The attempt of the ophthalmologist to predict the visual potential of the eye with a mature cataract is no simple task. Normally, if the eye accurately projects light and can perceive colors, the prognosis for visual improvement is excellent. However, a pathologic condition that prevents the eye from achieving excellent central vision may exist. Unanticipated macular degeneration or partial optic atrophy, for example, may be found after the cataract is removed.

The following information is helpful in estimating the visual potential of the eye with a mature cataract.

History

There is no more valuable information than an accurate report of an examination performed previously by another ophthalmologist. If an ophthalmologist examined the eye in the early stage of the cataract, valuable information regarding the fundus will be available. In the absence of such an examination the patient may be able to supply useful data concerning the vision of the eye before the cataract developed. He may state that the eye turned early in life and never saw well or that the eye was always very nearsighted. However, one should not write off an eye, since this information might merely indicate that a corrective lens or a stronger lens was required for this eye than for the "good" eye.

Light perception

If the eye has no light perception, one may safely assume that a favorable prognosis for visual improvement is nil.

Light projection

The ability to accurately project light is encouraging. It usually informs us that a large retinal detachment or an absolute visual field defect is not present. The test, however, tells us nothing about the condition of the macula.

Two-light discrimination

The ability to distinguish two lights close together is a good sign and informs us a little more about retinal function. The test is best performed with two transilluminator bulbs of equal intensity.

Color perception

If the patient can accurately report colors, it usually indicates that some macular function is present and that the optic nerve is relatively normal. If the patient cannot perceive colors, the prognosis is poor but not necessarily hopeless. Glaucomatous excavation of the disc, macular degeneration, and a vitreous hemorrhage may cause faulty color perception. One should not depend on normal color perception to indicate a normal macula. It is seldom that a patient with macular degeneration cannot pass the color test.

The possibility of congenitally deficient color perception must be considered. In such a case, the opposite eye will also be affected.

Entoptic visualization

The entoptic visualization test for estimation of visual potential was described originally by Eber[3] in 1922 and by Friedman[4] in 1931. The light of a transilluminator is pressed against the sclera through the skin of the eyelid while the eye remains closed. The light is gently moved to and fro. An alternate, and perhaps better, method is to have the patient cover the eye not being tested with his hand. He is asked to rotate his eyes so as to expose the temporal portion of the globe of the eye being tested. This eye is left open. The light bulb of the transilluminator is moved up and down close to the globe over the area of insertion of the lateral rectus muscle. The patient is asked to report what he sees. His response should be the equivalent of a pattern similar to the veins of a leaf. The ability to detect this image provides a favorable impression of retinal function. The claim that the patient will be able to detect a patch of choroiditis, his own retinal detachment, or a macular degeneration has proved, in my experience at least, to be somewhat overenthusiastic. However, the test is a good one, is easy to perform, and provides some important information about retinal function. Absence of the pattern is significant only if it is present in the fellow seeing eye.

Maddox rod test

Another reliable test similar in its purpose to light projection is the Maddox rod test. The patient is asked to fixate the light of a transilluminator head at a distance of $\frac{1}{3}$ of a meter through a Maddox rod in a trial frame or a hand-held Maddox rod with the opposite eye occluded. If he can perceive a vertical and horizontal bar of light, it indicates good retinal function. A break or distortion in the center of the bar of light may indicate a macular lesion. The test is somewhat more meaningful if it is performed with a red Maddox rod, since it tells us something about color perception. The Maddox rod should also be rotated so the various oblique meridians can be tested. I have found this to be one of the most useful of all tests for retinal function in any eye with an advanced cataract. Occasionally this test may fail in an eye with a totally opaque lens. The patient may report the line to be a string of beads or some equivalent of this. I am aware of a recent case in which the examiner only tested the vertical meridian and after removal of the cataract found a nasal retinal detachment with a large dialysis. Testing various meridians may reveal a retinal detachment or a glaucomatous field defect. The examiner should become very familiar with this test because ability to interpret the response of the patient will improve with experience. I use it on every patient before cataract extraction.

Afterimage transfer test

The afterimage transfer test has been mentioned previously and sometimes is possible in the presence of a mature cataract. But it is less useful for a patient with a mature cataract because it is often too complicated. The contralateral awareness of an afterimage gives some indication of retinal and optic nerve function. Its main use is to test the fixation pattern of the macula in amblyopic eyes. An eccentric transfer of the afterimage indicates that eccentric fixation exists in the amblyopic eye. It tells us little about the condition of the macula, since patients with macular degeneration show centric transfers.

Pupillary response to light

A vital test in a patient with a mature cataract is pupillary response to light. A brisk response to direct light and a similar pupillary reaction in the opposite eye indicate good optic nerve function. A positive Marcus Gunn pupillary response greatly dims the outlook for visual restoration.

Ultrasonography

The use of ultrasonography is becoming widespread and has a unique application in the preoperative examination of an eye with a mature cat-

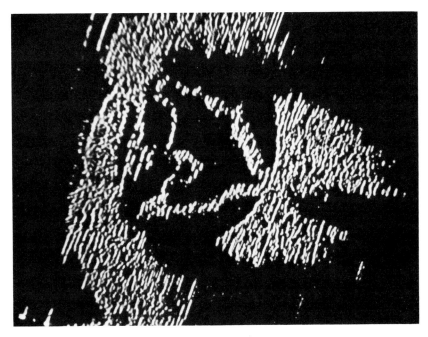

Fig. 1-1. B-scan ultrasonogram demonstrating presence of retinal detachment in eye with mature cataract. (Courtesy of Dr. E. Fineberg.)

aract. In concert with the tests just described, retinal detachment may be diagnosed (Fig. 1-1) as well as other pathologic conditions such as hemorrhage or a tumor within the eye. This method has become increasingly useful. I generally reserve it for patients with a very opaque lens in whom the responses to the previously described tests are questionable.

Electrophysiology

As utilized in most institutions, electrophysiology refers primarily to the electroretinogram (ERG) and the electro-oculogram (EOG). Both these techniques operate on the general principle of alteration of the electrical potential of the eye by illumination of the retina. Dense cataracts are therefore difficult to quantitate electrophysiologically because of the light filtering and scattering effects of the cataract.

The focal ERG has been evaluated in testing macular function. However, the stray light problem from the light-scattering effect of a cataract would militate against the use of this test in cataract cases. The ERG is usually absent in total retinal detachment. The classic use of the ERG is in hereditary degenerative retinal disease, with

retinitis pigmentosa[5] being the prototype. However, the clinician must obtain a history of night blindness or a family history to think of performing an ERG in these cases. Trauma should lead the clinician to order an ERG because of the possibility of detecting a retinal detachment or siderosis bulbi.[6]

The EOG is probably generated by the retinal pigment epithelium in conjunction with the photoreceptors.[7] The EOG light rise is probably generated at the biopolar cell layer. The EOG would be of less value than the ERG because good visual function for good fixation in the contralateral eye is necessary to accurately perform the test. In addition the light absorbance of the cataract is unpredictable and would interfere somewhat with the test. The EOG could be useful in those hereditary degenerative diseases that have a rather specific effect on the retinal pigment epithelium. The best examples in this group are Best's vitelliform macular degeneration, fundus flavimaculatus, the progressive form of retinitis punctata albescens, and extensive drusenosis.[8] However, the clinician would require a family history to suspect the diagnosis unless the EOG was used as a screening test.

Thus if used intelligently, electrophysiologic testing can add objectivity and increased accuracy in the diagnosis of disorders of retinal function in the face of a dense cataract.

PREPARATION OF THE PATIENT FOR SURGERY

There is no place in medicine where expertise in the art of medicine is more important than in the management of the patient who requires ocular surgery. The preparation of the patient for cataract surgery is nearly as important as the operation itself. It is significant that some ophthalmologists appear to harvest the crop of good patients, whereas others inherit the bad actors. Although there is a wide variance in behavior patterns among patients, it is generally the surgeon who makes the good actor. The introspective physician who is quick to recognize the emotional strengths and weaknesses of the patient on the initial office visit is generally most effective in clearing the barriers to a successful conclusion of the case. However, it is admitted that surgeons vary widely in their abilities to effectively combat the emotional obstacles in their patients.

The surgeon usually has a head start in the initial office visit. The patient has chosen the surgeon because of reputation in the community, because of the surgeon's management of friends or others in his family, or because of the recommendation of his personal physician. It is up to the surgeon to justify this initial confidence. Note how often a patient will speak glowingly of a physician saying, "My doctor takes the time to explain things," or simply, "My doctor talks to you." They rarely say, "My doctor eases my anxieties," but this is what they mean.

The surgeon, in preparing the patient for a cataract operation, must impart the impression that it is a team effort with the surgeon and the patient as the principal players but with the surgeon as the ultracompetent head coach. There is ample justification for minimizing the ordeal of surgery, although forthrightness in discussing the visual potential of the eye after surgery is mandatory. This is the basis of informed consent. This subject has become very complex in recent years. Unfortunately, most cases of legal litigation following a poor surgical result focus on improper informed consent. Therefore the surgeon must make an effort to properly inform the patient about possible complications in language understandable by the patient. This is done for two reasons: one, for the benefit of the patient so that he is placed in a position to make as intelligent a decision as possible in deciding whether he consents to have the surgery performed, and the other, for medicolegal reasons, so that a jury will agree that the surgeon has made a sincere effort to adequately inform the patient. It is a pity that there are no exact guidelines for proper informed consent. Many forms are available. They must be simple, in the language of the nonphysician, and not too long. There are also commercially available documents that include diagrams. These are signed by the patient and, preferable, the spouse or nearest of kin. I am in favor of a universal informed consent form composed by a joint committee of ophthalmologists and attorneys that can be used in all communities. I hope such a form will be forthcoming.

I personally find it rewarding to compliment the patient frequently on his behavior and cooperation. He will usually respond by saying, "Every doctor tells me that." He will then make a special effort to maintain this reputation. It is surprising how often the patient who appears frightened beyond description about the impending surgery turns out to be a model of cooperation during the operation. I regard with suspicion the actor who shrugs off everything and appears to whistle in the dark. He is less predictable.

Surgeons must never lose sight of the fact that they are dealing with the patient as a whole and not with just a particular ailment. Most elderly patients will accept the fact of the cataract as another sign of the aging process. However, the reaction in younger patients is often quite different. They may consider it a sign of premature deterioration in all parts of the body, or may merely react bitterly to its appearance. The surgeon can help by explaining that the premature development of a cataract is not much different from premature graying of hair and that one would not consider a person unhealthy who has gray hair in his twenties. I find it useful to state that there are no blood vessels in the human lens and therefore the cataract is not associated with any breakdown of the cardiovascular system. The surgeon must leave the impression that although we do not know the cause of most cataracts, we certainly do know that it is not a prelude to a progression of future deteriorations.

Some elderly patients will react to the cataract with a sense of despair. They feel that they are too old to undergo surgery and that they must resign themselves to impending blindness. The surgeon can help by explaining that cataract surgery is not like surgery in other parts of the body, that it is no more life-threatening than dental surgery, that patients even in the 90s can be helped, and that a past history of coronary artery disease or stroke is not a deterrent to a good visual result. It helps to have patients meet other patients in the office who have recently undergone surgery.

Especially among the elderly, old notions must be swept aside. They may remember the ordeal of a parent, a relative, or a friend who had cataract surgery many years previously and underwent prolonged bed rest and prolonged hospitalization. It helps to explain that cataract surgery has advanced a great deal. Bed rest is brief, ambulation is rapid, and hospitalization is short. I like to tell the patient that he will enter the hospital on a particular day, have surgery the next morning, leave the hospital the next morning and return to the office chair in which he is seated a day or two later. Patients like to hear this orderly procession of events.

Many patients dread having surgery while they are awake and ask, "Will I see the operation?" They say, "You will have to put me to sleep." Since I perform nearly all my cataract surgery with the aid of local anesthesia, I tell them that they will not see the operation, that they will be sedated, that I prefer to talk to them during the procedure, and that I want to avoid the occasional problems of general anesthesia such as vomiting. However, I emphasize that I am going to use the technique that I have found over the years to give me the best results and that any departure from this regime would be unwise. The patient's response to this is usually a simple "I am in your hands."

Of almost equal importance to the surgeon's management of the patient is the attitude of the surgeon's office staff. Employees should be friendly and sympathetic. An introspective office assistant who communicates well and recognizes the dreadful anxieties of the patient is of inestimable value to the surgeon. There is no place for gruffness, bad temper, or lack of courtesy. The surgeon does the patient an injustice by becoming indifferent to poor behavior on the part of office personnel. The role of office staff in instilling confidence and in allaying patients' fears is discussed more fully in Chapter 31.

Once the decision to perform surgery is made, the details of scheduling the hospitalization, the surgery, and the room accommodations may be left to the office assistant, who should be well versed in the surgeon's routine. The details of a private versus semiprivate room and of floor, group, or private duty nursing should be discussed. Unless there is some reason to deviate, my routine is to suggest a semiprivate room without private duty nursing. I find it convenient, especially when scheduling elective surgery well in advance, to give the patient or his family a sheet containing the following information. Every ophthalmologist will have personal variations.

POSTOPERATIVE INSTRUCTIONS

Patient

1. Remove the eye shield daily. If there are secretions, take a piece of absorbent cotton or a tissue and moisten with tap water and *gently* remove the secretions from the skin. DO NOT RUB OR APPLY ANY PRESSURE TO THE EYE! Apply the drops as directed. Then put the shield back on the eye, using two strips of clear tape. I recommend that you get Johnson & Johnson clear tape, 1/4 inch wide.
2. Use the medications as directed on the bottles.
3. Return to the office as directed.

Restrictions

You are not allowed to do any of the following things until permission is given by one of the physicians:

1. Absolutely no bending or stooping.
2. Do not sleep on the side of the operated eye.
3. Do not wash hair for 2 weeks.
4. No showers for 2 weeks. A bath is allowed daily if patient is assisted on entering and leaving the tub to prevent a fall.
5. No violent movements of any kind.
6. Do not lift anything weighing more than 5 pounds.

IN THE HOSPITAL

The surgery actually begins once the patient reaches his hospital room. After the laboratory tests previously described, a member of the house staff takes a medical history and performs a physical examination. Unusual findings are reported to the surgeon. If the patient is also under the hospital care of an internist, the latter will aid in the physical examination. This is certainly preferable.

I have found a routine cataract physician's order sheet convenient and efficient. This sheet contains instructions and orders that apply to all patients undergoing cataract surgery but allows for additions and deletions for a specific patient. Digitalis preparations and vasodilators are continued at their usual dosage. The surgeon must be certain that any anticoagulation therapy has ceased and that the prothrombin level is suitable for surgery. If the patient is diabetic, half the usual dose of insulin or oral therapy is given the morning of surgery because breakfast is omitted. I resume normal therapy the next day.

There is a wide variation in preference for premedication among ophthalmologists. Over the past 30 years I have learned to appreciate that the dangers of excess medication greatly exceed the problems of undermedication. In recent years, I have used very little analgesic and antiemetic therapy. I prefer to perform cataract surgery on a patient who is in fit condition to cooperate. If the proper surgeon-patient relationship has been established, the presence of the surgeon and the sound of the surgeon's voice will calm the patient. I have abandoned the use of barbiturates because of their unpredictable effect on elderly patients. I give every patient diazepam (Valium), 10 mg, by intramuscular injection 90 minutes before surgery. This makes it easier for the nursing personnel, an advantage in these days of nursing shortages. The incidence of nausea and vomiting that I now encounter has been reduced to virtual nonexistence.

Preanesthetic medication

Surgeons must establish for themselves a routine of preanesthetic medication that suits their requirements for intraocular surgery. It is impossible and impractical to present a complete list of these medications. New ones and variations of old ones appear with such frequency that the list will be incomplete and obsolete within a short time. Therefore examples of frequently employed medications and their modes of action will be outlined here.

A good regimen is to use a combination of drugs that potentiate each other and at the same time exert a lower total toxicity. Lundy[9] emphasized that a suitable combination of drugs is beneficial, because they mutually lessen the untoward effects of each other. This is safer than using one drug in large dosage.

The combination is usually chosen from groups of sedatives, analgesics, and antiemetics. Until the mid 1950s, the two drugs most frequently used by ophthalmologists in the United States to produce sedation and analgesia were pentobarbital sodium (Nembutal) and meperidine HCI (Demerol). Secobarbital sodium (Sodium Seconal) was third and chloral hydrate a distant fourth.[10]

The medications (and usual adult dose) available for use today are analgesics, sedatives, ganglionic blocking agents, atropine sulfate, and antiemetics.

Analgesics. *Meperidine HCl (Demerol),* 50 mg IM, causes little nausea, vomiting, and respiratory depression. It may rarely cause a severe hypotension. It is probably the best of the analgesic drugs.

Morphine sulfate, 15 mg IM, may be substituted for meperidine but causes more nausea, vomiting, and respiratory depression. It may also block the mydriatic effect of cycloplegic agents.

Sedatives. *Barbiturates* are useful drugs that have different rates of absorption. They will occasionally cause delirium and excessive agitation in elderly patients. Giving the same drug as a soporific the night before surgery helps determine which patients may become agitated on barbiturates. Pentobarbital sodium (Nembutal), 100 mg by mouth, is short acting and is probably the most useful for cataract surgery. Secobarbital sodium (Seconal Sodium), 100 mg by mouth, is also useful. It is shorter acting than Nembutal. Phenobarbital sodium (Luminal Sodium), 100 mg by mouth, is longer acting. Amobarbital sodium (Amytal Sodium), 100 mg by mouth, is also popular.

Nonbarbiturates, such as chloral hydrate, 500

mg to 2 g by mouth, are relatively safe, rapidly effective and reliable. The unpleasant taste and odor can be disguised by the use of the capsule form. They are contraindicated in patients with severe hepatic or renal disease.

Ganglionic blocking agents. *Promethazine HCl (Phenergan),* 25 mg IM or by mouth, not only interferes with neural transmission in autonomic ganglia but has hypnotic, antiemetic, analgesic, and antihistaminic properties.

Perphenazine (Trilafon), 5 mg IM, is almost identical in action with Phenergan.

Chlorpromazine HCl (Thorazine), 25 mg IM or by mouth, may cause a severe hypotension and should be used with caution.

These agents are becoming more popular and are used by many ophthalmologists today in place of sedatives or combined with smaller doses of sedatives.

Atropine sulfate. Atropine sulfate, 0.4 mg IM, suppresses vagal reflex activity and inhibits respiratory tract secretions. Secopolamine hydrobromide, 0.4 mg IM, may be substituted in cases of atropine sensitivity.

Antiemetics. Perphenazine (Trilafon) and promethazine (Phenergan), also ganglionic blocking agents, have been discussed. Dimenhydrinate (Dramamine), also an antihistamine, 50 mg, and prochlorperazine dimaleate (Compazine), 5 to 10 mg, can be taken IM or by mouth. Trimethobenzamide hydrochloride (Tigan), an antiemetic that acts on the chemoreceptor trigger zone, may be given 200 mg IM or 250 mg by mouth.

Antianxiety agents

Diazepam (Valium) has been increasing in popularity as a preanesthetic medication. Like other antianxiety agents, diazepam acts mainly on the central nervous system and has the ability to produce mild sedation in doses that are generally unlikely to cause soporific effects or to adversely affect the clarity of consciousness and the quality of psychomotor performance. For the past few years this has been my favorite preanesthetic agent. I give it to every patient, 10 mg IM. I use no other medication. Chlordiazepoxide (Librium), 50 to 100 mg IM, is probably just as effective. Surgeons should adopt a system or preanesthetic medication that most fits their needs.

Surgeons who are calm and well organized will generally prescribe less medication. Surgeons who perform better surgery only with an extremely quiet patient, will probably order more medication or resort to general anesthesia.

Hyperosmotic agents

Hyperosmotic agents have been employed to soften the eye preparatory to cataract surgery. The two agents that have become most popular in the United States for use in cataract surgery are glycerin administered orally and mannitol given intravenously.

Glycerin. *Osmoglyn* (Alcon) is a 50% solution of glycerin with unsweetened lime flavoring. It is dispensed in a 6-ounce plastic bottle.

Glyrol (Smith, Miller & Patch, Inc., New York) is a 75% solution of glycerin with citrated pineapple flavoring. It is dispensed in a 4-ounce brown glass bottle.

Osmoglyn is slightly more palatable because it is less viscous, but a greater amount must be ingested, since it is a 50% solution, whereas Glyrol is a 75% solution. The preparation is served in a glass containing cracked ice and drunk with a straw. It is given to the patient 90 minutes before surgery, simultaneously with the preanesthetic drugs. Its main advantages over other agents are its convenience, low toxicity, wide dosage range, and low diuretic effect. Many surgeons who have used it state that it causes vomiting in a high percentage of patients. This has not been my experience. I have found that if preanesthetic medication is used in low dosage, vomiting is uncommon. I have observed that the heavily sedated patient vomits more easily. Of course, in the patient with acute-angle closure glaucoma, nausea and vomiting are often present before the glycerin is given. The latter makes them worse. This is not a problem because urine flow rate is about one fifth of the flow rate with mannitol.

Mannitol. *Osmitrol* (Travenol Laboratories, Inc., Morton Grove, Ill.) as a 20% solution of mannitol is intended for intravenous administration. It is given in a dosage of 2 g/kg of body weight. Thus a 70-kg patient requires over 700 ml of intravenous fluid. In actual practice, probably half this amount is adequate. The larger amount involves some risk in the patient with a borderline cardiovascular status. It exerts a marked ocular hypotensive effect but often promotes a disturbing diuresis, which might require an indwelling catheter. It appears to be the agent of choice in the patient whose cataract surgery will be performed under general anesthesia. Mannitol may also be used during surgery, in which case 50 ml of 25% mannitol is given as a rapid bolus intravenously. Several other hyperosmotic agents are available, but they are less frequently used.

Mydriatics, antibiotics, and steroids

Mydriatic eye drops are administered starting 90 minutes before surgery. A variety of agents are available. The most frequently used are phenylephrine HCl (Neo-Synephrine) 10%, homatropine, hydroxyamphetamine hydrobromide (Paredrine Hydrobromide), cyclopentolate HCl (Cyclogyl HCl), and Cyclomydril (composed of cyclopentolate HCl, phenylephrine HCl, and povidone). My personal preference is for one drop of the last placed in the eye to be operated on every 2 minutes for four doses.

Some consider preparatory mydriasis to be a superfluous procedure, since the retrobulbar injection usually provides sufficient mydriasis for cataract extraction. This depends to some extent on the method of extraction and the state of the lens. Erisiphake extraction requires the largest pupil, whereas cryoextraction requires the least mydriasis. Forceps extraction by the tumbling technique requires a larger pupil than the sliding method. An intumescent lens with a tense capsule requires a larger pupil. I prefer to use a mydriatic routinely.

I do not use antibiotics systemically or locally as drops before surgery, although some ophthalmologists find them useful. This is a matter of preference for each surgeon to decide. However, there is little strong evidence at present that they are beneficial (p. 451). Currently, I inject 20 mg of gentamicin through the interior conjunctiva at the conclusion of the surgery.

Steroids, administered systemically, may be useful before surgery in special instances, but they may do more harm than good in routine cases.

REFERENCES

1. Jaffe, N. S., and Brock, F. W.: Some phenomena associated with amblyopia, Am. J. Ophthalmol. **36:**1075-1086, 1953.
2. Kestenbaum, A.: Clinical methods of neuro-ophthalmologic examination, ed. 2, New York, 1961, Grune & Stratton, Inc., p. 92.
3. Eber, S. I.: Autoophthalmoscopy. Subjective examination of the retina, Am. J. Ophthalmol. **5:**973-974, 1922.
4. Friedman, B.: A test for retinal function in cataractous patients, Arch. Ophthalmol. **5:**636-637, 1931.
5. Arden, G. B., and Fojas, M. R.: Electrophysiological abnormalities in pigmentary degenerations of the retina; assessment of value and basis, Arch. Ophthalmol. **68:**369-387, 1962.
6. Schmöger, E.: Elektroretinographie bei Siderosis und Chalkosis, Klin. Mbl. Augenheilk. **128:**158-166, 1956.
7. Arden, G. B., and Kelsey, J. H.: New clinical test of retinal function based upon the standing potential of the eye, Br. J. Ophthalmol. **46:**449-462, 1962.
8. Krill, A. E., and Klein, B. A.: Flecked retina syndrome, Arch. Ophthalmol. **74:**495-508, 1965.
9. Lundy, J. S.: Clinical anesthesia, Philadelphia, 1942, W. B. Saunders Co.
10. Atkinson, W. S.: Observations on anesthesia for ocular surgery, Ophthalmology (Rochester) **60:**376-380, 1956.

CHAPTER 2

Healing of the wound

Our understanding of the complex phenomena associated with the healing of ocular surgical wounds is far from complete because death after cataract surgery is relatively rare. Therefore much of our knowledge is derived from experimental observations in animal eyes. Too often conclusions are drawn from isolated case reports, which, although valuable, can only provide information on wound healing at a specific time after surgery. To understand the stages of healing of the cataract incision, previous investigators have made studies of animal eyes at frequent intervals after surgery. Fortunately, these conclusions are probably valid, since there is not a great deal of contradictory data provided by research in different animals. However, species differences do exist, and therefore greater efforts to obtain human material should be made.

It is ironic that cataract surgeons who studiously involve themselves in every detail of surgical technique and who attack surgical complications with a scholarly approach pay such little attention to the phenomenology of wound healing. They make an incision and expect it to heal. The physiology and histology of the healing of a cataract incision should be understood by all who initiate the process.

The patterns of wound healing will vary according to the location of the incision (corneal, limbal, or scleral), whether a conjunctival flap has been used, and if so, whether it is limbus- or fornix-based. The presence of sutures further alters the healing process. There are different responses to absorbable and nonabsorbable sutures. They are described on pp. 27 to 29. It must also be noted that most cataract incisions are located more toward the scleral side anteri-orly (superficial) and toward the corneal side posteriorly (deep). Thus the healing of the wound usually involves elements of scleral, limbal, and corneal repair.

CORNEAL INCISION

A corneal incision is often performed in the extraction of a lens from an eye that has previously undergone a filtering procedure for the control of glaucoma and in patients with certain types of blood dyscrasias. Some surgeons employ a corneal incision routinely.

Immediately after completion of the incision, the wound edges swell and become somewhat opaque because of imbibition of fluid by the injured corneal lamellae. There is a simultaneous outpouring of exudative material. Thus, as noted by Clarke[1] just before the turn of the century, these factors favor wound coaptation to the extent that the cohesion may be sufficient to withstand the intraocular pressure within 30 minutes of a penetrating wound. However, this union is not uniform along the entire length of the incision. Anterior and posterior triangles result because of retraction of the superficial and deep parts of the wound. The apices of these triangles point toward each other.

Anterior healing

The healing of the anterior triangle is like the reparative mechanism in a corneal abrasion. Healing is accomplished by two mechanisms:

1. Epithelial slide, by which the cells surrounding the epithelialized area migrate to cover the defect[2]
2. Mitotic multiplication of the epithelial cells surrounding the lesion[3]

The slide mechanism commences about an hour after injury.[4] Mitotic activity is observed uniformly around the lesion so that the growth near the center of the cornea is as rapid as that near the limbus.[5,6] Thus the anterior triangle is rapidly filled by epithelium, partly by epithelial slide and partly by mitotic multiplication of cells. It has been demonstrated that the anterior triangle is larger than the posterior triangle and the epithelial plug forms quickly and is well developed in 2 days in rhesus monkeys.[7]

The biochemical role of epithelium in wound healing is significant. Epithelial repair occurs at a much faster rate than stromal repair. The absence of corneal epithelium, however, markedly decreases the normal gain in tensile strength of corneal wounds during healing. This may be accounted for by at least two possibilities: First, oxygen necessary for the hydroxylation reactions in collagen formation gains entrance via the epithelium, and, second, epithelial cells may produce collagen. If, following injury, corneal epithelium is not available, then conjunctival epithelium will migrate in an attempt to provide a stromal covering. However, this epithelium differs biochemically from corneal epithelium. While corneal epithelium contains large amounts of glycogen, conjunctival cells are rich in mucin. Certain polygonal cells, probably of melanocytic origin, which are morphologically distinct from the other cells, have been identified in corneal epithelium. When epithelium is injured, the polygonal cells squeeze through intercellular spaces at the wound margin with ameboid movement. There is simultaneously a loosening of the regular epithelial basal cells, which then slide without losing their characteristic shape.

Epithelial cells elaborate various compounds that in turn influence stromal cells. How this inductive effect is mediated biochemically is unknown. There is evidence that epithelial cells may produce stromal collagen or its precursors. Once stromal collagen has been elaborated, the epithelium is important for production of collagenase, which is necessary for the remodeling of collagen.

Studies of the histogenesis of basement membrane suggest that it is produced by overlying epithelial cells. Bowman's membrane is composed of very fine collagenous fibers that appar-

ently are never replaced if damaged. Rather, an epithelial facet forms to fill the defect. Basement membrane failure after a wound is more significant. Recurrent epithelial erosions are related to inadequate basement membrane repair.

Posterior healing

The endothelial cells produce the collagen and polysaccharides of Descemet's membrane. The collagen is similar to stromal collagen in that it contains a high percentage of glycine and hydroxyproline. However, it differs from stroma by containing no sulfated proteoglycans. The laminated appearance of Descemet's membrane may be due to episodic secretions from endothelial cells. Another interpretation of electron microscopy studies permits the concept of a gradually increased density from endothelium to stroma (p. 553).

The filling of the posterior triangle occurs more slowly. Some[3,8] have noted the presence of a fibrin plug, presumably derived from the secondary aqueous. However, others[9,12] have not observed this plug in man and monkeys. It is not surprising to see this in rabbits, since the aqueous in these animals has a high fibrin content.

The endothelial lining of the cornea, although one cell thick, is metabolically complex and has a wide range of responses to injury. It is not only sensitive to direct and indirect trauma, it can also be seriously damaged by a great many agents that are innocuous to other tissues. The cells rearrange themselves by sliding, mitosis, and thinning. After several weeks the cells appear to be normal, although by specular microscopy they are enlarged, and the cell count is reduced.

Endothelial cells at the edge of the wound commence division within 24 hours in rabbits,[10,13,14] within about 3 days in monkeys,[7] and within 7 to 14 days in man.[15] In rabbits the regenerating endothelial cells assume a fusiform, fibroblast-like appearance, and form a multilaminar sheet. They contain a granular or fibrillar basement membranelike material and secrete a basement membranelike substance between them so that they are sandwiched within thin layers of Descemet's membrane.[16] The latter is apparent at 7 to 14 days as a thin, loose, irregular lamina adjacent to the endothelial cell.[9] This layer migrates over the defect from the cut and retracted Descemet's membrane.[10] The endothelial growth is sufficiently prolific so that it does not stop when the defective area is filled but continues to proliferate until a fusiform scar of cellular tissue is produced over the area of incision. Mitotic and amitotic cell divisions in all phases can be seen. The number of mitoses are greatest during the 24- to 36-hour period. Although mitosis practically disappears from the injured area after 5 days, amitoses are still present after 2 weeks, although the denuded area of stroma is covered in the first few days.[17] Mitoses are not seen in normal endothelium[18] and occur only under unusual circumstances. Amitosis appears to be the method of regeneration of corneal endothelium under normal conditions.[17] If the incisional wound is widespread, repair may be permanently incomplete, leaving unprotected an area of stroma that shows persistent swelling and edema.[19] If a large gape in Descemet's membrane is caused by the wound, stromal fibroblasts may participate in the healing process. They form a plug in the gape that shows no continuity with the curled Descemet's membrane and the endothelial cell layer. After 2 months a more compact Descemet's membrane of about one half the normal thickness covers the wound. The original Descemet's membrane at the wound edge shows no evidence of ultrastructural alterations. The regenerated endothelial cells now contain more mitochondria and less rough endoplasmic reticulum, suggesting a shift from Descemet's membrane synthesis to the metabolic activity required to maintain corneal clarity.[16]

If the posterior wound edges are in good apposition, the endothelial sheet covers it more rapidly, but a poorly apposed wound is bridged by a fibrous scar, which protrudes into the anterior chamber, is continuous with the stromal scar, and is more slowly covered by regenerated endothelium.[16] Endothelial cells are found within this scar.[13] Occasionally an exuberant fibroblastic response may occur, with the eventual production of a retrocorneal membrane (p. 541).

The cut edges of Descemet's membrane make no attempt at union and therefore probably do not reform over the wound. However, as noted before, a new basement membrane is elaborated by the proliferating endothelial cells, at first thin-

ner than the original membrane, then gradually thickening after several months, although rarely attaining full thickness. Of 18 aphakic eyes in patients 57 to 91 years old, Flaxel and Swan[15] found a thin regenerated Descemet's membrane in only three eyes. In all three, lens extraction had been performed more than 2½ years earlier. As mentioned previously, this regeneration of Descemet's membrane is in contrast to Bowman's membrane anteriorly.

Stromal healing

While collagen fibers form the structural meshwork of scar, ground substance is the most extensive component of the corneal stroma. Ground substance is crucial to the determination of fiber size and fiber arrangement. Ground substance consists of a protein core to which are covalently linked many long-chain linear polysaccharides made up largely of disaccharide repeating units. In the disaccharides, one sugar is always a hexosamine (either glucosamine or galactosamine) and the other a nonnitrogenous sugar (glucuronic acid or L-iduronic acid). The protein-carbohydrate combination that makes up the ground substance was formerly called mucopolysaccharides. New terminology has been internationally adopted. Currently, glycoproteins are referred to as proteoglycans, and the carbohydrate chains are called glycosaminoglycans. The proteoglycans normally found in the cornea are chrondroitin-4-sulfate and keratan sulfate. Biochemical studies of corneal wounds have demonstrated that initially all proteoglycans disappear. After 72 hours, chrondroitin-4-sulfate begins to be replenished from extracytoplasmic granules. After 1 month, keratan sulfate begins to reappear and gradually builds up to normal levels. The collagen fibrils that fill in a wound early, before keratan sulfate is available, are very fine and relatively weak. The proteoglycans typical of the cornea are produced only by keratocytes, or corneal fibroblasts. Wounds healed by fibroblasts not originating in the cornea do not produce either of the corneal proteoglycans and may account for an opaque scar.

It has been postulated that material in the ground substance forms polymeric chains that link the collagen fibrils together in a latticework arrangement. Dissolved proteins, salts, water, and cells are contained in this network by physicochemical forces. When the cornea is incised, the ground substance takes in water, which disrupts the collagen fiber arrangement and causes loss of corneal transparency.

Stromal healing is more complex than anterior and posterior healing. It appears to occur from without inward, but the process apparently proceeds less rapidly than originally thought. Purtscher[20] examined human eyes removed 9 and 14 days after cataract surgery and observed that scar tissue extended only to the middle of the incision by the fourteenth day. In cats, normally healing limbal incisions apparently do not attain their maximum tensile strength until at least 6 months after operation.[21] It is now known that the slowness of these reparative processes is such that at least 2 months are required for permanent union of the margins of the incision. The cellular and structural changes involved in stromal healing are more fully discussed on p. 23 under the topic of limbal incision.

While the epithelium covers the stromal defect, a simultaneous invasion of the stroma by polymorphonuclear leukocytes occurs within 24 hours of the incision. Their role is not fully understood, but according to Duke-Elder,[22] it is partly to bring phosphatase into this avascular tissue to supply the raw materials for the phosphorylation necessary for tissue repair. Because of the arrangement of the corneal lamellae, these cells become deformed and streamlined. They proceed in long rows in Indian file. The leukocytic infiltration lasts about 1 week. The leukocytic phase is shortly followed—48 hours after incision—by a macrophage invasion. They enter the cornea from the limbus and accumulate in and near the traumatized area.[23] The macrophage phase becomes more intense, reaching a peak at 7 days. Their role appears to be as scavengers for removal of cellular debris. They later become transformed into keratoblasts, forming new corneal fibers and probably corneal corpuscles.[22] Duke-Elder observed that they tend to become deformed into long, thin fusiform cells with tenuous elongated nuclei. The regenerated fibers do not form a perfect optic medium because although they are smaller than the normal corneal lamellae and are spindle shaped, they are laid down irregularly and run in nonparallel bundles.[22] This avascular form of healing was first studied by Donders[24] in 1847.

Robb and Kuwabara[25] noted in rabbit eyes that leukocytes were found to enter stromal tissue surrounding corneal incisions from the precorneal tear film as early as 5 to 6 hours after wounding. They originate in conjunctival vessels and reach the tear fluid by passing through conjunctival epithelium. Leukocytic concentration is greater near the limbus than the center of the cornea. Their study fully supported the vascular origin of polymorphonuclear cells in contradiction to the few authors[26-28] who still maintain that the origin of inflammatory cells is from in situ differentiation of tissue cells. Their observations also stressed the importance of the precorneal tear film as a carrier of inflammatory cells from conjunctival tissue to corneal wound.

Additional insight into the process of wound repair has recently been provided. The initial phase of wound repair is usually referred to as the "lag" phase. In 1955 Dunphy and Udupa[29] showed that this phase was in reality a period of intense biochemical activity and renamed it the "substrate" phase. This was characterized by a low collagen content and a low tensile strength of the wound and lasted 3 to 5 days. This phase was immediately followed by a sudden intense formation of collagen and increase in wound strength. Weimar[30,31] had previously concluded that the substrate phase represented a period during which the cells in the area of the repair were becoming reorganized and were developing their enzyme machinery preparatory to the synthesis of this new connective tissue. The cells of the connective tissue layer are about 95% fibrocytes. The remaining cells are histiocytes and occasional polymorphonuclear leukocytes.

After a corneal incision the fibrocytes themselves slowly develop into the active fibroblasts. In experiments in rats, Weimar and Haraguchi[32] clearly showed that in corneal wounds there is new enzyme formation, or activation, in the cells surrounding the injured area within short periods after injury to the cornea. This occurs in normally negative (for enzyme activity) connective tissue fibrocytes within 6 to 24 hours after injury. Their work indicated that the wound or injury itself may profoundly alter the enzyme activities of cells within its range of action and within a very short period after injury. This occurs during the lag phase.

The fibroblasts, which arise at least partly from fibrocytes at the wound edge, gradually develop large nucleoli and a large mass of new cytoplasm, which becomes oriented between 24 to 48 hours to the familiar spindle shape.[33,34] 5-Nucleotidase and succinic dehydrogenase, as well as the formalin-resistant oxidase, were shown by Weimar and Haraguchi[32] to be intensely active in this newly formed cytoplasm, although normal corneal fibrocytes were entirely negative. Somewhat later, about 4 days after injury, enzyme activity began in the basal cell layers of the epithelium adjacent to the active fibroblasts in the wound. This activation also occurs in the endothelial cells.

The new connective tissue derived from the stroma pushes the epithelial plug toward the surface and simultaneously fills out the posterior triangle so that the cornea gradually returns to normal layering. However, it is at least a month before this new connective tissue has fully consolidated.[20,35] The eventual contraction of this tissue, which unites the two lips of the wound, makes the scar diminish in extent and may even make the edges of Bowman's membrane, originally retracted, override each other and become convoluted.[22]

LIMBAL INCISION

To this point we have only considered incisions located within the cornea. However, the classical limbal incision made in cataract surgery shows a similar healing mechanism with some variations. The epithelial plug that fills the open anterior triangle in a corneal wound is partially replaced by a mass of highly vascularized granulation tissue derived from the episclera. When a conjunctival flap is employed, the epithelium is prevented from entering the anterior triangle. The latter is filled by a fibrinous exudate derived

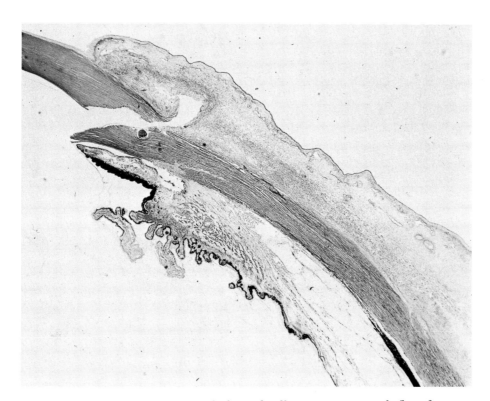

Fig. 2-1. Five days after surgery, newly formed collagenous tissue seals flap of conjunctiva and Tenon's capsule to sclera. Fibroblasts have not yet grown into stromal wound. Stromal wound separation occurred post mortem. (van Gieson's stain, ×22.) (From Flaxel, J. T., and Swan, K. C.: Arch. Ophthalmol. **81:**653-659, 1969.)

from the subconjunctival and episcleral vessels.[7] This coagulum rapidly causes adherence of the flap to the underlying tissues[36] and later becomes reinforced by an ingrowth of fibroblastic connective tissue and a variable number of vessels. The size of this granulation tissue plug depends on the degree of apposition of the lips of the wound. If this is defective, the granulation and fibrous tissue may not only fill the hiatus but may grow exuberantly and extend deeply into the wound and may even reach the anterior chamber.

An unusual opportunity to study limbal wound healing after cataract extraction was provided by Flaxel and Swan.[15] Eighteen aphakic eyes obtained post mortem from 11 patients were studied. The information, presented later, is highly significant because it not only describes human data but concerns histologic findings in eyes operated on with contemporary techniques.

Fibrin plug. Although Henderson[37] reported in 1907 that human limbal wounds after cataract extraction were sealed initially by a fibrin plug that formed between the wound edges, later and more recent findings dispute this.[7,8,20,36] In addition the retraction of the anterior and posterior edges of the incision to form triangles, as described previously with corneal incisions, was not observed.

Anterior healing

The most significant early finding in eyes operated on with a limbus-based flap including conjunctiva and Tenon's capsule was the firm attachment of the conjunctival flap at a time when the limbal wound edges were still ununited. In a human specimen obtained 25 hours after surgery, the flap was firmly adherent[36] to the sclera as a result of fibrovascular proliferation in the episcleral and subconjunctival connective tissue in the area operated on. In a 5-day postmortem specimen, collagen is present under the flap but is not yet seen bridging the stromal wound (Figs. 2-1 and 2-2). In 8- and 10-day specimens, the conjunctival flap is sealed even more securely to the underlying sclera by thicker collagenous fibers that assume an orientation parallel to the sclera (Fig. 2-3). At this stage the fibrovascular ingrowth of connective tissue barely extends between the outer edges of the underlying stromal wound (Fig. 2-4). In fact, in postmortem specimens ob-

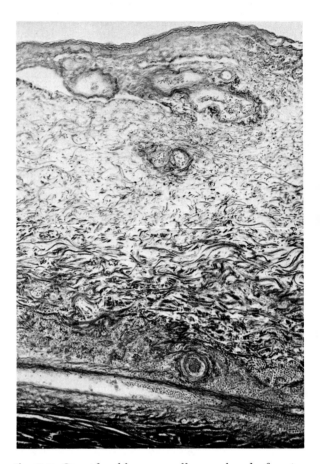

Fig. 2-2. Considerable new collagen already forming under conjunctival flap 5 days after surgery. (van Gieson's stain, ×425.) (From Flaxel, J. T.: Arch. Ophthalmol. **83:**436-444, 1970.)

tained within 2 weeks of cataract extraction, the stromal wounds invariably separate, whereas the conjunctival flap remains secure. Thus histologic findings substantiate clinical observations that the flap strongly supports the stromal wound in the critically important early postoperative period when it is still quite weak.

Posterior healing

Endothelial proliferation was not observed in a 5-day postmortem specimen, but changes in the cell nuclei are frequently observed. In 8- and 10-day specimens, endothelial cells with dark, flattened nuclei and attenuated cytoplasm are observed to cover stromal lamellae where Descemet's membrane is missing. These cells may

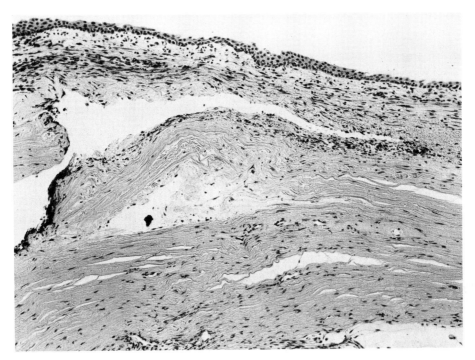

Fig. 2-3. Dense connective tissue sealing flap and aligned parallel to stromal lamellae 10 days after surgery. Stromal wound separation occurred post mortem. (Hematoxylin and eosin, ×150.) (From Flaxel, J. T., and Swan, K. C.: Arch. Ophthalmol. **81:**653-659, 1969.)

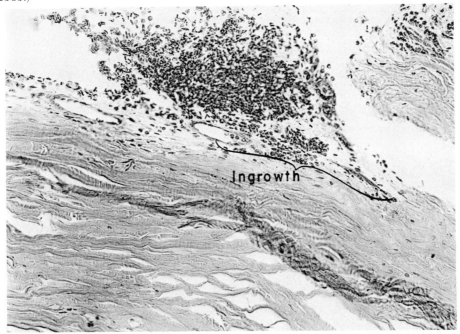

Fig. 2-4. Eight days after surgery, fibrovascular tissue barely extends into stromal wound. (Hematoxylin and eosin, ×255.) (From Flaxel, J. T., and Swan, K. C.: Arch. Ophthalmol. **81:** 653-659, 1969.)

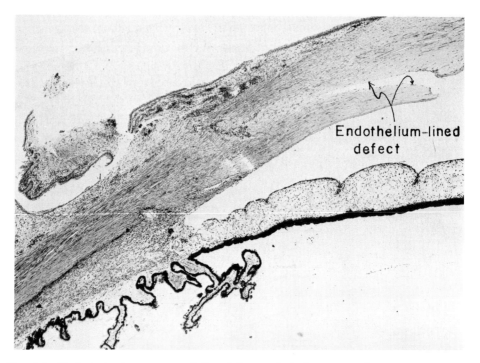

Fig. 2-5. Defect in inner wound lined by endothelium, 32 days after surgery. (Hematoxylin and eosin, ×39.) (From Flaxel, J. T., and Swan, K. C.: Arch. Ophthalmol. **81**:653-659, 1969.)

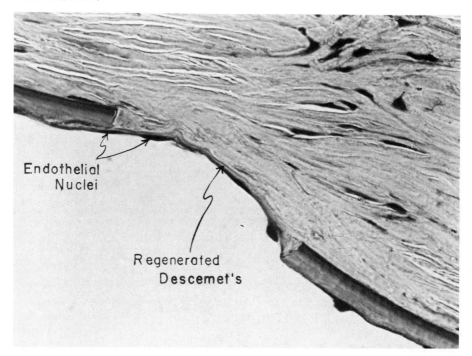

Fig. 2-6. Descemet's membrane partially regenerated in this specimen, 2½ years after surgery. Note flattened endothelial nuclei. (Hematoxylin and eosin, ×595.) (From Flaxel, J. T., and Swan, K. C.: Arch. Ophthalmol. **81**:653-659, 1969.)

even bridge over the incised edge of Descemet's membrane onto the edges of adjacent lamellae exposed by wound gaping (Fig. 2-5). All later specimens show endothelial repair. Areas of overriding of the wound edges become covered. However, even years after operation the endothelial cells in healed areas still retain the appearance of flattened nuclei and attenuated cytoplasm. In fact the endothelial cell counts in both the upper and lower angles remain significantly reduced. As mentioned previously, the new Descemet's membrane is elaborated by the proliferating endothelial cells, but it rarely gains full thickness (Fig. 2-6).

Stromal healing

Descemet's membrane very frequently shows no evidence of regeneration, although regeneration may be partially present in some specimens. Its incised ends remain bridged by endothelium.

As early as 1907, Henderson[37] showed that after cataract extraction, human limbal wounds healed by primary union resulting from an ingrowth of subconjunctival tissue into the wound

that begins by the third day and is well advanced by the seventh day. Purtscher[20] also made observations in the human eye and reported that the ingrowth of connective tissue reached the midportion of the stromal wound 14 days after surgery. Henderson[37] found it there by 7 days. Dunnington and Regan[38] reported that in monkeys the ingrowth reached the middle level in only 2 days. This does not indicate firm healing because, as observed previously, postmortem handling of specimens 2 weeks or sooner after cataract surgery easily disrupts the stromal wound, although the conjunctival flap remains sealed to the underlying sclera. The recent study of Flaxel and Swan[15] showed that the 15-day specimen was the earliest in which connective tissue ingrowth extended through the entire thickness of the wound (Figs. 2-7 and 2-8). Thus stromal wounds are sealed by an ingrowth of subepithelial connective tissue, whereas stromal fibrocytes are inactive and appear to play little or no role in wound healing. At first the cells and fibers run parallel to the incision, demonstrating weak union of the incised edges (Fig. 2-9). However,

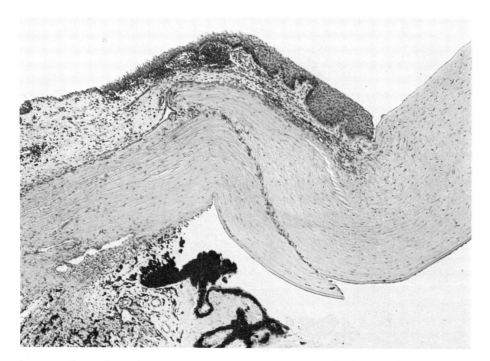

Fig. 2-7. Fifteen days after surgery, connective tissue extends through full thickness of stromal wound. (Hematoxylin and eosin, ×82.) (From Flaxel, J. T., and Swan, K. C.: Arch. Ophthalmol. **81:**653-659, 1969.)

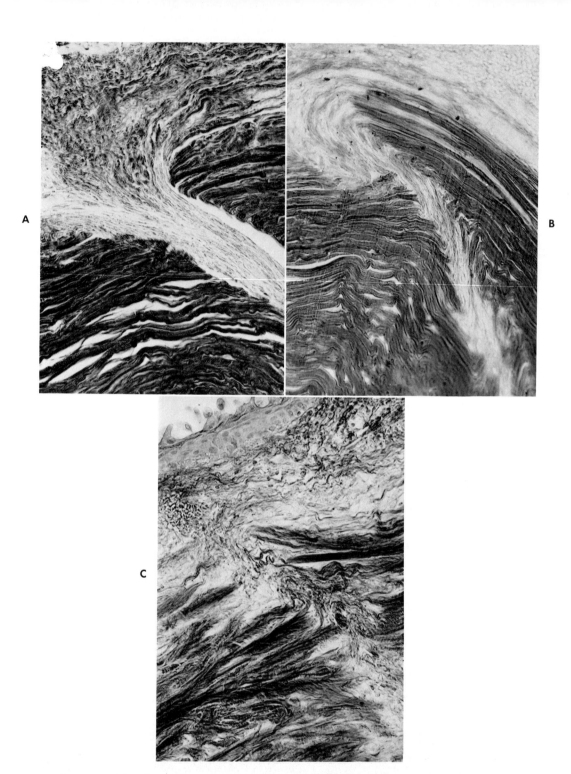

Fig. 2-8. A, Ten days after surgery, scanty collagen in ingrowth. **B,** Fifteen days after surgery, collagen in ingrowth (which now extends through full thickness of stromal wound) is moderately dense and actually bridges wound to unite incised lamellae. **C,** Forty-six days after surgery, collagen fibers bridging wound are still thin and irregularly aligned. (van Gieson's stain, ×425.) (From Flaxel, J. T.: Arch. Ophthalmol. **83:**436-444, 1970.)

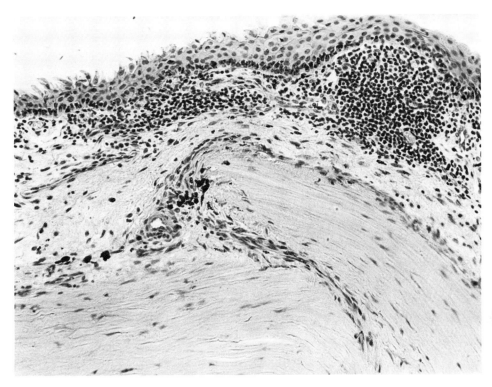

Fig. 2-9. Fifteen days after surgery, orientation of fibrovascular ingrowth parallel to incision, demonstrating weak union of incised edges. (Hematoxylin and eosin, ×255.) (From Flaxel, J. T., and Swan, K. C.: Arch. Ophthalmol. **81:**653-659, 1969.)

remodeling of the wound then occurs. This process is sufficiently slow so that in a well-closed incision the central portion of the stroma may show cells and fibers parallel to the corneal lamella after 2 months, but the anterior and posterior portions of the wound still demonstrate weak union. It may take as long as 2 years or more for full remodeling of the wound to occur (Fig. 2-10).

The process of wound remodeling is still poorly understood. Although fibroblasts in maturing connective tissue may either disappear or lose their proliferative capacity and become fibrocytes, the cells seem to retain some ability to synthesize mucopolysaccharide ground substance and collagen precursors.[39] This is in agreement with the current concept that wound remodeling may occur by deposition and resorption of collagen.[40,41] Hypercellularity and connective tissue ingrowth gradually disappear simultaneously with wound contraction. The prolonged period of wound remodeling and collagen maturation in

human limbal incisions (2 to 3 years) has been observed in other tissues.[42,43]

The practical points to be learned from this discussion are the importance of the conjunctival flap (in conjunction with sutures) for early wound support and the long delay in stromal wound healing. Since the subepithelial connective tissue is the prime source of healing for the flap and the underlying stroma, there should be minimal dissection, cauterization, irrigation, and sponging, which may destroy this tissue, incite excessive inflammation, and prolong healing.

SCLERAL INCISION

Healing of a scleral incision differs greatly from that of corneal and limbal incisions. When the sclera is incised, its fibers do not swell but rather tend to contract. There are no epithelial or endothelial surfaces to bridge across the gap, and the stromal cells of the sclera take little part, if any at all, in the healing of a wound so that heal-

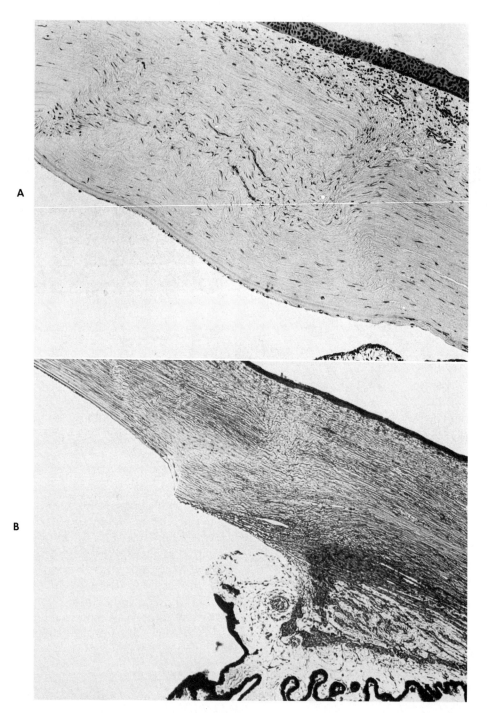

Fig. 2-10. A, Fifteen months after surgery, remodeling of stromal wound still incomplete. Ingrowth of connective tissue remains in outer part of stromal wound. (Hematoxylin and eosin, ×170.) **B,** Two and one half years after operation, stromal wound well remodeled. Dense subepithelial connective tissue resembles sclera. Endothelium bridges overriding inner wound edge. (Hematoxylin and eosin, ×71.) (From Flaxel, J. T., and Swan, K. C.: Arch. Ophthalmol. **81:**653-659, 1969.)

ing by primary intention does not occur. Instead, highly vascularized tissues on one side or the other, the episclera or the uvea, actively participate in the repair while the sclera itself plays a more or less passive role.

Within the first 24 hours after a scleral incision the region is invaded by leukocytes, which originate from all the vessels in the neighborhood. Their role is mainly phagocytic, since their function is to remove injured tissues. After 48 hours, in uncomplicated healing, the leukocytes have in large part disappeared, and the picture is dominated by the activity of histiocytes and vascular elements mainly derived from extrascleral tissues, particularly episclera and conjunctiva. The sclera[44] itself remains relatively inert, with the edges of the wound remaining clear cut while the proliferating fibrous tissue runs in between them at right angles.[45] Several weeks are necessary before wound remodeling progresses to the point when the fibers of the new scar run in the same direction as those of the normal sclera. The scar can always be distinguished from the normal tissue by the close packing of its fibers, their lack of regimentation bundles, and the absence of lymphatic spaces.[44] Scattered pigmentation of the scar because of inclusion of uveal chromatophores and pigment granules derived from the underlying uvea is frequently seen. The conjunctiva becomes fused to the scar.

Healing of a scleral incision therefore has been related to healing of the dermis of the skin by secondary intention.[46] What has been outlined here apparently indicates that a scleral incision does not heal as effectively as limbal and corneal incisions. However, when a scleral incision is used during cataract surgery, it usually does not remain scleral in its entire depth. It is usually beveled or made in planes so that the deeper portion assumes the characteristics of limbal or corneal wound healing.

Corticosteroids. Kirk[47] contributed clinical evidence that corticosteroids interfere with wound healing. Topical corticosteroids were used in one series of 250 cataract extractions but were omitted in a second series of 250 cataract extractions. When corticosteroids were eliminated, the incidence of postoperative filtering blebs dropped from 8.7% to 1.6%. In addition, the postoperative astigmatic error decreased.

ROLE OF SUTURES

Thus far there has been no consideration of the role of sutures in wound repair. Sutures, which bind the lips of the incision and facilitate the process of repair just described, modify the histologic appearance of wound healing. These modifications will vary with the kind of suture material used.

It is apparent that a complex sequence of reparative processes is initiated during the first several days after the cataract incision is made. Healing will be more effective and rapid if the edges of the wound are held in apposition during the first 4 to 5 days. This is the primary function of sutures. Immediately after the incision is made the strength of the sutured wound depends on the holding power of the tissues surrounding the suture rather than on the tensile strength of the suture.[48] Obviously if the tensile strength of the suture exceeds the holding power of the tissues, the suture is of little value and tends to cut through the wound edges.

Silk sutures

Silk sutures are used more frequently in cataract surgery than any other material. However, in recent years catgut has gained increasing popularity. There are marked differences in the histologic tissue responses to silk and catgut. Meade and Ochsner[49] termed healing around silk sutures "dry healing" and around gut "wet healing." The latter is caused by an outpouring of leukocytes and serum in an attempt to digest the suture material.

In general the effectiveness of sutures is determined by the duration of its tensile strength, the tissue response incited by the suture material, the rate at which it is absorbed (gut), and the degree to which it predisposes to infection.[38]

Dunnington and Regan[50] divided the response to silk sutures into the following three stages:

1. Rapid downgrowth of epithelium along the suture tract occurs. Within 2 to 3 days the entire tract is often outlined by surface epithelium.
2. Polymorphonuclear infiltration is relatively light during the first week but then increases, until at the end of the third week the suture is usually surrounded by an area of necrosis.
3. Fibroplastic proliferation in the vicinity of the suture is always decreased and in the presence of marked necrosis entirely absent.

The response to silk sutures is influenced by several factors. The greater the number of sutures, the more intense the cellular response. The intensity of reaction generally varies with the size of the suture. A suture placed too deeply invites cellular proliferation deep into the surgical wound, causing a weaker wound. A too tightly tied suture provides less support to the wound than a loosely tied suture because the tissues caught within a tight suture necrose and liquefy prematurely. This condition encourages the sutures to slough and provides a weaker wound.

Much of our knowledge regarding silk sutures has been derived from postmortem human material and animal experimentation using 6-0 silk. Finer silk and synthetic nonabsorbable materials are now available, and at least from a clinical point of view they appear to provide adequate support and definitely less ocular reaction.

Catgut sutures

Catgut sutures incite a characteristic tissue response, although there are differences between the response to plain and chromic catgut. Jenkins and co-workers[51] divided the cellular response to catgut into two phases:

1. In the leukocytic phase, an invasion of gut by polymorphonuclear cells occurs during the first 72 hours, more intense with plain gut. This subsides with the destruction of the gut.
2. The macrophagic phase occurs 5 to 7 days after operation and is associated with fibroblastic proliferation.

Generally if the leukocytic invasion is severe, the macrophage response is less marked because the suture material fragments are absorbed more quickly.

Dunnington and Regan's[50] well-known study of absorbable sutures in rhesus monkeys revealed that plain catgut incited a rapid polymorphonuclear cellular response, which was noted at the end of 48 hours. On the third postoperative day the suture began to fragment, and by the sixth day it had undergone marked disintegration. There was little tendency to epithelial downgrowth along the suture tract, presumably because of the early disintegration of the suture. At 1 week much of the suture had absorbed, although remnants remained surrounded by round cells, both polymorphonuclear leukocytes and macrophages. At this time fibroblastic proliferation was marked, and there was no evidence of necrosis. During the second week the cellular reaction subsided and the polymorphonuclear cells disappeared. This is in contrast to the response to silk sutures. Fibroblastic tissue became more prominent.

They found that mildly chromicized catgut incited a polymorphonuclear response less marked than that of plain catgut largely in the first 72 hours. During this time there was no fragmentation of the suture, and healing was evident only in the episcleral tissue. Between the fourth and sixth days there was little increase in the round cell infiltration, the suture tended to remain intact, and fibroblastic proliferation became evident. Epithelial downgrowth and necrosis were minimal. At 7 days there was an increase in macraphages surrounding the suture. At this time fragmentation and absorption of the suture occurred. During the second week the episcleral vessels became dilated and were more numerous. There was obvious perivascular cuffing by round cells. Firm healing was evident at the end of the second week. In the third week the cellular reaction disappeared except around residual suture shreds, which then formed the centers of small granulomas.

Jenkins and co-workers[51,52] and Haugaard and coworkers[53] found nearly a complete loss in tensile strength of plain catgut in 5 days. The former noted that the duration of tensile strength of chromic catgut varied inversely with the size of the suture. Chromic catgut sutures of small size retained their tensile strength longer than did larger sutures, possibly because of the lesser leukocytic reaction produced by them.

The rate of absorption apparently varies with the degree of the polymorphonuclear cellular response. Plain gut incites an early tissue response; therefore it is rapidly absorbed. Jenkins and co-workers[51,54] found plain catgut to be completely absorbed after 10 to 12 days, whereas chromic catgut absorbed more slowly and at a variable rate. They stated that if a chromic catgut suture retains its tensile strength for 10 days, it may take as long as 3 to 6 months to undergo complete absorption.

Fechner[55] studied seven postmortem eyes of

four patients who died between the twelfth and ninety-fourth days after cataract extraction. In all eyes, 6-0 chromic catgut sutures were used. He observed that the sutures could remain for as long as 3 months postoperatively. Absorption progressed from the conjunctiva into the depths of the corneoscleral lamellae. The suture tracts may remain open for a long period of time and therefore constitute minor reservoirs for infection. Histologically, the process of absorption presented two stages that were distinctly different. At first, mononuclear cells (lymphocytes, plasma cells, and macrophages) aggregated around and within the suture material. After 2 months a rather dense granulation tissue was found to have infiltrated the suture material. Giant cells were found in both phases. He observed no polymorphonuclear cellular response, but his earliest material was 12 days postoperative, whereas Dunnington and Regan[50] described this response within the first 72 hours.

There appears to be some discrepancy regarding epithelial downgrowth. Fechner[55] observed epithelial downgrowth into the suture tract. Kara[56] reported an eye with chromic catgut examined 4 days after surgery. Epithelialization had already taken place along with sutures. Christensen[57] stated that in two postsurgical specimens obtained after cataract extraction with a limbal-based flap and chromic catgut sutures, epithelium was found to extend along the suture tract in a manner very similar to that with silk. The growth was not exuberant; nevertheless it was present. McPherson[58] showed that epithelial downgrowth occurred around 6-0 chromic catgut sutures in the corneas of rabbits. Thus it appears that epithelial downgrowth may occur with catgut, but Dunnington and Regan's work[50] seems to indicate that the tendency for epithelial downgrowth is much greater with silk.

Any surgeon who has had wide experience with the use of catgut will attest to the wide variability of the absorption rate from patient to patient and even in individual sutures in the same eye. Part of this variability may be controlled by the manufacturer of the suture, but there are many factors beyond their control.

The following are some of the factors that determine the rate of absorption of catgut sutures.

Type of catgut. The United States Pharmacopeia[59] no longer designates absorption according to the number of days. Instead it uses the terms plain, mild chromic, medium chromic, and so on because of the great variability in the rate of absorption. Plain catgut absorbs more rapidly than does chromic catgut because the latter is treated in a chromic salt solution that coagulates the proteins and hardens the suture. The greater the degree of treatment, the longer the suture will remain in the tissues before becoming completely absorbed.

Location of the suture. Catgut sutures absorb more rapidly when inserted in vascularized tissue. Therefore corneal sutures tend to absorb more slowly.

Exposure of the suture. In my experience, when catgut sutures are not protected by a conjunctival flap, they disintegrate more rapidly. Thus, when a fornix-based conjunctival flap is used, the sutures at the nasal and temporal extremities of the wound fragment earlier than those covered by the flap. When the sutures are buried under a limbus-based flap, they persist longer; 7-0 chromic catgut sutures may be placed under such a flap. One can only speculate about the action of the eyelids causing earlier disintegration of exposed sutures.

Size of the suture. Smaller size catgut sutures cause less irritation and tissue reaction than do larger sutures. This delays absorption of the suture. However, most manufacturers chromicize each size of suture to the degree required to ensure an absorption rate approximately equal to that of all other sizes.

Effect of pharmaceuticals. Steroids applied topically are likely to retard suture absorption because of lessening of the inflammatory response. The effect of alpha-chymotrypsin is still unsettled. The role of the elevated intraocular pressure induced by the enzyme is likewise unsettled.

Presence of infection. Infection significantly hastens absorption because of the increased concentrations of proteolytic enzymes associated with leukocyte and macrophage invasions.[60,61]

Physical condition of the patient. Surgical gut is more rapidly absorbed in undernourished, old, debilitated, or anemic patients.[61] It is also absorbed more rapidly in certain neoplastic diseases and febrile diseases. A small rise of body temperature of about 2° may cause a fivefold increase in proteolytic enzyme concentration.[60]

Kind of tissue. The rate of absorption in ocular wounds differs from that seen in other parts of the body. Surgical gut is absorbed more rapidly in serous or mucous membranes than in muscle tissue. Also, the more aseptic the wound, the slower the absorption. For example, catgut is absorbed more rapidly in the cervix or vagina because of the presence of secretions with digestive action.[61]

It is now generally accepted that an absorbable suture in a wound may appear entirely intact yet may have lost nearly all its tensile strength. The tensile strength is usually lost long before it is absorbed. These observations have suggested that when exposed to tissue, an alteration of the molecular integrity of its collagen results that does not involve loss of its mass. These changes are probably caused by destruction of hydrogen bonds and partly by enzymatic attack on the backbone of the collagen polymer. At first only a few bands will be broken, but the loss of these bands will be sufficient to weaken the fiber appreciably. Subsequently, the tissue cathepsins break the collagen down to soluble polypeptides and possibly even constituent amino acids. These are metabolized like any other protein. At this stage disappearance of the suture can be noted.[60]

The tensile strength of sutures is evaluated on the basis of knot strength rather than on straight pull because when breaking occurs, it most often does so at the knot. The ability of a suture to resist the shearing stress imposed during knot tying is significant. The resistance of the suture to shearing stresses is always less than the resistance to longitudinal stress, and therefore the important measurement of suture strength is the so-called knot strength.[60] Standards for tensile strength are set up by the United States Pharmacopeia.

REFERENCES

1. Clarke, E.: Some experiments on the union of corneal wounds, Trans. Ophthalmol. Soc. U.K. **18**:307-313, 1898.
2. Ranvier, L.: Une théorie nouvelle sur la cicatrisation et la rôle de l'épithélium antérieur de la cornée dans la guérison des plaies de cette membrane, Compte Rendu Acad. Sci. **123**:1228-1233, 1896.
3. Weinstein, A.: Experimentelle Untersuchungen über den Heilungsprocess bei perforirenden Schnittwunden der Hornhaut, Arch. Augenheilk. **48**:1-50, 1903.
4. Friedenwald, J. S., and Buschke, W.: Mitotic and wound-healing activities of the corneal epithelium, Arch. Ophthalmol. **32**:410-413, 1944.
5. Rucker, C. W.: Regeneration of the cornea, Arch. Ophthalmol. **2**:692-698, 1929.
6. Benedict, W. L.: Excision of corneal leukoma, Arch. Ophthalmol. **11**:32-41, 1934.
7. Dunnington, J. H.: Healing of incisions for cataract extraction, Am. J. Ophthalmol. **34**:36-45, 1951.
8. Tooke, F.: The pathology of the corneal section and its complications in cataract extraction, Trans. Am. Ophthalmol. Soc. **13**:742-769, 1914.
9. Klouček, F.: The corneal endothelium, Acta Univ. Carol. [Med.] **13**:321-373, 1967.
10. Morton, P. L., and Ormsby, H. L.: Healing of endothelium and Descemet's membrane of rabbit cornea, Am. J. Opthalmol. **46(II)**:62-67, 1958.
11. Werb, A.: The postgraft membrane, Int. Ophthalmol. Clin. **2**:771-780, 1962.
12. Dunnington, J. H.: Normal healing of the cataract incision. In Haik, C. M., editor: Symposium on diseases and surgery of the lens, St. Louis, 1957, the C. V. Mosby Co., p. 26.
13. Maruyama, T., Haruyama, S., and Kitano, S.: Studies on the burn of the cornea. Report III. Autoradiographic observation. Acta Soc. Ophthalmol. Jap. **71**:1112-1122, 1967.
14. Stocker, F. W.: The endothelium of the cornea and its clinical implications, ed. 2, Springfield, Ill., 1971, Charles C Thomas, Publisher.
15. Flaxel, J. T., and Swan, K. C.: Limbal wound healing after cataract extraction. A histological study, Arch. Ophthalmol. **81**:653-659, 1969.
16. Inomata, H., Smelser, G. K., and Polack, F. M.: Fine structure of regenerating endothelium and Descemet's membrane in normal and rejecting corneal grafts, Am. J. Ophthalmol. **70**:48-64, 1970.
17. Binder, R. F., and Binder, H. F.: Regenerative processes in the endothelium of the cornea, Arch. Ophthalmol. **57**: 11-13, 1957.
18. Cogan, D. G.: Applied anatomy and physiology of the cornea, Ophthalmology (Rochester) **55**:329-359, 1951.
19. Heydenreich, A.: Die Hornhautregeneration. Sammlung zwangloser Abhandlungen aus dem Gebiete der Augenheilkunde, Suppl. 15, Halle, 1958, Carl Marhold Verlag.
20. Purtscher, E.: Histologische Frühuntersuchungen nach intracapsulärer Staroperation. (Wundheilung, postoperative Aderhautabhebung and Glaskörperhernie), Graefe Arch. Ophthalmol. **144**:669-697, 1942.
21. Gliedman, M. L., and Karlsen, K. E.: Wound healing and wound strength of sutured limbal wounds, Am. J. Ophthalmol. **39**:859-866, 1955.
22. Duke-Elder, S.: Textbook of ophthalmology. Vol. VI. Injuries, St. Louis, 1954, The C. V. Mosby Co., pp. 5963-5993.
23. Paufique, L., Sourdille, G. P., and Offret, G.: Kératoplasties. Les graffes de la cornée, Paris, 1948, Masson & Cie, Editeurs (Rapport Société Francaise d'Ophtalmologie).
24. Donders, F. C.: Onderzoekingen over afpelling en rege-

neratie van het hoornvlies. Nederl. Lancet 2(series 3): 197-226, 1847-1848.

25. Robb, R. M., and Kuwabara, T.: Corneal wound healing. I. The movement of polymorphonuclear leukocytes into corneal wounds, Arch. Ophthalmol. 68:636-642, 1962.

26. Grawitz, P. B.: In welcher Minimalzeit kann die Hornhaut in situ Gewebeleukocyten bilden? Graefe Arch. Ophthalmol. 164:151-155, 1961.

27. Lassmann, G.: Uber die Entstehung von Leukozyten aus Hornhautkörperchen, Mikroskopie 13:373-380, 1959.

28. Pau, H.: Woher stammen die Leukocyten in der lädierten Hornhaut? Graefe Arch. Ophthalmol. 159:540-559, 1958.

29. Dunphy, J. E., and Udupa, K. N.: Chemical and histochemical sequences in the normal healing of wounds, N. Engl. J. Med. 253:847-851, 1955.

30. Weimar, V.: Effect of amino acid, purine, and pyrimidine analogues on activation of corneal stromal cells to take up neutral red, Invest. Ophthalmol. Vis. Sci. 1:226-232, 1962.

31. Weimar, V.: Activation of corneal stromal cells to take up vital dye neutral red, Exp. Cell Res. 18:1-14, 1959.

32. Weimar, V. L., and Haraguchi, K. H.: The development of enzyme activities in corneal connective tissue cells during the lag phase of wound repair. I. 5-Nucleotidase and succinic dehydrogenase, Invest. Ophthalmol. Vis. Sci. 4: 853-866, 1965.

33. Weimar, V.: The transformation of corneal stromal cells to fibroblasts in corneal wound healing, Am. J. Ophthalmol. 44(part 2):173-182, 1957.

34. Weimar, V.: The sources of fibroblasts in corneal wound repair, a quantitative analysis, Arch. Ophthalmol. 60:93-109, 1958.

35. Maggiore, L.: Ricerche istologiche con deduzioni cliniche sui processi riparativi normali e anormali della ferita corneale e sul decorso ed esito delle varie complicanze negli occhi operati di cataratta, Ann. Ottal. 68:561-615, 641-667, 721-758, 881-913, 1940; 69:1-26, 65, 1941.

36. Flaxel, J. T.: Histology of cataract extractions, Arch. Ophthalmol. 83:436-444, 1970.

37. Henderson, T.: A histological study of the normal healing of wounds after cataract extraction, Ophthalmol. Rev. 26: 127-144, 1907.

38. Dunnington, J. H., and Regan, E. F.: The effect of sutures and of thrombin upon ocular wound healing, Am. J. Ophthalmol. 35:167-177, 1952.

39. Dunphy, J. E.: The fibroblast, a ubiquitous ally for the surgeon, N. Engl. J. Med. 268:1367-1377, 1963.

40. James, D. W., and Newcombe, J. F.: Granulation tissue resorption during free and limited contraction of skin wounds, J. Anat. 95:247-255, 1961.

41. Abercrombie, M.: Wound contraction, contracture and remodeling. In Levenson, S. M., and others, editors: National Research Council, Committee on Trauma: Wound Healing; proceedings of a work shop . . . 5-8 December, 1963; Washington, D.C., 1966, National Academy of Sciences.

42. Verzar, F., and Willenegger, H.: Das Altern des Kolla-gens in der Haut und in Narben, Schweiz, Med. Wschr. 91:1234-1236, 1961.

43. Jackson, D. S.: Some biochemical aspects of fibrogenesis and wound healing, N. Engl. J. Med. 259:814-820, 1958.

44. Duke-Elder, S.: System of ophthalmology. Vol. VIII. Diseases of the outer eye. Part 2. Cornea and sclera, St. Louis, 1965, The C. V. Mosby Co., p. 997.

45. Renard, G., Leliévre, A., and Naneix, G.: La cicatrisation des plaies de la sclérotique, Arch. Ophthalmol. 12:5-18, 1952.

46. Swan, K. C.: Some contemporary concepts of scleral disease, Arch. Ophthalmol. 45:630-644, 1951.

47. Kirk, H. Q.: Corticosteroids as a cause of filtering blebs after cataract extraction, Am. J. Ophthalmol. 77:442-444, 1974.

48. Howes, E. L., and Harvey, S. C.: Tissue response to catgut absorption, silk and wound healing; correlation with tensile strength, Int. J. Med. Surg. 43:225-230, 1930.

49. Meade, W. H., and Ochsner, A.: The relative value of catgut, silk, linen and cotton as suture materials, Surgery 7:485-514, 1940.

50. Dunnington, J. H., and Regan, E. F.: Absorbable sutures in cataract surgery, Arch. Ophthalmol. 50:545-556, 1953.

51. Jenkins, H. P., Hrdina, L. S., Owens, F. M., Jr., and Swisher, F. M.: Absorption of surgical gut (catgut): Duration in the tissues after loss of tensile strength, Arch. Surg. 45:74-102, 1942.

52. Jenkins, H. P., and Hrdina, L. S.: Absorption of surgical gut (catgut). II. Pepsin digestion tests for evaluation of duration of tensile strength in tissues, Arch. Surg. 44: 984-1003, 1942.

53. Haugaard, G., Thoennes, C. A., and Hall, M. J.: A study of the absorption characteristics of surgical gut, Surg. Gynecol. Obstet. 83:521-527, 1946.

54. Jenkins, H. P., and Hrdina, L. S.: Absorption of surgical gut (catgut). I. Decline in tensile strength in tissues, Arch. Surg. 44:881-895, 1942.

55. Fechner, P. U.: The histology of 6-0 mild chromic gut sutures in cataract wounds, Am. J. Ophthalmol. 59: 1019-1034, 1965.

56. Kara, G. B.: Histologic appearance of an eye four days after cataract extraction, Arch. Ophthalmol. 49:285-292, 1953.

57. Christensen, L.: Epithelization of the anterior chamber, Trans. Am. Ophthalmol. Soc. 58:284-300, 1960.

58. McPherson, S. D., Jr.: The use of absorbable sutures in surgery of the cornea, Am. J. Ophthalmol. 51:118-140, 1961.

59. The Pharmacopeia of the United States of America (The United States Pharmacopeia), ed. 16, Bethesda, Md., 1960.

60. Van Winkle, W., Jr.: Physical, chemical and biologic properties of absorbable collagen sutures, Somerville, N.J., Ethicon, Inc.

61. The production and quality control of Davis and Geck surgical gut sutures, Danbury, Conn., B-150-R, 1962, Davis and Geck.

CHAPTER 3

Surgical technique

An increasing variety of cataract extraction methods is being employed, depending on the needs of the patient and the training of the surgeon. The main techniques in use today are the following:

1. Standard intracapsular cataract extraction (ICCE)
2. Standard extracapsular cataract extraction (ECCE)
3. Phacoemulsification (Chapter 6)
4. Intraocular lens implantation with any of the first three (Chapter 5)
5. Penetrating keratoplasty with any of the first three (Chapter 9)
6. Glaucoma surgery with any of the first three (Chapter 9)

Each of these methods has a seemingly endless number of variations. Each surgeon develops a preference; it is really a personal affair. It is beyond the scope of this book to consider in depth all of these variations. It is hoped that a discussion of the important principles of each step of the procedure will be applicable to these variations. Therefore it is with an apology for the unavoidable lack of completeness that this chapter is presented.

Surgeons in training and those most recently trained perform intraocular surgery with the aid of a microscope. However, a significant percentage of surgeons operate with the aid of surgical loupes that magnify from two to six times. Some techniques cannot be safely performed without the microscope. However, most of the surgical techniques described in this chapter can be performed with loupes or a microscope.

ANESTHESIA

Surgeons who prefer general anesthesia for patients undergoing cataract extraction should have available a competent anesthesiologist versed in the special requirements for intraocular surgery. Supplemental orbicularis muscle akinesia and retrobulbar block may be included. The techniques and agents used for general anesthesia in cataract surgery are beyond the scope of this book and are not considered. Except for the rare patient whose behavior is such that general anesthesia is mandatory, I personally find local anesthesia entirely satisfactory and preferable.

After the preparation of the skin with one of the numerous disinfectants available for this purpose (I prefer Betadine solution swabsticks from The Purdue Frederick Company, Norwalk, Conn., the povidone-iodine solution being antiseptic and germicidal), oxygenation of the patient is provided by means of a sterile, disposable nasal catheter (Fig. 3-1). The oxygen input is set at 6 to 8 liters per minute. If bleeding vessels are thermally cauterized, the oxygen supply should be temporarily suspended to lessen the chance of a flash fire. For this reason compressed air is often substituted for oxygen. In addition to the value of the air supplied, the sensation of air entering the nostrils provides a psychologic benefit for the draped patient.

There are numerous methods of draping the region about the eye. I personally find the lightweight, plastic sheet supplied by 3M Company (St. Paul, Minnesota) satisfactory (Fig. 3-2). Since accidental pressure against the patient's opposite eye by the hand of the surgical assistant may cause the patient to move at an inopportune time, this eye is covered with an aluminum or plastic

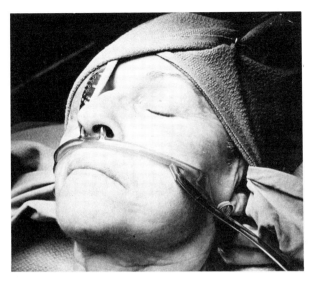

Fig. 3-1. Oxygenation provided by means of sterile, disposable nasal catheter. Opposite eye is covered with shield to prevent accidental pressure against globe during surgery.

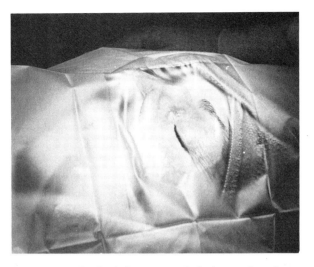

Fig. 3-2. Method of draping with lightweight, plastic sheet supplied by 3M Company, St. Paul, Minnesota.

eye shield, which is covered in turn by the drape sheet (**Fig.** 3-1).

Akinesia of the orbicularis oculi

To prevent the squeezing action of the eyelids during cataract extraction, temporary paralysis of the orbicularis muscle is effected by one of the following methods utilizing a solution of lidocaine (Xylocaine) 2% to 4% (or procaine 2%) with epinephrine 1:100,000 and hyaluronidase, 150 units per 20 ml of anesthetic solution.

Van Lint akinesia[1] (Fig. 3-3) is obtained by infiltration anesthesia in the region of the terminal branches of the facial nerve.

Several milliliters of the anesthetic mixture are injected 1 cm temporally to the lateral canthus down to bone, using a 1.5 inch, 22- or 25-gauge, disposable needle. The surgeon slightly withdraws and redirects the needle along the inferior orbital margin, injecting several milliliters as it advances to the middle third of the orbital margin. The needle is then withdrawn to the site of the original puncture without being removed completely. It is redirected superiorly, and several milliliters are injected along the superior orbital margin until the middle third is reached. Pressure is then exerted over the injected area to distribute the solution and reduce swelling.

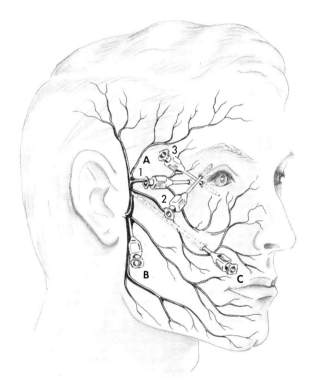

Fig. 3-3. Akinesia of orbicularis oculi. **A,** Van Lint akinesia. **B,** O'Brien akinesia. **C,** Atkinson akinesia.

Modification of Van Lint akinesia (Fig. 3-4) is made by injection of the anesthetic mixture in a vertical direction for a distance of 3 to 4 cm about 1 cm temporal to the lateral canthus. The mixture is then injected subcutaneously along the entire extent of both eyelids. The region of the lateral canthus is included to obtain sensory anesthesia in the event a lateral canthotomy is performed. Pressure over the injected area will distribute the anesthetic as well as flatten the tissues.

The *O'Brien akinesia technique*[2] (Fig. 3-3) obtains a paresis of the orbicularis muscle by blocking the facial nerve at the proximal trunk of the nerve. The condyloid process of the mandible is palpated just in front of the tragus of the ear by

asking the patient to open and close his mouth. The process is felt to slip forward under the finger during this movement. By use of a 1-inch, 27-gauge, disposable needle inserted to the center of the condyloid process at a depth of 1 cm, several milliliters of the anesthetic mixture are injected. The needle should not be inserted into the joint.

Atkinson akinesia[3] (Fig. 3-3) involves an injection made along the inferior edge of the zygomatic bone and then upward across the zygomatic arch toward the top of the ear. The injection is begun at the inferior edge of the zygomatic bone at a point slightly posterior to a vertical line drawn from the lateral margin of the orbit. A 1.5-

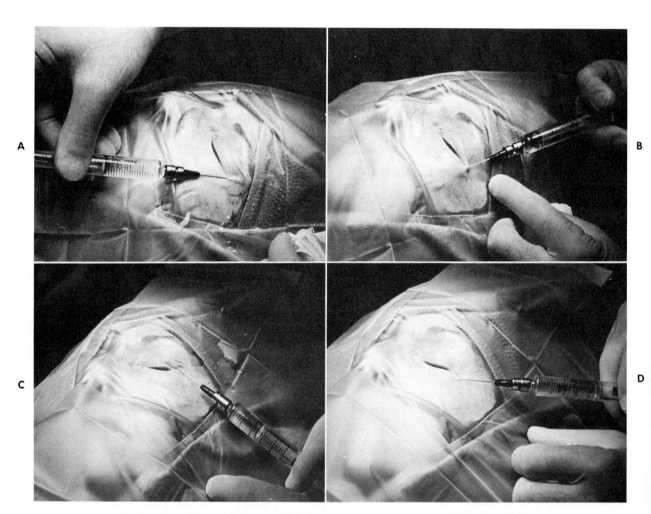

Fig. 3-4. Modification of Van Lint akinesia. **A,** Injection superiorly 1 cm temporal to lateral canthus. **B,** Injection inferiorly. **C,** Injection upper eyelid. **D,** Injection lower eyelid.

inch, 23-gauge needle with a rounded point is used to inject the anesthetic mixture as it advances close to the bone and then across the zygomatic arch to a point just in front of the top of the ear. A total of about 3 ml is injected.

The landmarks are easy to find, and the lower branches of the facial nerve supplying the lips and lower muscles of the face are seldom blocked. However, the claim that ballooning of the eyelids is unnecessary and no longer considered an advantage, since hyaluronidase aids in rapid diffusion of the anesthetic.

Alcohol block is used in patients with a severe facial tic or blepharospasm, since prolonged akinesia of the orbicularis muscle may be advisable. Ethyl alcohol, 25% to 40%, mixed with procaine or lidocaine (Xylocaine) may be injected after a preliminary injection of the anesthetic mixture.

Retrobulbar injection

The intraocular pressure is measured by use of a sterile, autoclavable Schiøtz tonometer.

The anesthetic solution is prepared by dissolving the contents of a 1 ml ampule of hyaluronidase (150 units) in a 20 ml bottle of 2% lidocaine hydrochloride (Xylocaine HCl) with epinephrine 1:100,000. Lidocaine has become more popular than procaine for ophthalmic surgery. Mepivicaine (Carbocaine) is also being used more frequently. It is employed as a 2% solution to which hyaluronidase is usually added. The rapidity of its onset time of ocular anesthesia and akinesia is comparable to that of lidocaine, and it may have a slightly more prolonged effect. In case of allergy to procaine, lidocaine, or mepivicaine, one agent may be substituted for another. Some ophthalmologists prefer a longer-acting agent. Bupivicaine (Marcaine) is ideally suited for this. It is usually used as a 0.75% solution combined with hyaluronidase. Its main disadvantage is its highly variable and often prolonged onset time of akinesia. Its prolonged action is beneficial for long surgical procedures such as scleral bucklings and some vitrectomies, but it is impractical for cataract surgery when used alone. To retain its prolonged postoperative effect and overcome its prolonged onset time, some surgeons use a combination of Bupivicaine and mepivicaine as follows: A mixture of 2 ml of 0.75% Bupivicaine and 2% mepivicaine combined with hyaluronidase is used. One instance in which a prolonged effect is undesirable is with an intraocular lens implantation. The pupil may redilate once the patient leaves the operating room. This may cause a dislocation of an iris-supported intraocular lens.

Two to 4-ml of the anesthetic mixture is inject-

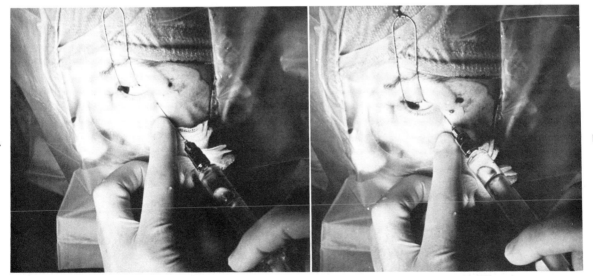

Fig. 3-5. Retrobulbar injection. **A,** Injection made at junction of lateral and middle thirds of inferior orbital rim. **B,** Needle directed toward optic nerve. Solution injected as needle advances.

ed into the muscle cone in the following manner by use of a 1.5-inch, 22- or 25-gauge needle. Although some surgeons prefer to use a dull-tipped needle to avoid perforating vessels in the orbit, this is unnecessary if the solution is injected as the needle penetrates the orbit (Fig. 3-5). The patient is instructed to look up and to the left for the right eye or up and to the right for the left eye. The injection is made through the skin at the junction of the lateral and middle thirds of the inferior orbital rim. The needle is directed toward the optic nerve. If the tip of the needle strikes the floor of the orbit as it is inserted, it is withdrawn slightly and redirected more superiorly toward the orbital apex (Fig. 3-6). The injection can be made in the same manner through the inferior cul-de-sac, if preferred. To be certain that the patient's eye is directed properly during the injection, it is useful to retract the upper eyelid with an eyelid retractor, as shown in Fig. 3-5.

Pressure should be exerted over the closed eyelids for approximately 30 seconds to ensure hemostasis and satisfactory distribution of the anesthetic solution. The effectiveness of the akinesia is tested by asking the patient to move his eye up, down, left, and right. If necessary, the individual rectus muscles may be injected with additional anesthetic solution to obtain more complete immobility of the globe.

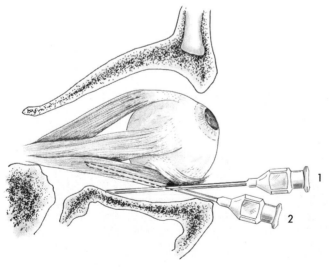

Fig. 3-6. Retrobulbar injection. If tip of needle strikes floor of orbit as it is inserted (*1*), it is withdrawn slightly and redirected more superiorly (*2*).

The most frequent complication of the retrobulbar injection is an orbital hemorrhage. This is detected by increasing proptosis, tightness of the lids, conjunctival ecchymosis, and elevated intraocular pressure. In such instances it is mandatory to postpone the surgery. I have learned from sad experience that the intraocular pressure may occasionally be lowered to what would ordinarily be a safe level for cataract surgery. This might encourage the surgeon to continue with the operation. However, any space-occupying mass in the orbit such as a hemorrhage will likely cause forward propulsion of the vitreous, even though the eye is soft. It is prudent to reschedule the surgery in spite of any inconvenience or disappointment to the patient. I generally wait at least 1 week before operating again. The optic nerve may be punctured by using a needle that is thin and sharp and longer than 1.5 inches. It is also possible to perforate the globe, especially when using a very sharp disposable needle. This accident occurs most frequently in highly myopic eyes.

Some surgeons feel they can lessen the risk of a retrobulbar hemorrhage or puncture of the optic nerve by using a variation of the classic method of performing the retrobulbar injection. The patient is instructed to look downward. The injection is performed with a 1.5-inch 25-gauge needle just medial to 12 o'clock through the superior cul-de-sac. The needle penetrates to about one half to two thirds of its full length. Another variation is to penetrate the orbital septum between the globe and the medial wall of the orbit until the tip of the needle strikes bone. It is then retracted slightly, and the anesthetic mexture is injected.

Another tragic complication of a retrobulbar injection is closure of the central retinal artery. This has been observed following retrobulbar hemorrhage resulting from a closed head injury, from ocular contusion, and as a complication of blepharoplasty. On the basis of the observation of closure of the central retinal artery during retrobulbar hemorrhage in three patients who had been scheduled for photocoagulation treatment, it has been suggested[4] that this complication may also occur while preparing for any intraocular surgery. It was observed that the central retinal artery is closed off during the retrobulbar hemorrhage as the eyeball reaches maximal proptosis and the orbit cannot accommodate more blood, thus transmitting the increased pressure to the globe. When the retinal circulation cannot be visualized, as in cataract surgery, a lateral canthotomy should be performed or enlarged immediately on diagnosis of retrobulbar hemorrhage to maintain retinal circulation and prevent retinal anoxia.

DIGITAL PRESSURE

Digital pressure is exerted against the closed eyelids (Fig. 3-7) for at least 5 minutes, if by this time the intraocular pressure registers 12 scale units or more (4.9 mm Hg or less) with the 5.5 g weight of the autoclavable Schiøtz tonometer (Fig. 3-8). Otherwise, pressure is applied for up to a total of 10 minutes with the fingers or the heel of the hand. Some consider steady pressure better than massage because there have been reports of dislocation of the lens with the latter. I have never recognized such a case. I perfer intermittent massage with release of pressure every 30 seconds to ensure against a vascular occlusion.

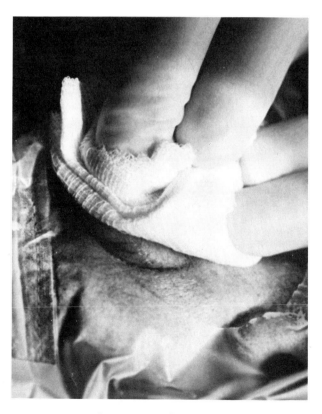

Fig. 3-7. Digital pressure.

During this interval the pressure is measured. I have found that those eyes whose intraocular pressure can be massaged to a scale reading of 12 or greater within 2 minutes or less usually have a markedly dehydrated vitreous. If it requires at least 5 minutes to achieve this hypotony, a more dangerous situation exists. If necessary, a lateral canthotomy is performed. Frequently, the intraocular pressure will fall considerably after the canthotomy (Fig. 11-6). If the intraocular pressure remains unsatisfactory, a posterior sclerotomy is performed.

Although the use of digital pressure is a most important factor in lowering the intraocular pressure, it does not ensure against operative loss of vitreous if other factors such as pressure against the open globe, unsatisfactory akinesia, and so on have not been eliminated. However, it lessens the effects of these other factors.

The pressure of the globe may be estimated by tactile sensation or by corneal indentation with the tip of a muscle hook. However, I would not perform intraocular surgery without using a tonometer as a guide to the intraocular pressure of the eye.

Various new techniques of applying continuous ocular pressure have been described. Whether or not they are more effective and as safe as digital pressure is not known. The benefits of digital pressure and of these variations in methods of ocular and orbital compression and their modes of action in achieving a soft eye are discussed on p. 257.

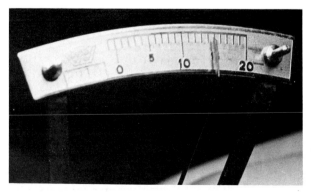

Fig. 3-8. Satisfactory hypotonia occurring after digital pressure. Fifteen scale units with 5.5 g weight, using autoclavable Schiøtz tonometer.

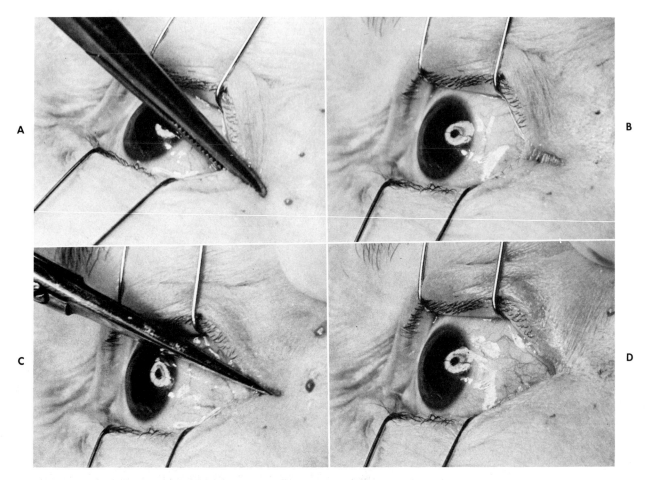

Fig. 3-9. Lateral canthotomy. **A,** Hemostat supplied to outer canthus. **B,** Hemostat removed. **C,** Canthus cut with scissors. **D,** Canthotomy completed.

LATERAL CANTHOTOMY

Lateral canthotomy is performed to increase surgical exposure and to reduce pressure of the outer canthus on the globe. Thus it is necessary in a very deep set eye, in an eye with a short palpebral fissure, in exophthalmos, in high myopia, and so on.

A hemostat is applied to the outer canthus for about 5 seconds. The clamp is angulated slightly upward to coincide with the lateral raphe of the orbicularis oculus (Fig. 3-9, A and B). The canthus is then cut with scissors (Fig. 3-9, C and D). It is not as important to make a wide skin incision as it is to cut the tight band under the skin, which presses on the globe. If bleeding occurs, the bleeding.vessel may be crushed with the hemo-

stat, it may be cauterized, or pressure may be exerted against the lateral canthus.

It is not necessary to suture a small lateral canthotomy, but a large canthotomy should be sutured to avoid a postoperative ectropion of the lateral portion of the lower eyelid. I perfer 7-0 chromic catgut or a synthetic absorbable suture, which I have found entirely satisfactory even though this material is generally not used to suture skin in other parts of the body. There is, of course, no objection to silk or nylon sutures.

SEPARATION OF THE EYELIDS

Exposure of the operative field is accomplished by separating the eyelids but not at the expense of increasing the intraocular pressure by creating pressure on the globe. There are several factors that determine the degree of exposure, such as a deep set eye, a short palpebral fissure, microphthalmos, exophthalmos, a large globe as in high myopia, and orbital abnormalities.

As discussed on p. 261, the most effective method of avoiding pressure on the globe involves the use of separate upper and lower lid retractors, such as those recommended by Desmarres. However, because this involves the use of a trained, alert assistant throughout the entire procedure, this technique has not gained widespread popularity.

Ideal exposure is obtained with the eyelids well away from the globe and the tarsus in its normal plane. Eyelid sutures and small marginal lid clamps (Castroviejo) provide excellent exposure but may cause pressure on the globe because of eversion of the tarsus. The eyelid speculum is convenient, but most of them do not permit independent control of each eyelid. Occasionally, maximum separation of the eyelids will cause elevation of intraocular pressure. Lessening the retraction of the lower lid, independent of the upper lid, will reduce this tendency. This is possible only with separate upper and lower lid retractors or eyelid sutures.

The main source of pressure from a speculum is from the weight of the central, or screw, end of the speculum. This danger may be lessened by placing a cotton pledget between the screw end of the instrument and the lateral orbital margin. Some of these shortcomings have been minimized by the Guyton-Park or Maumenee-Park lid speculum.

My preference over the past 30 years has been for separate upper and lower eyelid retractors made of malleable stainless steel (Fig. 3-10). The curved end of the retractor fits behind the tarsus. It is sufficiently broad so that the notch type of retraction seen with a single eyelid suture is avoided. The curved portion of the retractor, which fits behind the eyelid, is approximately the same length as the tarsus, therefore there is no bending or folding of the tarsus. The retraction is in the direct plane of action of the lids. These is no pressure on the globe, and satisfactory exposure is obtained (Fig. 3-11). A No. 1 nylon suture is tied to the end of the retractor. I have kept this in place on some retractors for over 2

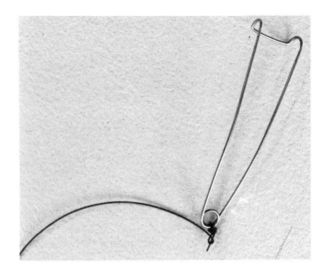

Fig. 3-10. New model Jaffe lid retractor (Storz E-997).

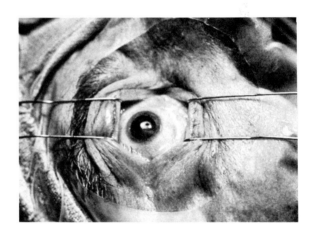

Fig. 3-11. Retraction of eyelids in direct plane of action of eyelids. Eyelids make no contact with globe. No annoying screws or locks on retractors.

years, since the suture may be autoclaved. There are no annoying screws or locks. The retractors are easily and readily removed.

It will come as a surprise to some surgeons to note the marked change in intraocular pressure in going from a one-piece wire speculum such as the blepharostat designed by Colybri to the separate eyelid retractors just described (Figs. 11-3 and 11-4).

The intraocular pressure should be checked again after the eyelids are retracted. Occasionally the pressure will rise because of excessive retraction. Since I use separate upper and lower eyelid retractors, it is convenient for me to lessen the degree of retraction of the lower eyelid or to remove this retractor completely.

Sutures are commonly used to retract the eyelids. They have the advantage of permitting independent retraction of the upper and lower eyelids, but they may cause inversion of the tarsus so that its upper end presses against the globe.

Superior rectus suture

A suture placed beneath the tendon of the superior rectus muscle is useful to keep the globe rotated downward, to retract a fornix-based conjunctival flap from the limbus, and to aid in lifting a deeply set globe from the orbit.

The superior rectus, or bridle suture, is placed by grasping the conjunctiva, Tenon's fascia, and the underlying superior rectus muscle with forceps approximately 10 mm from the limbus at 12 o'clock (Fig. 3-12). To facilitate this maneuver, the globe is rotated downward by placing a muscle hook in the inferior fornix or by grasping the globe at the superior limbus with another pair of forceps. I prefer Lester forceps (2 × 3 teeth) to grasp the muscle. As a test of whether an adequate grasp of the muscle tendon is obtained, the globe is rotated downward. The structures included in the teeth of the forceps are lifted slight-

ly as the needle passes beneath them. If the maneuver is properly performed, the suture will pass under the muscle just behind its insertion. This procedure must never be taken lightly or performed carelessly; I have seen cases where the sclera was perforated by the needle.

When a fornix-based conjunctival flap is used, it may be helpful to place the suture directly under the muscle tendon without including the conjunctiva. This applies to those cases where a posterior incision through the sclera or a beveled incision commencing 1.5 to 2 mm behind the limbus is preferred, because the conjunctiva may interfere with the preparation of the incision or the placement of the sutures, especially if fine suture material is used. If a midlimbal or anterior limbal incision is used, this method of retracting the conjunctiva by the superior rectus suture has no special advantage. The technique consists of preparing the fornix-based flap in the usual manner. The conjunctiva and Tenon's fascia are undermined in the 12 o'clock position to permit access to the insertion of the superior rectur muscle. The conjunctival flap is lifted upward by

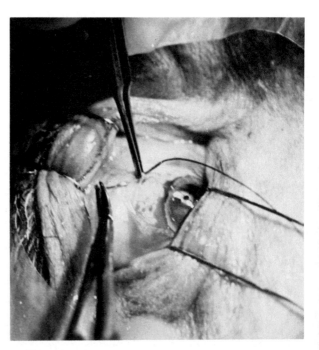

Fig. 3-13. Superior rectus suture placed after retraction of fornix-based conjunctival flap. Suture serves as bridle as well as effectively keeping cut edge of flap away from area of limbal incision.

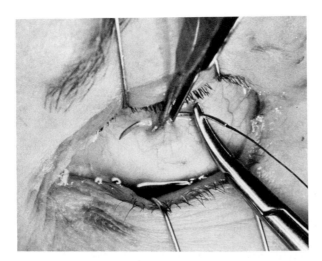

Fig. 3-12. Superior rectus (bridle) suture placed by grasping conjunctiva, Tenon's fascia, and underlying superior rectus muscle with forceps approximately 10 mm from limbus at 12 o'clock.

grasping it at its cut margin with forceps. A second pair of forceps is slid under the flap along the globe until the region of the superior rectus tendon is reached. The latter is grasped, and the globe is rotated up and down to test whether the muscle tendon is included in the teeth of the forceps. The flap is released and a suture is inserted beneath the tendon, behind its insertion, with the free hand (Fig. 3-13). The suture serves as a bridle and effectively keeps the cut edge of the conjunctival flap well away from the limbus.

The superior rectus suture should never be clamped into position while the globe is open. This will cause marked gaping of the wound during the incision and will invite prolapse of vitreous during the extraction of the lens. It is best left resting on the drape sheet over the forehead or loosely placed under the instrument that retracts the upper eyelid. Some surgeons have informed me that it is difficult to clamp nylon sutures to the head and chest drape if they are of the new paper disposable types. For this I recommend using sterile tape to secure the nylon suture to the forehead and cheek. The superior rectus suture is wrapped under one of the stainless steel arms of the eyelid retractor, which will hold it loosely in place (Fig. 3-14).

POSTERIOR SCLEROTOMY

There are rare situations when a posterior sclerotomy is useful before making the cataract incision. I may resort to it when vitreous was lost during surgery on the first eye or when a marked gaping of the wound occurs at any point during the surgery. I may use it when the intraocular pressure cannot be lowered to at least 10 Schiøtz scale units with a 5.5 g weight.

The technique is made simple by using a 25-gauge Rizzuti-Spirizzi cannula needle (Fig. 17-9). This needle has a tiny keratome tip. The sclera is exposed in the superior temporal quadrant at a point 5 mm from the limbus. The cannula needle is attached to a 2 ml syringe and is passed through the sclera and pars plana at this point and directed superiorly and posteriorly where the retrovitreal space is usually found (Fig. 17-9). Aspiration pressure is exerted on the syringe as the cannula passes into the vitreous. A sudden gush of fluid will enter the syringe when the retrovitreal space is reached. Aspiration of as little as 0.25 ml of fluid will make the globe mushy soft. No attempt is made to remove formed vitreous. A 25- or 27-gauge disposable needle may be substituted because of its sharpness.

CONJUNCTIVAL FLAP

Although there are some surgeons who routinely perform a cataract extraction through a corneal incision without the use of a conjunctival flap and claim good results, most surgeons employ some form of conjunctival covering over the operative wound. There are two type of common-

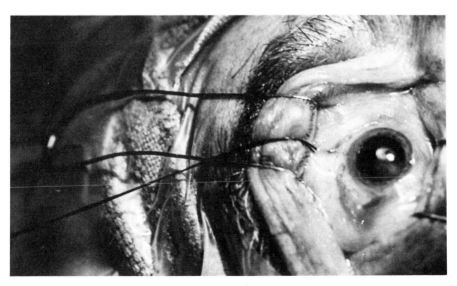

Fig. 3-14. Superior rectus suture held in place by eyelid retractor.

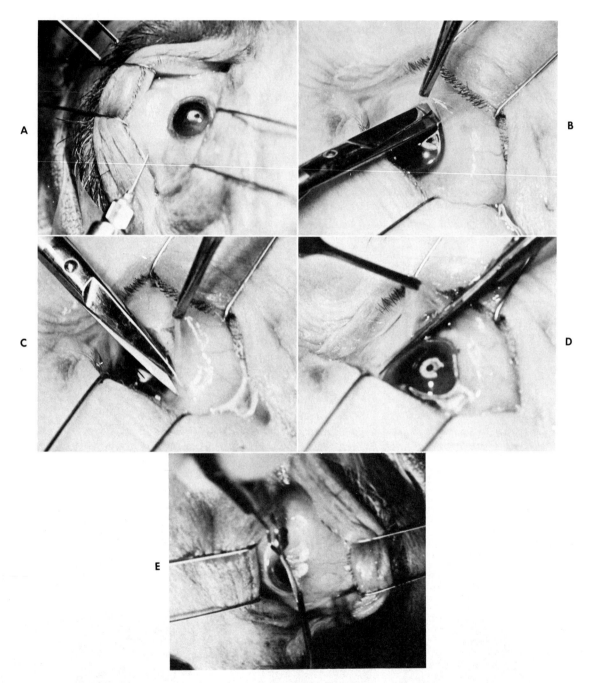

Fig. 3-15. Preparation of fornix-based conjunctival flap. **A,** Subconjunctival injection of anesthetic mixture. **B,** Peritomy and undermining at 12 o'clock. **C,** Dissection temporally. **D,** Dissection nasally. **E,** Testing mobility of flap.

ly used conjunctival flaps—fornix based and limbus based.

Fornix-based flap (Fig. 3-15)

To facilitate dissection of the flap, a subconjunctival injection of the anesthetic solution is performed over the upper half of the globe. The conjunctiva is grasped with forceps, and a small buttonhole incision is made with sharp-tipped scissors or razor knife at any location along the junction of the conjunctiva and cornea. The conjunctiva is undermined in both directions, separated from the cornea by scissors section, and cut flush with the globe so that no tags of conjunctiva are left. Since such tags have a cut proliferating edge of conjunctival epithelium that may enter the incision and facilitate an epithelial invasion of the anterior chamber, the conjunctiva should be incised as closely as possible to its corneal attachment. The incision is extended from 4 to 8 o'clock.

It is not necessary to undermine Tenon's fascia to the upper fornix. Since the fascia usually commences slightly posterior to the conjunctivocorneal border, it is possible to fashion a thin conjunctival flap that can be easily drawn down over the wound without incorporating much of the fascia. Extensive undermining of conjunctiva and fascia to the upper fornix is not recommended because it usually causes excessive bleeding and may cause some ptosis of the upper eyelid. The flap is tested by pulling it down to be sure that it will cover the wound. If it cannot, it should be freed to a greater degree. It is better to make this test at this point rather than at the end of the operation. After closure of the operative wound the flap is anchored at 4 and 8 o'clock. It should cover the entire wound, usually extending one fifth of the way down the cornea, without buckling the globe. If the flap is not easily drawn down because of fibrinous adhesions or inadequate dissection, it must be mobilized further before final anchorage.

A fornix-based flap retracts to the limbus in 1 to 3 weeks. It may not retract completely, but it usually retracts to the point where an anterior limbal incision and its sutures may be bared. This probably represents the main disadvantage, since the wound and sutures may become exposed too early in the postoperative period. If

catgut sutures are used, they may disintegrate and disappear too early because of mechanical agitation by the upper eyelid. If wound healing is defective, the interior of the eye may be unprotected against external contamination. This situation as a possible cause of late postoperative endophthalmitis (vitreous wick syndrome) is discussed on p. 441. The exposure of the sutures may cause sufficient discomfort to the patient to sure of the sutures depends to some degree on the location of the incision. Anterior incisions provide greater exposure. Less discomfort seems caused by 8-0 or 9-0 silk sutures, even if exposed. Greater discomfort, especially if the knots are exposed, is caused by 10-0 nylon. When the incision is mid- to posterior-limbal, the fornix-based flap usually covers the sutures permanently.

A fornix-based flap has undeniable advantages. It is easy to prepare and requires a simpler technique than does a limbus-based flap. It permits a greater variety of incision sites, including a corneal incision when indicated. It makes the incision and suture placement easier. It allows a much better view of instruments in the anterior chamber. Buttonholing of the flap near the limbus is of little importance, since it is easily corrected. Finally, a fornix-based flap makes certain postoperative complications such as iris prolapse, wound gape, or a too deeply placed suture easier to manage, since it can be freed by slight undermining and drawn over the wound again.

Limbus-based flap (Fig. 3-16)

To facilitate preparation of the flap, a subconjunctival injection of the anesthetic solution is performed over the upper half of the globe, although the flap may be dissected without it. The line of incision may be varied from 2 to 7 mm from the limbus. I prefer a width of 3 mm. The conjunctiva is incised down to the sclera anywhere along the intended line of incision. It is then extended to 4 and 8 o'clock, maintaining the same distance from the limbus. The flap is then retracted down over the cornea. Tenon's fascia is dissected free by using sharp-pointed scissors. There are numerous instruments available to bare the limbus. I prefer to use a Bard-Parker No. 15 scalpel blade or a No. 64 Beaver blade to clean off residual fascia from the sclera. If the curved portion of the blade is used, the conjunctival flap

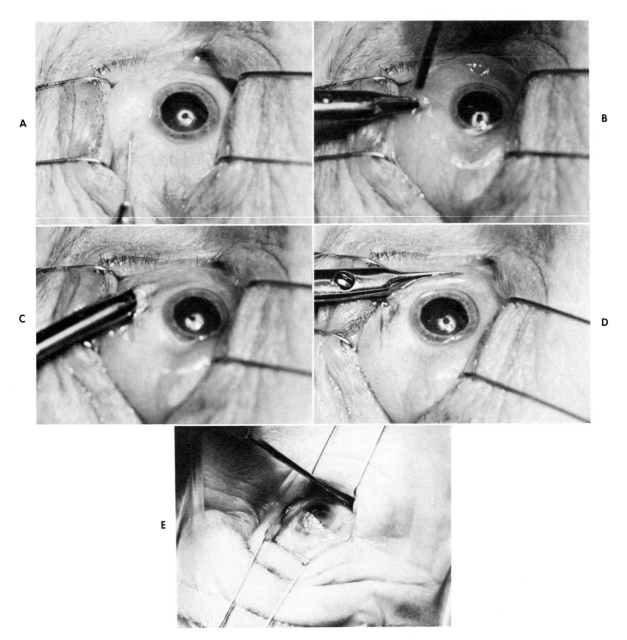

Fig. 3-16. Preparation of limbus-based conjunctival flap. **A,** Subconjunctival injection of anesthetic mixture. **B,** Conjunctiva incised down to sclera at 12 o'clock. **C,** Conjunctiva undermined nasally. **D,** Conjunctival incision. **E,** Flap retracted over cornea to expose limbal region.

is not likely to be buttonholed. If it is, the conjunctival rent may be sutured later to avoid exposure of a buried suture. As described earlier, bleeding may be controlled with cautery or epinephrine packs.

The limbus-based flap may be sutured by using absorbable or nonabsorbable material in either a continuous or interrupted manner. It is not important to close the conjunctival incision perfectly. Two to four anchoring sutures are sufficient to ensure that the flap does not retract over the cornea postoperatively.

Preparation of a limbus-based flap when adhesions exist from prior surgery may be difficult. In such cases a fornix-based flap may be indicated. If an anterior limbal incision is preferred, the limbus-based flap must be meticulously dissected to adequately expose the intended line of incision. More posteriorly placed incisions are easier to work with when using this type of conjunctival flap.

The disadvantages of the limbus-based flap are the difficulty of preparing it in patients with a very friable conjunctiva, the difficulty in visualizing instruments within the anterior chamber during enlargement of the wound, and the difficulty in inserting sutures without incorporating subconjunctival tissue in the incision. With this type of flap the sutures may be buried completely or tied externally. When the latter is done, a narrow flap is easier to work with. Of course, sutures may also be brought through a fornix-based flap and tied externally. However, because they must be tied near the edge of the cut conjunctiva, the risk of epithelial invasion of the anterior chamber may be increased. With a limbus-based flap it is more difficult to deal with certain complications such as an iris prolapse. Postoperative wound blebs are substantially more frequent with a limbus-based flap (see tabulated results).

There are several important advantages to this type of flap. It remains anchored in its usual position at the limbus, and its cut edge is well away from the incision. It provides coverage in case of wound separation, iris prolapse, or vitreous prolapse. This flap undoubtedly affords protection against intraocular infection. Catgut sutures may be completely buried and thus are protected from mechanical agitation. There is a growing tendency to bury ultrafine nonabsorbable sutures under such a flap. The patient's comfort is increased when the knots of the sutures are covered by conjunctiva.

My own experience with fornix- and limbus-based flaps leads me to conclude that when well performed, they do not influence the incidence of epithelial downgrowth and have no bearing on the amount of postoperative astigmatism.

The incidence of postoperative conjunctival blebs with both types of flaps was studied in 452 cases. The following results were tabulated:

Flap	Number of cases	Number of blebs	Blebs (%)
Limbus	90	9	10.0
Fornix	362	10	2.8

In both series, fine suture material such as 9-0 virgin silk and 10-0 nylon was used. This probably accounts for a higher percentage of blebs, but the proportion of blebs between the two kinds of flap compares favorably with that reported by Christensen and Rundle.[5] These blebs tend to disappear after some time, but the larger ones may persist. The blebs associated with fornix-based flaps are definitely smaller than those with limbus-based flaps, and they tended to disappear more readily. If they cause foreign body irritation or ocular hypotony with visual loss, they should be repaired.

It should be pointed out that the type of conjunctival flap does not influence the incidence of wound leak but rather how the leak is manifested. Wound leaks result in a filtering bleb much more frequently with a limbus-based flap because the flap heals rapidly and permits a closed space for aqueous filtration. A flat anterior chamber is more likely with a fornix-based flap, since aqueous can leak out of the wound and escape between the cut edge of the conjunctiva and the cornea.

HEMOSTASIS

Hemostasis is essential after the conjunctival flap has been completed. Actively bleeding vessels will interfere with the surgical incision and will fill the anterior chamber with blood, making intraocular visualization impossible. In common usage is a disposable Hildreth thermal cautery unit. Light cautery is applied to the bleeding vessels. The high-intensity units that are useful for cautery sclerostomy (p. 233) should not be used for this because they cause excessive scleral tissue shrinkage.

The most satisfactory method for obtaining hemostasis is the Wet-Field Coagulator (Mentor Division of Codman, Randolph, Mass.). This offers precision, speed, and minimal tissue trauma. The wet field enhances the low-temperature, low-voltage operation of the forceps. The standard forceps has fine tips. Both tips are separated

2 to 3 mm, and they must both be in contact with the sclera. The field is continually irrigated during coagulation. The power setting is 20 to 25. I prefer the coaptation forceps, which has coarser tips. A setting of 35 is used.

Epinephrine-soaked cellulose sponges are pressed against the exposed limbal area for 30 seconds to 1 minute.

The most troublesome bleeding vessels are found at 3 and 9 o'clock. They can be avoided by making the incision closer to the cornea at these points. However, if blood continues to flow into the anterior chamber in spite of all these techniques, the incision should be temporarily closed, and the anterior chamber irrigated free of blood and then filled completely with air. This will usually cause cessation of bleeding within 1 to 3 minutes. Surgery should not be continued until all bleeding has ceased.

INCISION
Location

Before discussing the various locations for the placement of the cataract incision, some knowledge of the surgical anatomy of the limbus is helpful.

The anterior boundary of the limbus is located at the most anterior point where a limbus-based flap can be reflected. A bump marks this location. Just posterior to this there is a slightly blue area about 1 mm wide that blends with a whitish area also about 1 mm wide. The junction of the blue and white areas overlies the end of Descemet's membrane or Schwalbe's line. The blue portion of the limbus overlies clear cornea, whereas the white portion overlies the trabecular meshwork (Fig. 3-17).

Kasner[6] has likened the surgical anatomy of the limbus to a tennis court. The junction of the blue and white areas is the net that overlies Schwalbe's line. The anterior baseline (bump) overlies the termination of Bowman's membrane. This is the anterior border of the limbus. The posterior baseline overlies the scleral spur, or root, of the iris. This is the posterior border of the limbus (Fig. 3-17). Thus a cataract incision may be posterior limbal, commencing over the trabecular meshwork; it may be midlimbal, commencing over Schwalbe's line; it may be anterior limbal, commencing just posterior to the termination

of Bowman's membrane. In addition the incision may be scleral or corneal (Fig. 3-18). There are wide variations in the appearance of the limbus in different individuals, with some caused by postinflammatory conditions such as trachoma or congenital anomalies such as scleralization. Since the limbal zone is wider in the vertical meridians and narrower in the horizontal meridians, the cornea has the appearance of an ellipse whose largest dimension is horizontal (Fig. 3-19).

It should be obvious that one can only accurately describe the location of the cataract incision if it is made in the vertical meridan and perpendicular to the wall of the globe. For example, a scleral incision may be made perpendicularly so that it reaches the ciliary body, but an incision commencing at the same location may be so beveled that it enters the anterior chamber anterior to Schwalbe's line. The various locations of incisions are shown in Fig. 3-18.

Types

The cataract incision may proceed from the outer surface of the globe to the anterior chamber in a perpendicular plane or else it may be made in several planes. Some of the possibilities are as follows (Figs. 3-20 to 3-22):
1. Perpendicular
2. Beveled
3. Markedly beveled
4. Perpendicular-beveled
5. Beveled-perpendicular
6. Four-plane
7. Three-plane

A perpendicular incision is made into the anterior chamber with a scalpel or razor blade. The wound is enlarged with scissors having blades rotated so that perpendicular cuts are made. Such an incision is easy to suture, but it also lends itself to gaping more readily than other types of incisions. In addition the distance from the superficial surface of the incision to the anterior chamber is the shortest of all incisions.

A beveled incision may be made with a keratome, a cataract knife, a rounded scalpel blade, a No. 64 Beaver blade, and a razor blade. When made ab externo, the wound is enlarged with scissors having blades rotated so that beveled cuts are made. This is probably the most frequently used incision. It is relatively easy to su-

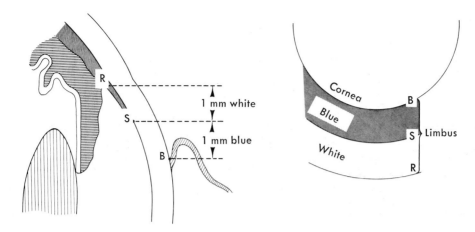

Fig. 3-17. Surgical anatomy of limbus. *Left,* Surgical limbus is approximately 2 mm wide. Anterior limbal border overlies Bowman's membrane, *B.* A 1 mm blue zone terminates at point overlying Schwalbe's line, *S.* A 1 mm white zone terminates at posterior limbal border, which overlies scleral spur, or iris root, *R. Right,* Modified after Kasner's analogy between surgical limbus and tennis court. Net represents midlimbal area and overlies Schwalbe's line, *S.* Anterior blue zone overlies clear cornea and extends from Bowman's membrane, *B,* to Schwalbe's line. Posterior white zone overlies trabecular meshwork and extends from Schwalbe's line to scleral spur, or iris root, *R.* (Note reversed positions of R-S-B in each illustration.)

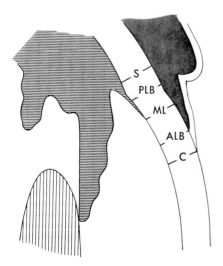

Fig. 3-18. Variety of locations of cataract incisions. *C,* Corneal; *ALB,* anterior limbal border; *ML,* midlimbal; *PLB,* posterior limbal border; *S,* scleral.

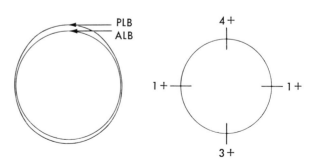

Fig. 3-19. Width of limbal zone is greatest superiorly, slightly less inferiorly, and least horizontally. *Right,* Relative widths of zones. *ALB,* Anterior limbal border; *PLB,* posterior limbal border.

ture and probably affords better protection than a perpendicular incision.

A markedly beveled incision may be made with numerous instruments, but the enlargement of the wound must be made with scissors having blades that permit a very beveled section. The best instrument for this is that designed by José Barraquer (Fig. 3-23). It permits an incision that is 135 degrees to the plane of the sclera and cor-

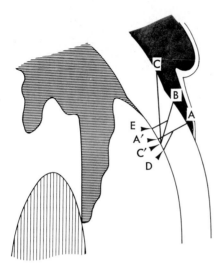

Fig. 3-20. Types of cataract incision. *A-A'*, Perpendicular; *B-C'*, beveled; *C-C'*, markedly beveled; *A-D*, perpendicular-beveled; *B-E*, beveled-perpendicular.

nea. This is probably the most difficult incision to suture, since the posterior bite must be relatively superficial because of the marked beveling and the thinness of the anterior lip of the incision. It is also difficult to preplace sutures before the incision. This incision, when mastered, permits an excellent closure and lends itself well to closure with fine sutures buried under a limbus- or fornix-based flap. I recall that such an incision was used without sutures in clear cornea in infants and children in the older technique of linear cataract extraction.

A perpendicular-beveled incision is made by preparing a perpendicular groove to a depth of at least one half the thickness of the wall of the globe by use of a rounded scalpel blade, a No. 54 guarded Beaver blade, a No. 64 Beaver blade, a razor blade, or one of many other instruments designed for this purpose. The sutures may be preplaced or postplaced. The anterior chamber is entered anywhere along the groove, and the incision is enlarged with scissors held at an angle to the wall of the globe according to the amount of bevel desired. My preference in making the initial groove is for a No. 54 guarded Beaver blade, which is a No. 64 Beaver blade with a protective guard preset to expose 0.5 to 0.75 mm of the tip of the blade. This ensures against accidental entry into the anterior chamber while making the

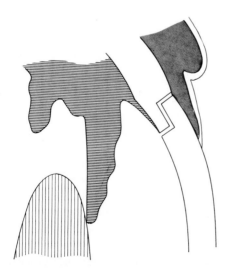

Fig. 3-21. Four-plane incision. *First* plane is conjunctival flap, *second* plane is superficial perpendicular incision through half the thickness of limbus, *third* plane is lamellar dessection 1 to 2 mm toward cornea, and *fourth* plane is deep perpendicular incision into anterior chamber.

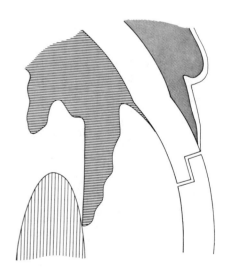

Fig. 3-22. Three-plane incision. Similar to four-plane incision except made in clear cornea without use of conjunctival flap.

groove. A disadvantage is that it is impossible to see the exact point of contact at the limbus with the tip of the blade because of the thickness of the protective guard. However, considerable accuracy is attained with experience. The sclera is fixated at 12 o'clock, 3 to 4 mm from the limbus. A right-handed surgeon commences the groove at the surgeon's left extremity of the intended incision. Firm pressure is exerted against the globe as the blade is moved in an uninterrupted, curvilinear sweep to the right extremity. The blade should be moved slowly to the right and firm pressure exerted, since there is no danger of entry into the anterior chamber. I prefer to enter the anterior chamber through the groove with a No. 75 L or M (large or medium) Beaver blade. This is equivalent to a razor blade fragment. In most instances the blade can complete the incision to the right. The blade should be held in a beveled plane. It should not be moved to the right until its tip is clearly seen in the anterior chamber. Otherwise it is possible to dissect the cornea or cause a detachment of Descemet's membrane. The incision is then completed to the left using the José Barraquer scissors described earlier.

A beveled-perpendicular incision is made by initially preparing a beveled groove, penetrating the anterior chamber perpendicularly, and en-

larging with perpendicular cuts. This is more difficult technically than the perpendicular-beveled incision.

The four-plane incision is made by first preparing a limbus-or fornix-based conjunctival flap (first plane). A perpendicular groove is made in the sclera or limbus to half the thickness of the wall of the globe extending approximately 180 degrees (second plane). A lamellar dissection is then made extending 1 to 2 mm toward the cornea. This can be done with a pyriform knife, a Beaver No. 66 lamellar dissection blade, or scalpel blade (third plane). The anterior chamber is entered perpendicularly at the anterior end of the third plane. The incision is then completed by a perpendicular section with scissors (fourth plane). By this technique the deeper layers of the wound are cut to form a small flange or flap valve. It is obvious that gaping of the wound is prevented, since the flange is forced toward the cornea. It is also easy to avoid placing the sutures too deeply, and they are more safely removed, since the deep part of the incision is offset from the sutures (if larger sutures are used). This type of incision was introduced by Dobree,[7] who referred to it as a "flanged incision", and Swan,[8] who recommended it for peripheral iridectomy and cyclodialysis. He termed it a "half-lap incision." This is an excellent incision but probably the most difficult of all to execute properly.

The three-plane incision was introduced by Gormaz,[9] who based it on Wheeler's halving principle in the sense that the superficial part of the incision does not coincide with the deeper part. This incision is no different from the four-plane incision except that it is made in clear cornea without the use of a conjunctival flap.

Extent

A corneal incision must be made larger than a scleral incision to provide the equivalent working space in the anterior chamber. By the same reasoning, an anterior limbal incision must be larger than a posterior limbal incision (Fig. 3-24). A larger incision is required for the tumbling method of forceps extraction than for the sliding technique and also for an erisiphake extraction by the open-sky method. If there is any question about the extent of the incision required, it is better to err on the side of a larger section.

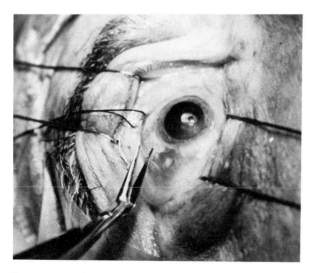

Fig. 3-23. José Barraquer corneoscleral scissors, which permits a markedly beveled incision 135 degrees to plane of sclera and cornea.

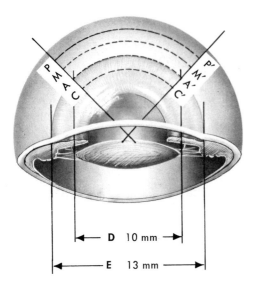

Fig. 3-24. Extent of incision varies with location. A 90 degree incision made at anterior limbal border, *A-A'*, will have amplitude of 10 mm, *D*, and will just barely permit passage of lens. A 90 degree corneal incision, *C-C'*, will have smaller amplitude, whereas midlimbal, *M-M'*, and posterior limbal, *P-P'*, incisions have larger amplitudes. Posterior limbal incision has amplitude of 13 mm, *E*.

Point of entry

Most cataract incisions are made superiorly. However, occasionally the incision must be moved to another location. For example, in an eye with a large filtering bleb a variety of alternative incisions are possible (Fig. 3-25). The location of a corneal scar or an anterior-segment pathologic condition might likewise indicate a change of the location of the incision from the normal.

The most versatile type of incision is an ab externo section with scissors enlargement. It can be applied to almost every situation and therefore should be mastered by every surgeon. However, there is nothing more artful than a well-performed full incision made by a von Graefe knife. It is a dying art because far fewer surgeons now use this technique. It requires a normal-depth anterior chamber. The zonules must be intact so that subluxation of the lens or vitreous loss will not occur during the incision. It requires considerable training and dexterity and therefore has been replaced by simpler techniques that achieve comparable results. The best technique for a shallow anterior chamber is an ab externo

incision with scissors enlargement. A rounded scalpel blade or a Beaver No. 64 blade is preferable to a sharp-pointed instrument such as a razor blade or a keratome.

Although surgeons generally select a location for the incision that they have found successful, variations are occasionally indicated. A corneal incision without a conjunctival flap is frequently substituted to avoid a functioning filtering bleb. It may also be used in patients who show bleeding tendencies as in hemophilia and other blood dyscrasias. On the contrary a scleral incision is employed by some surgeons in patients with Fuchs' dystrophy to avoid damaging the corneal endothelium. This incision is made entirely ab externo. The surgeon should also be prepared to vary the point of entry into the anterior chamber if there is a degenerative pannus, a pterygium, or other pathologic condition that would interfere with the healing of the incision in the usual location. Most surgeons who use microscopes enter the anterior chamber close to the 12 o'clock position. Enlargement is usually performed with right and left scissors. Surgeons who use loupes may enter the anterior chamber at any convenient location. For example, if the point of entry is at the right extremity of the intended incision, enlargement proceeds in one direction only (Figs. 3-26 and 3-27).

Ab externo incision. The ab externo incision may be made with any one of several instruments. The plane of entry of the cutting instrument into the anterior chamber is varied according to the type of incision used. The point of entry may be at any convenient location between 3 and 9 o'clock. For example, the incision may be made at 12 o'clock, and the enlargement proceeds to the left and right.

Secure fixation of the globe must be maintained during the incision. This may be accomplished with Castroviejo forceps with 0.12 to 0.5 mm teeth, which easily grasp the sclera. Scleral fixators with 0.3 or 0.5 mm teeth function by engaging the sclera and twisting to the right or left (according to the surgeon's preference). It is released by twisting in the opposite direction (Fig. 3-26). The Barraquer-Lloberas forceps permits a firm grasp at three points with minimum trauma to the conjunctiva. It is usually used in the 6 o'clock position just beyond the limbus. No mat-

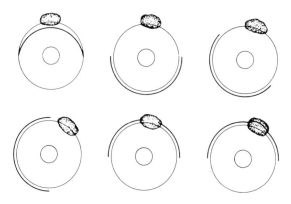

Fig. 3-25. Possible incision sites in presence of large filtering bleb.

ter which instrument is used for fixation, it is important that the globe be gently pulled out of the orbit to ensure that the instrument does not indent the globe and thus increase the intraocular pressure during the incision.

The incision into the anterior chamber may be made with any one of the following instruments.

Keratome. The keratome is available in a variety of widths and curves. It is first directed toward the center of the globe (Fig. 3-28). When the tip appears in the anterior chamber, the puncture is completed with the keratome rotated parallel to the iris.

Razor blade. A piece of a sharp razor blade held in a blade breaker may be used to enter the anterior chamber. A No. 75 Beaver blade and a Superblade (Medical Workshop of Holland) with

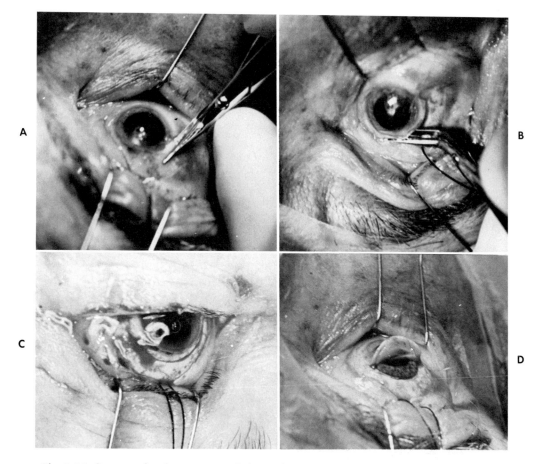

Fig. 3-26. Corneoscleral incision with fornix-based conjunctival flap. **A,** Scissors inserted through keratome incision. **B,** Beveled incision. Stop device used to prevent scissors from closing completely. **C,** Completed beveled incision. **D,** Cornea retracted.

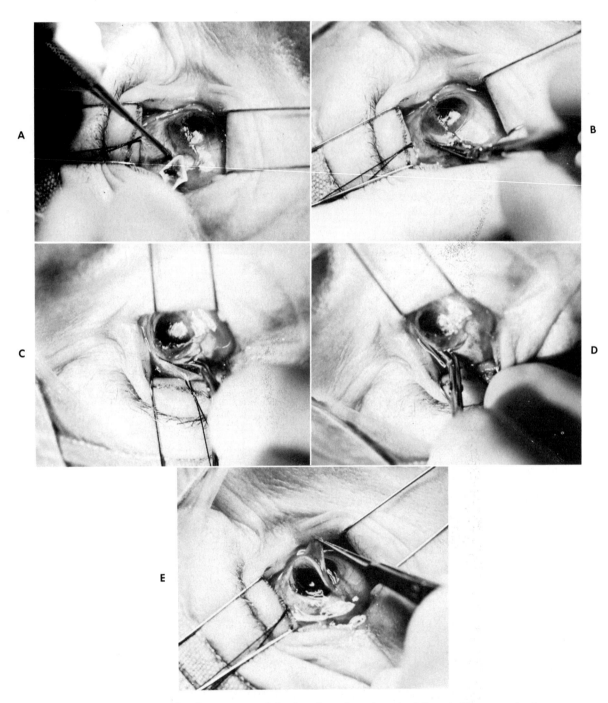

Fig. 3-27. Corneoscleral incision with limbus-based conjunctival flap. **A,** Keratome incision temporally. **B** to **D,** Scissors section. **E,** Cornea retracted by grasping flap.

a 30-degree–angled tip are similar to a razor blade fragment. The incision is enlarged slightly as the blade is withdrawn, or it may be completed to one or both sides of 12 o'clock. This is more easily performed along a preplaced groove.

Scalpel. A curved blade such as the Bard-Parker No. 15 perforates the globe by making several back and forth horizontal motions with the scalpel. It is easier to gain entry in a perpendicular direction than in a beveled plane. It is probably the best instrument to use in the presence of a shallow anterior chamber. Other instruments with a rounded cutting edge such as the Desmarres scarifier and the Beaver No. 64 blade serve as well.

The enlargement of the incision is made with scissors that are designed to cut in one direction. Some of them are designed with a stop device between the handles to prevent the blades from closing completely so that the incision can be completed without withdrawing from the anterior chamber and without producing uneven edges (Figs. 3-26 and 3-27). The Castroviejo scissors have the lower blade, the one in the anterior chamber, 1 mm longer than the upper blade so that it remains in the anterior chamber each time the scissors are closed. The inclination of the section is determined by the angulation of the scissors produced by the surgeon.

Ab interno incision. The classical von Graefe knife incision is much more difficult to master and gives rise to more complications than the ab externo incision just described. It may be performed with a fornix- or limbus-based conjunctival flap. The width of the limbus-based flap is more difficult to control if it is made simultaneously with the incision. Some surgeons prefer to prepare the flap first and then proceed with the knife section. The incision may be made with or without a preplaced groove.

To make the von Graefe knife incision and conjunctival flap in one maneuver, one should be certain that the conjunctiva is freely movable over the sclera. This is tested by lifting the conjunctiva with forceps in various locations. Since the conjunctiva is usually more adherent at 3 and 9 o'clock, it is easier to make this incision from 9:30 to 2:30 o'clock. If a reliable assistant is available for fixation, the surgeon has one hand available to manipulate the conjunctiva. Fixation is made with forceps at 6 o'clock. It is important for the assistant to exert gentle traction on the globe, pulling it out of the orbit and slightly downward to avoid pressure on the eyeball during the incision. The incision is usually begun on the temporal side by piercing the conjunctiva approximately 5 mm from the limbus. The tip of the knife then enters the anterior chamber 0.5 mm from the limbus. The blade is passed across the anterior chamber parallel to the iris and a counterpuncture is made 0.5 mm outside the limbus on the nasal side. To obtain a large conjunctival flap on this side, the surgeon gently lifts the conjunctiva with forceps until the tip of the knife emerges 5 mm from the limbus. At this juncture there usually occurs an escape of some aqueous, which aids in lifting the conjunctiva. The incision is advanced by sweeping the knife upward on the nasal side in a counterclockwise direction. A second upward sweep is then made on the temporal side, rotating in a clockwise direction. With practice the second sweep is then made on the temporal side, rotating in a clockwise direction. With practice the second sweep can com-

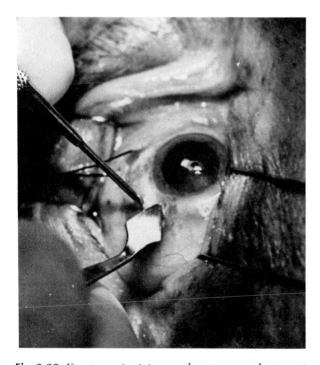

Fig. 3-28. Keratome incision made at temporal extremity of intended incision. Globe fixated with twist-grip scleral fixator.

plete the corneoscleral incision. If necessary, a third sweep on the nasal side may be made (Fig. 3-29). The conjunctival flap is completed by lifting the conjunctiva and sweeping the knife back and forth. To facilitate the preparation of the flap in case of minor adhesions, a preliminary subconjunctival injection of the anesthetic solution may be made.

The blade of the knife must be kept flat at all times. Inadvertent rotation may cause premature emptying of the anterior chamber, making it difficult to complete the incision without cutting the iris. The incision must be kept approximately 0.5 mm from the limbus throughout. It is important to keep the cutting edge of the blade against the nasal and temporal punctures at all times. There is a tendency in going from the first to the second sweep to allow the tip end of the knife to lose contact with the incision (Fig. 3-30). This favors an irregular incision. Pressure must not be exerted against the globe at any time by the surgeon, the assistant, the eyelid retractors, or the lateral canthus. If the knife accidently enters the anterior chamber with the cutting edge facing

downward instead of upward, it should be removed. If the anterior chamber has not flattened, the knife may be reinserted properly. If most of the aqueous has escaped, the anterior chamber may be reformed with balanced salt solution and another knife incision attempted. In this situation it may be advisable to proceed in another manner. A conjunctival flap is prepared, either fornix- or limbus-based, and the incision is enlarged with scissors.

When one contemplates the number of accidents that may occur during a von Graefe knife incision, it is not surprising that older surgeons used to pass on the dictum that "as the section goes, so goes the operation." The surgeon has less visible control over the incision than with an ab externo and scissors-enlarged incision. It is more difficult to place the incision at the exact location desired. It is impossible to vary the amount of the bevel or to make a four-plane, a perpendicular-beveled, or a beveled-perpendicular incision without first preparing a conjunctival flap.

An ab interno incision may be made after a pre-

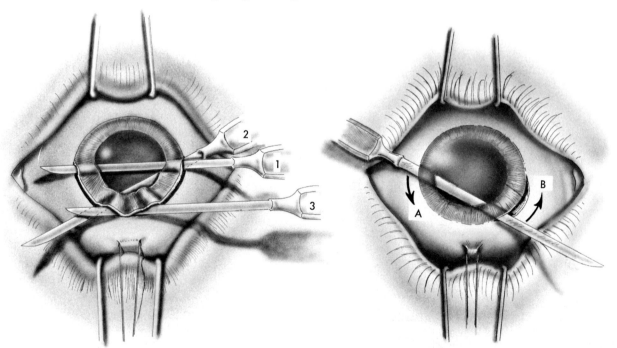

Fig. 3-29. Ab interno incision. *1,* Knife enters anterior chamber on temporal side and counterpuncture is made on nasal side. *2,* Incision is advanced by sweeping knife upward on nasal side in counterclockwise direction. *3,* Second upward sweep is made on temporal side in clockwise direction.

Fig. 3-30. In going from first sweep to second sweep, *A,* knife must be kept in contact with incision and must not lose contact, *B,* as shown. Drawing shows surgeon making incision with left hand.

liminary fornix- or limbus-based flap is prepared. If the surgeon desires, a 3 to 9 o'clock groove may be made, preplaced sutures inserted in the groove, and the knife incision made through the groove. With practice, great proficiency may be developed. It is not difficult to make the counterpuncture through the prepared groove, especially since the conjunctiva does not impair visibility.

Complications of the incision

Ab externo incision

Complications related to the flap. The conjunctiva is very thin and friable in some elderly patients. It may be perforated during the preparation of the flap, especially in the horizontal meridian. Small perforations are insignificant, unless they occur at the site of a suture that is intended to remain buried in situ under the flap. In such cases the perforation may be sutured at the conclusion of the operation. If a large perforation occurs, this portion of the conjunctiva may be trimmed and converted into a fornix-based flap with the residual portion of the flap remaining limbus-based (Fig. 3-31). Occasionally, the amount of conjunctiva that has to be sacrificed includes the entire width of the limbus-based flap. In such an instance the conjunctiva distal to the original conjunctival incision is mobilized and pulled down over the incision. To provide greater mobility, a counter incision in the fornix parallel to the limbus may be made. The fornix-based flap is sutured to the inferior conjunctiva in

the horizontal meridian, to the cornea, or both, depending on its location (Fig. 3-32). The fornix-based flap should not be dissected excessively if a troublesome postoperative ptosis of the upper eyelid is to be avoided. A thin conjunctival flap that disturbs the underlying Tenon's capsule very little is desirable. It should be tested for wound coverage by drawing it down over the cornea before the anterior chamber is entered. If the conjunctiva is fragile it may fragment easily when it is sutured in place after the wound is closed. To avoid this, a horizontal incision in the conjunctiva above, approximately 10 mm from the limbus, may provide the necessary mobility of the flap. An alternate approach is to make horizontal conjunctival incisions at 3 and 9 o'clock to permit the conjunctiva to be pulled down without tension (Fig. 3-33).

Injury to the cornea, iris, and lens. Injury to the cornea, iris, and lens is more likely to occur if the anterior chamber is entered with a sharp-tipped instrument such as a keratome or a piece of a razor blade than if a blade with a round surface (a No. 64 Beaver blade or a No. 15 Bard-Parker scalpel blade) is used. However, it may occur with any dull instrument, since the anterior chamber may be penetrated abruptly. If the anterior chamber empties before the cutting instrument is withdrawn, the iris and lens move forward and may be damaged if the surgeon attempts to enlarge the incision while removing the blade. The tip of the keratome may strike the lens if the heel of the blade is not depressed as it

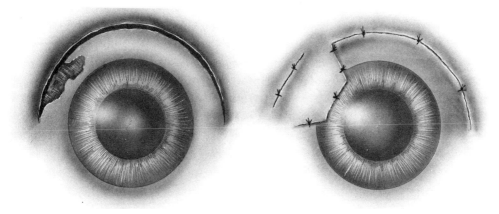

Fig. 3-31. Repair of perforated limbus-based flap by converting this portion into fornix-based flap with residual portion remaining limbus based.

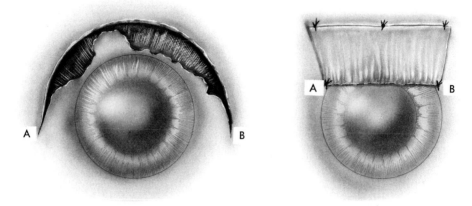

Fig. 3-32. If most of limbus-based flap must be sacrificed because of widespread laceration, conjunctiva distal to original conjunctival incision is mobilized and pulled down over incision.

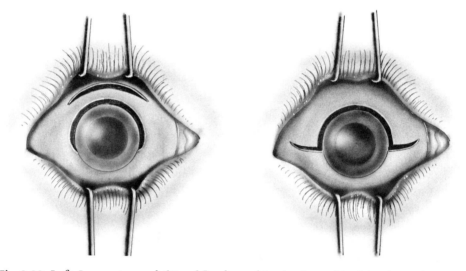

Fig. 3-33. *Left,* Increasing mobility of flap by making horizontal incision in conjunctiva above, approximately 10 mm from limbus. *Right,* An alternate approach is to make horizontal conjunctival incisions at 3 and 9 o'clock.

enters the anterior chamber. On the other hand, if the tip points too much anteriorly, it may strike the back of the cornea. This is rare but is more likely to occur if the keratome is used in an eye with a shallow anterior chamber. I have seen the tip of a dull razor blade enter the eye abruptly and cause immediate loss of vitreous. The enlargement of the incision with scissors may cause detachment of Descemet's membrane if the tip of the scissors blade does not enter the anterior chamber easily. The blades should not be closed

unless the instrument is freely movable, otherwise corneal splitting will result. If the surgeon exerts pressure on the globe with the scissors during enlargement, the iris will prolapse and may be cut. This is most likely to occur if the globe is not hypotonic. This may also occur if the scissors are not sharp. No more than gentle traction on the superior rectus suture should be exerted during the enlargement of the incision, since this encourages prolapse of intraocular contents.

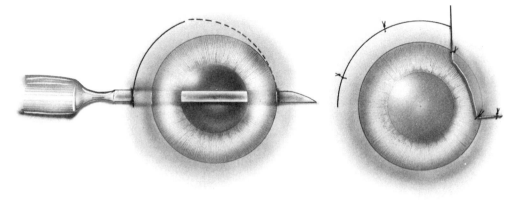

Fig. 3-34. If part of ab interno incision is left without conjunctival flap, it may be corrected by preparing small fornix-based flap to cover this area.

Irregularity of the incision. Dentate irregularities and defective coaptation may result if the blades of the scissors cut to their tips. This can be prevented by making short cuts without closing the scissors completely. Scissors with a stop device that prevents the tip from meeting or scissors with the lower blade (in the anterior chamber) longer than the upper blade (outside the anterior chamber) will prevent full cutting. The tips of the scissors should be slightly rounded so that the iris within the eye and Tenon's fascia outside the eye are not caught as the scissors advance during the enlargement.

Excessive bleeding. Bleeding may be encountered during the preparation of the conjunctival flap or during the incision into the anterior chamber. Bleeding vessels may be gently cauterized, but excessive cauterization, especially near the limbus, should be avoided. As stated on p. 45 wet-field coagulation is the best method to obtain hemostasis without excessive tissue trauma. As the wound is enlarged toward 3 and 9 o'clock, the incision should be directed closer to the cornea to avoid the larger episcleral vessels. One minute of pressure exerted against the superior limbus with an epinephrine-soaked cellulose sponge provides additional hemostasis.

Ab interno incision

Inadequate fixation. An ab interno incision is impossible to make without good fixation. The fixation forceps or scleral fixator must engage the episclera or sclera because the conjunctiva is usually too mobile or too fragile to control the globe adequately for a good knife section. Fixation must not be made too far from the limbus. Fixation of the globe must be properly performed so that pressure is not made against the globe during the incision, otherwise the lens, iris, and even vitreous may be pushed forward, making completion of the incision impossible.

Inadequate conjunctival flap. It is possible to leave part of the incision without a conjunctival flap if the puncture or the counterpuncture with the knife is made too close to the cornea. This may be corrected by preparing a small fornix-based flap to cover this area (Fig. 3-34). An inadequate or irregular flap may be created if the conjunctiva is adherent to the underlying sclera as a result of previous surgery, previous inflammation, or other conditions. This can be prevented by testing the freedom of the conjunctiva with forceps before the incision is made. These problems can also be avoided by preparing the flap before the incision. The complications of preparing the limbus-based or fornix-based conjunctival flaps before making the incision have been described earlier.

Inadequate incision. It is possible to make the incision too corneal, too scleral, or irregular by not keeping the blade of the knife parallel to the plane of the iris or by misjudging the point of puncture or counterpuncture. A corneal incision will make it more difficult to cut the iris near its root in performing a sector or peripheral iridectomy. It makes it more difficult to grasp the lens near its upper pole with capsule forceps and

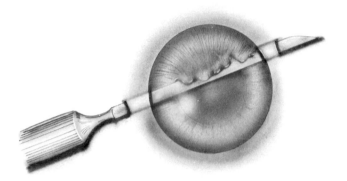

Fig. 3-35. Premature loss of anterior chamber because of failure to keep blade of knife parallel to iris may result in cutting iris.

more difficult to perform zonular stripping under direct observation. If the incision is too corneal, it may be too small for an erisiphake extraction. A too scleral incision will cause excessive bleeding because of the presence of large scleral vessels at the horizontal meridian. The incidence of postoperative hyphema will be higher. It favors the formation of peripheral anterior synechias. Wound healing in the sclera is less satisfactory than limbal healing (p. 25). Since the incision may go directly through angle drainage structures, conjunctival blebs may readily result. The iris root or ciliary body may be cut and excessive bleeding caused during or after surgery. As mentioned earlier, if the tip end of the knife loses contact with the incision in changing directions from one sweep to the next, an irregular incision may result (Fig. 3-30). Excess bleeding from the margins of the incision should not be cauterized, since shrinkage and retraction may result, which favor a filtering wound. Epinephrine packs are more suitable. Excess bleeding from the iris root or ciliary body may be controlled by irrigation with balanced salt solution or by placing air in the anterior chamber.

A premature loss of the anterior chamber from failure to keep the blade of the knife parallel to the iris may result in cutting the iris (Fig. 3-35) or damaging the lens. If the iris is engaged by the knife or if it folds over the knife, it is best to remove the knife from the anterior chamber and complete the incision with scissors. If the knife enters the anterior chamber with the cutting edge facing downward, it should be removed

immediately. The anterior chamber may be deepened by instillation of fluid. If the knife can be reinserted through the same opening, the incision may proceed as originally planned. However, it may be safer to enlarge the incision with scissors.

Incision in special situations

Presence of filtering bleb from previous glaucoma surgery. If the bleb is nonfunctioning, it may be disregarded. The location of the incision need not be varied from the surgeon's preferred site. The conjunctiva is scarred in this area, and a decision must be made regarding the conjunctival flap. A fornix-based flap is less complicated in this situation. More than average bleeding should be anticipated.

If the bleb is functioning, the location of the incision should be changed. A popular incision is one made in clear cornea just below the inferior edge of the bleb. The approach to the anterior chamber is ab externo or ab interno. In the former situation a blade with a round edge such as the No. 64 Beaver blade or the Bard-Parker No. 15 scalpel blade is preferred to a sharp-pointed tip such as a fragment of a razor blade. The iris is often not available to protect the lens if a previous sector iridectomy or an iridencleisis was previously performed. I prefer a beveled incision made at an angle of 45 degrees and to stay as close to the limbus as possible. The enlargement is made with scissors held at the same angle. A knife incision is relatively easy to make in this situation.

It is important not to make the amplitude of the incision too small, since a corneal incision must extend further than a limbal incision. I do not bevel the incision excessively when it is corneal because the deep portion of the incision would be well within Schwalbe's line where endothelial proliferation and Descemet's membrane secretion may occur along vitreous strands or zonular fibers (Descemet's tubes). Also, the closer the incision to the edge of the pupil, the greater the tendency to astigmatism. In this regard I prefer to extend the incision below the horizontal meridian to 8 and 4 o'clock. This extension tends to neutralize some of the astigmatism against the rule created by the corneal incision above by causing some flattening of the horizontal meridian of the cornea (p. 93). Silk sutures are preferable to catgut sutures; the latter are likely to fragment early because of the lack of a conjunctival covering over them. The sutures should remain in place at least 4 weeks before removal. I prefer 8-0 silk for this incision.

If the bleb is very cystic and extends well down over the cornea, the site of the incision should be changed to an inferotemporal, a temporal, or an inferior incision (Fig. 3-25). In these locations the incision need not be corneal. A conjunctival flap is used. I prefer to make the incision exactly as I would a routine superior incision. Incisions made through the bleb or passed sclerally superior to the bleb are cumbersome and of dubious value.

Blood dyscrasia. Some hemophiliacs have undergone successful cataract surgery employing a purely corneal incision. The incision should be placed 1.5 to 2 mm within the limbus. Silk sutures are preferred to catgut sutures.

Endothelial dystrophy of the cornea. McLean[10] has recommended making a deep scleral section to avoid corneal injury in this situation. I prefer a posterior limbal section in all patients with moderate-to-severe cornea guttata and those with Fuchs' dystrophy. The incision should be made about 180 degrees in amplitude because this large an incision requires less bending of the cornea during the remainder of the operation (p. 340). A sector iridectomy facilitates the lens extraction by minimizing the maneuvers required within the anterior chamber.

SUTURE TECHNIQUE

The surgeon should become familiar with different techniques because no one technique fits every situation.

The most frequently employed postplaced suture is a radial edge-to-edge suture that is placed through the middle third of each border of the incision. With the increasing popularity of very fine sutures (particularly 10-0 nylon), there is a growing trend to place the sutures very deeply, to the level of Descemet's membrane or even full thickness of the wound margins.[11] Each bite should be 0.5 to 1 mm in length. The surgeon should strive to place the sutures equidistant apart, insert them to the same depth, make them as radial as possible, and tie them with the

same degree of tension. The number of sutures will depend on the diameter of the material and the length of the incision. One cannot deny that the use of the surgical microscope has improved suture placement and should be learned by the student surgeon. An experienced surgeon, however, may or may not benefit greatly from such a change in technique.

It may be difficult to postplace an exactly radial suture if the wound gapes from forward displacement or collapses from excessive retraction of the intraocular contents. In the latter situation the anterior chamber may be inflated with air after the placement of a single suture. This makes wound apposition more suitable for accurate suturing (Fig. 3-36). Another technique consists of making several radial marks with a fine toothpick dipped in sterile methylene blue. When the incision is completed, the edges of the wound can be accurately aligned by suturing the blue-stained edges together (Fig. 3-37). If a suture is not placed radially, it will cause lateral displacement of the wound edges (Fig. 3-38).

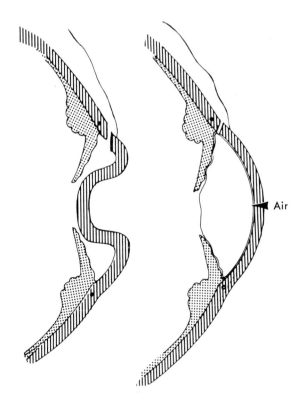

Fig. 3-36. Facilitation of insertion of postplaced sutures by inflating anterior chamber with air.

The ideal depth of large suture (6-0 or 7-0) placement is the middle third or the wound margins. A too superficial suture may slough out too soon and may cause posterior gaping of the wound (Fig. 3-39). A too deeply placed suture may reach the anterior chamber and provide a path for escape of aqueous. Necrosis of the deeper layers of the wound may result from the crushing effect of the suture, which will then penetrate the anterior chamber (Fig. 3-40). Deep necrosis of the wound does not result from 10-0 nylon; it may from silk or catgut.

If the suture is placed at different depths on the two sides of the wound, wound apposition suffers (Fig. 3-41). If the length of the bite on both sides is unequal, wrinkling may occur when the suture is tied (Fig. 3-42). Wrinkling may also occur if the bites are too long on both sides, especially if the sutures are tied too tightly.

The sutures must be tied sufficiently tight to

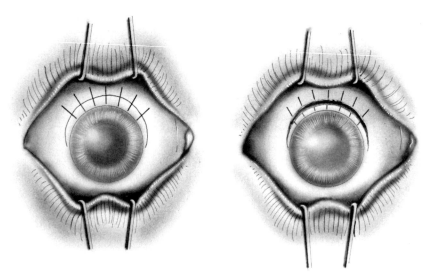

Fig. 3-37. Radial marks made across groove with methylene blue. When incision is completed, edges of wound can be accurately aligned by suturing blue-stained edges together.

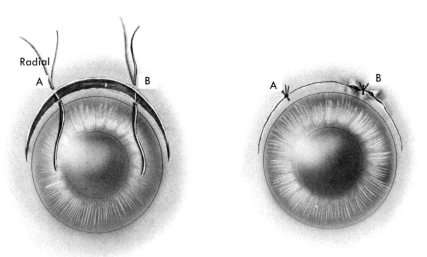

Fig. 3-38. Radial suture, *A*, provides accurate alignment of wound edges. Nonradial suture causes lateral displacement, *B*.

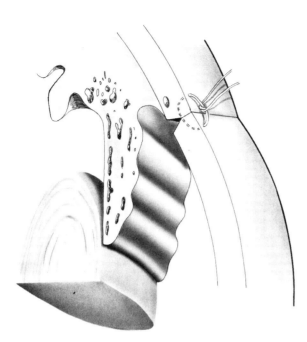

Fig. 3-39. Too superficial suture may cause posterior gaping of wound.

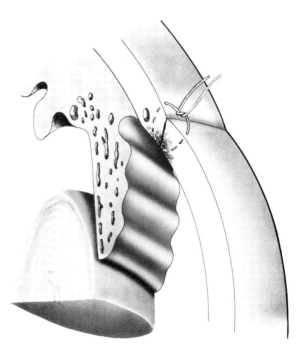

Fig. 3-40. Too deeply placed suture may cause necrosis of deeper layers of wound.

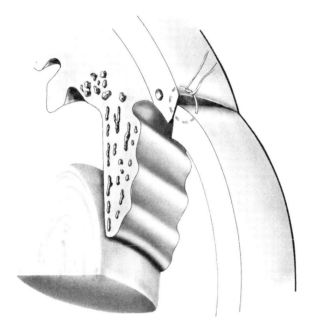

Fig. 3-41. Faulty wound apposition because of suture placed at different depths on two sides of wound.

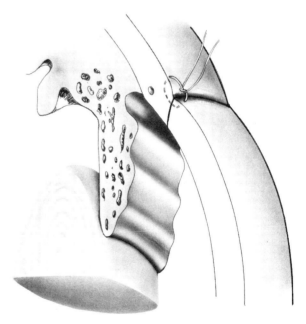

Fig. 3-42. Unequal length of bites on two sides of wound may cause wrinkling and buckling.

unite the wound edges but not so tight that necrosis and posterior gaping occur (Fig. 3-43). With experience, the surgeon learns to tie with optimum tightness. Excessive wrinkling of the cornea will be apparent if the suture is tied too tight-

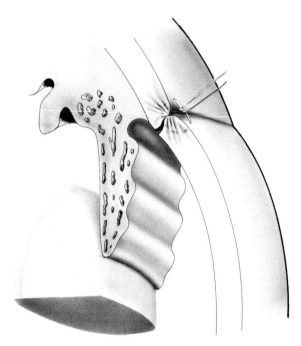

Fig. 3-43. Wrinkling, necrosis, and posterior gaping of wound because of too tightly tied suture.

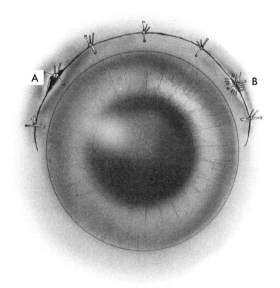

Fig. 3-44. *A,* Loosely tied suture. *B,* Tight suture.

ly, and fluid will escape from the anterior chamber when it is re-formed if the suture is tied too loosely (Fig. 3-44). Visualization of the wound edge is important when using fine sutures because it is difficult to "feel" the proper degree of tightness of the knot. In this instance it is wise to repressurize the anterior chamber before the sutures are tied. I use a single 7-0 silk suture at 12 o'clock to retract the cornea. After the lens is extracted, this suture is tied. The entire anterior chamber is filled with air. This creates good wound apposition. The preplaced and postplaced sutures are then tied. Repressurizing the eye reduces the tendency to tie the sutures too tightly and to cause excessive wound compression (Chapter 4). After the suturing has been completed, most of the air bubble is replaced by balanced salt solution.

Preplaced sutures with limbus-based flap

A preliminary groove is prepared as previously described. It may be made along the entire length of the intended incision or only in two or more places where sutures are to be inserted. The sutures are placed before the anterior chamber is entered. They may be entirely subconjunctival or transconjunctival. In the former the needle is grasped with the needle holder relatively close to the tip. The globe may be fixated in several ways. I prefer using forceps with fine teeth (0.12 mm). The corneal edge of the groove margin is grasped, and the needle is passed directly under the forceps or just to one side by initially penetrating the outer layers of the cornea perpendicularly and then curving the needle so that its tip appears in the groove. Fixation of the scleral edge of the groove margin is then made as the needle passes across the groove, penetrates the scleral edge, and emerges from the scleral portion of the partial incision. I prefer to take an 0.5 mm bite in the anterior part and a 1 mm bite in the posterior part of the wound except where a markedly beveled incision is made. In this case a 1 mm bite is taken in both edges of the incision because the corneal margin is relatively thin. The limbal zone and sclera should be cleaned of all fascia to avoid the annoying tendency of this tissue to become incorporated in the groove as the suture is pulled through the edge of the incision. The suture is tied in the following manner to keep the knot on the scleral side of the incision and prevent the cut ends from pointing upward through the overlying conjunctiva. A double surgeon's knot is made first. Both arms of the suture are pulled toward the surgeon at an angle of 45 degrees, diverging as the knot is secured. The knot is then squared and a granny made in the third and last tie. When using fine suture material such as 9-0 virgin silk or 9-0 and 10-0 nylon, a triple surgeon's knot is necessary in the first tie to prevent the knot from slipping. Some surgeons preplace all the sutures in the preliminary groove, but most preplace some and add additional sutures after the lens is extracted. The conjunctival incision is then closed with two or three sutures. It is not necessary to meticulously close this incision. There is a growing trend to permanently bury the newer finer sutures. Of course, absorbable sutures lend themselves best to this technique, since the knots are protected to some degree from the action of the upper eyelid by the overlying conjunctiva. Nylon sutures are cut flush with the knot. They usually do not untie because of the "memory" of this material. It can be stretched considerably while being tied (to increase by about one third its length), although this is to be avoided. The suture may then be grasped with fine tying forceps and rotated so that the knot is buried in the suture track, although this is not always possible. It prevents the knot or ends of the suture from working through the conjunctiva and becoming irritating. The 9-0 silk suture should not be cut too close to the knot because it may untie. The ends of this suture material rarely irritate the patient.

The sutures may be placed transconjunctivally by passing the needle through the corneal edge of the incision external to the insertion of the limbus-based flap and directing it through the edge of the groove under the flap. After the scleral bite is taken, the needle is passed through the base of the flap and tied externally.

Preplaced sutures with fornix-based flap

A preliminary groove is prepared at the location of preference along the entire length of the intended incision or in two or more places where preplaced sutures are to be inserted. The sutures are inserted in the same manner as described earlier for buried subconjunctival sutures. If the surgeon prefers to incorporate any of the incisional sutures to pull down the fornix-based flap, the ends should be double armed so that both needles can be brought through the conjunctiva near its cut end. They are tied externally. I prefer to bury sutures under a fornix-based flap no matter what suture I use. The flap is pulled down separately and anchored at 3 and 9 o'clock. The flap covers the upper one fifth to two fifths of the cornea. If the incision is made sufficiently scleral, the flap usually covers the sutures permanently. Otherwise, suture removal in the case of large nonabsorbable sutures becomes necessary. Fine material such as 9-0 silk, 9-0 nylon, or 10-0 nylon need not be removed if exposed unless it is irritating to the patient.

Preplaced sutures without a conjunctival flap

Preplaced sutures without a conjunctival flap are generally used in corneal incisions. However, with limbal incisions, some surgeons prefer to peritomize the conjunctiva and allow it to retract and remain in this position after the entire wound is closed. A preliminary groove is placed along the entire incision or in two or more places where sutures are to be inserted. I must caution against the use of absorbable sutures to close such an incision. Without the protection of overlying conjunctiva, they tend to fragment early, thus placing the wound in jeopardy.

Postplaced sutures

Postplaced sutures are inserted after the incision is made. Approximation is more difficult and less accurate than with preplaced sutures. If radial marks are made in several locations before the incision is made or if the surgical microscope is used, wound apposition approaches or is equal to that seen with preplaced sutures without the microscope. It is more difficult to place the suture at the proper depth or to place it at equal depths on the two sides of the incision than when a preliminary suture groove is prepared. However, the experienced surgeon is handicapped little by these drawbacks. As stated earlier, repressurizing the anterior chamber with a bubble of air facilitates accurate suturing. If the sutures are buried under a limbus-based flap, the sclera must be meticulously cleaned of fascia because this is more difficult to do after the incision is made than with a preliminary groove. There is an annoying tendency for fascia and subconjunctival tissue at the edge of the flap to be drawn into the suture track by the suture. This occurs much more readily with 8-0 and 9-0 virgin silk than with 10-0 nylon. The flap may be retracted over the cornea by a sponge or smooth forceps during the suturing. Postplaced sutures may be placed before the lens extraction, after the lens extraction, or some before and some after. It is best to tie the knots on the scleral side of the incision, as described previously, since the conjunctival flap is thicker here than at its anterior edge.

Special suture techniques

A variety of continuous sutures have been described. In all these techniques, 10-0 monofilament nylon is used. It would be impractical to describe them all, but the following are those used most commonly at present:

1. Shoelace suture. A scleral bite is taken at one end of the incision. Radial bites are then taken until the opposite end is reached. The suturing is then reversed and continued to the starting point where the last bite passes through the corneal edge of the incision. After the suture loops are tightened, the suture ends are tied in the groove of the incision (Fig. 3-45).

2. Troutman suture (Fig. 4-6). The suture is cut in half. One portion is tied at 9:30 o'clock, from which point it is continued nearly to 12 o'clock. The other half is anchored at 2:30 o'clock and continued nearly to 12 o'clock. The two halves are tied to each other at 12 o'clock.

3. Willard suture (Fig. 4-6). A 3 mm transverse scleral bite is taken 1.5 mm posterior to the line of incision at 12 o'clock. The right end of the suture continues to the left and the left end to the right. The sutures are finally anchored at 2:30 and 9:30 o'clock.

4. Over-and-over suture (Fig. 4-7). The suture is anchored to the sclera at one end of the incision and continued to the opposite end where it is again anchored in the sclera.

5. Continuous interlocking suture (Fig. 3-46). This is similar to the over-and-over suture except that each suture bite is locked. The continuous portion should be closer to the cornea than to the sclera because this is the shortest circumference. If placed on the scleral side of the wound, it

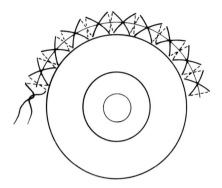

Fig. 3-45. Shoelace suture.

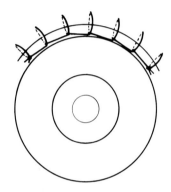

Fig. 3-46. Continuous interlocking suture.

could loosen if slippage to the corneal side occurs.

Except for the continuous locking suture, none of the suture bites are locked in these techniques. Before the final tying and anchoring of the suture, the tension should be equalized as much as possible along the entire path of the suture. There is a tendency to pull too tightly, especially at the points of final anchorage. This is discussed in Chapter 4. As stated earlier, it is helpful to place a single suture of 7-0 silk at 12 o'clock and tie it after the lens is extracted. The anterior chamber is filled with air so that the lips of the wound are more exactly approximated. This prevents tying too tightly as is more likely with a collapsed anterior chamber (Fig. 3-36). Most of the air can be removed and replaced with fluid after completion of the suturing. The continuous sutures are intended to remain permanently buried under a limbus- or fornix-based flap. They may be removed if placed entirely corneally.

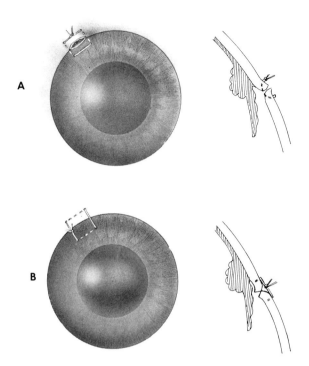

Fig. 3-47. A, Vertical mattress suture tends to cause eversion of wound. **B,** Horizontal mattress suture causes inversion and posterior gaping of wound.

However, this should be delayed for at least 6 months.

Track sutures are intermediate between preplaced and postplaced sutures. Before the incision is made, a suture of greater width such as 4-0 silk is passed through the limbal area in several locations. When the incision is made, the sutures are cut. They are left in place, serving as tracks for the passage of finer sutures. This procedure is facilitated if the latter are swaged onto a blunt needle. The cut track suture is withdrawn as the finer suture is passed through the track. The track suture may be coated with fluorescein or methylene blue to outline the track.

Mattress sutures are less commonly used now than formerly. A transverse or horizontal mattress suture is placed by taking horizontal, equal, and parallel bites of cornea and sclera. They are usually unsatisfactory because they unite the wound only superficially and have a tendency to cause inversion and posterior gaping of the wound (Fig 3-47). Vertical mattress sutures are more effective, since radial bites are taken

through both lips of the wound a slight distance apart. However, since they pass across the incision only within the tissues, the wound edges tend to become everted (Fig. 3-47). Some surgeons place one or more vertical mattress sutures before the incision and convert them into radial sutures to close the wound.

The variations in techniques of suturing the cataract wound are legion. It would be impractical to describe them all. The most commonly used methods as well as various personal preferences will now be discussed.

COMMON TYPES OF WOUND CLOSURE
Postplaced sutures

There are two kinds of postplaced sutures — those inserted after the incision has been completed and those placed after the cataract has been extracted.

Buried sutures pass through the edges of the incision without involving the conjunctival flap. They are covered by a limbus- or fornix-based flap that is sutured independently (Fig. 3-48).

Exteriorized sutures pass through the conjunctival flap as well as through the edges of the incision. They are tied externally to the conjunctival flap (Figs. 3-49 and 3-50). They are usually used with a limbus-based flap, but some surgeons pass one or more sutures through a fornix-based flap and tie them so that the knot lies externally a short distance from the cut end of conjunctiva.

Exposed sutures are usually those that are placed entirely within the cornea without a conjunctival covering (Fig. 3-51). Some surgeons place sutures at the limbus but peritomize the conjunctiva and allow it to retract so that the sutures remain exposed. A fornix-based flap, which initially covers sutures buried under it, may retract so that the sutures become exposed.

Preplaced sutures

Preplaced sutures are generally set into a groove that outlines the incision (Fig. 3-52). The sutures are placed before the anterior chamber is opened. A popular technique consists of placing two or more sutures in the preliminary groove and then placing the remainder after the lens extraction. The sutures may be buried, exteriorized, or permitted to remain exposed, as with postplaced sutures.

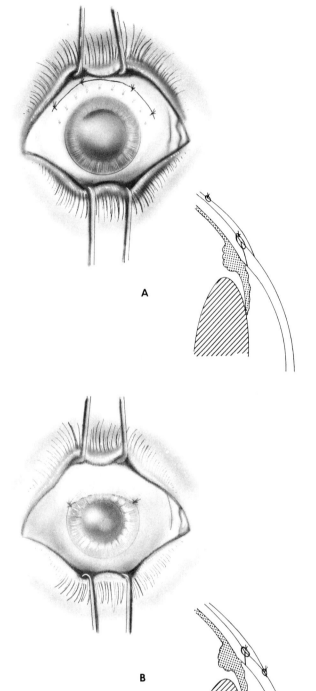

A

B

Fig. 3-48. Buried sutures with, **A,** limbus-based flap and, **B,** fornix-based flap.

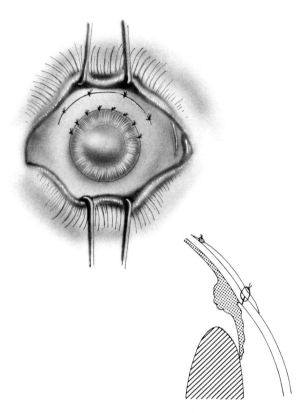

Fig. 3-49. Exteriorized sutures with limbus-based flap.

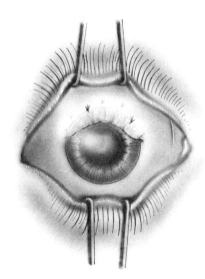

Fig. 3-50. Partly buried and partly exteriorized sutures with fornix-based flap.

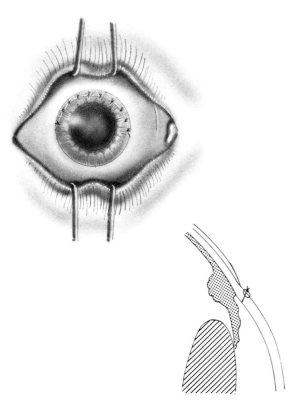

Fig. 3-51. Exposed sutures with corneal incision.

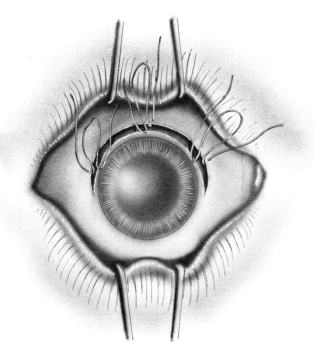

Fig. 3-52. Sutures preplaced in groove.

Track sutures

Track suture technique consists of preplacing sutures without making a preliminary groove. The sutures are cut during the incision, and tracks are created for the insertion of other sutures in the preformed tracks. The technique appears to be cumbersome and time consuming but has attracted many surgeons in some parts of the country.

IRIS SURGERY DURING CATARACT EXTRACTION

Some form of iris opening is an important part of the cataract extraction because it is a safeguard against the occurrence of iris prolapse and pupillary block. However, because of improvements made in wound closure, wound leak is now much less frequent. When it does occur, an unequal pressure gradient is created between the anterior and posterior chambers. The higher pressure in the latter pushes the iris toward the dehiscence in the surgical wound. If not an iris prolapse, a pupillary block may result, since the vitreous moves forward against the iris and may interfere with the communication of aqueous between the posterior and anterior chambers. The presence of a surgically made iris opening affords some protection against these two occurrences. However, it is not an absolute guarantee. When wound healing is uncomplicated and pupillary block is absent, as is usually the case, the creation of a surgically made iris opening may appear unnecessary. However, wound leak is unpredictable, making the creation of an alternate iris opening a recommended safeguard. This view is not universally shared; some excellent cataract surgeons feel that the high quality of modern sutures and closure techniques make iris surgery unnecessary. It is not yet known whether this is a justified omission.

Aside from its benefits in aiding postoperative aqueous humor dynamics, iris surgery serves other ends. A sector iridectomy or radial iridotomy may also serve an optical purpose, as in the case of corneal scars. Either technique may also facilitate lens delivery in the presence of a small pupil resulting from prolonged use of miotics or posterior synechias. An inferior radial iridotomy may prevent an updrawn pupil in case of operative loss of vitreous or chronic iridocyclitis. Iris surgery may also facilitate examination of the peripheral fundus postoperatively when retinal detachment is anticipated.

No matter which technique of iris surgery the surgeon employs, the instruments used should be carefully selected. The scissors should have blunt tips to avoid injury to the corneal endothelium and the lens capsule. The forceps should have no teeth. This type causes less iris atrophy and does not catch the iris when released. Forceps with teeth may cause an accidental iridodialysis when the surgeon removes them from the eye without realizing the teeth have caught the iris. In addition, an inadvertent cyclodialysis cleft may be created.

It is remarkable how little the iris bleeds when cut. This is probably caused by an axon reflex, although Babel[12] attributed it to the elasticity of the iris stroma and the peculiar double-walled structures of its vessels. Bleeding may be prevented by avoiding the iris root. Bleeding can usually be controlled by irrigating the anterior chamber with balanced salt solution. Air injection into the anterior chamber is also useful but rarely necessary. The operative procedure should be delayed until all bleeding has ceased.

Peripheral iridectomy

Peripheral iridectomy is the excision of a small piece of iris near its base. One or more of these openings in the iris may be made by grasping the iris near its base with very fine forceps without teeth. A small, full-thickness piece of iris is excised with fine scissors by cutting either parallel or perpendicular to the plane of the incision. The former results in a larger opening, the latter in a smaller one. This may be done under direct observation with the cornea retracted or with the surgeon grasping the iris and drawing it out over the sclera with the cornea in place. It is more difficult to perform a truly peripheral iridectomy when a corneal incision is made. The opening in the iris need not be truly basal. It is probably most effective when made 1 or 2 mm from the base. The surgeon must check that the excision of iris is full thickness, since a schisis may be obtained, leaving the pigment epithelium behind.

A peripheral iridectomy preserves the round pupil. Thus miosis is retained in glaucomatous eyes, photophobia is less, the cosmetic appearance is better, and the iris above serves as a protective barrier against vitreous when the latter is lost at surgery or when a postoperative rupture of the anterior hyaloid membrane occurs. Offsetting these advantages to a degree are the slightly greater difficulty in examining the peripheral fundus, the greater incidence of pupillary block, and the greater chance of occlusion of the pupil by postoperative inflammation.

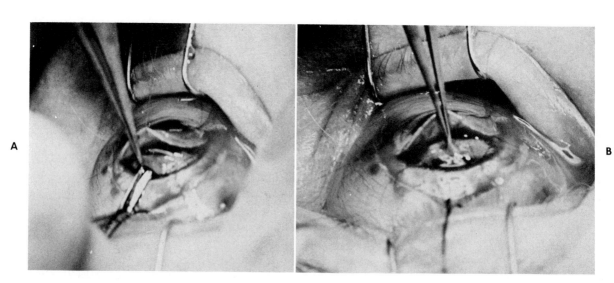

Fig. 3-53. Peripheral iridotomy. **A,** Iris grasped with Hoskins No. 19 forceps. Transverse incision made in periphery of iris. **B,** Two peripheral iridotomies shown.

Peripheral iridotomy

Peripheral iridotomy is the incision of full-thickness iris near its base. It is performed by grasping a small portion of iris with forceps near its base, gently drawing it upward, and making a transverse cut in the iris between its base and the forceps (Fig. 3-53). A small scissors incision made in this manner will provide an opening as large as an iridectomy, since that cut is made against the grain of the iris fibers. A longitudinal cut in the direction of the iris fibers will not provide a gaping wound, and it closes more easily. The surgeon should exercise caution to grasp iris only and pull it up sufficiently so that lens capsule is not cut with the scissors. The tips of the scissors should be rounded rather than sharp. The iridotomy should be performed under direct visualization. It is technically easier to perform than a peripheral iridectomy, especially in the presence of a corneal incision.

The advantages and disadvantages are identical to those of a peripheral iridectomy.

Sector iridectomy

Sector iridectomy is the excision of a sector of iris from its sphincter to its base. It may be performed under open-sky visualization or by grasping the iris near its sphincter and drawing it out of the eye. A narrow sector opening is obtained by grasping the iris very close to its sphincter. A

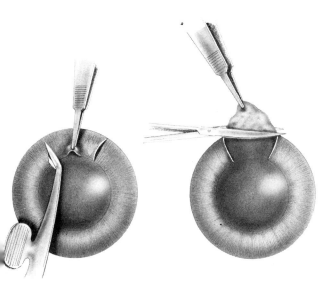

Fig. 3-54. Sector iridectomy. Two radial incisions are made from sphincter to base, and included iris sector is resected at its base.

wider opening occurs when the iris is grasped midway between its sphincter and base. The portion of iris is exteriorized and excised with scissors that cut parallel to the corneoscleral incision or perpendicular to it. In the latter case the tips of the scissors should be directed toward 12 o'clock rather than 6 o'clock. It has been recommended that an iridodialysis be created before the iris sector is excised. This is unnecessary and may be dangerous because a very large iridodialysis may occur and excess bleeding may result.

The surgeon can perform a perfectly symmetrical iridectomy to the exact size desired by the following technique: The cornea is retracted. The iris is grasped near its sphincter and gently lifted. Two radial incisions are made from the sphincter to the base, and the included iris sector is resected at its base (Fig. 3-54).

A sector iridectomy is performed to facilitate delivery of the lens in the case of a small, rigid pupil or one bound down by posterior synechias, to provide better postoperative visualization of the fundus where retinal detachment is more likely or was repaired before the cataract surgery, to lessen the chances of pupillary occlusion in cases of chronic iridocyclitis, to allow greater evacuation of lens debris in an extracapsular extraction, and for optic reasons in the presence of a central corneal opacity.

It leaves the patient with a wider pupillary aperture, which causes greater photophobia, is less desirable cosmetically, and, according to some contact lens experts, makes contact lens correction less effective.

Radial iridotomy

Radial iridotomy is a radial incision through the sphincter and a portion of iris. It is usually placed inferiorly but may be performed in any location. It is performed by inserting one blade of the deWecker-Barraquer or straight iris scissors under the iris and cutting to the desired extent (Fig. 3-55). To avoid injury to the corneal endothelium and lens capsule, blunt-tipped scissors should be used. It is performed by visualization through the cornea. A radial iridotomy facilitates extraction of the lens through a pupil that cannot be dilated adequately and may serve an optical function in the presence of a central corneal opacity. It also prevents an updrawn pupil in

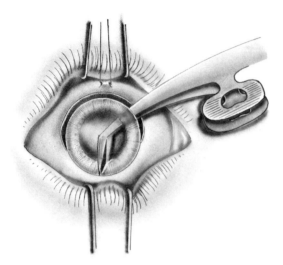

Fig. 3-55. Radial iridotomy.

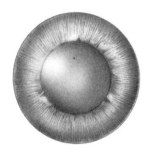

Fig. 3-56. Three small sphincterotomies placed in eye with small pupil resulting from prolonged miotic therapy.

case of operative loss of vitreous or postoperative iridocyclitis. In the same manner it is useful when employing a corneal incision in an eye with posterior synechias after a filtering procedure.

Sphincterotomy

Sphincterotomy is a tiny incision through the sphincter muscle of the iris. It is usually performed in more than one location, but generally sphincterotomies placed at 4:30 and 7:30 o'clock are adequate (Fig. 3-56). If further dilation is desired, an additional incision may be made at 12 o'clock. If the incisions are too large, permanent pupillary dilation will result. Its most frequent indication is in eyes with small pupils, resulting

from prolonged miotic therapy, when lens extraction through a round pupil is desired. Peripheral iridectomy or iridotomy is performed along with the sphincterotomies.

Iridodialysis

Iridodialysis is the intentional separation of the iris root from its attachment over a small distance to create a peripheral iris opening. The iris is grasped at its base with forceps and pulled away from its insertion. Too often, the iris will pull away excessively, leaving an unsightly large opening and a distorted pupil. The iridodialysis opening is used by some surgeons to deliver the lens. Bleeding is more likely to occur than with the other techniques described earlier. However, more serious is the inadvertent separation of the scleral spur, which creates a communication between the anterior chamber and the suprachoroidal space. The ensuing hypotonia and its consequences are discussed in Chapter 12. The technique of iridodialysis offers no advantages over other methods, may cause more complications, and probably should be abandoned.

EXTRACAPSULAR CATARACT EXTRACTION

In this section, extracapsular cataract extraction refers to surgery performed with a standard size incision. It does not refer to phacoemulsification (Chapter 6), phacofragmentation, or any other kind of extracapsular procedure in which a 3 mm incision may be used. The type of planned extracapsular extraction performed by a surgeon who uses loupes differs from that which can be performed by a surgeon trained in the use of the surgical microscope. This will be apparent during the description of the techniques.

The young ophthalmologist rarely has an opportunity to learn the technique of a planned extracapsular cataract extraction with a standard incision. Experience with such an operation generally stems from a mishap during an intended intracapsular cataract extraction. The accidental rupture of the lens capsule may then require an unplanned extracapsular extraction.

The intracapsular cataract extraction is still the preferred method in the United States. However, there is a definite trend toward the extracapsular cataract extraction, which appears to be stronger each year. The following is a list of alleged advantages of the extracapsular over the intracapsular method of cataract extraction. It will be readily apparent that some of these are highly questionable, although others appear reasonable.

1. Retention of an avascular membrane between the vitreous and the anterior chamber. This presumably lowers the incidence of retinal tears.

2. Less likelihood of a redetachment in patients who have had previous retinal detachment surgery and who require cataract extraction.

Some clinicians assume that the posterior capsule (even with a capsulotomy) keeps the vitreous from bulging forward, thus lessening vitreous shock. There are no valid statistics currently available to support this premise, but it appears promising enough to warrant further investigation.

3. Greatly reduced endophthalmodonesis.

4. Preservation of a barrier between the aqueous and vitreous and protection of the retina from the possible toxic constituents of the aqueous. These two alleged advantages have been cited as a protection of the retina against the development of cystoid macular edema.

Endophthalmodonesis refers to the relative mobility of certain intraocular structures such as the iris or an intraocular lens compared to immobile structures such as the cornea and sclera. The greatest degree of endophthalmodonesis occurs with an iris-supported intraocular lens in conjunction with an intracapsular cataract extraction. An anterior chamber angle-supported lens with an intracapsular cataract extraction is associated with much less endophthalmodonesis. A difference in the incidence of cystoid macular edema between an iris-supported and an angle-supported lens implant has not yet been demonstrated.

As to a barrier protecting the retina from toxic constituents of the aqueous, these constituents have not yet been positively identified, and it is unknown whether the intact posterior capsule and surrounding zonular apparatus are impermeable to them.

5. Where operative loss of vitreous is likely. This is an advantage that may be valid, but it will not be realized until the surgeon becomes fully familiar with the technique of the extracapsular cataract extraction.

6. Preservation of a membrane anterior to the vitreous in the event a secondary lens implant is indicated. Therefore, if a routine cataract extraction is performed in anticipation of postoperative contact lens wear and the management of the contact lens proves unsuccessful, a secondary lens implant becomes much less hazardous. I predict that this will influence many surgeons as extended wear contact lens becomes more popular. This is a valid advantage that should appeal to many cataract surgeons.

7. In corneal dystrophy, protection of the endothelium from vitreous touch by preservation of the posterior capsule. This is undoubtedly true; but this becomes less of an advantage when one considers that an extracapsular cataract extraction probably causes more endothelial cell loss than an intracapsular extraction, according to most studies.

8. In aphakic penetrating keratoplasty, greater safety and technical ease with an intact posterior capsule. Most corneal surgeons would consider this a highly valid advantage.

9. In young, active, and athletic individuals, less possibility with the posterior capsule of postoperative rupture of the anterior hyaloid membrane with incarceration of vitreous in the operative wound; the architecture of the vitreous is more likely to be maintained. Similarly, if a postoperative wound dehiscence should occur, the posterior capsule may prevent vitreous from gaining access to the wound. This advantage may also be valid if the first eye suffered corneal edema from vitreocorneal adherence. The preservation of a posterior capsule may prevent this complication in the second eye.

10. Less risk of a cystoid macular edema if the first eye suffered a significant cystoid macular edema after an intracapsular procedure. While the evidence that the posterior capsule lessens the risk of this complication has not absolutely been proven, reports supporting this view are appearing (Chapter 18). At this time, I would favor an extracapsular cataract extraction with preservation of an intact posterior capsule in this situation if surgery on the second eye becomes necessary.

It must be emphasized that there is no overwhelming agreement among ophthalmologists that these advantages are valid ones. However, an extracapsular lens extraction is often performed for the foregoing reasons, however meritorious they may be.

Technique

Planned extracapsular cataract extraction using loupes. The pupil must be fully dilated. If this is not possible, a sector iridectomy is necessary. Toothed capsule forceps such as those designed by Schweigger are inserted into the anterior chamber with the closed jaws placed over the center of the lens. The jaws of the forceps are

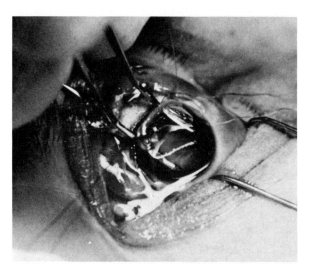

Fig. 3-57. Capsulectomy with toothed (Schweigger) forceps.

opened wide and pressed against the anterior capsule of the lens (Fig. 3-57). A moderately large piece of capsule is grasped between the jaws as the forceps are closed. The teeth of the forceps should be very sharp, otherwise an excessively large piece of anterior capsule that might include some of the posterior capsule will be removed. The forceps are then moved back and forth horizontally and vertically to be sure the engaged piece of capsule is free of the remainder of the lens. Otherwise the entire lens may follow the forceps as it is removed from the eye. For the same reason, alpha-chymotrypsin should not be employed in an extracapsular cataract extraction. The nucleus of the lens is delivered by pressing against the limbus at 6 o'clock with an instrument such as a muscle hook or a lens expressor while a lens spoon or wire loop presses firmly against the posterior lip of the wound (Fig. 3-58). Gentle irrigation of the anterior chamber with balanced salt solution is performed. If there is no tendency for the intraocular contents to bulge forward, large pieces of anterior capsule and cortex that cannot be irrigated from the eye may be removed with smooth forceps. It is best not to be overzealous with this procedure, since vitreous may be lost. Postoperative mydriasis is maintained until most of the residual lens cortex has become absorbed.

The nucleus of the lens may be removed by other methods. A sharp pick or a disposable 27-

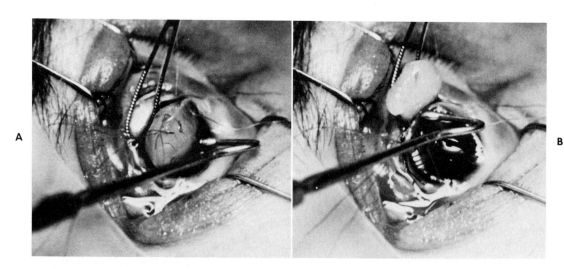

Fig. 3-58. A, Pressure exerted at limbus at 6 o'clock with tip of muscle hook. Wire loop slid between edge of incision and lens at 12 o'clock. **B,** Completed extracapsular extraction.

gauge needle may be inserted to effectively pull the nucleus from the eye. A cryoprobe may also be used to extract the lens nucleus. These techniques are useful in cases where vitreous bulge is evident, since external pressure against the globe is not required.

Planned extracapsular cataract extraction using a surgical microscope. A variation of the extracapsular cataract extraction technique that occupies a role between the method just described and phacoemulsification is gaining popularity. It is best performed with the aid of a surgical microscope. A small ab externo incision is made at 12 o'clock. An anterior capsulectomy is performed in one of several ways. One popular method is to bend a 22- or 23-gauge disposable needle at its tip and attach it to an irrigation flow solution bottle. It may also be attached to the irrigating handpiece of an automated unit. Another employs a Kelman cystotome (Storz Instrument Co. Catalogue No. E-141-1). The "Christmas tree" type of capsulectomy is described on p. 193. The capsule is excised as it is withdrawn from the anterior chamber. Another method employs a "can opener" anterior capsulectomy. Punctures are made in the anterior capsule at each hour of the clock just within the border of the dilated pupil (Fig. 3-59). The portion of the anterior capsule within the punctures is easily freed. After the capsule is open, the nucleus of the lens is freed from the surrounding cortex by using the vertical and lateral seesaw maneuvers described on p. 193. It is not necessary to dislocate the lens nucleus into the anterior chamber, although this is preferable. The nucleus can be prolapsed into the anterior chamber with the Kelman cystotome because it has a sharp point and a dull posterior curve that will usually engage the nucleus rather than tear through it. For this reason, this cystotome can perform the "Christmas tree" capsulectomy. It engages the capsule and does not puncture it at the point of initial contact. It tears the capsule only after the tip of the cystotome has been drawn a few millimeters toward the limbal incision. The bent 22-gauge needle will perforate the capsule on initial contact and therefore is suitable for a "can opener" type of capsulectomy. The latter can also be performed with the Kelman cystotome.

The incision is enlarged to 120 to 130 degrees. The lens nucleus is then expressed from the eye in the manner just described. If the lens nucleus is brought into the anterior chamber, a simple method of expression is used. A Pearce or Knolle irrigating vectis is slid under the lens nucleus while pressure is exerted posteriorly. An assistant irrigates while the surgeon handles the vectis. The irrigation lifts the nucleus away from the cortex and aids its exit from the eye. This vectis is shaped like a wire loop. The nucleus may also be

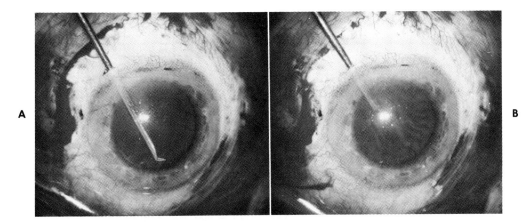

Fig. 3-59. A, Twenty-two–gauge needle with tip bent to form cystotome. **B,** Circular anterior capsulectomy in "can-opener" pattern. (From Jaffe, N. S., et al.: Pseudophakos, St. Louis, 1978, The C. V. Mosby Co.)

delivered from the posterior chamber. In this case the nucleus is usually separated from the surrounding cortex at 12 o'clock only, or all around. Pressure is exerted against the sclera just outside the limbus at 12 o'clock. When the superior nucleus is seen, it may be lifted out of the eye by a sharp needle or by sharp pointed forceps held by an assistant. There are many variations in the method of removing the lens nucleus. Most surgeons choose the method according to the situation at the time of surgery, for example, according to the size of the pupil.

Some of the larger cortical remnants are gently irrigated from the eye. The incision is closed with the three sutures. The remainder of the cortical material is aspirated by a technique of aspiration-irrigation. This is satisfactorily accomplished by one of the many available aspiration-irrigation needles. One example is the O'Gawa needle (Storz Instrument Co. Catalogue No. E-4916-20), which consists of two different sized hypodermic needles soldered together and blunted (Fig. 3-60). The size of the irrigating bore is that of a 23-gauge needle, and the aspirating bore is 20 gauge. The irrigation occurs through the side part of the needle while the as-

piration is through the tip of the needle. A needle such as this permits separate control of aspirating and irrigating flow volumes so that irrigating volume can be delivered at a rate sufficient to replace that lost through the aspirating channel and from leakage around the needle. It also permits the surgeon to aim the irrigation stream from the needle tip in a direction that would not wash away lens material from the aspirating orifice. The unit, including the tubing, can be stream autoclaved, since the two halves of the irrigating channel are connected by silicone rubber (Silastic) tubing, size 0.020 by 0.037 inches. This technique permits gravity flow of Ringer's lactate solution into the eye from an infusion stand setup. The input drip is moderately slow. The surgeon places the aspiration bore adjacent to cortical remnants. When the surgeon is satisfied with the degree of aspiration, the wound is closed with fine sutures.

Other methods of removing the cortical remnants from the eye. Some of these methods involve simple aspiration in a closed system. The incision is temporarily closed with sutures. The residual cortex is aspirated with a fine cannula (usually 23 gauge) with a side opening. The

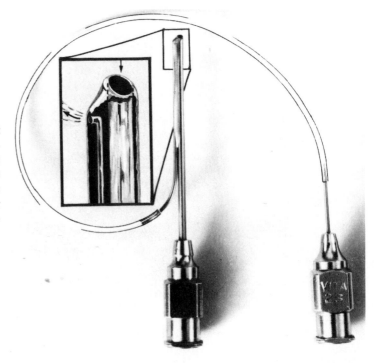

Fig. 3-60. Double-bore O'Gawa cataract aspiration unit with inset to show magnification of needle tip. Each needle hub is attached to 10 ml syringe. Surgeon controls aspirating syringe while assistant handles irrigating syringe to keep anterior chamber formed. (From O'Gawa, G. M.: Am. J. Ophthalmol. **64:**970-972, 1967.)

chamber is kept from collapsing by replacing aspirated fluid with irrigation of fluid. This is a push-pull type of action. A simple technique is that used by Simcoe.[13] After the capsulotomy is done and the nucleus removed, the incision is closed with temporary sutures, and the anterior chamber is filled with balanced salt solution. A 13 mm long blunt, curved 23-gauge cannula with a side port opening near the tip (Storz Instrument Co., Catalogue No. E-4969) is attached to a silicone anterior chamber irrigating bulb with Luerlock adaptor (Fig. 3-61). The bulb is filled with balanced salt solution. Light squeeze pressure is maintained on the bulb as the cannula is introduced through the incision, across the anterior

chamber (with the side aperture facing away from the posterior capsule), and into the cortex contained in the capsular fornix. The squeeze is released, and the plastic bulb expands to resume its normal shape. The cortex is then pulled toward the center of the anterior chamber by the slight suction (Fig. 3-62). The cortex is then released by gentle pressure on the silicone bulb. This sequence is repeated in all quadrants (Fig. 3-63). When considerable cortex accumulates in the anterior chamber, the cannula is withdrawn almost to the wound lip (Fig. 3-64). The loose cortical material is irrigated out of the eye as the posterior wound lip is slightly depressed by the tip of the cannula.

For those surgeons who have access to the phacoemulsification unit, the residual cortical material is very effectively removed by using the nonultrasonic handpiece and tip, which performs only irrigation and aspiration (Fig. 3-65). The wound is temporarily closed with sutures. A 3 mm opening is required at the 11 o'clock position

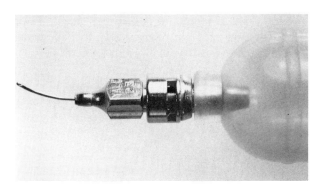

Fig. 3-61. Cortex extractor cannula with bulb and Luerlock adaptor. (From Simcoe, C. W.: J. Am. Intraocul. Implant Soc. **3:**194-196, 1977.)

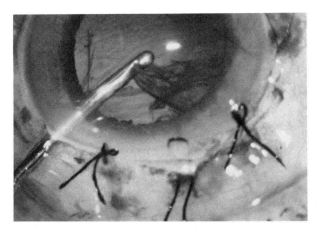

Fig. 3-62. Cortex being stripped out of capsular fornix. (From Simcoe, C. W.: J. Am. Intraocul. Implant Soc. **3:** 194-196, 1977.)

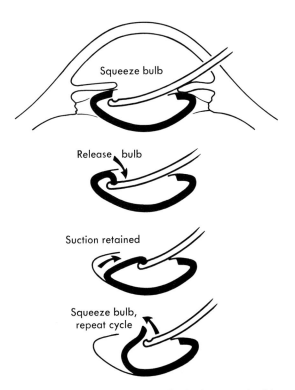

Fig. 3-63. Steps in Simcoe method of removal of lens material. No true aspiration employed. (From Simcoe, C. W.: J. Am. Intraocul. Implant Soc. **3:**194-196, 1977.)

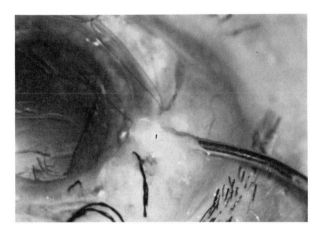

Fig. 3-64. Cortex evacuation from anterior chamber around cannula. (From Simcoe, C. W.: J. Am. Intraocul. Implant Soc. **3:**194-196, 1977.)

for a right-handed surgeon to introduce the tip (Fig. 3-66).

When all the cortex has been removed, the posterior capsule can be polished with a sandblasted irrigating device such as the Kratz scratcher (Fig. 3-67). It may also be polished with the 0.2 or 0.3 mm tip of the irrigation-aspiration handpiece of the Cavitron unit under low suction power. This may be used with all the techniques described here, but it requires a surgical microscope.

The problems associated with retained lens material in the past made extracapsular cataract extraction in adults practically obsolete. These difficulties are discussed in Chapter 24. However, these methods are far more sophisticated than those used in the past. The planned extracapsular extraction procedure described here should not be compared with the planned extracapsular extraction involved in phacoemulsification, for reasons outlined in Chapter 6.

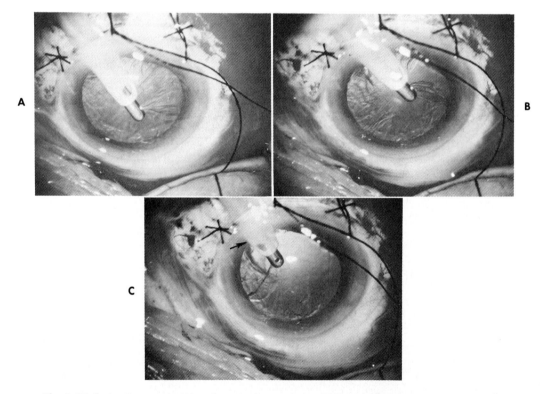

Fig. 3-65. Irrigation-aspiration of cortical remnants. **A,** Cortex drawn into aspirating device. **B,** Clear posterior capsule visible as cortex is aspirated. **C,** Note cortex being drawn into aspirating aperture. Anterior chamber is kept formed by irrigation through plastic sleeve on tip *(arrow)*. (From Jaffe, N. S., et al.: Pseudophakos, St. Louis, 1978, The C. V. Mosby Co.)

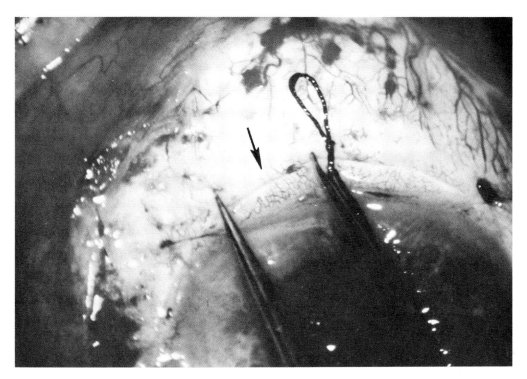

Fig. 3-66. Incision temporarily closed, leaving 3 mm opening *(arrow)* for irrigation-aspiration tip. (From Jaffe, N. S., et al.: Pseudophakos,. St. Louis, 1978, The C. V. Mosby Co.)

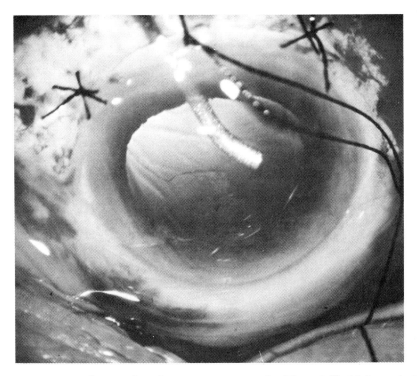

Fig. 3-67. Kratz scratcher used to clean posterior capsule. (From Jaffe, N. S., et al.: Pseudophakos, St. Louis, 1978, The C. V. Mosby Co.)

CATARACT ASPIRATION

The favored surgical technique of management of congenital and juvenile cataracts has decidedly turned from discission and linear extraction to aspiration. Lens aspiration is an ancient technique practiced by Antyllus[14,15] in the second century. Although others[16-20] reported it in the literature during the past century, it was Scheie[20] who deserves the major credit for its reintroduction. It is likely to increase in popularity because it is ideally suited to current trends of surgery under microscopic control.

The discission technique, although still applicable to certain kinds of cataracts such as membranous cataracts, does too little. It opens the anterior capsule of the lens and stirs up the lens material. It depends entirely on the eye to absorb the retained lens remnants. Pupillary block glaucoma, secondary pupillary membranes, fibrovascular vitreous membranes, and retinal detachment are not infrequent results. Linear extraction, essentially an extracapsular method, succeeds in more effectively removing the lens material but proves to be associated with a high incidence of operative loss of vitreous. A relatively large incision is dangerous in a young eye because of low scleral rigidity. The globe collapses when opened, and additionally, the vitreous and posterior capsule move forward with the capsulectomy. It was not surprising that attempts at intracapsular extraction would be made after the introduction of alpha-chymotrypsin. After some experience with this method, Girard[22] concluded that the intracapsular method in infants and children was not recommended. The problems he encountered may be listed as follows:

1. Problems encountered at the time of surgery
   a. Increased intraocular pressure under general anesthesia
   b. Decreased scleral structural rigidity of infants and children
   c. Presence of lenticular vitreal adhesions
   d. Occasional failure of alpha-chymotrypsin to produce complete zonulysis
2. Problems encountered postoperatively
   a. Increased intraocular pressure in the postoperative period
   b. Difficulty in patient control

With increasing popularity of lens aspiration, the method has been applied boldly to older patients up to 40 years old. Although the method is simple, there are numerous techniques currently in practice:

1. Aspiration by suction alone
2. Aspiration by alternate suction and irrigation—"push-pull"
3. Simultaneous aspiration and irrigation through a double-barreled needle (Fuchs, Fink, O'Gawa, and so on)
4. Simultaneous aspiration and irrigation by separate needles introduced through separate openings
5. Preliminary ripening followed by aspiration several days later

Although this technique can be performed with a surgical loupe, this is undoubtedly one of the situations in which the surgical microscope serves its greatest usefulness. No matter which technique is followed, the anterior capsule of the lens must first be opened. This is best accomplished with a knife needle (Barkan knife) whose blade is smaller than its shaft so that the anterior chamber does not empty while the knife is manipulated within the eye. I prefer to enter the globe just outside the limbus (using a small fornix- or limbus-based conjunctival flap) for two reasons. First, the blade can be kept closer to parallel with the iris, thus avoiding the posterior capsule, and second, incisions central to the termination of Schwalbe's line may result in Descemet's tubes (Chapter 28). Some surgeons make a wide incision in the anterior capsule and then stir up and whip the lens for several minutes. Others simply make a cruciate or V-shaped incision without stirring the lens or they make a single incision. The important point is that these maneuvers are safe as long as the anterior chamber is not lost. Otherwise, the posterior capsule and the anterior face of the vitreous will be incised. Greater leeway is permitted when the surgery is performed under microscopic control. As the knife is removed, the incision is slightly enlarged to permit the introduction of the aspirating needle.

There are many needles in current use that serve well for aspiration. Short needles are less clumsy to utilize under the microscope. They range from a thin-walled, 18-gauge needle to a thick-walled, 23-gauge needle. It is surprising how well a fine needle performs in this procedure. If the needle fits snugly in the incision, the anterior chamber remains adequately deep for aspiration without accompanying irrigation. The plunger in the syringe to which the needle is attached should work smoothly. A moistened glass syringe performs better than a disposable plastic syringe. The tip of the needle should be blunt. Gass[23] uses a 22-gauge needle with a side opening, as well as a needle with an opening at the tip. If the needle is beveled, it should enter the anterior chamber with the opening facing the vitreous. It is then rotated so that all aspiration is performed with the opening facing the corneal endothelium. Under microscopic control the surgeon can easily rotate the opening to aspirate isolated bits of tenacious lens material. A satisfactory method is to break up and remove the cataractous portion of the lens with push-pull jets of balance salt solution and then aspirate the remaining clear cortex by suction alone. There is no need to rush. The surgeon should attempt to remove as much lens material as possible without damaging the vitreous face. If a posterior subcapsular or a posterior polar cataract that cannot be aspirated is present, the needle is removed from the anterior chamber, and the wound is sutured. The chamber is re-formed and a discission may then be performed. At the conclusion of the aspiration procedure, it is a good practice to make a second needle puncture and sweep a 1 mm spatula across the wound to ensure that no strands of capsule, zonules, or vitreous are caught in it. If the posterior capsule has been ruptured and vitreous is present in the anterior chamber, the wound is closed, an inferior limbal incision is made, a bubble of air is placed in the anterior chamber, the pupil is constricted with acetylcholine solution, and the sweep maneuver is performed under the air bubble. Vitreous may initially be removed through the first incision by use of cellulose sponges to exteriorize it. Air is then placed in the anterior chamber, and the remainder of the procedure is performed as just outlined.

The disadvantages of a double needle are that an assistant is necessary, and the incision into the anterior chamber must be larger. The Fink needle requires an assistant to force fluid into the eye while the surgeon directs the needle in the anterior chamber. The Fuchs syringe does not require an assistant but is much too cumbersome for fine control and requires a larger incision.

Another method is to use two pediatric scalp vein sets, which come with 23-gauge needles and polyethylene tubes attached to them. One needle is placed into the anterior chamber and is controlled by an assistant who keeps the anterior chamber filled with balanced salt solution. The other needle enters the anterior chamber at a different location and is used by the surgeon for aspiration.

Phacoemulsification is ideally suited for congenital and juvenile cataracts, since they can be easily removed by aspiration alone.

The performance of a preliminary ripening procedure, followed several days later by aspiration, appears less necessary now that aspiration may be accomplished under microscopic control. The need for two separate anesthesias and parental anxiety are definite disadvantages.

There is still some controversy about how to manage the iris during an aspiration procedure. In most instances an iridectomy is unnecessary. However, if the pupil dilates very poorly before surgery, as occasionally occurs in rubella, one may be prudent by performing an iridectomy. A small opening is made with a Graefe knife at the superior limbus. An iris hook is used to pull a portion of the iris out of the wound where it is excised. This may be repeated inferiorly as well. This is the Franceschetti iridectomy. The capsulotomy and aspiration may then be performed through the superior incision. Pupillary block is much less of a problem now that it is possible with the aid of the microscope to remove practically all of the lens material.

Two other situations where the aspiration technique is useful are in the patient with a senile cataract who has an unplanned extracapsular cataract extraction with considerable retained lens material and in traumatic cataracts. In the former a lens aspiration will clear the pupil sufficiently so that the patient does not have to go through a convalescence that may last several months. In the latter, if there is a gaping corneal wound and a ruptured lens capsule, the wound should be closed first, the anterior chamber re-formed, and aspiration performed as described earlier. If vitreous is present in the wound, a partial anterior vitrectomy should be performed first. It is essential to free the anterior chamber of all material that can give rise to a destructive fibroplastic reaction. It is poor policy to close the wound and wait for the lens to absorb.

It is essential to keep the pupil dilated for several months after lens aspiration. This must be impressed on the parents, who play an important role in the postoperative management of these children.

The optimum time for surgery in congenital cataracts and the optic correction of the aphakia are still controversial subjects. It is agreed that it is important to avoid deprivation amblyopia. Early surgery may accomplish this, but the exact age at which surgery must be performed to avoid amblyopia is not known. This is probably sometime during the first year. If the surgery is performed at age 3 to 4 years, permanent amblyopia is almost certain to develop. If the cataract occurs at age 4 to 6 years, deprivation amblyopia rarely develops. Despite successful surgery, the visual result may be very disappointing because of retinal or optic nerve damage, deprivation amblyopia, or anisometropic amblyopia.

The effectiveness of the optic correction of the aphakia is still unknown. The use of contact lenses is worth a trial if cooperative parents are available. The use of lenses in the first year of life is usually considerably easier than in the second to fourth years. The approximate refractive error and corneal K readings can be obtained in the anesthetized infant. In the child with rubella, the refractive error is usually approximately +30.00 D. It may be wise to overcorrect this amount by several diopters to permit close vision in the infant. After a year or two, close to 50% of the hyperopia may be gone. Therefore it is necessary to refract these children every 4 to 6 months. This form of management is undertaken at many centers today, and before long the true value of this arduous regimen should be known.

Intracapsular cataract extraction

The intracapsular cataract extraction is still the method of choice among most ophthalmologists for patients over the age of 30. However, an increasing number of surgeons at this time are turning to phacoemulsification in patients whose lens nuclei are not too sclerotic. To achieve an intracapsular cataract extraction, ophthalmologists have at their disposal numerous methods that have been thoroughly described in previous books on cataract surgery. However, because of modern advances such as methods of inducing ocular hypotony, enzymatic zonulysis, and improved suture material, these methods have been modified to work in harmony with these improvements. The cryoextraction technique has gained such wide popularity and acceptance in recent years that it has practically made obsolete all other methods of intracapsular cataract extraction. This poses a dilemma for the young ophthalmologist who must learn techniques that are practiced today with lessening frequency. Formerly, a resident ophthalmologist would become familiar with capsule forceps in one series and the erisiphake in another, tumble some lenses, and slide others. It is becoming increasingly difficult to find teachers who still practice these techniques.

Since the cryo method can be applied to virtually all situations where an intracapsular extraction is indicated, why learn any other procedure? A cryoextractor may not be available or else it may fail to perform. The complete cataract surgeon should be able to meet this situation by substituting another technique.

Cryoextraction

After Krawicz introduced the technique of cryoextraction of cataracts and demonstrated its practicality, several prominent ophthalmologists in this country and abroad predicted that the method would not replace more conventional techniques in the average case. They were wrong. Cryoextraction has gained such wide popularity in a few years that it has become the procedure of choice in all cases where an intracapsular cataract extraction is desired.

Its main advantage is that a cryoextractor provides the firmest possible grip on the lens capsule. This is accomplished by forming an ice ball that includes the capsule and a portion of the underlying cortex and nucleus attached to the cryoprobe as a single physical unit. It is obvious that this ensures a lowered incidence of capsule rupture. It is an effective technique for intumescent or hypermature cataracts and subluxated and dislocated lenses. It permits a cataract extraction through a relatively small pupil as well as a smaller incision if this is desired. It is also much easier to grasp the lens in a deep set eye with a cryoextractor than with capsule forceps or an erisiphake.

The cryoextractor units available range from simple, sterile, disposable ones to complicated, permanent units with bulky, plastic pipelines. Some are equipped with a heating element that operates in case of inadvertent adherence of the cryoprobe to the cornea or iris. In the others such a mishap is overcome by directing a stream of balanced salt solution to the site of adherence. The most popular coolants in the United States are carbon dioxide and freon.

Technique. Enzymatic zonulysis is used by many surgeons but may be superfluous with the cryoextraction method in all patients over 50. I still use it in every intended intracapsular lens extraction, regardless of age.

Unless a sector iridectomy has been performed, some method of retracting the iris is necessary. The least traumatic is by use of a cellulose sponge. Iris forceps without teeth may also be used. They have the advantage of minimal iris trauma and no pressure against the ciliary process. I prefer Hoskins No. 19 forceps. They also aid in separating the zonules. However, since they provide a V-shaped pupillary aperture with the apex pointing toward the surgeon, it is rela-

tively easy for iris to adhere to the cryoprobe. Numerous iris retractors that provide a more adequate pupillary opening for delivery of the lens are available. They are made of plastic or stainless steel. The handle may be in line with the direction of iris retraction, or it may be at a right angle to it (Fig. 3-68). With the latter the two hands of the surgeon are separated from each other by a more convenient distance. These instruments aid in separating the zonules as the superior pole of the lens is pulled upward. Their main disadvantage is that they are more traumatic to the iris, and it is possible to massage the heads of the ciliary processes by excessive retraction. Although it is possible to mold a soft lens through a relatively small pupil, the surgeon must exercise good judgment with a hard lens and a rigid iris sphincter. It may not be possible to accurately predict the softness of the lens, but the rigidity of the iris. If the inferior portion of the pupil is pulled upward during iris retraction so that the aperture remains small, it is unwise to attempt a lens extraction without enlarging the opening by a sector iridectomy or one or more sphincterotomies. If retraction can be accomplished without an exaggerated upward displacement of the pupil and with an adequate aperture, sphincteric rigidity is probably not sufficient to interfere with cryoextraction.

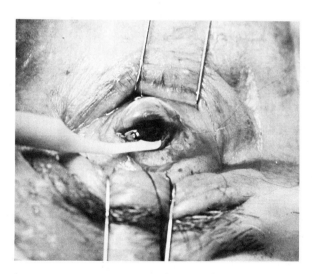

Fig. 3-68. Iris retraction with Rosenbaum-Drews retractor.

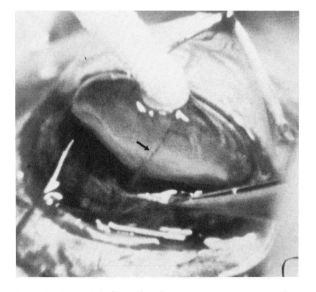

Fig. 3-69. Zonular fiber fundle *(arrow)* incorporated in cryoprobe ice ball.

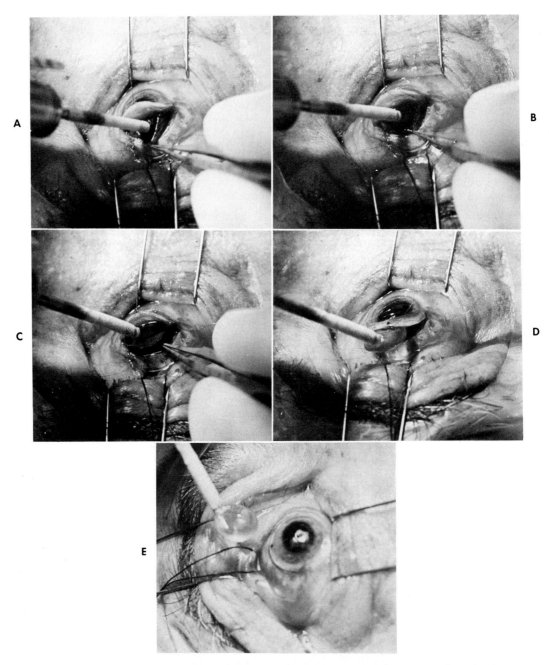

Fig. 3-70. Cryoextraction with Mark II cryostylet. **A,** Lens rotated to surgeon's right. Iris retracted with Hoskins No. 19 forceps. **B,** Lens rotated to surgeon's left. **C,** Lens lifted. **D,** Lens slid out of eye. **E,** Extraction completed.

The iris retractor (or sponge or forceps) is held in one hand and the cryoextractor in the other hand. The cornea is retracted by an assistant who grasps the conjunctival flap at 12 o'clock or a suture placed in the anterior lip of the incision. The surface of the lens is dried with a cellulose sponge. The cryoprobe is placed on the lens warm. It is placed midway between the anterior pole and the superior equator. If placed too close to the equator, it may include the zonular lamella (Fig. 3-69). Excess pull on the ciliary body will result. If applied at the anterior pole, traction is exerted on the entire zonule at one time, making release of one portion of the zonular lamella more difficult. A satisfactory ice ball usually forms within a few seconds of activation. If excess moisture is present over the lens, ice forms between the tip of the cryoprobe and the lens, making the cryoadhesion less effective. The cryoprobe tip temperature need be only $-19°$ C, but some instruments permit temperatures down to $-40°$ C. Excess freezing may rupture the posterior capsule or cause intraocular inflammation. However, if the cataract is completely mature or liquefied, the cryoprobe should remain in contact with the lens for a longer period of time before the extraction commences. This permits transmission of the ice ball to the deeper part of the lens and enables the surgeon to handle the probe and lens more as a single unit. This is unnecessary with an incomplete cataract, since the freezing temperature spreads more readily throughout the lens. If a disposable instrument that has no heating element is used, the frosted tip should be wiped clean with a finger before being applied to the lens.

When a satisfactory adhesion becomes apparent, the following three different movements aid in releasing the lens from the zonular lamella (Fig. 3-70).

1. Rotary movements, clockwise and counterclockwise
2. Rocking movements, alternately elevating the temporal and nasal equators of the lens
3. Elevation of the superior equator

Surgeons may use only one of these movements or a combination to free the lens. They usually learn a technique that performs best for them. It is important to pull slightly upward while rotating the lens. When rocking the lens, one equator is elevated, but the opposite equator must not be depressed into the vitreous.

As soon as the zonular attachments begin to separate, the lens can be pulled temporally or nasally and slid out of the eye. The instrument used for iris retraction may be used to strip the zonular fibers. This should be done very carefully. The delivery of the lens should not be forceful or excessively rapid, otherwise ciliary body trauma might occur. External pressure is usually not necessary. If the lens does not separate easily from the zonular lamella, the iris retractor or for-

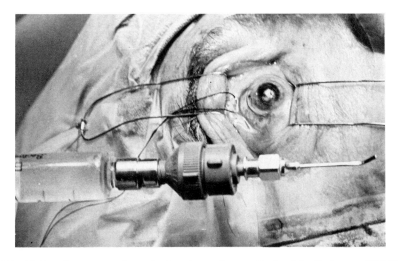

Fig. 3-71. Alpha-chymotrypsin solution in syringe attached to Swinnex-13 Millipore filter unit (Millipore Corporation, Bedford, Mass.).

Table 3-1. Comparison of lens extraction techniques

	Forceps	Erisiphake	Cryoprobe
Incision	Tumbling requires larger incision than sliding does	Larger incision than forceps Open sky requires largest incision	Smallest incision
Lens capsule	Small bite Weakest grasp Greatest incidence of capsule rupture Tense capsule – difficult Wrinkled capsule – better	Large bite Better grasp Less rupture Easier Worst	No capsule fold necessary Best grasp Least rupture Best Best
Zonules	Initiates localized separation of zonules more easily Good for resistant zonules Less danger of including zonules in grasping capsule	Localized separation more difficult Zonules stretch all over simultaneously Worst Least danger	Initiates localized separation Best Most danger
Technique	Requires most skill Most difficult to apply to lens Must squeeze forceps throughout except for cross-action forceps Instrumentation most simple Least manipulation of iris Slow delivery of lens Cornea least traumatized May tumble or slide	Less skill required Less difficult Not necessary More complicated More manipulation Faster delivery Most traumatized May tumble or slide	Least skill required Least difficult Not necessary Most complicated Most manipulation Fastest delivery Less traumatized May only slide
Principal advantage	Simplicity; less need for assistant	Simplicity; less need for assistant	Lowest incidence of capsule rupture
Principal disadvantage	Capsule rupture	Corneal damage unless open-sky technique with large incision is used	Requires assistant; instrumentation more cumbersome; inadvertent freezing of ocular structures

ceps may be removed after the lens is pulled free of the iris. In this way the zonules can be visualized and stripped with a zonule stripper. Zonular stripping under direct visualization is neither necessary nor desirable in every case. It may cause vitreous rupture.

If the cryoprobe adheres to the iris, cornea, or a suture, the contact should be released promptly by activating the heating element or directing a stream of balanced salt solution to the site of adhesion. The probe should not be pulled free, otherwise the cornea may be permanently injured, the iris may be torn, or an iridodialysis or a cyclodialysis may be created. The cryoprobe may be safely reapplied after drying the surface of the lens.

Forceps extraction

The two most commonly employed methods of lens extraction with forceps are by tumbling and sliding. To avoid rupture of the lens capsule, the delivery must be slower and traction gentler than with cryoextraction. Alpha-chymotrypsin is of greater usefulness with forceps extraction than with cryoextraction. I prefer to use it in all patients, although its greatest usefulness is in patients under 60 years of age. One milliliter of the enzyme diluted 1:5000 or 1:10,000 is irrigated through the iridotomy openings and the pupil.

After 1 minute the anterior chamber is irrigated with balanced salt solution. Because of the startling particulate contamination of alpha-chymotrypsin solutions (Chapter 22), the enzyme is irrigated into the eye through a disposable, presterilized, Millipore filter unit (Fig. 3-71).

Tumbling. Capsule forceps are introduced under the iris with the cups closed to a point slightly lower than midway between the anterior pole and the inferior equator where the capsule is thickest. The blades are opened 3 to 4 mm, and slight pressure is made against the capsule as a fold of capsule is grasped. Most capsule forceps are made so that the cups meet on the capsule side but not on the iris side to avoid catching iris between the cups. It is not always easy to be sure the lens capsule has been grasped adequately in the tumbling technique. The handle of the forceps is depressed slightly as the end holding the capsule is elevated. Tenting of the lens capsule becomes apparent if a proper grasp has been obtained.

The first movement is to gently tilt the inferior pole upward. This places the inferior zonule under tension. Gentle pressure is applied at the limbus at 6 o'clock with a lens expressor, muscle hook, or one of the numerous instruments available for this purpose. The grasping end of the forceps is then moved to the left while the inferior

Table 3-2. Comparison of tumbling and sliding

Tumbling	Sliding
Facilitates passage of lens through pupil, especially if dilation is poor	
Facilitates separation of posterior lens capsule from vitreous	
Tumbling lens acts as a barrier between vitreous and the incision	
Poor technique for a flat, hard lens, since the capsule may rupture at the inferior border and the superior border may indent the vitreous	
More difficult to visualize grasp of lens	Better view of hold on lens
	Easier to grasp lens capsule
	Permits zonular stripping under direct visualization
Requires larger incision	Smaller incision required
More corneal trauma	Less corneal trauma
Unsafe in presence of wound gape	Preferred in presence of gaping wound
Requires less mydriasis	Requires greater mydriasis
	Exposure of hyaloid superiorly from the beginning of the procedure

pole of the lens is still elevated. Pressure is applied at the limbus from 6 to 9 o'clock. The forceps are then moved to the right, and pressure is applied at the limbus from 3 to 6 o'clock. Pressure should not be made too far below the limbus because of the danger of vitreous prolapse. The surgeon should then feel the lower pole of the lens dislocate. Tumbling of the lens is continued by tilting the capsule forceps back with the heel of the forceps as the center of rotation. As slow upward traction is made, the expressor follows the lens upward by gentle pressure through the cornea. As the lens emerges from the wound, the superior zonules are usually placed on stretch. They may be separated by lateral motion of the

capsule forceps. In resistant cases the zonular fibers may be separated with the lens expressor instrument.

Sliding (Fig. 3-72). The grasp of the capsule near the superior pole is best made under direct observation. The cornea is retracted by an assistant. The superior portion of iris is gently retracted with a cellulose sponge or smooth forceps. The superior pole of the lens may be tilted upward by applying pressure against the limbus at 6 o'clock. The lens may be grasped with the cups of the capsule forceps held in a horizontal or vertical position. The grasp is made slightly superior to a midway point between the anterior pole and the superior equator. If the grasp is made hori-

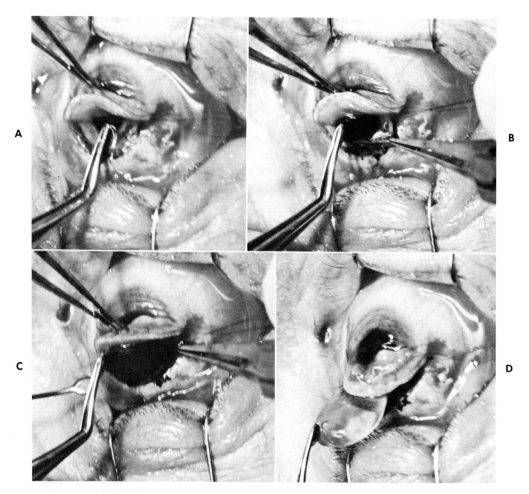

Fig. 3-72. Forceps extraction by sliding technique. **A,** Superior pole of lens rotated to surgeon's right. **B,** Lens rotated to left. **C,** Zonules stripped on right with Hoskins No. 19 forceps while lens is rotated extremely to left. **D,** Lens removed from eye.

zontally, the surgeon is better able to visualize the zonules because the hand holding the forceps is out of the way.

The first movement is a tilting of the superior pole of the lens upward. This places the zonules on stretch. The forceps are then moved to the left and right until the zonullar lamella begins to separate. The lens is then slid out of the eye in the direction where the zonular lamella first separates. This technique is ideally suited for zonular stripping under direct observation. As the superior pole of the lens is tilted to the left, the zonules on the right are placed on stretch and easily stripped with an instrument. The superior pole is then tilted in the opposite direction as the zonular stripping proceeds.

A variation in the sliding technique is the Verhoeff method. A sector iridectomy is performed. Verhoeff capsule forceps, or some modification of them, each having the cups set at right angles to the shaft, are used to grasp the true equator of the lens above. If the pupil is to be left round, the iris must be retracted. Some models of these forceps have an iris retractor set in the lower blade. The extraction proceeds in the same manner described for the sliding technique.

The grip on the capsule is obviously much weaker than with a cryoprobe; thus the incidence of capsule rupture is higher. The maneuvers involve a combination of traction and pressure with or without mechanical stripping of the zonules. With the tumbling technique the corneal endothelium is more vulnerable to trauma by the capsule forceps. It also requires a larger incision than the sliding technique. It is easier to tumble a lens through a small pupil than to slide it through. Tumbling facilitates separation of the lens capsule from the anterior hyaloid membrane. In the sliding technique the vitreous face is exposed from the beginning of the procedure. In the case of a hard, flat lens, sliding is safer than tumbling. Forceps are usually ineffective for an intumescent lens. If there is any tendency to gaping of the wound, sliding is safer than tumbling.

Phacoerysis

An erisiphake may be used instead of capsule forceps, either to slide or tumble the lens. Some cataract surgeons prefer this technique for all extractions, and it has a decided advantage over capsule forceps in the case of an intumescent lens. The instruments designed for this purpose vary from a simple suction cup attached to a rubber or silicone bulb to a motorized vacuum apparatus. The former is operated by hand, whereas the latter has an adjustable valve and gauge and may also incorporate a dwell or bypass valve to eliminate suction at the erisiphake until it is in complete contact with lens capsule.

Tumbling. With this method, phacoerysis may be performed by open-sky technique or without corneal retraction. The erisiphake is introduced through the lateral side of the incision to the lower part of the lens. In the case of a hand-operated erisiphake, the air in the bulb is replaced with balanced salt solution. The solution is expelled from the bulb, and pressure is released to allow suction to grasp the lens capsule. However, the air may be expelled before the instrument enters the anterior chamber and then applied to the lens capsule dry while the bulb is squeezed firmly. The pressure is then released to grasp the lens capsule. The delivery of the lens then proceeds as follows. With a motorized vacuum apparatus the erisiphake cup is passed through the pupil, and gentle contact is made with the lens capsule. The vacuum pressure should be about 30 cm Hg for an average lens, 45 to 55 cm Hg for young patients, and as little as 5 to 15 cm Hg for an intumescent lens. As soon as suction is created, the equatorial diameter of the lens is reduced because of partial prolapse of the anterior lens capsule into the cup of the instrument. At the same time, tension is increased on the zonular fibers to facilitate their separation from the lens. The vacuum pressure is increased slightly. The erisiphake is raised slightly. The inferior pole is then rotated slightly upward by rotating the handle between the fingers. Pressure is exerted at the lower limbus to aid in zonular rupture. As soon as the lens is freed, it is easily tumbled out of the eye. The superior pole of the lens must not be depressed into the vitreous as the inferior pole is elevated. With gentle pressure through the cornea, the instrument used for counterpressure follows the lens during the tumbling maneuver.

Sliding. Sliding is best performed by using the open-sky technique. The cornea is retracted by an assistant. The anterior capsule of the lens is dried with a cellulose sponge. The erisiphake cup is passed through the pupil and applied gently to the anterior lens capsule, slightly eccentrically toward the superior pole. When suction is achieved, the lens is lifted slightly and the superior pole is tilted slightly upward in a reverse tumbling maneuver. The inferior pole must not be depressed into the vitreous. The zonules are thus placed on stretch. The lens may be rotated slightly in the plane of the iris or rocked by alternately elevating the nasal and temporal equators. These maneuvers may be augmented by direct stripping of the stretched zonules with the surgeon's free hand. As the lens is removed from the eye, the cornea is permitted to follow.

REPOSITIONING OF THE IRIS

Immediately after delivery of the lens, the surgeon's attention should be directed toward repositioning of the iris, toilet of the anterior chamber, and closure of the wound. The drama of cataract surgery does not terminate with the removal of the lens from the eye. Many of the serious postoperative complications are related to faulty restoration of the anterior chamber.

The following outlines the various situations that may be encountered and measures suggested to remedy them:

1. Air fills the anterior chamber. This expresses satisfactory ocular hypotony. The air usually reposits the iris and aids in identifying the peripheral iris openings or margins of sector iridectomy.

2. Air passes behind the iris, pushing its superior portion into the wound. Since this also indicates a very soft eye, the cornea may be safely retracted and several drops of balanced salt solution irrigated into the anterior chamber. The air will be displaced by the fluid, and the iris will simultaneously slide back into place within the eye.

3. The anterior chamber is flat, but there is no gaping of the wound. The peripheral iris openings or the basal portion of the sector iridectomy are difficult to identify. The preplaced sutures should be pulled up to close the wound. Air is placed in the anterior chamber through a Millipore filter (p. 446). This measure usually reposits the iris and brings the margins of the wound into perfect apposition.

4. The iris is adherent to the wound because of fibrinous adhesions. This condition is frequently encountered if there has been troublesome seepage of blood into the anterior chamber during the surgery. If filling the anterior chamber with air does not reposit the iris completely, an iris repositor may be used to gently stroke the iris back into place. If there is no evidence of gaping of the wound, I prefer to lift the cornea and break the fibrinous adhesions by pulling the iris back into the anterior chamber with Hoskins No. 19 forceps. When this has been accomplished, the anterior chamber is filled with air.

5. There is a marked bulge of vitreous without rupture of the anterior hyaloid membrane. The iris is wedged between the vitreous and the wound. The peripheral iris openings are not visible. The preplaced sutures should be pulled up gently without attempting to close the wound completely. The vitreous may begin to settle back after several minutes. By a combination of placing acetylcholine and air in the anterior chamber and gently stroking the iris into place with a repositor, the situation is usually remedied. It is difficult to keep air in the anterior chamber while the vitreous pushes forward. Acetylcholine is often ineffective in this situation. Repositioning of the iris is dangerous. It is important not to be hasty. Closing the wound temporarily helps tampon the bulging vitreous and encourages its retraction. It then becomes less difficult to institute one or more of these suggested maneuvers.

6. Formed vitreous has been lost. At this time I would favor partial anterior vitrectomy, removing formed vitreous from the superior angle, the face of the iris, and the pupillary area according to the technique described on p. 268. Acetylcholine aids in constricting the pupil.

COMPLETION OF THE SURGERY

Once the iris has been satisfactorily reposited, the wound is closed permanently. Preplaced sutures are pulled up and tied. Additional sutures are placed according to the surgeon's preferred technique. If all sutures are to be placed after extraction of the cataract, it may be helpful, as mentioned earlier, to fill the anterior chamber with balanced salt solution or air to improve wound apposition. This filling is particularly

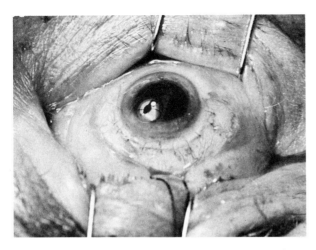

Fig. 3-73. Markedly beveled incision sutured with 10 interrupted 10-0 nylon sutures.

helpful in cases of extreme hypotonia where the cornea collapses inward. If air is used, some of it should be aspirated by using a 27- or 30-gauge cannula. The remainder of the anterior chamber should be filled with balanced salt solution. After all the sutures are in place, the wound should be tested for leaks by stroking the cornea and the scleral portion of the wound with the tip of a muscle hook. Additional sutures are inserted as needed (Fig. 3-73).

If a fornix-based conjunctival flap is used, it is anchored at 3 and 9 o'clock (Fig. 3-74). I prefer 7-0 chromic catgut suture for this. This is especially important if sutures are intended to remain permanently under the flap. If a limbus-based flap is used, it is secured by two to four interrupted sutures, just sufficient to prevent it from flapping back over the cornea (Fig. 3-75). Some surgeons

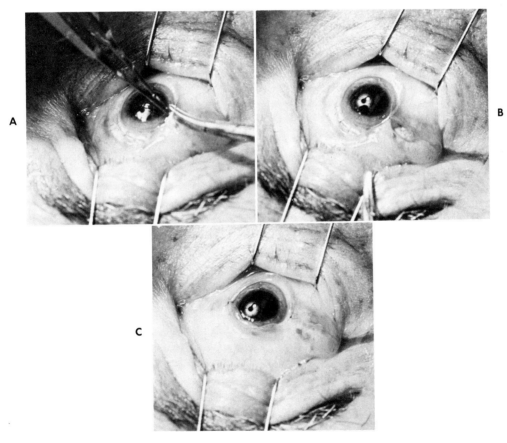

Fig. 3-74. Suturing of fornix-based conjunctival flap. **A,** Suture (7-0 chromic catgut) inserted in temporal portion. **B,** Temporal suture completed. **C,** Completed suturing of flap.

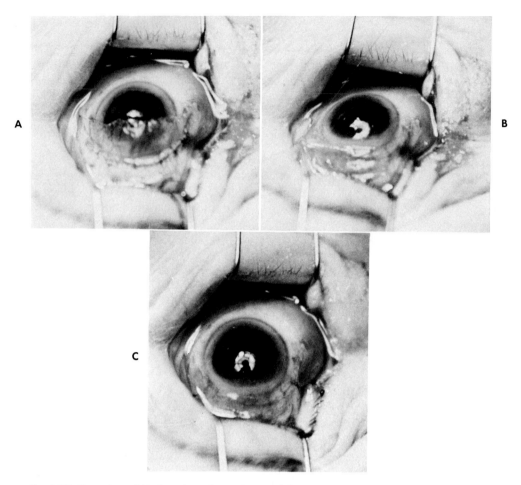

Fig. 3-75. Suturing of limbus-based conjunctival flap. **A,** Corneoscleral incision closed; conjunctival flap retracted over cornea. **B,** Interrupted (7-0 chromic catgut) suture placed. **C,** Flap secured with three interrupted sutures.

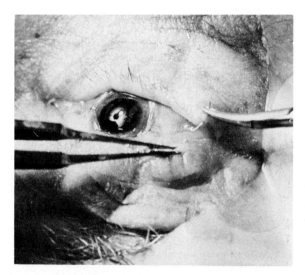

Fig. 3-76. Lateral canthotomy sutured.

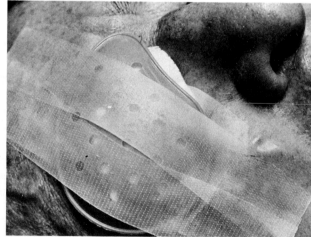

Fig. 3-77. Ocular dressing and protective plastic shield in place.

close conjunctival flaps, both fornix-based and limbus-based, with the coaptation forceps of the Wet-Field Coagulator (p. 45). If a sizable lateral canthotomy is performed, it is closed with one or more interrupted sutures (Fig. 3-76). Here again I find 7-0 chromic catgut satisfactory. A small canthotomy does not require closure. An antibiotic ointment such as chloramphenicol is placed in the eye. An eye pad is placed over the eye, and this in turn is covered by a plastic or an aluminum eye shield (Fig. 3-77). The opposite eye is not occluded. There is a growing trend to place the shield over the eye without the eye pad beneath it.

REFERENCES

1. Van Lint, A.: Paralysie palpébrale temporaire provoquée dans l'opération de la cataracte, Ann. Ocul. **151:**420-424, 1914.
2. O'Brien, C. S.: Local anesthesia in ophthalmic surgery, Trans. Sect. Ophthalmol. A.M.A. **78:**237-253, 1927.
3. Atkinson, W. S.: Anesthesia in ophthalmology, Springfield, Ill., 1955, Charles C Thomas, Publisher (American Lecture Series, No. 251).
4. Kraushar, M. F., Seelenfreund, M. H., and Freilich, D. B.: Central retinal artery closure during orbital hemorrhage from retrobulbar injection, Ophthalmology (Rochester) **78:**OP65-69, 1974.
5. Christensen, R. E., and Rundle, H. L.: Repair of filtering blebs following cataract surgery, Arch. Ophthalmol. **84:**8-11, 1970.
6. Kasner, D.: Important aspects of surgical anatomy of the limbal area. In Welsh, R. C., and Welsh, J., editors: The new report on cataract surgery, Miami, 1969, Miami Educational Press, pp. 106-107.
7. Dobree, J. H.: Scalpel and scissors. A flanged incision for cataract extraction, Br. J. Ophthalmol. **43:**513-520, 1959.
8. Swan, K. C.: Surgical anatomy in relation to glaucoma. In Clark, W. B., editor: Symposium on glaucoma, Transactions of the New Orleans Academy of Ophthalmology, 1957, St. Louis, 1959, The C. V. Mosby Co., pp. 38-52.
9. Gormaz, B. A.: Corneal "flap" incision for cataract operation, Br. J. Ophthalmol. **42:**486-493, 1958.
10. McLean, J. M.: Atlas of cataract surgery, St. Louis, 1965, The C. V. Mosby Co.
11. Troutman, R. C., and Eve, F. R.: Deep suturing of corneal incisions, Am. J. Ophthalmol. **4:**16-22, 1974.
12. Babel, J.: L'iridectomie sous l'angle de l'anatomie, de la physiologie et de la pathologie, An. Inst. Barraquer **3:**137-145, 1962.
13. Simcoe, C. W.: Simplified extracapsular extraction, J. Am. Intraocul. Implant Soc. **3:**194-196, 1977.
14. Garrison, F. H.: Introduction to the history of medicines, ed. 4, Philadelphia, 1929, W. B. Saunders Co., p. 109.
15. Chance, B.: Ophthalmology (Clio Medica, vol. 20), New York, 1939, Paul B. Hoeber, Inc., p. 22.
16. Derby, H.: In Buck, A. H., editor: Reference handbook of the medical sciences, New York, 1885, Wood & co., vol. 1, pp. 791-808.
17. Teale, R. L.: Cited in Dean, F. W.: Cataracts: operation for congenital and juvenile, Ophthalmology (Rochester) **31:**261-270, 1926.
18. Blaess, M. J.: Removal of cataract by aspiration, Arch. Ophthalmol. **19:**902-911, 1938.
19. Wolfe, O. R., and Wolfe, R. M.: Removal of soft cataract by suction; a new double-barreled aspirating needle, Arch. Ophthalmol. **26:**127-128, 1941.
20. Rodriguez Barrios, R., and Martinez Recalde, E.: Direct suction of congenital and juvenile cataracts, Arch. Oftal. B. Air. **32:**169-176, 1957.
21. Scheie, H. G.: Aspiration of congenital or soft catracts: A new technique, Am. J. Ophthalmol. **50:**1048-1056, 1960.
22. Girard, L. J.: Experiences with intracapsular cataract extraction in infants and children. In Welsh, R. C., and Welsh, J., editors: The new report on cataract surgery, Miami, 1969, Miami Educational Press, pp. 444:446.
23. Gass, J. D. M.: Lens aspiration using a side-opening needle, Arch. Ophthalmol. **82:**87-90, 1969.

CHAPTER 4

Postoperative corneal astigmatism

Although the ophthalmic surgeon has been concerned with postoperative corneal astigmatism because it is an integral part of the postoperative refractive error in aphakia, there has been much confusion in explaining the pathophysiology of postoperative changes in corneal curvature.

Fig. 4-1 illustrates that the vertical corneal meridian is more steeply curved than the horizontal meridian in astigmatism with the rule (corrected by plus cylinder axis 90 degrees). The opposite is true in astigmatism against the rule (corrected by plus cylinder axis 180 degrees). In an eye whose cornea requires a plus correcting cylinder at 45 degrees, the 45 degree meridian is more steeply curved than the 135 degree meridian.

□This chapter is taken in part from Jaffe, N. S. and Clayman, H. M.: The pathophysiology of corneal astigmatism after cataract extraction, Ophthalmology (Rochester) **79**:OP 615-630, 1975.

Since the turn of the century, it has been observed that astigmatism after cataract extraction is generally of the against-the-rule variety, which is caused by some degree of flattening of the corneal meridian at a right angle to the direction of the incision. That is to say, when the incision is made above, in its usual location, a postoperative flattening of the vertical meridian results. This is the basis for surgical procedures designed to reduce corneal astigmatism. For example, Sato[1] performs a "posterior half-incision," the midpoint of which is placed on the meridian of the cornea where the refractive power of the eye is greatest. The effectiveness of the procedure is greatest when the incision is made tangential to the pupil. Corcostegui Moliner[2] reported that the reduction of refraction in the meridian of greatest curvature is greater the larger the amplitude of the keratotomy, the more tangential the incision is to the cornea, and the closer it is to the pupil.

In the study of astigmatism, it is important to

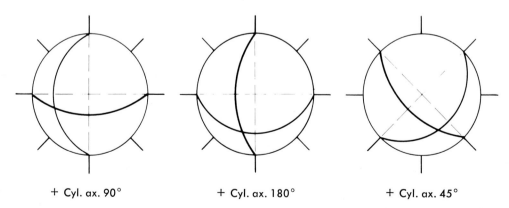

+ Cyl. ax. 90°   + Cyl. ax. 180°   + Cyl. ax. 45°

Fig. 4-1. *Left,* Astigmatism with rule. *Center,* Astigmatism against rule. *Right,* Oblique astigmatism. Cylindric notation represents corrective cylinder, not eye cylinder.

distinguish between astigmatism determined by keratometry and that determined by retinoscopy or manifest refraction. This is pertinent to the higher degrees of astigmatism found after intraocular lens implantation than after routine cataract surgery. For example, if the corneal astigmatism is identical to two different eyes following cataract extraction, and if one eye is aphakic and the other pseudophakic, the former will require in the cataract spectacle a cylinder smaller than that in the spectacle required by the pseudophakic eye. This is entirely related to the effectivity of lenses and is unrelated to other factors in the pseudophakic eye such as tilting of the lens implant, more sutures, tighter sutures, increased use of postoperative steroids, and so on. In the aphakic eye, the spherical equivalent of the 're-fraction is a strong plus sphere unless the eye was highly myopic preoperatively. The higher the plus sphere and the larger the vertex distance of the spectacle lens, the smaller the spectacle cylinder. The same reasoning applies to the pseudophakic eye. If the residual refractive error is a plus spherical equivalent, the cylinder in the prescribed spectacle is smaller than if the residual refraction is a minus spherical equivalent. If there is zero residual spherical equivalent refraction, the cylinder will be identical to the corneal astigmatism. Since most surgeons tend to overcorrect when using an intraocular lens, the spectacle prescribed is usually a minus lens with a higher cylinder than is required for an aphakic eye if the corneal astigmatism is the same in both eyes. In general, in hyperopia, as in aphakia, the spectacle cylinder is usually smaller than the corneal astigmatism, whereas in myopia the spectacle cylinder is usually larger than the corneal astigmatism.

The formula for effectivity correction is as follows:

$$R_s = \frac{R_c}{1 + vR_c}$$

where

   R_s = The spectacle refraction in diopters
   R_c = The refraction at the cornea in diopters
   v = The vertex distance in meters

The larger the vertex distance, the more effective a plus lens and the less effective a minus lens.

The amount of postoperative astigmatism has been reduced considerably from the days of unsutured incisions. With the popularization of corneoscleral sutures and improved methods of performing the incision and closing it, the degree of postoperative astigmatism has shown a steady decline. In addition, there have been recent radical changes in the techniques of incision and closure and in the availability of new suture materials. These have been accompanied by significant changes in the amount of postoperative astigmatism and in the direction of its axis. Meticulous wound closure and uncomplicated healing of the incision have been considered responsible for these improved optic results. However, as a result of observations made over a period of more than 30 years, I have concluded that this is only partially factual. I have reached the following impressions regarding postoperative astigmatism:

1. Incisions made very anteriorly (e.g., corneal) result in more postoperative astigmatism than those made more posteriorly. The axis of the astigmatism is dependent on the suture technique employed (see following discussion).

2. The smaller the amplitude of the incision above, the less the effect on the horizontal meridian. Incisions that end at or beyond the horizontal meridian tend to neutralize some of the changes in the vertical meridian.

3. Separation of the wound (filtering bleb) has surprisingly little effect on the amount of postoperative astigmatism when the incision is scleral but causes considerable astigmatism when the incision is more anterior.

Documentation of these impressions is supplied by a study of 662 cataract extractions divided into three series, each employing a different incision. The study occurred over a 20-month period between March 1966 and November 1967. The surgery was performed jointly by my associate, Dr. David S. Light, and myself. The type of incision in each series is shown in Fig. 4-2.

Series 1. An anterior limbal 140-degree incision was made in two planes as follows: A groove was made along the entire length of the incision at an angle of 75 degrees to the plane of the

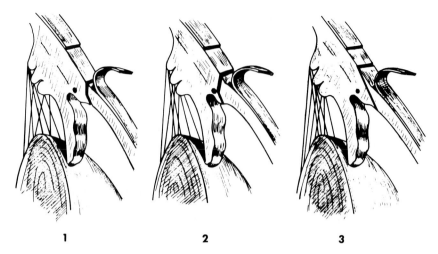

1   2   3

Fig. 4-2. Series 1, Anterior limbal incision. Series 2, Midlimbal to posterior limbal incision. Series 3, Markedly beveled incision commencing in sclera. Conjunctiva is reflected similarly in all three series to demonstrate location of incision.

globe. The anterior chamber was entered at any part of the groove with a piece of razor blade, scalpel blade, or keratome at an angle of 45 degrees. Scissors enlargement was then performed at an angle of 45 degrees. In all cases, 7-0 silk sutures were used. Two to five sutures were placed across the groove before the anterior chamber was entered, the remainder after the lens extraction. An average of eight sutures were used per case. A fornix-based conjunctival flap was used throughout.

Series 2. A midlimbal to posterior limbal 180-degree incision was made in two planes, as just described. In every case, 7-0 silk and a fornix-based conjunctival flap were used.

Series 3. A markedly beveled 180-degree incision was made 3.5 mm behind the anterior limbal border at 12 o'clock and gradually tapered toward the limbus at 3 and 9 o'clock. The anterior chamber was entered at 9 o'clock position with a keratome. Using scissors designed by Barraquer that permit a markedly beveled incision at an angle of 135 degrees (Fig. 3-23), enlargement proceeded clockwise to 3 o'clock. At 12 o'clock the incision was located in the sclera 3.5 mm behind the anterior limbal border, and at 3 o'clock it was located exactly at the limbus. The scissors have a spring handle, blunt tips, and straight blades. Because of the angulation, the blades are kept parallel to the iris during the enlargement. A stop device

prevents the tips of the scissors from closing completely. Thus the entire incision may be made without withdrawing the scissors from the anterior chamber and without producing ragged edges. The incision resembles that made with a Graefe knife. In about half the cases, 9-0 virgin silk sutures were used and in the other half 10-0 monofilament nylon. A limbus-based conjunctival flap was used in 129 eyes of this series, and a fornix-based conjunctival flap was used in 147 eyes.

• • •

Although ophthalmometer readings were obtained preoperatively and postoperatively in every case, the series were considered sufficiently large that only postoperative keratometer (*K*) readings were recorded. The fallacy of this reasoning is emphasized later in this chapter. The results are shown in Table 4-1 and Figs. 4-3 to 4-5.

The differences observed are highly significant. The average astigmatism in series 1 was 3.5 times that in series 3, whereas the astigmatism in series 2 was double that in series 3. However, an equally enlightening point is the change in the axis of the astigmatism in the three series. There is a marked trend away from astigmatism against the rule in going from series 1 (95%) to series 3 (36%). The percentage of eyes showing no astigmatism and astigmatism with the rule rises sharp-

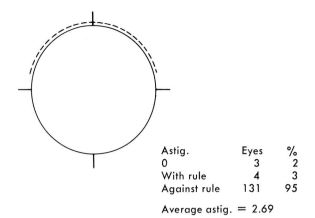

Astig.	Eyes	%
0	3	2
With rule	4	3
Against rule	131	95

Average astig. = 2.69

Fig. 4-3. Results in series 1. Incision shown as dotted line.

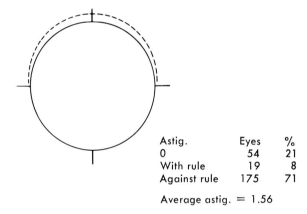

Astig.	Eyes	%
0	54	21
With rule	19	8
Against rule	175	71

Average astig. = 1.56

Fig. 4-4. Results in series 2. Incision shown as dotted line.

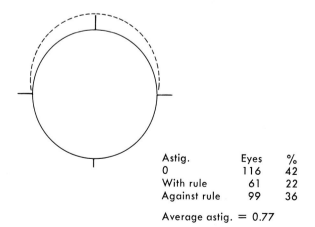

Astig.	Eyes	%
0	116	42
With rule	61	22
Against rule	99	36

Average astig. = 0.77

Fig. 4-5. Results in series 3. Incision shown as dotted line.

Table 4-1. Astigmatism after cataract extraction involving three types of incisions

	Series 1	Series 2	Series 3
Number of eyes	138	248	276
Average astigmatism (diopters)	2.69	1.56	0.77
% Eyes no astigmatism	2	21	42
% Eyes astigmatism with the rule	3	8	22
% Eyes astigmatism against the rule	95	71	36

ly from 5% in series 1, to 29% in series 2, to 64% in series 3.

Twenty-one postoperative filtering blebs occurred in the three series. Fourteen of them occurred in the 129 eyes in series 3 in which a limbus-based flap was used (10.8%). In the remaining 533 eyes in the three series in which a fornix-based conjunctival flap was used, there were only seven filtering blebs (1.3%). However, four of these occurred in series 3. Thus most of the filtering blebs (18) occurred in series 3 in which a scleral incision and 9-0 virgin silk and 10-0 nylon sutures were used. Whereas one might expect a greater amount of postoperative astigmatism in eyes with filtering blebs, the average astigmatism in the 13 cases in series 3 was only 0.46 D compared to 0.77 D in the entire 276 eyes in series 3. However, the remaining three blebs were found in series 2, and the average astigmatism of these was 3.85 D. None were found in series 1.

In series 3 a limbus-based flap was used in 129 eyes, a fornix-based flap in 147 eyes. The average astigmatism in the former was 0.70 D, 0.85 D in the latter. The difference is probably not significant. The amount of astigmatism and the axis were similar in those eyes in which 9-0 silk was used and those in which 10-0 nylon was used.

A curious sidelight to these series was observed in another in which 7-0 chromic catgut was used under a fornix-based flap. The incision was made in the same manner as that described in series 3 (a markedly beveled incision commencing well back in the sclera). The average postoperative astigmatism in 75 eyes was 2.52 D. Of these, 81% had astigmatism against the rule, 11% had astigmatism with the rule, and 8% had no astigmatism. A special effort was made to pull the flap well down over the cornea to protect the catgut sutures from mechanical agitation by the eyelids. This was successful in most cases; the sutures were visible and intact under the flap for at least 1 month after surgery. Despite this protective covering, the average astigmatism was 3.3 times greater than that recorded in series 3 where the incision was identical, but the wound was closed with 9-0 silk or 10-0 monofilament nylon.

To add further to our knowledge of the pathophysiology of corneal astigmatism after cataract extraction, a more recent series of 1557 cataract extractions utilizing a variety of suture materials and techniques of incision and closure was analyzed. This series included cataract extractions performed during a 64-month period between November 11, 1968, and March 5, 1974, in patients ranging in age from 44 to 94 years. In every case, preoperative and postoperative keratometry was recorded using the American Optical Company ophthalmometer. Postoperative readings were taken 5 to 7 weeks after surgery.

The following suture techniques were employed:

A. Continuous, all using 10-0 monofilament nylon
  1. Willard
  2. Troutman
  3. Over-and-over
  4. Locking
B. Interrupted
  5. 10-0 monofilament nylon
    a. Posterior, ½ depth
    b. Anterior, ¾ depth
  6. 9-0 virgin silk
    a. Posterior, ½ depth
    b. Anterior, ¾ depth
  7. 7-0 silk
  8. 7-0 chromic catgut
  9. 7-0 chromic collagen

A fornix-based conjunctival flap was used in all cases except for 7-0 collagen when a limbal-based flap was used.

The anterior chamber was entered at 9:30 o'clock in all eyes and the incision was enlarged to the surgeon's left, markedly beveled, and

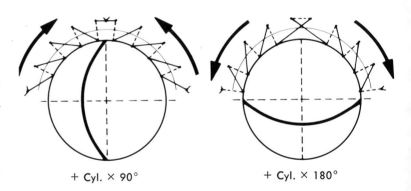

Fig. 4-6. *Left,* Troutman continuous suture commences at 2:30 and 9:30 o'clock and terminates at 12 o'clock, where suture is anchored. *Right,* Willard suture commences with transverse scleral bite at 12 o'clock and continues to 2:30 and 9:30 o'clock (as shown), where each half is anchored. Typical postoperative corrective astigmatic lens is shown. (From Jaffe, N. S., and Clayman, H. M.: Ophthalmology [Rochester] **79:**OP 615-630, 1975.)

+ Cyl. × 90°   + Cyl. × 180°

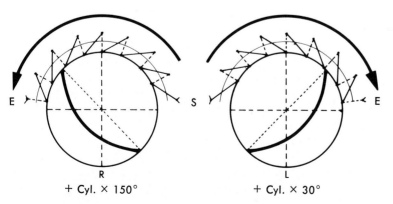

+ Cyl. × 150°   + Cyl. × 30°

Fig. 4-7. Over-and-over continuous suture (as performed in this study) commences on nasal side of either eye (*S*) and terminates on temporal side (*E*), where it is anchored. Typical steepest meridian is shown, as well as typical corrective astigmatic lens. (From Jaffe, N. S., and Clayman, H. M.: Ophthalmology [Rochester] **79:**OP 615-630, 1975.)

placed at the posterior limbal border except for the midlimbal incisions in one of each of the 10-0 nylon and 9-0 silk, interrupted suture series. When using 7-0 silk and 7-0 chromic catgut, a midlimbal to posterior limbal incision was made in two planes, and a superficial 75-degree groove was completed by a beveled entry into the anterior chamber.

The Willard suture (Fig. 4-6) commenced by taking a 3 mm horizontal scleral bite 3 mm from the anterior limbal border. The left extremity of the suture was inserted in a continuous manner to the surgeon's right and the right extremity to the surgeon's left. The suture was secured and tied at 2:30 and 9:30 o'clock.

The Troutman suture (Fig. 4-6) commenced at 2:30 and 9:30 o'clock in a continuous manner to 12 o'clock where the two halves of the suture were tied to each other.

The over-and-over suture (Fig. 4-7) commenced on the nasal side of each eye (2:30 o'clock in the right eye and 9:30 o'clock in the left eye). The suture was inserted in a continuous manner and was finally secured and tied temporally (9:30 o'clock in the right eye and 2:30 o'clock in the left eye).

The continuous interlocking suture (Fig. 3-46) commenced at either extremity of the incision and continued to the opposite extremity. The suture was locked after each bite.

These four continuous sutures were inserted to three fourths of the depth of the wound margins.

The 10-0 monofilament nylon and 9-0 interrupted suture series were divided into two separate parts. In one series the incision was made at the posterior limbal border to slightly posterior to it. The sutures were inserted at approximately one half the depth of the wound margins. In a later series a midlimbal incision was used, and the sutures were inserted to a depth of about three fourths of the wound margins.

THE NEED FOR PREOPERATIVE AND POSTOPERATIVE KERATOMETRY

The disparity between postoperative astigmatism and the calculated surgically induced change and the subsequent need to calculate these changes are emphasized in Tables 4-2 and 4-3. In Table 4-2, postoperative K (K_3) is considerably greater than the surgically induced

astigmatism (K_2). In Table 4-3, K_2 is much greater than K_3. In the former the surgeon has not deformed the corneal curvature as much as would be indicated by postoperative keratometry. In the latter the effect on corneal curvature is excessive compared to the postoperative K findings. It is obvious therefore that to estimate the effect on corneal curvature induced by cataract surgery, one must calculate the difference between preoperative and postoperative keratometry. This is not a simple task, since the axes are usually obliquely related to each other. To my knowledge, there have been no published series reporting exact quantitative differences between preoperative and postoperative corneal curvature. It is simple to calculate the difference if the axes are

Table 4-2. Larger postoperative K (K_3) than calculated change (K_2)*

Suture	Postoperative K (K_3)	Calculated change (K_2)
Willard	$-2.50 \times 20°$	$-0.50 \times 25°$
Troutman	$-4.25 \times 160°$	$-2.75 \times 175°$
Over-and-over	$-2.50 \times 35°$	$-0.87 \times 160°$
Continuous locking	$-3.50 \times 100°$	$-0.75 \times 85°$
10-0 nylon	$-2.75 \times 170°$	Zero
9-0 silk	$-3.25 \times 10°$	$-0.50 \times 105°$
7-0 silk	$-1.75 \times 105°$	$-0.25 \times 80°$
7-0 chromic catgut	$-3.50 \times 100°$	Zero
7-0 chromic collagen	$-4.25 \times 20°$	$-0.75 \times 5°$

*The cylindric values represent the corrective cylinder required to eliminate the astigmatic error.

Table 4-3. Smaller postoperative K (K_3) than calculated change (K_2)*

Suture	Postoperative K (K_3)	Calculated change (K_2)
Willard	$-2.00 \times 75°$	$-4.25 \times 75°$
Troutman	$-2.50 \times 10°$	$-4.87 \times 5°$
Over-and-over	$-0.25 \times 75°$	$-2.50 \times 130°$
Continuous locking	$-2.00 \times 80°$	$-4.50 \times 100°$
10-0 nylon	Zero	$-4.00 \times 80°$
9-0 silk	Zero	$-1.75 \times 115°$
7-0 silk	$-0.50 \times 90°$	$-2.00 \times 85°$
7-0 chromic catgut	Zero	$-3.25 \times 90°$
7-0 chromic collagen	Zero	$-1.75 \times 135°$

*The cylindric values represent the corrective cylinder required to eliminate the astigmatic error.

90 degrees apart. For example, if preoperative keratometry reveals +1.00 D × 90°, and the postoperative finding is +1.00 D × 180°, there has been a net change of +2.00 D × 180° induced by surgery. However, it is much more complicated if the axes are greater or less than 90 degrees apart and if the amplitudes of astigmatism also differ. There is also some spherical change introduced, but this is ignored in these calculations, since we are solely concerned with the changes in astigmatism.

METHODS OF CALCULATION OF DIFFERENCE BETWEEN PREOPERATIVE AND POSTOPERATIVE KERATOMETRY

The calculations in this series of 1557 cataract extractions were performed by three different methods, to my knowledge the first time they have been applied to a series of cataract extractions. A fourth method is added.

Vector method

The vector method is based on a variation of a technique[3,4] of finding the sum of oblique cylinders in which the cylinder is represented on a graph by a vector. A vector provides two pieces of information — amplitude and direction. The problem of finding the sum of two obliquely crossed cylinders can be solved by treating the component powers of the two cylinders as vectors in a vector diagram, but in so doing the vectors representing the cylindric powers are directed at angles twice the actual angles of orientation before the eye.[5] Such a graphic plot representing the resultant of two planocylindric lenses with axes at different angles is shown in Fig. 4-8. In this illustration, cylinder K_1 axis ϕ_1 is added to cylinder K_2 axis ϕ_2. The angles are represented on the graph at twice their angles. The resultant cylinder K_3 axis ϕ is shown. To find K_3, a parallelogram is made by constructing line $K_1 - K_3$, which is parallel and equal in length to line $0 - K_2$ and line $K_2 - K_3$, which is parallel and equal in length to line $0 - K_1$. An example of such a construction is shown in Fig. 4-9.

GIVEN: $K_1 = 2.00 \times 25°$
$K_2 = 1.50 \times 85°$

FIND: K_3

K_1 is represented on the graph as a line 2.00 units long at the 50-degree meridian ($2 \times 25°$). K_2

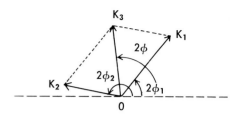

Fig. 4-8. Graphic representation of resultant (K_3) of 2 plano-cylindric lenses with axes at different angles. Represents sum of oblique cylinders, using vector method. K_1 is added to K_2 to get sum, K_3, by constructing parallelogram as shown. Axes of astigmatism are doubled, and final axis is divided by 2. (From Jaffe, N. S., and Clayman, H. M.: Ophthalmology [Rochester] **79:**OP 615-630, 1974.)

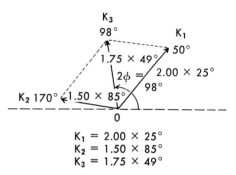

$K_1 = 2.00 \times 25°$
$K_2 = 1.50 \times 85°$
$K_3 = 1.75 \times 49°$

Fig. 4-9. Cylinder K_1 is added to cylinder K_2 to get resultant cylinder K_3, by constructing parallelogram as shown. K_3 is shown at axis 98 degrees. Angle is divided by 2 to get 49 degrees. (From Jaffe, N. S., and Clayman, H. M.: Ophthalmology [Rochester] **79:**OP 615-630, 1975.)

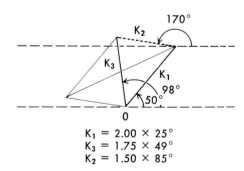

$K_1 = 2.00 \times 25°$
$K_3 = 1.75 \times 49°$
$K_2 = 1.50 \times 85°$

Fig. 4-10. Modification of parallelogram technique by construction of triangle. Since we already know preoperative corneal astigmatism (K_1) and postoperative corneal astigmatism (K_3), we find surgically induced change (K_2) by drawing line connecting end of K_1 to end of K_3. Axis of K_2 is determined by placing protractor at end of K_1 and dividing angle by 2. (From Jaffe, N. S., and Clayman, H. M.: Ophthalmology [Rochester] **79:**OP 615-630, 1975.)

is plotted as a line 1.50 units long at the 170-degree meridian (2 × 85°). The parallelogram is completed. Line K_3 is 1.75 units long at 98 degrees. Thus the sum of cylinders K_1 and K_2 in this example is K_3, which is 1.75 D × 49° (98 ÷ 2)°. This method has been illustrated by Ogle.[5]

This is not exactly the problem we encounter in cataract surgery. We know the preoperative corneal astigmatism (K_1) and the postoperative corneal astigmatism (K_3). We must calculate what is added to K_1 by the surgery to get the result K_3. This surgically induced cylinder is called K_2. It should be obvious at this juncture—and will be even more apparent later—that K_3 (postoperative corneal cylinder) may differ greatly from K_2 (surgically induced cylinder). It should also be obvious that K_2 is the only meaningful measure of what the surgeon does to corneal curvature.

To calculate K_2 by the vector method, a simple variation of the parallelogram is presented that requires the construction of a triangle. This is shown in Fig. 4-10. Using the same values as in Fig. 4-9, K_1 (preoperative corneal astigmatism) and K_3 (postoperative corneal astigmatism) are represented at double their axis angles. K_2 (surgically induced astigmatism) is found by plotting a line connecting the end of K_1 with the end of K_3. A line is plotted parallel to the base line so that the direction of K_2 can be measured with a protractor. In this illustration the angle is 170

degrees. Thus, K_2 = 1.50 D × 85°. This angle must always be measured around the end of K_1, not K_3.

Another example is illustrated in Fig. 4-11.

GIVEN: K_1 = 3.00 D × 25°
         K_3 = 1.50 D × 100°

FIND: K_2

The ends of the line connecting K_1 and K_3 is 4.36 units long. The direction of this line measured around the end of K_1 is 220 degrees. Thus K_2 (surgically induced astigmatism) is 4.36 D × 110°. Note the large difference in the amplitudes of astigmatism K_2 and K_3. It illustrates the folly of using K_3 to assess a surgical technique.

In these calculations, it makes no difference whether one uses positive or negative cylinders as long as the signs are kept the same in each calculation.

Rectangular coordinates

A highly precise method of calculating K_2 employs rectangular and polar coordinates. It will be recalled that any point may be represented on a graph by rectangular and polar coordinates. If x represents the abscissa on the graph (the distance to the right or left of the origin) and y represents the ordinate (the distance above or below the origin), any point may be represented by x and y. The abscissa (x) is positive if it is to the right of

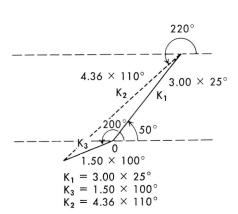

K_1 = 3.00 × 25°
K_3 = 1.50 × 100°
K_2 = 4.36 × 110°

Fig. 4-11. Vector method of finding K_2. K_1, Preoperative corneal astigmatism; K_2, postoperative corneal astigmatism; K_2, surgically induced astigmatism. (From Jaffe, N. S., and Clayman, H. M.: Ophthalmology [Rochester] **79:**OP 615-630, 1975.)

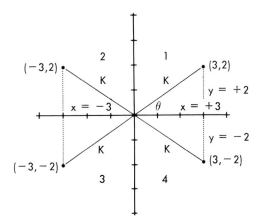

Fig. 4-12. Rectangular coordinates of K values of identical amplitudes are shown. Coordinates show different algebraic signs, since axes of Ks differ so that each K lies in one of the four quadrants. (From Jaffe, N. S., and Clayman, H. M.: Ophthalmology [Rochester] **79:**OP 615-630, 1975.)

the origin and negative if to the left. The ordinate (y) is positive if it lies above the origin and negative if it lies below the origin. Fig. 4-12 shows the rectangular coordinates of points in all four quadrants when they lie 3 units to the right $(+3)$ or 3 units to the left (-3) of the origin and 2 units above $(+2)$ the origin or 2 units below (-2). The amplitude of the astigmatism (K) is represented on the rectangular graph as K and in a direction at twice its angular axis. This doubled angle is represented by θ. It follows (Fig. 4-13) that

$$\cos \theta = x/K \text{ and } x = K \cos \theta$$
$$\sin \theta = y/K \text{ and } y = K \sin \theta$$

In this way we determine the x,y coordinates for K_1 (preoperative corneal astigmatism) and K_3 (postoperative corneal astigmatism). Thus the coordinates are represented as follows:

$$K_1 = (x_{K_1}, y_{K_1})$$
$$K_3 = (x_{K_3}, y_{K_3})$$

The rectangular coordinates for K_2 (surgically induced corneal astigmatism) are calculated by subtracting the x and y coordinates of K_1 from those of K_3. Thus

$$K_2 = K_3 - K_1$$
$$= (x_{K_3} - x_{K_1}, y_{K_3} - y_{K_1})$$
$$= (x_{K_2}, y_{K_2})$$

Amplitude

$$\cos \theta = x/K \qquad x = K \cos \theta$$
$$\sin \theta = y/K \qquad y = K \sin \theta$$

$$K_1 = x_{K_1}, y_{K_1} \qquad K_3 = x_{K_3}, y_{K_3}$$

$$K_2 = \begin{cases} x_{K_3} - x_{K_1}, y_{K_3} - y_{K_1} \\ x_{K_2}, y_{K_2} \text{ (quadrant)} \end{cases}$$

$$K_2 = x_{K_2}^2 + y_{K_2}^2 \text{ Pythagoras}$$
$$K_2 = \sqrt{x_{K_2}^2 + y_{K_2}^2}$$

K_1 = Preoperative astigmatism
K_3 = Postoperative astigmatism
K_2 = Surgically induced astigmatism

Fig. 4-13. Calculation of amplitude of K_2 (surgically induced astigmatism) by rectangular coordinates method. (From Jaffe, N. S., and Clayman, H. M.: Ophthalmology [Rochester] 79:OP 615-630, 1975.)

Since we are dealing with a right triangle in which K_2 represents the hypotenuse, x the side adjacent to θ, and y the side opposite θ, K_2 may be calculated as follows by applying the Pythagorean theorem:

$$K_2^2 = x_{K_2}^2 + y_{K_2}^2$$
$$K_2 = \sqrt{x_{K_2}^2 + y_{K_2}^2}$$

This provides the amplitude of the surgically induced astigmatism. The axis of this astigmatism is calculated as follows (Fig. 4-14):

$$\tan \theta = y/x \text{ and } \theta = \arctan y/x$$

If θ is negative, add 360 degrees to make the angle positive. Determine in which quadrant K_2 is located by its rectangular coordinates (x,y). If θ is in the correct quadrant, divide by 2 to determine the axis of K_2, since all angles were previously doubled. If θ is in the wrong quadrant, add 180 degrees and divide by 2.

Example: Fig. 4-15

GIVEN: $\quad K_1 = 3.00 \text{ D} \times 25°$
$\qquad\qquad K_3 = 1.50 \text{ D} \times 100°$

FIND: $\qquad K_2$

SOLUTION: $\quad K_1 = (x_{K_1}, y_{K_1})$
$\qquad x_{K_1} = 3.00 \cos 50° = 1.93$, since $\cos 50° = 0.64$
$\qquad y_{K_1} = 3.00 \sin 50° = 2.30$, since $\sin 50° = 0.77$

$\qquad K_3 = (x_{K_3}, y_{K_3})$
$\qquad x_{K_3} = 1.50 \sin 200° = -1.41$, since $\cos 200° = -0.94$
$\qquad y_{K_3} = 1.50 \sin 200° = -0.51$, since $\sin 200° = -0.34$

$\qquad K_2 = (x_{K_3} - x_{K_1}, y_{K_3} - y_{K_1})$
$\qquad\quad = (-1.41 - 1.93, -0.51 - 2.30)$
$\qquad\quad = (-3.34, -2.81)$

Axis

$$\tan \theta = y/x$$
$$\theta = \arctan y/x$$
$$\frac{\theta}{2} = \text{axis}$$

Fig. 4-14. Calculation of axis of K_2 by rectangular coordinates method. If θ is negative, add 360 degrees. If θ is in wrong quadrant, add 180 degrees. (From Jaffe, N. S., and Clayman, H. M.: Ophthalmology [Rochester] 79:OP 615-630, 1975.)

Thus the rectangular coordinates of K_2 place it in quadrant 3 (Fig. 4-12), since both the abscissa and ordinate are negative.

$$K_2 = \sqrt{(-3.34)^2 + (-2.81)^2}$$
$$= 4.36$$

$$\tan \theta = y_{K_2}/x_{K_2}$$
$$\theta = \arctan -2.81/-3.34 = 40°$$

However, 40 degrees lies in quadrant 1. Therefore, add 180 degrees to θ and divide by 2. Therefore,

$$\theta = (40° + 180°) \div 2 = 110°$$
$$K_2 = 4.36 \text{ D} \times 110°$$

Example: Fig. 4-16

GIVEN: $K_1 = 1.50$ D $\times 90°$
           $K_3 = 7.00$ D $\times 135°$

FIND: K_2

SOLUTION: $x_{K_1} = 1.50 \cos 180° = -1.5$, since
           $\cos 180° = -1.0$

           $y_{K_1} = 1.50 \sin 180° = 0$, since
           $\sin 180° = 0$

           $x_{K_3} = 7.00 \cos 270° = 0$, since
           $\cos 270° = 0$

$$y_{K_3} = 7.00 \sin 270° = -7.0, \text{ since}$$
$$\sin 270° = -1.0$$

$$K_2 = (x_{K_3} - x_{K_1}), (y_{K_3} - y_{K_1})$$
$$= (0 - [-1.5]), (-7.0 - 0)$$
$$= (1.5, -7.0)$$

Thus the rectangular coordinates of K_2 lie in quadrant 4 (Fig. 4-12), since the abscissa is positive and the ordinate negative.

$$K_2 = \sqrt{(1.5)^2 + (-7.0)^2}$$
$$= 7.16$$

$$\tan \theta = y_{K_2}/x_{K_2}$$
$$\theta = \arctan -7.0/1.5 = -78°$$

Add 360 degrees to θ to make it positive.

$$\theta = (-78° + 360°) \div 2 = 141°$$
$$K_2 = 7.16 \text{ D} \times 141°$$

Law of sines and cosines

These trigonometric functions serve for the solution of any triangle for the explicit determination of the remaining parts of a triangle of which any three independent parts are known (Fig. 4-17).

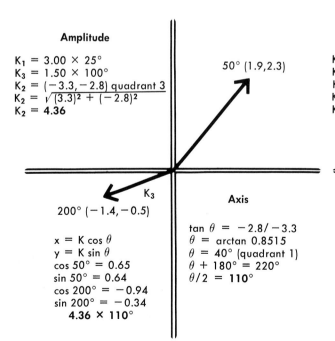

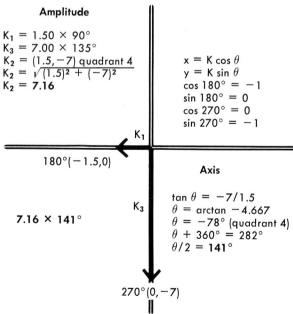

Fig. 4-15. Calculation of K_2 by rectangular coordinates method. (From Jaffe, N. S., and Clayman, H. M.: Ophthalmology [Rochester] **79**:OP 615-630, 1975.)

Fig. 4-16. Calculation of K_2 by rectangular coordinates method. (From Jaffe, N. S., and Clayman, H. M.: Ophthalmology [Rochester] **79**:OP 615-630, 1975.)

Law of cosines

$$K_2^2 = K_1^2 + K_3^2 - 2K_1K_3 \cos k_2$$

Law of sines

$$\frac{K_1}{\sin k_1} = \frac{K_2}{\sin k_2} = \frac{K_3}{\sin k_3}$$

Fig. 4-17. Law of cosines and sines applied to triangle where K_1 (preoperative astigmatism), K_2 (surgically induced change), and K_3 (postoperative astigmatism) represent the three sides of a triangle, as in Fig. 4-11. Angles opposite their respective sides are represented by k_1, k_2, and k_3. (From Jaffe, N. S., and Clayman, H. M.: Ophthalmology [Rochester] **79:**OP 615-630, 1975.)

$$
\begin{aligned}
K_2^2 &= K_1^2 + K_3^2 - 2K_1K_3 \cos k_2(k_2 = 200° - 50° = 150°) \\
&= 3.00^2 + 1.50^2 - 2(3.00)(1.50) \cos 150° \\
&= 11.25 - 9 \cos 150°(\cos 150° = -0.866) \\
&= 11.25 + 7.794 \\
&= 19.044 \\
K_2 &= 4.36
\end{aligned}
$$

Fig. 4-18. Finding K_2 by law of cosines. Illustration uses same values as in Fig. 4-11, using vector method. (From Jaffe, N. S., and Clayman, H. M.: Ophthalmology [Rochester] **79:**OP 615-630, 1975.)

$$\frac{K_3}{\sin k_3} = \frac{K_2}{\sin k_2} \qquad \sin k_3 = \frac{K_3 \sin k_2}{K_2}$$

$$\arcsin \frac{K_3 \sin k_2}{K_2} = k_3$$

$$\arcsin \frac{1.50 \sin 150°}{4.36} = k_3$$

$$\arcsin \frac{1.50 \times 0.50}{4.36} = k_3$$

$$\arcsin 0.172 = k_3$$
$$k_3 = 9.9°$$

Fig. 4-19. Finding angle k_3 by law of sines. Refer to Fig. 4-11. As described in text, axis of K_2 can be determined once k_3 is found. (From Jaffe, N. S., and Clayman, H. M.: Opthalmology [Rochester] **79:**OP 615-630, 1975.)

The problem illustrated in Fig. 4-11 may be solved by trigonometry, as shown in Figs. 4-18 and 4-19.

The amplitude of K_2 (surgically induced astigmatism) is found by the law of cosines, and angle k_3 (the angle opposite side K_3) is found by the law of sines.

To calculate the axis of K_2 (surgically induced astigmatism), refer again to Fig. 4-11. The angle of K_1 is 50 degrees. Its supplementary angle is 130 degrees. This is added to angle k_3 (9.9 degrees). To complete the circle we require 220 degrees. Thus the axis is 110 degrees, since all angles were previously doubled. These values coincide with those calculated by the vector and rectangular coordinates methods.

The vector method requires graph paper, a ruler, and a protractor. Trigonometric functions may be calculated by any of the many currently available calculators for this purpose or by using trigonometric function tables available in most trigonometry textbooks.

A rapid method of calculating surgically induced astigmatism (K_2) involves the use of a programmable calculator such as the TI 59 (Texas Instruments, Lubbock, Texas). A program that can be placed by the user on a magnetic tape is supplied by the company.

The surgically induced change in corneal curvature (K_2) in the series of 1557 eyes was calculated in every case by the vector and rectangular coordinates techniques. The calculations were then verified by computer analysis. Since exact objective measurements of corneal astigmatism were used, it is to be expected that the astigmatism induced by surgery in this series would appear greater than that usually reported. The American Optical Company Micro-Ophthalmometer was used for all keratometric measurements. Postoperative K values were obtained 5 to 7 weeks after surgery.

Lensometer

The lensometer method is a variant of Rubin's[6] method of adding cylinders in a lensometer. To subtract cylinder 2 from cylinder 1, merely change the sign of cylinder 2, keeping the axis the same. Thus one may use cylinders from the trial lens set, combine the two at the correct axis on the lensometer, and read the answer in the instrument. Thus let us suppose we want to subtract a +2.00 cyl. ×70° from a +2.00 cyl. × 40°. The +2.00 cyl. × 70° is changed to −2.00 cyl. × 70°. The two cylinders are then combined on the lensometer, and the answer is read as +2.00 cyl. × 10°. This technique is not as easy as it sounds: Since most lensometers do not have a protractor scale, it is difficult to know the exact position in which we put the cylindrical axes. However, the cylinders may be placed in a trial frame (calibrated as to degrees), and then the trial frame is placed in the lensometer. The answers are never as exact as true calculations, but they are close enough. This method is made even simpler by using one of the automated lensometers currently available.

PREOPERATIVE CORNEAL ASTIGMATISM IN PATIENTS BEFORE SURGERY FOR SENILE CATARACT

This study presented an opportunity to evaluate the type of preoperative corneal curvature one might expect to find in patients at an age range when cataract surgery is usually performed. It is generally reported that corneal astigmatism is usually performed. It is generally reported that corneal astigmatism is with the rule in young eyes, and that there is a shift toward against-the-rule astigmatism with advancing age.[7] The rea-

son for this is unclear. It has been suggested that the upper and lower eyelids compress the upper and lower portions of the cornea, thus increasing the curvature of the vertical corneal meridian. This effect is lessened with increasing rigidity of the globe. Furthermore, elevations of intraocular pressure have been associated with a shift toward against-the-rule astigmatism. Even a chalazion has been known to affect corneal curvature.

In this series of 1557 eyes in patients aged 44 to 94, the following distribution was recorded.

Astigmatism	No. eyes	%	Diopters
With the rule	466	30.0	1.15
Against the rule	662	42.5	1.02
Zero	402	25.8	
45°	16	1.0	
135°	11	0.7	
TOTAL	1,557	100.0	0.64

SUMMARY OF RESULTS

In summarizing the astigmatism induced by the various techniques in this series of 1557 eyes, it was found that in most instances there was a characteristic with-the-rule or against-the-rule astigmatism induced by a particular technique. This is demonstrated in Table 4-4. With-the-rule astigmatism was associated with the following: Troutman continuous suture (6:1), 10-0 nylon interrupted suture with a midlimbal incision and

Table 4-4. Summary of 1557 eyes in all series[*]

Suture	No.	K_2[†] (axis included)	K_2[‡] (without axis)	C:VS[§]	P[‖]
Troutman	138	−2.28 × 179°	2.97	6:1	0
Willard	134	−1.16 × 109°	2.58	1:2	0.0002
Over-and-over	52		2.70		
Continuous locking	72	−2.07 × 95°	2.35	1:15	0
10-0 nylon, posterior, 1/2	390	−0.12 × 145°	1.43	1:1	0.3509
10-0 nylon, anterior, 3/4	123	−1.27 × 172°	2.13	4:1	0
9-0 silk, posterior, 1/2	124	−0.17 × 110°	1.38	1:1	0.2722
9-0 silk, anterior, 3/4	146	−1.17 × 176°	2.19	3:1	0
7-0 silk	88	−0.94 × 85°	1.61	1:3	0.0007
7-0 chromic catgut	208	−2.21 × 93°	2.76	1:11	0
7-0 chromic collagen	82	−0.31 × 161°	1.89	8:5	0.1406

[*]From Jaffe, N. S., and Clayman, H. M.: Ophthalmology (Rochester) **79:**OP615-630, 1975.
[†]Average cylindric correction of surgically induced astigmatism with axis taken into account.
[‡]Average of corrective K values without axis.
[§]Ratio of with-the-rule to against-the-rule astigmatism.
[‖]Assumption is made that there is an equal chance of getting with-the-rule or against-the-rule astigmatism. The chance of this being true expressed in this column.

deeply inserted sutures (4:1), and 9-0 silk interrupted suture with a midlimbal incision and deeply inserted sutures (3:1). Against-the-rule astigmatism was associated with the following: Willard continuous suture (2:1), continuous locking suture (15:1), 7-0 silk (3:1), and 7-0 chromic catgut (11:1). A more even distribution was found with the following: 10-0 nylon and 9-0 silk interrupted sutures with a posterior incision and less deeply placed sutures and 7-0 chromic collagen covered by a limbal-based conjunctival flap. The over-and-over continuous suture always commenced on the nasal side of the globe and terminated on the temporal side. The steepest corneal meridian was usually found to lie between 90 degrees and the temporal extremity of the incision. This occurred in 16 of 20 right eyes and 28 of 32 left eyes.

EXPLANATION OF RESULTS

How can one explain these results? It is suggested that the results are determined by one of two mechanisms:

1. Wound gape
2. Wound compression

Larger sutures that are removed (7-0 silk) and those that tend to disintegrate early (7-0 catgut) permit the wound to gape, thus increasing the circumference of the globe in the meridian perpendicular to the line of incision. This causes a flattening of the vertical meridian and, hence, astigmatism against the rule. There is also some increase in curvature of the horizontal meridian.

Finer sutures such as 10-0 monofilament nylon and 9-0 silk, which are intended to remain in situ, tend to compress the wound. This tendency is increased if the incision is made more anteriorly and if the sutures are inserted more deeply. Wound compression results in a shortening of the vertical meridian of the globe. This increases the curvature in the vertical meridian and, hence, astigmatism with the rule. There is also some flattening of the horizontal meridian[8] but to a lesser degree than the increased curvature in the vertical meridian.

The Willard and Troutman continuous sutures appear similar at first glance because both are anchored at 2:30, 9:30, and 12 o'clock. However, the Troutman suture commences at the two hori-

zontal extremities of the incision and is finally anchored in the vertical meridian. The Willard suture commences at the most vertical extremity of the wound and is finally anchored at the two horizontal extremities. Most surgeons have a compulsion to pull up the sutures tightest at their termination to ensure an airtight closure. This tends to cause greatest wound compression near their final points of anchorage, that is, 12 o'clock for the Troutman and 2:30 and 9:30 o'clock for the Willard suture. The ratio of with-the-rule to against-the-rule astigmatism was 6:1 with the Troutman and 1:2 with the Willard suture. Since the final securing of the over-and-over continuous suture occurs on the temporal side, it was not surprising that the steepest corneal meridian was found between 90 and 180 degrees in the right eye and between 0 and 90 degrees in the left eye. This was also attributed to greatest wound compression near the terminal portion of the suture.

It was apparent in this study that moving the incision closer to the cornea and inserting the sutures to a deeper level, as is possible and even desirable with finer sutures (especially 10-0 monofilament nylon), tended to increase astigmatism with the rule. Using 10-0 monofilament nylon interrupted sutures placed more superficially in a more posteriorly situated incision gave a with:against ratio of 1:1. Moving the incision closer to the cornea and placing the sutures more deeply changed the ratio to 4:1. Comparable figures were obtained for interrupted 9-0 silk sutures: a change from 1:1 to 3:1. This is attributed to greater wound compression.

Especially if the incision is more anterior, 7-0 chromic catgut sutures covered by a fornix-based conjunctival flap, tend to disintegrate more readily and permit some wound gaping. The with:against ratio was 1:11. When another absorbable suture, 7-0 chromic collagen, was buried under a limbal-based flap, the with:against ratio was 8:5. The incision was also placed slightly more posteriorly. This increased protection provided to the suture probably caused less wound gaping.

The preponderance of against-the-rule astigmatism (ratio 3:1) when using 7-0 silk is probably due to wound gaping. These relatively large sutures are generally removed 3 to 4 weeks postoperatively when the healing of the incision is histologically incomplete.

These studies showed that the closer the incision is to the cornea, the greater the induced astigmatism, whether due to wound gape or wound compression.

The factors that appear to increase wound compression are the following:

1. Fine sutures such as 10-0 nylon and 9-0 silk used to close relatively anterior incisions
2. Deeply inserted fine sutures
3. Wide suture bites
4. Tightly tied sutures
5. Greater number of sutures
6. Overlapping of the wound

Wound gape is favored by the opposites of these factors. The effect of the location of the incision on corneal curvature is probably related to the delayed wound healing observed with anterior incisions.[9]

It should be emphasized that the astigmatic error revealed by keratometry is greater than the spectacle cylinder required. In aphakia, since the nodal point of the eye has been moved forward, the optical effect of the corneal curvature is never so strong as indicated by the keratometer. Thus the keratometer does not give the cylinder required for correcting spectacles, but the value of the cylinder that when placed on the cornea would correct the astigmatic curvature of its anterior surface. When the lenses are worn 13 to 15 mm from the eye, their effective value is very different. Thus a hyperopic correction (as in aphakia) induces a lower final correcting cylinder than the keratometer reading would indicate, while a myopic correction increases the final correcting cylinder value found with the keratometer. In the average aphakic eye with a $+12.00$ D refractive error, the reduction in the K finding would be about 25%. Thus if keratometry reveals 4.00 D of corneal astigmatism, the spectacle cylindric correction would be 3.00 D.

EFFECT OF CUTTING SUTURES

The concept of wound compression is adequately defended in our series by the results of removing or cutting a suture in the steepest corneal meridian. The effect of this is shown in Tables 4-5 to 4-8. Thus an effective method of re-

ducing or eliminating the wound compression caused by 10-0 monofilament nylon and 9-0 virgin silk is the removal of one or more interrupted sutures in the meridian of greatest corneal curvature or in the severing of a continuous suture in the area of the steepest corneal meridian. In most instances the change in corneal curvature is observed immediately by keratometry and is more dramatic with nylon than silk. The following results illustrate how much wound compression and subsequent increased corneal curvature can be caused by these sutures. An eye with a Troutman continuous suture had a K reading of $-12.00 \times 180°$ 9 weeks postoperatively. The terminal knot was cut at 12 o'clock. The K reading was immediately reduced to zero. An eye with a Willard continuous suture had a K reading of $-7.00 \times 135°$ 7 weeks postoperatively. The suture was cut at the 45-degree meridian (steepest corneal meridian), and the K reading immediately changed to $-0.50 \times 90°$ (an induced change of $-7.00 \times 50°$). An eye with interrupted 9-0 silk sutures had a K reading of $-6.00 \times 180°$ 3 weeks postoperatively. Three sutures at 10, 11, and 12 o'clock were removed. The K reading changed to $-1.50 \times 90°$ (an induced change of $-7.50 \times 90°$). An eye with an over-and-over continuous suture had a K reading of $-7.00 \times 175°$ 3 weeks postoperatively. The suture was cut, and a section between 11 and 1 o'clock was removed. The K reading immediately changed to zero. With few exceptions, cutting a suture in the meridian of steepest corneal curvature is an effective method of reducing high degrees of corneal astigmatism due to wound compression. The rule to be remembered is to cut the suture in the axis of the correcting plus cylinder. This technique cannot be used in instances of astigmatism due to wound gape.

Some patients showed a tendency to large amounts of postoperative astigmatism in both eyes whether or not the same suture technique was used in the two eyes. Conversely, other patients exhibited little tendency to postoperative corneal astigmatism no matter which technique was used for each eye. This is demonstrated in Tables 4-9 and 4-10. It is assumed that this tendency or lack of tendency to global deformation is a characteristic peculiar to certain eyes.

Table 4-5. Effect of cutting Troutman suture

Postoperative K*	Weeks	New K*	Δ†	Remarks
−12.00 × 180°	9	Zero	−12.00 × 90°	Cut at 12
−4.00 × 180°	10	−1.00 × 90°	−5.00 × 90°	Cut at 12
−10.75 × 5°	7	−6.00 × 10°	−4.95 × 90°	Cut at 12
−9.00 × 20°	7	−0.50 × 25°	−8.50 × 110°	Cut at 11-12
−6.00 × 160°	12	−1.50 × 105°	−7.35 × 70°	Cut at 12-2
−6.00 × 180°	11	−0.50 × 180°	−5.50 × 90°	Cut at 12
−8.00 × 180°	6	−3.50 × 60°	−10.20 × 80°	Cut at 12

*Cylindric values represent corrective cylinder required to eliminate astigmatic error.
†Calculated change in postoperative K as result of cutting suture.

Table 4-6. Effect of cutting Willard suture

Postoperative K*	Weeks	New K*	Δ†	Remarks
−3.00 × 155°	3	−4.50 × 85°	−7.00 × 75°	Cut at 65°
−6.00 × 90°	6	−6.00 × 90°	Zero	Cut at 3 and 9
−5.00 × 105°	9	−5.00 × 105°	Zero	Cut at 3 and 9
−7.00 × 135°	7	−0.50 × 90°	−7.00 × 50°	Cut at 45°
−7.00 × 140°	7	−1.00 × 55°	−8.00 × 50°	Removed 90°-180°

*Cylindric values represent corrective cylinder required to eliminate astigmatic error.
†Calculated change in postoperative K as result of cutting suture.

Table 4-7. Effect of cutting 9-0 silk suture

Postoperative K*	Weeks	New K*	Δ†	Remarks
−2.50 × 65°	6	−2.50 × 120°	−4.10 × 140°	2 sutures at 10 and 11
−6.00 × 180°	3	−1.50 × 90°	−7.50 × 90°	3 sutures 11, 12, and 1
−3.50 × 180°	3	−1.00 × 110°	−4.31 × 95°	1 suture at 12
−4.00 × 130°	5	−0.75 × 165°	−3.81 × 35°	3 sutures at 1 and 2
−5.50 × 130°	8	−1.00 × 125°	−4.50 × 40°	1 suture at 2
−8.00 × 180°	2½	−4.00 × 55°	−10.00 × 80°	3 sutures at 11, 12, and 1 (slight wound gape)
−6.50 × 10°	8	−2.50 × 45°	−6.10 × 90°	2 sutures at 10 and 11

*Cylindric values represent corrective cylinder required to eliminate astigmatic error.
†Calculated change in postoperative K as result of cutting suture.

Table 4-8. Effect of cutting suture — miscellaneous

Suture	Postoperative K*	Weeks	New K*	Δ†	Remarks
Over and over	−7.00 × 175°	3	Zero	−7.00 × 85°	Cut 11-1
Over and over	−4.00 × 145°	6	−2.00 × 120°	−3.12 × 70°	Cut 1-2
10-0 nylon	−8.00 × 175°	9	−2.50 × 95°	−10.50 × 85°	1 suture at 12
7-0 collagen	−7.50 × 165°	6	−4.00 × 75°	−4.00 × 65°	2 sutures 12 and 1

*Cylindric values represent corrective cylinder required to eliminate astigmatic error.
†Calculated change in postoperative K as result of cutting suture.

Table 4-9. Bilateral high cylinder*

First eye		Second eye	
Suture	Δ†	Suture	Δ†
Willard	$-3.50 \times 75°$	10-0 nylon	$-6.00 \times 30°$
Willard	$-4.25 \times 75°$	9-0 silk	$-3.00 \times 55°$
Willard	$-4.25 \times 115°$	Troutman	$-3.25 \times 165°$
Willard	$-4.75 \times 105°$	7-0 collagen	$-3.00 \times 105°$
Willard	$-3.25 \times 90°$	7-0 catgut	$-4.12 \times 100°$
Troutman	$-4.50 \times 175°$	10-0 nylon	$-3.00 \times 180°$
10-0 nylon	$-6.25 \times 170°$	9-0 silk	$-3.25 \times 180°$
10-0 nylon	$-8.00 \times 175°$	7-0 catgut	$-3.50 \times 60°$
9-0 silk	$-3.00 \times 30°$	7-0 catgut	$-5.50 \times 80°$
9-0 silk	$-4.25 \times 160°$	7-0 collagen	$-4.00 \times 85°$
7-0 catgut	$-5.00 \times 60°$	Continuous locking	$-3.00 \times 100°$
7-0 catgut	$-4.00 \times 115°$	7-0 silk	$-5.00 \times 70°$
10-0 nylon	$-5.25 \times 160°$	10-0 nylon	$-3.50 \times 155°$
9-0 silk	$-5.00 \times 145°$	9-0 silk	$-4.00 \times 45°$
7-0 catgut	$-5.50 \times 80°$	7-0 catgut	$-5.00 \times 120°$

*The cylindric values represent the corrective cylinder required to eliminate the astigmatic error.
†Δ represents the calculated surgically induced change in astigmatism.

Table 4-10. Bilateral low cylinder*

First eye		Second eye	
Suture	Δ†	Suture	Δ†
Willard	$-0.50 \times 95°$	10-0 nylon	Zero
Willard	$-1.00 \times 95°$	9-0 silk	$-0.75 \times 180°$
Willard	Zero	7-0 catgut	$-1.00 \times 95°$
Troutman	$-0.75 \times 30°$	10-0 nylon	$-1.00 \times 90°$
9-0 silk	$-0.75 \times 180°$	7-0 catgut	$-0.25 \times 180°$
9-0 silk	$-1.00 \times 45°$	7-0 collagen	Zero
9-0 silk	$-0.37 \times 175°$	Troutman	$-1.00 \times 80°$
10-0 nylon	$-0.50 \times 75°$	7-0 catgut	$-1.00 \times 90°$
10-0 nylon	Zero	9-0 silk	Zero
10-0 nylon	$-1.00 \times 120°$	Over and over	Zero
7-0 catgut	$-0.75 \times 60°$	7-0 silk	$-0.25 \times 105°$
10-0 nylon	Zero	10-0 nylon	Zero
9-0 silk	Zero	9-0 silk	Zero
7-0 catgut	$-0.37 \times 155°$	7-0 catgut	$-1.00 \times 60°$

*The cylindric values represent the corrective cylinder required to eliminate the astigmatic error.
†Δ represents the calculated surgically induced change in astigmatism.

CLINICAL APPLICATION OF FINDINGS: THE CONTROL OF POSTOPERATIVE ASTIGMATISM

This study suggests that from a variety of suture techniques the surgeon may choose one that will not exaggerate a preexisting corneal astigmatism and that might reduce it. For example, if an eye has 2.00 D of corneal astigmatism with the rule, one would not use a Troutman suture. Willard continuous, 7-0 chromic catgut, or 7-0 silk sutures would probably lessen the astigmatic error. The surgeon may also choose a technique that will lessen large amounts of preoperative corneal astigmatism. For example, if the preoperative corrective cylinder is $-6.00 \times 45°$, the steepest corneal meridian is at 135 degrees (the axis of the plus cylinder). The surgeon may elect to use interrupted 10-0 nylon or 9-0 silk sutures and tie them tightest in the vicinity of the 45-degree meridian. Two alternatives would be to use 7-0 chromic catgut or 7-0 silk between 90 and 180 degrees and 10-0 nylon or 9-0 silk between 0 and 90 degrees or to use an over-and-over continuous suture commencing on the side of the steeper corneal meridian and terminating on the side of the flatter corneal meridian.

It is not suggested that these represent the most effective methods of altering preoperative astigmatism. Troutman's wedge resection[8] might be more effective. It is performed by excising a crescentic wedge of limbal tissue through 60 to 90 degrees, its greatest width—1.5 mm—centered on the flat meridian. For example, if preoperative keratometry indicates 40 D $\times$ 30° and 46 D $\times$ 120°, the wedge resection would be centered at the 30 degree meridian. By thus shortening the circumference of the globe in this meridian, the flat meridian is steepened. Since the eyeball is basically a plastic sphere, some flattening of the opposing steeper meridian takes place. This procedure reduces the excess preoperative astigmatism and also shortens the axial length of the globe (greater hyperopia). In the example given, suppose the postoperative finding after such a wedge resection (without making a full cataract incision) was 42 D $\times$ 95° and 40 D $\times$ 5°. The calculated induced change by the wedge resection is 4.96 D $\times$ 39°. Moreover, there is a decided tendency for the cornea to resume its preoperative curvature over long periods of time. This is more emphatic with postoperative wound compression than wound gape. In addition, nylon sutures, whether placed in an interrupted or in a continuous manner, tend to show variations in their effect on corneal curvature.

Surgical keratometer

An exciting approach to the control of postoperative corneal astigmatism is by adjusting the tying tension of the sutures during surgery. The astigmatism is monitored by a surgical keratometer such as that designed by Troutman or Terry. This technique has an advantage over the conventional square knot, which is very difficult to tension properly. Furthermore, what appears as a tight suture may change considerably when the remaining sutures are placed. Terry[10] has suggested a method by which interrupted sutures could be individually adjusted after all the sutures are placed. The technique involves the use of a slide knot that resembles a lariat where the loop passes through the corneoscleral incision. The friction of the knot holds the suture tension while the additional sutures are adjusted.

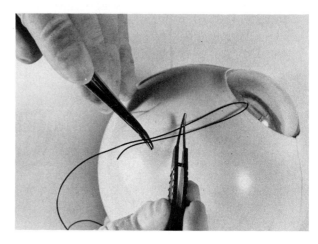

Fig. 4-20. Suture is placed through cornea and sclera, and both ends are grasped with instrument held in left hand. (From Terry, C.: J. Am. Intraocul. Implant Soc. **3:**197-198, 1977.)

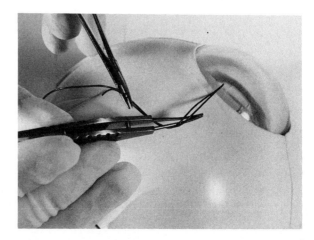

Fig. 4-21. Tying forceps in right hand is placed on top of both arms of suture to form "T." (From Terry, C.: J. Am. Intraocul. Implant Soc. **3:**197-198, 1977.)

The adjustable suture knot is easily tied with standard microsurgical instruments. The suture is placed through the cornea and sclera, and both ends are grasped with an instrument in the left hand (Fig. 4-20). The short end of the suture is positioned near the tip of the instrument in the left hand so that it may be easily grasped later. The tying forceps in the right hand is placed on top of both arms of the suture to form a "T" and then hooked under to grasp the prepositioned short end (Figs. 4-21 and 4-22). Pulling this end free of the instrument in the left hand forms the knot (Fig. 4-23). Pulling on the short end with the instrument in the right hand lengthens the loop and loosens the suture (Fig. 4-24). Pulling on the long end with the instrument in the left hand tightens the suture (Fig. 4-25). The short end is cut shorter to reduce the suture clutter. The sutures are all placed with this slide knot to approximate the wound edges, and the anterior chamber is formed with air or fluid to reconstruct the surgical dome. The sutures are precisely adjust-

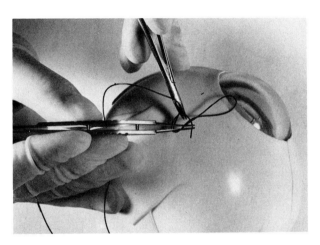

Fig. 4-22. Tying forceps is then hooked under to grasp prepositioned short end of suture. (From Terry, C.: J. Am. Intraocul. Implant Soc. **3:**197-198, 1977.)

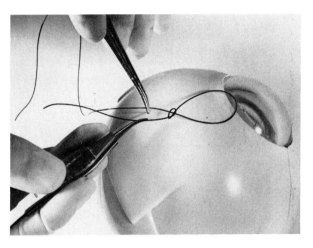

Fig. 4-23. Pulling short end of suture free of instrument in left hand forms knot. (From Terry, C.: J. Am. Intraocul. Implant Soc. **3:**197-198, 1977.)

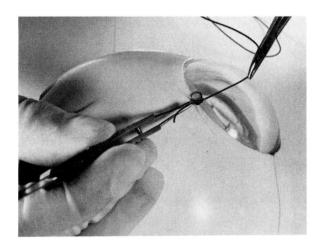

Fig. 4-24. Pulling short end with instrument in right hand lengthens loop and loosens suture. (From Terry, C.: J. Am. Intraocul. Implant Soc. **3:**197-198, 1977.)

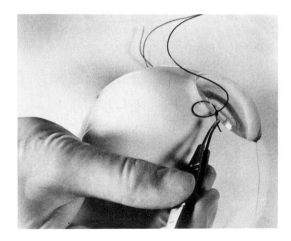

Fig. 4-25. Pulling long end with instrument in left hand tightens suture. (From Terry, C.: J. Am. Intraocul. Implant Soc. **3:**197-198, 1977.)

ed so as not to distort the cornea. A standard square knot permanently locks the suture. With deeply placed nonabsorbable radial sutures of equal tension, the corneal curvature will not significantly shift postoperatively.

REFERENCES

1. Sato, T.: Posterior half-incision of cornea for astigmatism, Am. J. Ophthalmol. **36:**462-466, 1953.
2. Corcostegui Moliner, A.: Surgical treatment of astigmatism, Arch. Soc. Oftal. Hisp.-Am. **16:**750-760, 1956.
3. Stokes, G. G.: 19th Meeting of the British Association for the Advancement of Science, 1849, London, 1850, Transactions of the Sections, p. 10.
4. Southall, J. P. C.: Mirrors, prisms, and lenses: a textbook of geometrical optics, ed. 3, New York, 1940, Macmillan Publishing Co., Inc., pp. 320-326. Reprinted 1964, New York, Dover.
5. Ogle, K. N.: Optics, an introduction for ophthalmologists, Springfield, Ill., 1968, Charles C Thomas, Publisher.
6. Rubin, M. L.: Optics for clinicians, ed. 2, Gainesville, Fla., 1974, Triad Scientific Publishers.
7. Duke-Elder, S.: System of ophthalmology. Vol. V. Ophthalmic optics and refraction, St. Louis, The C. V. Mosby Co., 1970, p. 279.
8. Troutman, R. C.: Microsurgical control of corneal astigmatism in cataract extraction, Ophthalmology (Rochester) **77:**OP 563-572, 1973.
9. Heller, M. D., Irvine, S. R., Straatsma, B. R., and Foos, R. Y.: Wound healing after cataract extraction and position of the vitreous in aphakic eyes as studied post mortem, Trans. Am Ophthalmol. Soc. **69:**245-262, 1971.
10. Terry, C.: The differentially adjustable slide knot, J. Am. Intraocul. Implant Soc. **3:**197-198, 1977.

CHAPTER 5

Intraocular lens implants

HISTORY

The history of intraocular lenses has been exciting, often frustrating, but finally rewarding. There have been abortive attempts at intraocular lens implantation dating back to the early eighteenth century. However, the modern era began with observations made during World War II. The canopy that covered the British Spitfire fighter plane was made of a plastic material known as polymethylmethacrylate (Perspex). When shattered by enemy gun fire, fragments of this material occasionally lodged within the eyes of fighter pilots. The apparent lack of reactivity to this substance by the eye was impressive. In 1949, Harold Ridley was inspired by a comment made by a medical student who exclaimed while observing Ridley close the incision after an intracapsular cataract extraction that he had forgotten to replace the diseased lens with a new one.[1]

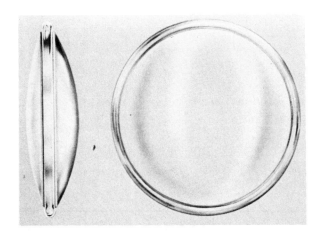

Fig. 5-1. Ridley posterior chamber lens.

Accordingly, Ridley implanted his first intraocular lens into the posterior chamber of the eye of a 45-year-old woman after an extracapsular cataract extraction on November 29, 1949. Because of an error in optic calculation, the patient became highly myopic (-18.00 D sphere -6.00 D cylinder $\times$ 120°), but corrected visual acuity was 20/60. His second attempt, on August 23, 1950, led to a similar result. The design of the lens was then changed (Fig. 5-1), but it could still only be used after an extracapsular lens extraction. The operation had to be carried out as a one-stage procedure because adhesions developing between the iris and the posterior capsule made it impossible to insert a lens of suitable power as a secondary procedure. The first Ridley lens implanted in the United States was by W. Reese of Philadelphia on March 17, 1952. Although numerous successes were achieved (Fig. 5-2), the long-term results were mostly disappointing due to downward decentration, anterior dislocation, and posterior dislocation. The procedure was therefore abandoned.

Because of difficulties encountered with secure fixation of the Ridley posterior chamber lens, anterior chamber angle-fixated lenses were designed. It seems incredible today that so many excellent ophthalmologists were so blinded to the delicacy of the corneal endothelium that they expected these lenses and their immediate good results to last a lifetime. Baron[2] implanted the first angle-supported lens on May 13, 1952. The design of the subsequent lenses varied according to whether the supports were rigid or elastic. The most frequently used implant with rigid supports was designed by Strampelli[3,4] (Fig. 5-3). He implanted his first such lens on September 28, 1953.

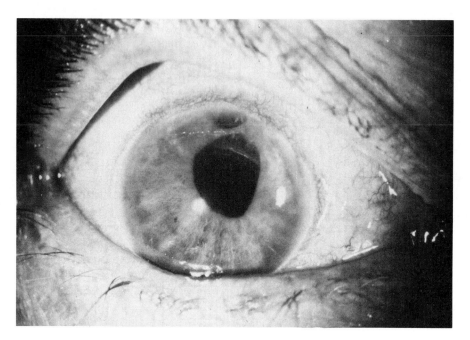

Fig. 5-2. Ridley posterior chamber lens in eye of 62-year-old patient 19 years after its implantation. Note upper edge of pseudophakos in pupillary area. Pupil is eccentric. Vision with correction is 20/40.

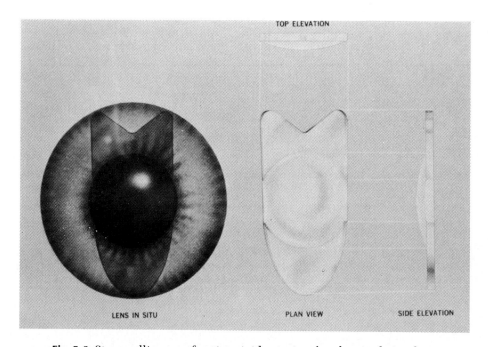

Fig. 5-3. Strampelli nonperforating rigid anterior chamber angle implant.

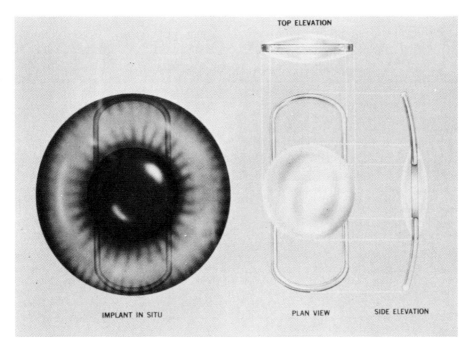

Fig. 5-4. Dannheim nonperforating elastic anterior chamber angle implant.

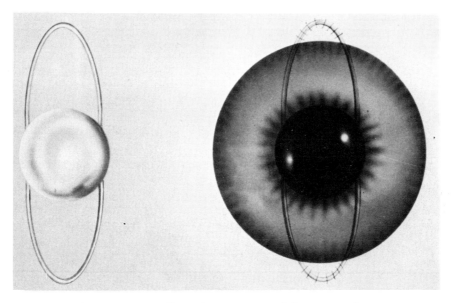

Fig. 5-5. Strampelli perforating external fixation implant.

Because of the rigid supports, this lens was difficult to center and to fixate ideally. Dannheim[5] attempted to solve these problems by using elastic supporting loops designed to stabilize the optic portion by means of pressure in the chamber angle (Fig. 5-4). Because of the high incidence of postoperative complications (mainly late corneal edema), various lenses were designed that modified the haptic portion, since this appeared to be the source of the problems. Strampelli[6-9] resorted

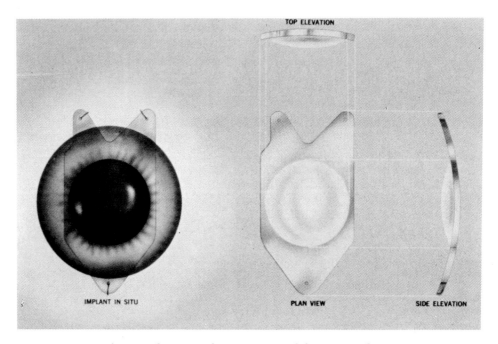

Fig. 5-6. Choyce perforating external-fixation implant.

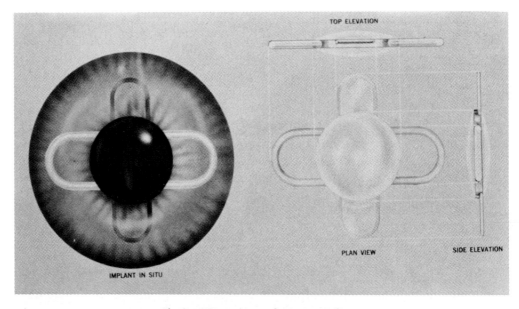

Fig. 5-7. Epstein iris-fixation implant.

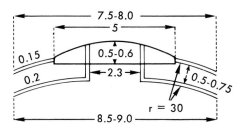

Fig. 5-8. Schematic of modern Binkhorst 4-loop iris-clip implant. Note relatively short anterior haptics and posterior curvature of both anterior and posterior nylon haptic supports.

to external fixation in 1956 (Fig. 5-5). Choyce also used one of these modifications (Fig. 5-6). In spite of numerous modifications, complications did not lessen appreciably. An example of this disastrous episode in implant surgery is the experience of Barraquer. He implanted 493 angle-supported lenses between 1954 and 1960 but eventually found it necessary to remove approximately 250 of these.[10] However, Choyce persisted in his use of angle-supported lenses and now uses a version called Mark VIII and a newer model called Mark IX. It is to his credit to have proven that, with really sophisticated supports, the corneal endothelium could be avoided and

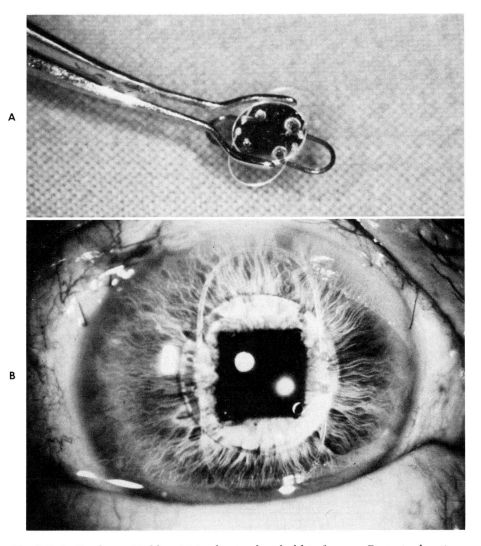

Fig. 5-9. A, Fyodorov-Binkhorst iris-clip implant held in forceps. Posterior haptic supports are dyed dark color. **B,** Fyodorov-Binkhorst iris-clip implant in situ.

the incidence of corneal endothelial breakdown consequently could be lowered significantly. Because so many excellent surgeons were involved in this disappointing period, the feeling spread throughout the world that implant surgery was adventuresome and fraught with potential disaster for the eye. It is understandable that a bias against later innovations and implant surgeons developed.

A revival of enthusiasm for lens implant surgery occurred when lenses that depended on the iris for support were designed. The major credit for this renewed interest belongs to Binkhorst, whose experience with Ridley's original posterior chamber lens and the ill-fated angle-supported lenses paralleled that of others. Epstein and Binkhorst independently directed their efforts to the iris diaphragm as a support for the implant. Epstein[11] designed an iris-supported lens shaped like a collar stud and used it with an extracapsular lens extraction after June 1953. He later abandoned the collar stud principle and developed

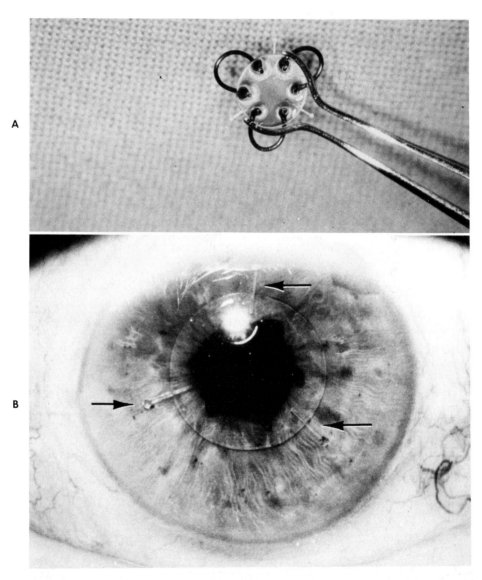

Fig. 5-10. A, Fyodorov "sputnik" implant held in forceps. Note three posterior loops dyed dark color and three anterior sticks with rounded knob at end. **B,** Hexagonal pupil (4 mm) in aphakic eye with Fyodorov lens. Three supporting sticks *(arrows)* anterior to iris.

his Maltese cross lens, a pupillary plane lens that at first had all solid supports and later two solid supports (placed posterior to the iris) and two fenestrated supports (placed anterior to the iris) (Fig. 5-7). Epstein did not report his work until 1959. In the meantime, Binkhorst developed his iris-clip lens in 1957 and used it for the first time on August 11, 1958.[12] He has used it ever since (with an intracapsular lens extraction), although variations in the shape, length, and insertions of the supporting loops have been made. The implant has four Supramid (nylon 6) loops, the optic portion and the two anterior loops on one level and the two posterior loops on a different level (Fig. 5-8). The entire optic portion rests in a pre-

pupillary position. The iris-clip lens avoids fixation in the posterior chamber and in the chamber angle. Thus the most important complication arising from positioning the implant behind the iris—dislocation—was greatly lessened. In addition, the possibility of corneal damage—the most important complication of angle-supported lenses—was greatly lessened.

Federov[13] used a modification of the iris-clip lens in 1964. The anterior and posterior loops were oriented 90 degrees to each other (Fig. 5-9). Since 1968,[14] he has used another modification with three posterior loops and three antennae, which are extensions with a small round knob at the end of each, placed anteriorly to the iris. This

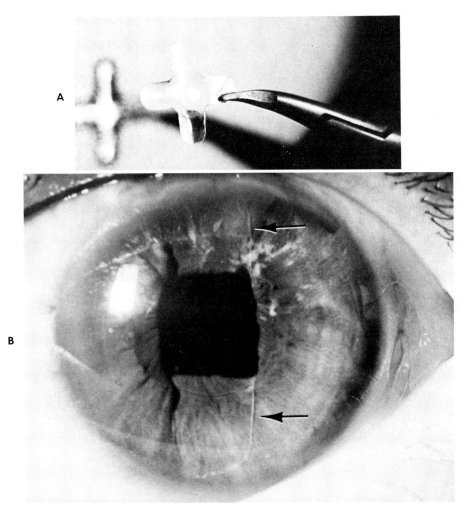

Fig. 5-11. A, Copeland iris-plane in needle holder. **B,** Square pupil (4 mm) in aphakic eye with iris-plane lens. Solid haptics (*arrows*) anterior to iris.

has been termed the "sputnik" lens (Fig. 5-10).

Another pupillary plane lens, the Copeland iris-plane lens, was first used in 1968.[15,16] It is shaped like the original Epstein lens except that the haptics are all solid, and the entire implant is much thinner (Fig. 5-11). It is unique among currently used iris-supported lenses, since the entire implant, optic and haptic portions, is made of one material, polymethyl methacrylate. The supports of other commonly used implants are made

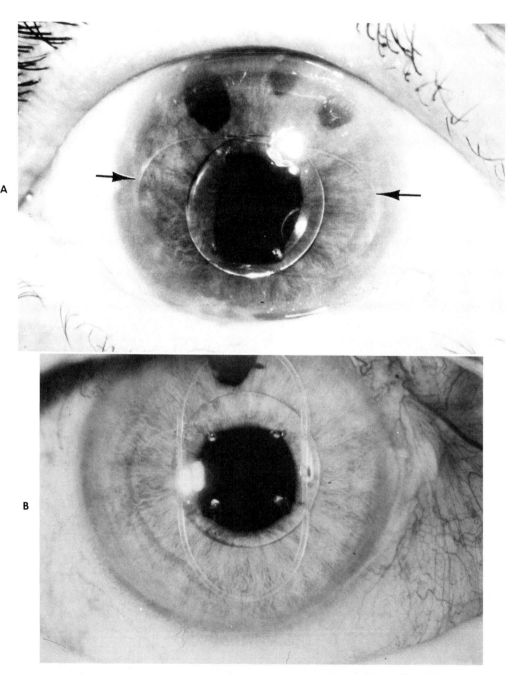

Fig. 5-12. A, Older method of Binkhorst 4-loop iris-clip implant in situ. Nylon loops (*arrows*) anterior to iris. **B,** New method of implantation of Binkhorst 4-loop iris-clip implant.

of other materials such as nylon, platinum, and platinum-iridium.

To prevent the occasional dislocation of the iris-clip lens, Worst[17] began, in February 1969, to suture one of the anterior loops to the iris. Binkhorst[18-20] changed his surgical technique so that the iris-clip lens was placed in the vertical, rather than the horizontal, position (Fig. 5-12).

This made it possible to connect both upper loops (anterior and posterior) in a peripheral iris coloboma with a monofilament Perlon suture (transiridectomy fixation) (Fig. 5-13). He commenced this technique in March 1970. Worst developed an implant with an enlarged lens body and two holes in the upper segment through which to pass a monofilament Perlon suture. This

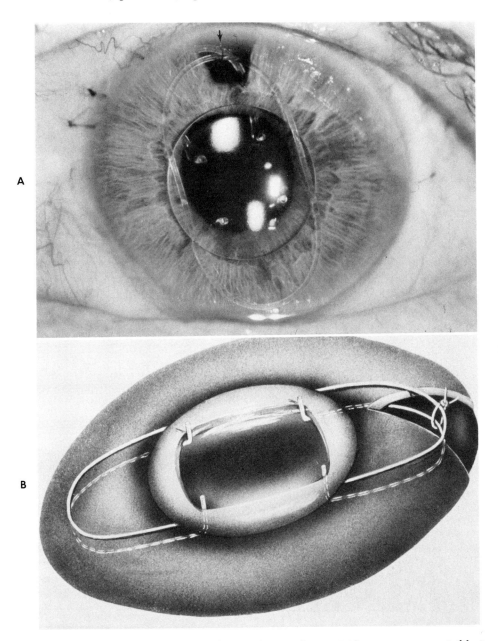

Fig. 5-13. A, Binkhorst 4-loop iris-clip implant with transiridectomy suture visible in peripheral iridectomy *(arrow).* **B,** Drawing of transiridectomy suture technique.

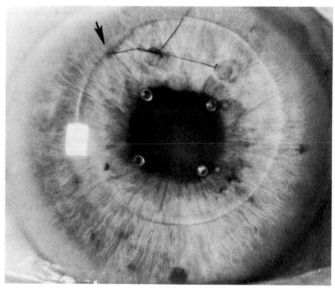

Fig. 5-14. Worst 2-loop Medallion implant in situ. Note iris suture *(arrow).*

lens contained a pair of loops that pass behind the iris in the horizontal position. There are no anterior loops (Fig. 5-14). This implant, known as the Medallion lens, was inserted for the first time on December 18, 1970.[21] Worst later developed a modification of this lens by mounting a finger-like, platina extension at the edge of the lens body. A transiridectomy hooking technique is used (safety pin principle). The haptic supports are placed in the vertical position with this implant. The Medallion lens may be used with an intracapsular or extracapsular lens extraction.

The possibility of capsular support as originally used by Ridley had been abandoned until December 1963, when Binkhorst inserted an iris-clip lens after an extracapsular extraction of a traumatic cataract. In this technique the anterior loops were removed (Fig. 5-15). A 2-loop irido-

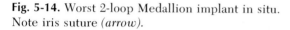

Fig. 5-15. Binkhorst 2-loop iridocapsular implant made from 4-loop implant by cutting off anterior loops *(arrows).*

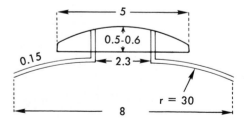

Fig. 5-16. Schematic of modern Binkhorst 2-loop iridocapsular implant. Supporting loops are made of platinum-iridium.

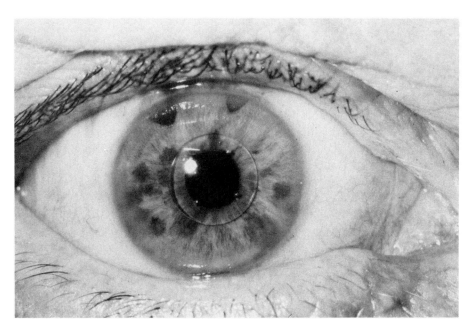

Fig. 5-17. Binkhorst 2-loop iridocapsular implant in situ.

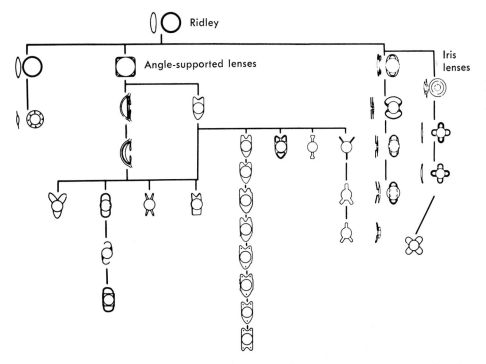

Fig. 5-18. Diagram of history of intraocular lenses: first generation, posterior chamber lenses; second generation, angle-supported lenses; third generation, iris- and capsule-supported lenses. (From Roper-Hall, M. J.: Ophthalmology [Rochester] **81:**OP67-69, 1976.)

capsular lens containing only posterior loops (Supramid) was designed and used for the first time on September 16, 1965.[22] An iridocapsular lens that substituted two platinum-iridium loops for the two Supramid loops was used for the first time on October 27, 1965 (Fig. 5-16). This implant is only used after an extracapsular lens extraction. True capsular fixation of the loops to the posterior lens capsule and residual cortex is obtained (Fig. 5-17). Thus the fixation is independent of the iris, and the name "iridocapsular" is something of a misnomer.

The furious pace of technologic advance in implant design has continued in recent years. The iris is no longer considered the only reliable intraocular structure for fixation of a pseudophakos. There has been a significant trend to return to anterior chamber angle-supported and posterior chamber lenses. (It is curious that this trend should occur to challenge the depressing history of the Ridley posterior chamber lens and the numerous anterior chamber angle-supported lenses of the 1950s.) Such a proliferation of lens implants has occurred that a family tree of intraocular lenses (Fig. 5-18) can be constructed, based on the three locations of fixation within the eye. This furious pace is attributable as much to improved lens design as to improve surgical technique. These are discussed later.

THEORY OF PSEUDOPHAKOS
Comparison of current methods of optic correction of aphakia

Since a spectacle lens and a contact lens are safe appliances because they can be removed if defective, what accounts for the current popularity of intraocular lenses? This is easily explained by examining the three available methods of optic correction of aphakia.

1. Spectacle lens in front of the eye
2. Contact lens on the eye
3. Intraocular lens inside the eye

Spectacle lenses were better accepted 30 years ago than today for two reasons. First, no other method of optic correction was available. Second, cataract surgery was rarely performed before the cataract was mature, or nearly so, in one eye and vision markedly reduced in the second eye, so that the improvement in vision appeared dramatic to the patient and therefore his psychologic adjustment to aphakia was easier. With the advent of the intracapsular cataract extraction and its subsequent sophistication, cataract extraction is often performed earlier. In addition, surgery is being performed on older patients, who adapt to the handicaps of spectacle lenses with less facility.

Woods[23] outlined the disadvantages of spectacle lenses in aphakia after having personally undergone cataract extraction in both eyes.

1. Magnification of image size by about 25%. On first receiving the aphakic spectacles, the aphakic patient is immediately astounded by the increase in the size of familiar objects. If aphakic in one eye only and still having some fair residual vision in the second eye, the attempt at binocular vision produces a superimposed diplopia. Useful binocular vision is impossible until the second eye is operated on. However, even if binocularity is restored by surgery on the second eye, the magnification of familiar objects causes false spatial orientation. This results in a series of minor domestic tragedies such as overturned tumblers, spilled ink, and crashed flower vases.

2. Spherical aberration. The aphakic patient suddenly finds himself in a parabolic world. Ocular movements cause this parabolic world to squirm like a writhing snake. Straight lines are transformed into curves. A pincushion distortion occurs.

3. Poor coordination of manual movements. The new visual imagery causes incessant clumsiness with simple tasks such as sharpening a pencil, carving a turkey, or placing a key in a lock.

Fortunately, the patient who is newly aphakic can be assured that the three most obvious difficulties—false orientation, spherical aberration, and lack of coordination—can be partly overcome with time, practice, and good aspheric spectacles. There are two other problems so difficult to overcome that they must be endured.

4. Restriction of visual field (Figs. 5-19 and 5-20). The visual field of the normal, uncorrected aphakic eye does not differ from that of the normal phakic eye if appropriately large test objects are used. The peripheral restriction of the visual field results from the use of aphakic spectacles. There are three causes of this reduction in field:

   a. Small size of aphakic lenticular spectacles
   b. Ring scotoma
   c. Unrefracted field of vision outside spectacle lens

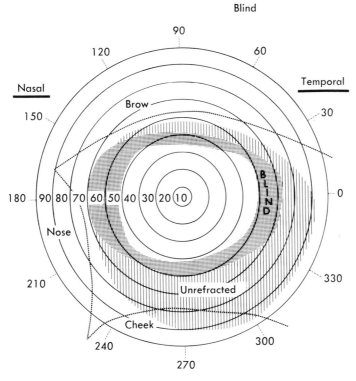

Fig. 5-19. Effect of aphakia spectacle lens on visual field. (From Dabezies, O. H., Jr.: Contact and Intraocular Lens J. **2:**8-13, 1976.)

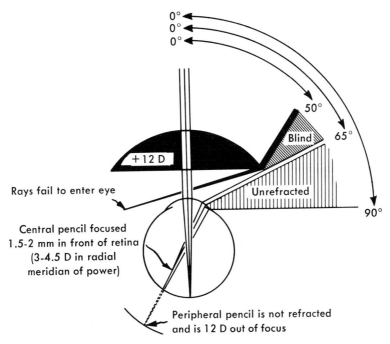

Fig. 5-20. Spectacle lens–corrected aphakia. Refraction of peripheral rays by high-plus nonapheric spectacle lens creates ring scotoma from 50 to 65 degrees. (From Dabezies, O. H., Jr.: Contact and Intraocular Lens J. **2:**8-13, 1976.)

The usual small size of the average aphakic lenticular spectacle moves the ring scotoma more centrally and leaves a greater amount of unrefracted visual field outside the spectacle lens.

The ring scotoma is inherent in high-diopter convex lenses. It takes the general shape of the spectacle lens, is about 12 to 15 degrees wide, and surrounds the refracted visual field. The edge of an aphakic spectacle can be considered a base in prism that bends light rays toward its base. Because of the considerable prismatic effect at the periphery of the spectacle lens, a ray in the area of 50 to 63 degrees from central fixation strikes the periphery of the lens, is bent 13 degrees to the base, fails to pass into the eye, and therefore is not seen (Fig. 5-21). This "blind" area completely circumscribes the restricted field of the aphakic eye. It is not a true scotoma of the eye but rather an optically produced defect in the visual field due to the prismatic effect at the periphery of the lens. The ring scotoma is not stationary. Its movements are initiated by movements of the eye. It is well known by all aphakic patients who wear spectacles that, in ordinary group conversation, faces pop in and out of the

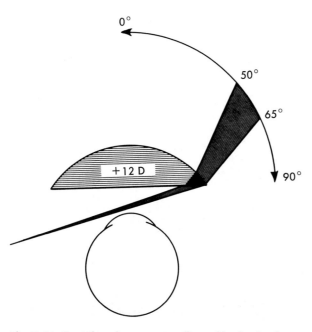

Fig. 5-21. Peripheral prismatic effect of high-plus lens. Rays from 50 to 65 degrees fail to pass into eye. (From Dabezies, O. H., Jr.: Contact Intraocular Lens J. 2:8-13, 1976.)

blind area with the annoying insolence of a jack-in-the-box. Welsh[27] referred to this as the roving ring scotoma, a term descriptive enough to be popularly accepted in spite of Linksz's[26] observation that "it is obviously the eye rather than the scotoma that does the roving."

To understand the jack-in-the-box phenomenon, consider a patient wearing aphakic spectacles gazing directly ahead through the center of the lens (Fig. 5-22). The center of the refractive field of view corresponds to the optic axis of the spectacle lens. The ring scotoma extends from 50 to 65 degrees of the visual field. If the eye rotates temporally (Fig. 5-23) (the head is not rotated), and fixates on an object 30 degrees from the original optic axis, the eye is now gazing through the midperiphery of the spectacle lens. Objects formerly located at 30 to 50 degrees in the original, straight-ahead field are deflected by the prismatic effect of the spectacle lens (base in effect) so that they no longer enter the eye. The blind area (ring scotoma) has moved centrally and lies 30 degrees lateral to the new optic axis. At the same time, objects formerly hidden inside the ring scotoma now appear. In summary, in the straight-ahead position, the blind area begins approximately 50 degrees from the optic axis. When the patient shifts the gaze 30 degrees laterally, the blind area now begins 30 degrees from the optic axis. This shifting centralward of the blind area causes the jack-in-the-box phenomenon.

The other major cause of the complaint of poor side vision is that the visual field, extending from the temporal 65 degrees to the most peripheral portion of the visual field at 85 degrees, is unrefracted, since light rays from this area are too far peripheral (temporal to the spectacle frame) to enter the spectacle lens. However, the unrefracted rays do pass into the eye. The resultant peripheral vision that surrounds the ring scotoma is very blurred but is nevertheless helpful to the patient in establishing overall space orientation.

The plight of the spectacle-corrected aphakic patient was humorously described in a paper entitled "Cadillacs, Volkswagens, and Aphakic Corrections."[24] The author, a bilaterally aphakic ophthalmologist, made the following observations regarding the ring scotoma. With 3 mm pupils, wearing 45 mm aspheric lenses at a vertex distance of 12 mm and a spectacle lens power of

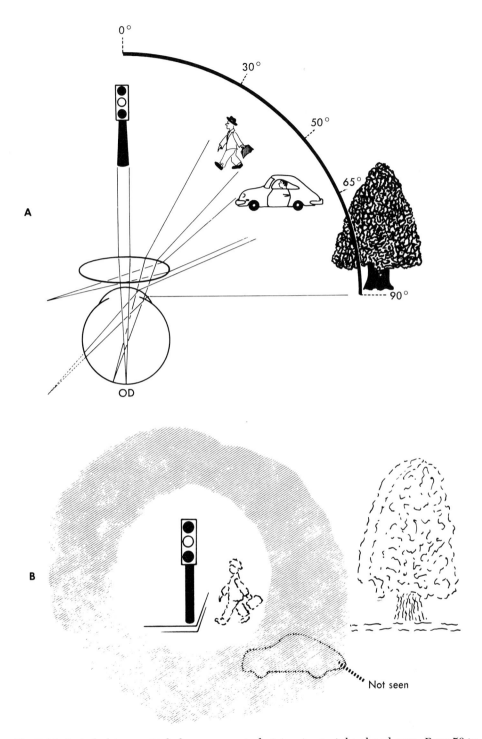

Fig. 5-22. A, Aphakia spectacle lens–corrected vision in straight-ahead gaze. Rays 50 to 65 degrees fail to enter eye. Rays 65 to 90 degrees are unrefracted by spectacle glass. **B,** View seen by patient. Ring scotoma (optically blind area). (From Dabezies, O. H., Jr.: Contact and Intraocular Lens J. **2:**8-13, 1976.)

OD + 10.00 + 0.75 × 20° = 20/10, OS + 8.50 + 1.00 × 160° = 20/10, the scotoma measured 15 degrees using a 1-degree test object at 330 mm. The position of the scotoma was between 40 and 55 degrees. Experimenting in his parking lot, he found that this scotoma obscured a Cadillac at 45 ft (13.5 m) and a Volkswagen at 40 ft (12 m). A person was completely obscured at 4 ft (1.2 m).

A means of simulating the plight of aphakic patients was suggested.[6] A −14 D contact lens is placed on the cornea and a +12 D spectacle is worn in front of the eye. This will convince any ophthalmologist that the adjustment to aphakic spectacles is not a minor problem.

5. Continual adjustment of aphakic spectacles. The glasses must be accurately centered and ad-

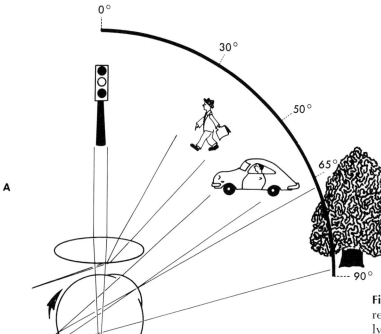

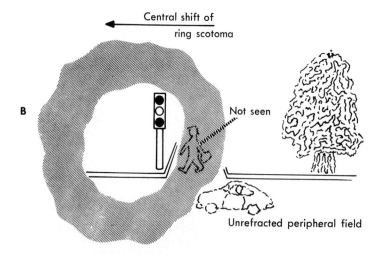

Fig. 5-23. **A,** Aphakia spectacle lens–corrected vision when gaze is directed laterally. Rays 30 to 50 degrees fail to enter eye. Rays 50 to 90 degrees are unrefracted, since they fail to enter spectacle glass. **B,** View seen by patient. Due to central shift of ring scotoma, person disappears. When gaze returns centrally, person reappears (jack-in-the-box phenomenon). (From Dabezies, O. H., Jr.: Contact Intraocular Lens J. **2:**8-13, 1976.)

justed. Since the optically active aphakic patient uses only the optic center of the lens, any maladjustment of the pupillary distance introduces at once a prismatic error that greatly reduces visual efficiency. A fraction of a millimeter in the vertical adjustment produces a similar error. In addition, small variations in vertex distance introduce relatively large errors of refraction. As any optician will attest, the spectacle-corrected aphakic patient occupies much valuable time with incessant requests for spectacle adjustments.

Contact lenses, for patients who can wear them, are far less visually disabling than aphakic spectacles and safer than intraocular lenses in that they can be discontinued with less difficulty. Linksz[26] cited the following advantages:

1. No significant magnification (only about 7%)
2. No appreciable spheric aberration; no pincushion distortion
3. No ring scotoma, jack-in-the-box phenomenon, or roving ring scotoma, and therefore full peripheral vision

There are other advantages: There is practically no false spatial orientation. They are effective for some superficially scarred corneas that produce irregular astigmatism. They are comfortable in eyes after cataract extraction, probably because of the reduced corneal sensitivity.

In general, they are more practical in the younger aphakic patient than in the elderly. This is their main disadvantage. Most elderly patients do not possess the manual dexterity required to insert and remove them. Patients with infirmities such as rheumatoid arthritis, parkinsonism, hemiplegia, or senility have similar problems with them. Many elderly patients live alone in somewhat less than adequate hygienic conditions. Experience has shown that most unilaterally aphakic elderly patients discard their contact lenses relatively soon, and the others do not use them for longer than a few years. Elderly bilaterally aphakic patients usually find contact lenses even more difficult to manage, since they must use aphakic spectacles to initiate the process of insertion and sometimes removal. However, they wear them more faithfully than unilaterally aphakic patients, probably because the poor vision of two uncorrected aphakic eyes produces better motivation. Although a 60-year-old patient

may satisfactorily manage contact lenses even with advancing age, a 70-year-old patient usually experiences frustration in learning how to manage them.

Most ophthalmologists have found contact lens correction of the unilaterally aphakic child (as a result of trauma) to be disappointing. Amblyopia and ocular deviation are rarely prevented. On the other hand, there is growing evidence that intraocular lenses may be far superior in this situation, as subsequent discussion will explain.

Soft or semisoft (silicone) contact lenses may prove to be more applicable in elderly patients if technologic sophistication increases so that the lenses can be worn for long periods. Although possible for some patients, this goal has not yet been routinely achieved.

Intraocular lenses provide many advantages over spectacles and contact lenses. The elimination of perceptual problems was discussed in connection with contact lenses and requires no repetition. Image size disparity is reduced still further. A comparison of 30 unilaterally aphakic adult patients wearing a contact lens with 30 unilaterally aphakic adult patients with an intraocular iris-clip implant showed an average retinal image size increase of 6.99% in the former group and 1.92% in the latter.[28] The figure of 1.92% was later corrected by Colenbrander[29] to 0.20% minification. The difference became clear in computing the average of cases with magnification and cases with minification. The AO Space Eikonometer was used for all measurements. An average visual acuity of 0.8 in the operated eye was found in both groups. The patients using contact lenses were considerably younger (49.6 years) than those with implants (67.7 years). Using the Wirt stereopsis test, the contact lens group recorded an average of 45.7% and the implant group 81.8%, in spite of the 18.1 years difference in their average ages.

Since the intraocular lens is intended to remain in situ permanently, it eliminates all the difficulties of inserting and removing contact lenses encountered by elderly patients and those with infirmities such as parkinsonism.

An intraocular lens may be advantageous for those working in unusual environments (cattle ranchers, miners) and for those whose visual requirements for occupation must be fulfilled (pilots, members of the armed services, and so on).

The potential for prevention of amblyopia in young children who suffer a traumatic cataract is high. Ophthalmologists have been frustrated in their attempts to prevent amblyopia in these children. In children 2 to 7 years of age, it is extremely difficult to employ a contact lens following removal of the traumatic cataract. Binkhorst and Gobin[22] fitted 10 of 22 unilaterally aphakic children with contact lenses and reported that suppression or diplopia developed in all cases. Van Balen[30] found that only 3 of 15 unilaterally aphakic children under the age of 14 could be treated adequately with a contact lens. A comprehensive report of the techniques and perspectives of lens implants in children, including an orthoptic analysis of all treated cases, was presented by Bierlaagh and co-workers,[31] who treated 29 patients less than 15 years of age who had unilateral pseudophakia after lens injury. The patients were divided into three groups according to the age at which injury occurred. They represented a consecutive series of cases of traumatic cataract treated by lens implant. The causes of the cataract were contusion of the eye as well as perforating injury with or without an intraocular foreign body. A few patients had very severely damaged anterior segments. During a follow-up period of 1 to 9 years, a complication was seen only once, and that was in a severely damaged eye in which a band-shaped keratopathy developed as a result of the injury and repeated subsequent surgical interventions. All other eyes were doing well in spite of corneal scarring and other posttraumatic pathology and an occasional inevitable case of amblyopia. Twenty-three of the 29 eyes had 0.5 vision or better, and only one eye had less than 0.1 vision. The summary of orthoptic evaluation of all patients revealed that in every age category, the final result far exceeded that of any other known method of treating these difficult problems.

The disadvantages of an intraocular implant center on the surgery itself. The surgery requires education in the proper selection of cases, the choice of surgical procedure, and the technique of the surgery itself. This is a formidable responsibility for the surgeon. It has not been statistical-

ly determined that implant surgery leads to more complications than routine cataract surgery does. However, if this proves to be the case, it must then be determined if the previously mentioned disadvantages of other forms of optic correction of aphakia outweigh any greater risk involved in the implantation of an intraocular lens. It is apparent that implant surgeons and their patients are sufficiently happy with their surgical results so that the procedure appears to be gaining in popularity. The specific disadvantages of operative and postoperative complications of implant surgery will be considered later.

ANISEIKONIA

The subject of aniseikonia appears to be a central theme in the various methods of the optic correction of aphakia. Much has been written on the limit of tolerance of image size disparity for comfortable binocular vision. Most ophthalmologists consider 5% to 8% to be the limit.

Patients wearing a spectacle lens are not usually disturbed by aniseikonia, since image size disparity is so great (22% to 35%) that binocular fusion in unilaterally aphakic patients is impossible. They use only one eye, either with aphakic spectacles or without, for all visual activities. Patients who use a contact lens on the aphakic eye do not possess the binocular visual efficiency of those with an intraocular lens. The degree of aniseikonia may exceed tolerable limits for some but apparently not for others.

If iseikonia is the aim in unilateral implantations, Binkhorst[20] attempts to make the posterior focal length of the uncorrected pseudophakic eye equal to that of the uncorrected fellow eye. Thus the corneal power of the eye to be operated on (corrected with the spectacle correction of the fellow eye) and the axial length of the fellow eye are decisive. The latter has to be corrected because of the forward displacement of the second principal plane in the pseudophakic eye compared with its position in the phakic eye. In the schematic pseudophakic eye, compared with the schematic phakic eye, this displacement is -0.657 mm, corresponding with a -1.69 D anisometropia.

There are several formulas and convenient nomograms for the selection of a suitable power lens.

PREOPERATIVE SELECTION OF OPTIC POWER OF PSEUDOPHAKOS*
Estimations of intraocular lens power based on the basic refraction of the eye

Most patients who undergo lens implant surgery in the United States receive implants whose power is estimated from the basic refraction of the eye (spherical equivalent). Experience has shown that when the basic refraction is accurate, a reasonable prediction of implant power is possible. However, there are many pitfalls in estimating the basic refraction. A reliable history of the refractive status before the onset of cataract is not always available. If lenticular myopia occurs, it is irrelevant to the basic refraction. If a reliable history is not available, it is impossible to assess the degree of myopia attributable to the crystalline lens. An old pair of spectacles may yield misleading information. The patient may have a high degree of unilateral myopia that is not reflected in the spectacle lenses. Conversely, there may be a high degree of unilateral hypermetropia or astigmatism not corrected because of the high degree of anisometropia or because of amblyopia. Therefore additional history is required. An inquiry should be made about the patient's vision in youth. Were glasses required for distance vision? Were reading glasses required during the usual presbyopic years? It would be useful to know that the patient did not require glasses to see the blackboard during school years or to drive an automobile, or that the first pair of glasses were for close vision at the age of 45 and that later in life he needed glasses for distance but not for reading. This is typical of emmetropia, which gives way to lenticular myopia in later life.

There are other sources of possible error. The power of the lens is unrelated to the refraction. The normal range of powers of the crystalline lens has been established, and the absence of correlation between the power of the crystalline lens and the refraction has been emphasized.[32,33] The main components of the refraction of the eye—power of the cornea, depth of the anterior chamber, power of the lens, and axial length of the eye—show relatively little correlation in emmetropia as well as in ametropia. Sorsby has

reported the following values for these major components in 107 emmetropic eyes:

	Corneal power (D)	Lens power (D)	Anterior chamber depth (mm)	Axial length (mm)
Range	39.0-47.6	15.5-23.9	2.5-4.2	22.3-26.0
Mean	43.1	19.7	3.5	24.2
Standard deviation	1.62	1.62	0.34	0.85

It is evident then that the emmetropic eye is a finely correlated functional apparatus built of widely varying components. Therefore the removal from the eye of a crystalline lens whose power is at either extreme of the range (15.5 to 23.9 D) may alter the refraction by significantly different amounts. Thus an error is possible if it is assumed that a standard power pseudophakos exists that will retain emmetropia in an emmetropic eye after lens implantation. Mean values for corneal power, lens power, and anterior chamber depth may be found in extreme refractive errors. Thus corneal power may be 43.1 D in an eye with +10 D hypermetropia or −10 D myopia. One or more of the other components of the refraction must vary from their mean values to create these extreme refractive errors. The only exception is that the mean value for axial length is rarely seen in extreme refractive errors.

To achieve emmetropia or the preoperative basic refractive error, the power of the pseudophakos should be less than that of the crystalline lens, since the pseudophakos is in a more forward position than the crystalline lens. This means that the equivalent planes of the pseudophakic eye are further forward than those of the phakic eye.

An 18 D intraocular lens tends to restore the basic refraction, that is, the refraction prior to the development of the cataract. It then becomes necessary to estimate the lens power required to achieve a desired postoperative refractive error. It is incorrect to assume a 1:1 relationship; that is, a +19 D pseudophakos placed in an emmetropic eye does not result in 1 D of residual spectacle myopia. Since the residual refractive error is corrected by a spectacle lens worn at a vertex distance of about 12 mm, a change in lens power within the eye has a slightly different effectivity.

A satisfactory rule is to add 1.25 D to 18 D for

---

*This discussion is modified from Jaffe, N. S., et al.: Pseudophakos, St. Louis, 1978, The C. V. Mosby Co.

each diopter of hypermetropia to be corrected and to subtract 1.25 D from 18 D for each diopter of myopia to be corrected. Stated in another way, given the basic refraction, we add to or subtract from 18 the number of diopters of hypermetropia or myopia to be corrected times 1.25. This also tells us that for each diopter of intraocular lens power change only 0.8 D change in the basic refraction results (see p. 129).

This method is not foolproof even if the basic refraction is accurately known (no small task in itself). Recall that Sorsby's survey of emmetropic eyes revealed a mean crystalline lens power of 19.7 D with a standard deviation of 1.62. Thus an error of some magnitude could result from assuming a lens of average power. A thorough analysis of biometric data reveals that for each diopter of basic refraction to be changed, 1.1 to 1.4 D must be added to or subtracted from 18 D. Therefore using the 1.25 rule may lead to additional error. It is also possible that further sophistication in biometric technology will prove the 18 D value for achieving the basic refraction to be erroneous. However, at our current state of knowledge, if the basic refraction is known with a reasonable degree of accuracy, a target error of greater than 2 D will rarely occur.

Basic refraction (D)	Emmetropizing pseudo-phakos power (D)
+5.00	24.25
+4.00	23.00
+3.00	21.75
+2.00	20.50
+1.00	19.25
0.00	18.00
−1.00	16.75
−2.00	15.50
−3.00	14.25
−4.00	13.00
−5.00	11.75

Estimations of intraocular lens power based on sophisticated measurements

It is theoretically possible to reach a highly accurate estimate of intraocular lens power by making sophisticated measurements of the various components of the basic refraction and incorporating the data into one of several formulas. The degree of accuracy of this method is still unsettled. There are no large documented series

published that support, on a clinical level, the dependability of this approach. There are inherent errors in the precision of the testing equipment and some unavoidable changes in this data postoperatively. This will be discussed later. In spite of these drawbacks, this method has great merit. It is impossible for a highly myopic eye (axial myopia) to escape detection. In addition, further application of this technique will lead to greater accuracy.

The feasibility of adapting the power of the intraocular lens to each individual depends on three measurements: (1) refracting power of the cornea, (2) depth of the anterior chamber or, more accurately, distance between the anterior surface of the cornea and the anterior surface of the pseudophakos at the optic axis, and (3) axial length of the eye, or distance from the anterior surface of the cornea to the fovea.

Refracting power of the cornea. The refracting power of the cornea is measured with the keratometer or ophthalmometer. To obtain a spheric equivalent, the two principal meridians are averaged. One popular formula utilizes the dioptric power, and another uses the radius of curvature of the anterior corneal surface. It should be recalled that, in contradistinction to the ophthalmoscope and the retinoscope, the keratometer measures the radius of curvature of a reflecting surface rather than the dioptric power of a refracting surface. If the dioptric power appears on the dial of a particular keratometer, it is only because an arbitrary overall index of refraction of the interface has been adopted. There are some sources of error that can be minimized. The average of at least three readings in each principal meridian is recorded. Some keratometers have a fixation light that can be seen by a patient with a nearly mature cataract. With some it is necessary to improvise to obtain central fixation. Another possible source of error is postoperative change in corneal curvature. Although surgically induced astigmatism can be considerable on occasion, there is usually little change in average corneal curvature with modern techniques of wound incision and closure. One suggested formula[34] allows for a slight postoperative flattening of the cornea by using a refractive index of 4/3 for the cornea. This compensates for a postoperative increase of about 0.08 mm in the radius of corneal curvature. Kera-

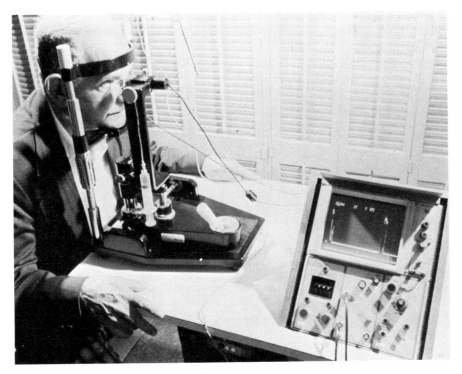

Fig. 5-24. Determination of axial length by A-scan ultrasonography using Digital Biometric Ruler. (From Sonometrics Systems, Inc., 2067 Broadway, New York, N.Y. 10023.)

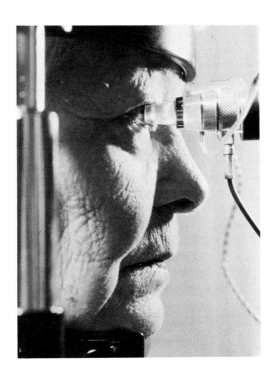

tometric measurement errors are rarely of high magnitude. An error of 0.1 mm in radius curvature results in a refractive error of approximately 0.5 D.

Anterior chamber depth. Estimation of anterior chamber depth is subject to more variability than the other measurements. A constant decrease in anterior chamber depth with age has been consistently reported and has been attributed to increasing lens thickness. This decreased depth is of less importance in the aphakic state, where anterior chamber depth averages about 4 mm. However, this measures the distance between the anterior corneal surface and the anterior iris surface at the pupillary border. The formulas for intraocular lens power utilize the corneal vertex distance of the pseudophakos, which is about 0.5

Fig. 5-25. Coupling device (filled with fluid) makes contact with cornea in much the same manner as an applanation tonometer. (From Sonometrics Systems, Inc., 2067 Broadway, New York, N.Y. 10023.)

mm less. Therefore many currently used methods employ an empiric value of 3.5 mm for anterior chamber depth. This can be a source of considerable error, especially in highly hypermetropic eyes. For this reason, some surgeons routinely subtract 2 to 3 D from calculations between 23 and 26 D for emmetropia and 1 to 2 D from calculations between 21 and 23 D. I use an empiric value of 3.2 mm for iris-supported implants and 3.5 for a posterior chamber implant. An accurate measure of axial anterior chamber depth can be made preoperatively by the Jaeger method, with an attachment to the Haag-Streit or the Zeiss slit lamp.

Axial length. Axial length measurements currently employ ultrasonography. The equipment is expensive. Biometric techniques employ A-scan ultrasonography. Various methods of providing the sound coupling path between the transducer and the eye are available according to the equipment used. This may be a Steri-Drape water bath, a contact lens, or a crystal transducer that resembles the prism of an applanation tonometer (Figs. 5-24 and 5-25). A high degree of accuracy in estimating axial length is mandatory if this is used in calculating intraocular lens power. An error of 1 mm leads to a miscalculation of 2.5 to 3.5 D, which is considerable. If an ultrasound frequency of 20 MHz or more is used, it may be possible to achieve an accuracy of about 0.1 mm. Aside from instrument error, another possible source of error is a change in axial length postoperatively. This is probably not highly significant, but it has not yet been investigated fully.

Formulas for calculating intraocular lens power. There are several formulas available for calculating the power of the intraocular lens. Their differences are based on a few minor variables resulting from voids in our complete understanding of the optic system of an eye containing an intraocular lens.

Colenbrander[35] has studied such a system and has offered a formula for arriving at the power of an iris-clip lens required to give a sharp image on the retina without the use of spectacles, that is, the power of the iris-clip lens required to produce emmetropia. The formulas to be presented use similar symbols to designate the various components of such an optic system. Colenbrander's formula is

$$D = \frac{n}{a - d - 0.00005} - \frac{n}{\dfrac{n}{Dc} - d - 0.00005}$$

D = Refracting power of the iris-clip lens in diopters

n = Refractive index of aqueous and vitreous (1.336)

d = Distance from the anterior surface of the cornea to the anterior surface of the iris-clip lens at the optic axis

a = Axial length of the eye

Dc = Refracting power of the cornea in diopters

The reader is referred to Colenbrander's article for the derivation of his formula.

Fyodorov and co-workers[36] have offered the following formula:

$$D = \frac{n - a\,Dc}{(a - d)\,1 - \dfrac{d\,Dc}{n}}$$

Richard Binkhorst[34] has suggested the following formula:

$$D = \frac{1336(4r - a)}{(a - d)(4r - d)}$$

r = Radius of curvature of the anterior surface of the cornea in millimeters

Binkhorst has made available an Intraocular Lens Power Calculation Kit that describes a variety of calculations that can be made on a relatively inexpensive programmable calculator. Once the basic measurements of corneal curvature, axial length, and anterior chamber depth have been made, several complex calculations can be performed in a matter of seconds.

Goals of preoperative estimation of lens power

Although it is often desirable, emmetropia may not be the ideal postoperative refraction in all patients who undergo intraocular lens implant surgery. To appreciate this the implant surgeon should have a basic understanding of the altered optics in an eye with an intraocular lens. This involves the principles of telescopic magnification. The intraocular implant lens occupies a more anterior position than the crystalline lens. Thus if the intraocular lens does not have enough refracting power to restore emmetropia, there will be a resulting hypermetropic pseudophakic refraction. This deficit in the refracting power of the intraocular lens plus the required hypermetropic spectacle correction form a Galilean telescope. Each diopter of spectacle correction represents an image size magnification of 2%. Conversely, if the intraocular lens has an excess of refracting power and thus renders a previously emmetropic eye myopic, an inverted Galilean telescope is introduced. Each diopter of myopia required causes an image size minification of 2%. Another factor must be considered. The iris-clip and Medallion lenses cause an image size magnification of 3.25%, the iridocapsular lens slightly less, and the iris-plane lens possibly the least. Thus it can be easily seen that if residual hypermetropia is significant, the image size can exceed that caused by contact lens correction of aphakia.

It has been stated[34] that when a 0.5 mm thick convexoplano lens, its anterior vertex 3.5 mm from the anterior vertex of the cornea, is substituted for the lens of the schematic eye, the magnification of the retinal image would be 3.25% if the eye is made emmetropic. To restore the original image size, the eye would have to be made 1.7 D myopic with the correction placed at the anterior focus. Similarly the axially ametropic schematic eye would have to be made 1.7 D more myopic, or less hypermetropic, to restore the original image size, again with the spectacle corrections at the anterior focal points.

C. D. Binkhorst[37] has described a method for determining the iseikonic pseudophakos for the schematic eye. Iseikonia between the schematic pseudophakic eye and the schematic phakic eye exists when the focal lengths of both eyes are identical. The following relationship is used for the focal length:

$$f_E = \frac{fc\, f_L}{f_L + fc^1 - d}$$

f_E = Anterior focal length of complete eye (-17.055 mm)
fc = Anterior focal length of cornea (-23.227 mm)
fc^1 = Posterior focal length of cornea (31.031 mm)
d = Distance of first equivalent plane of pseudophakos from second equivalent plane of cornea (3.5506 mm)
f_L = Focal length of pseudophakos

The value for d is calculated by assuming a corneal vertex distance (v) of 3.5 mm. The second equivalent plane of the cornea equals -0.0506 mm. Therefore the distance (d) of the first equivalent plane of the pseudophakos from the second equivalent plane of the cornea equals 3.5506 mm.

The focal length of the schematic iseikonic pseudophakos (f_L) turns out to be 75.921 mm, which gives a radius of the anterior surface (r_1) of 8.751 mm and an equivalent power of the pseudophakos (FL) of 17.6 D. In arriving at these figures, note that

$$r_1 = \left(\frac{1.49 - 1.336}{1.336}\right)$$

and

$$FL = \left(\frac{1.449 - 1.336}{r_1}\right)$$

Therefore a pseudophakos with power of 17.6 D at a corneal vertex distance of 3.5 mm is iseikonic with Gullstrand's schematic crystalline lens of 19.11 D.[38]

Since the pseudophakos is in a more forward position than the crystalline lens, the equivalent planes of the pseudophakic eye are further forward than those of the phakic eye. If the focal lengths are the same, this results in a more forward position of the posterior focal point and plus ametropia.

For the schematic pseudophakic eye one can calculate the anterior displacement of the second equivalent plane and the correlated myopia as follows: the distance of the second equivalent plane of the pseudophakos from its posterior surface is

$$(-n_1)\left(\frac{t}{n_2}\right)\left(\frac{FL^1}{FL}\right) = 0.448 \text{ mm}$$

in which t is the center thickness of the pseudophakos (0.5 mm), n_1 is the refractive index of the aqueous (1.336), n_2 is the refractive index of the pseudophakos (1.490), and FL^1 equals FL. The corneal vertex distance of the second equivalent plane of the pseudophakic eye is therefore $3.552 - 2.607 = 0.945$ mm.

Compared with the corneal vertex distance of the second equivalent plane of 1.602 mm in Gullstrand's schematic phakic eye, the second equivalent plane of the schematic iseikonic eye is in a 0.657 mm more forward position. Calculation with Newton's object image relation ($x \times$

$x^1 = f \times f^1$) shows that this corresponds with a 1.69 D myopia at the anterior focal point.

These estimations are for the schematic eye that represents the mean values of the components of refraction. However, as discussed previously, the components of the refracting system of the eye have been shown to have a normal distribution with considerable variation. For example, one eye may be emmetropic with a relatively long axial length but a flatter than average cornea. Another may have a shorter than average axial length, an average corneal curvature, but a crystalline lens of high refracting power. The possibilities are considerable in emmetropia as well as in ametropia. It should then be apparent that the 3.25% magnification of the retinal image is an average figure for the emmetropic eye. Taking the total variation of the components of emmetropic eyes into account, this range would be from 2.6% to 3.9%. Likewise there would be a range of myopia, from 1.15 to 2.35 D, with the correction at the anterior focus required to restore the original image size in previously emmetropic eyes.[34] The same range of magnification would apply for ametropia if the intraocular lens were meant to restore the original ametropia, and the range within which these eyes would have to be made more myopic or less hypermetropic would be the same. These figures must be varied slightly according to whether an iris-clip, iridocapsular, or iris-plane lens is used.

Ideally there should be neither anisometropia nor anieseikonia. However, from this discussion it is apparent that, with currently used intraocular lenses, *there can be no isometropia without aniseikonia and no iseikonia without anisometropia.*

The method just described to achieve iseikonia by changing the refraction of the pseudophakic eye a certain amount to the myopic side is subject to some errors, since it does not take into account the variation of the components of the refracting system of the eye. C. D. Binkhorst[37] has shown that his method of using a standard 19.5 D pseudophakos is subject to these errors and has suggested a method of producing iseikonia based on data obtained from both eyes. This will especially be more accurate in cases of anisometropia, whether absolute or relative. Absolute anisometropia, which refers to unequal refraction of the two eyes, is particularly common in the higher degrees of refractive errors. Relative anisometropia, which refers to equal refraction of the two eyes but with differences in their components, would remain unrecognized unless the components of both eyes are determined.

R. D. Binkhorst[34] has described a method that takes the variation of the components of the two eyes into account in the calculation of the intraocular lens power required to produce iseikonia in unilateral pseudophakia. As stated earlier by C. D. Binkhorst,[37] the aim is to equalize the focal lengths of the two eyes. The calculation is carried out in three steps:

1. In the first step the focal length of the crystalline lens in the fellow eye is determined with the following formula:

$$F = \frac{(a - ACD - 2.21)\left(\dfrac{1336}{Dc + Rc} - ACD - 2.08\right)}{\dfrac{1336}{Dc + Rc} - a + 2.21 - 2.08}$$

F = Focal length of the crystalline lens in millimeters
a = Axial length in millimeters
ACD = Anterior chamber depth in millimeters
Dc = Dioptric power of the cornea
Rc = Refraction at the cornea in diopters
2.08 and 2.21 = Respective schematic values for the distances of the anterior and posterior principal planes for the crystalline lens from its anterior vertex in millimeters

Given the thickness and the refractive indexes of a lens and the surrounding medium, the location of the principal planes depends almost entirely on the ratio of the radii of curvature. The power of the lens has a negligible influence. The value for Rc, the refraction at the cornea, can be found in a table of contact lens powers corresponding to the spectacle refraction at various vertex distances, or it can be calculated as follows:

$$Rc = \frac{Rs}{1 - vRs}$$

Rs = Spectacle refraction in diopters
v = Vertex distance in meters

2. With the value for the focal length of the crystalline lens *(F)*, the anterior focal length of the fellow eye can now be calculated:

$$F_1 = \frac{1000\,F}{Dc(F - [ACD + 2.08]) + 1336}$$

F_1 = Anterior focal length of fellow eye in millimeters

3. The pseudophakic eye must be given the same focal length. This is accomplished by calculating the intraocular lens power as follows:

$$D = \frac{1336\left(\dfrac{3r}{F_1} - 1\right)}{4r - d}$$

D = Dioptric power in aqueous of the intraocular lens

F_1 = Anterior focal length in millimeters

r = Radius of curvature of the anterior surface of the cornea in millimeters

d = Distance between the anterior vertex of the cornea and the intraocular lens in millimeters

The refractive index used for the cornea is 1.3375 for the fellow eye and 4/3 for the eye to be made pseudophakic.

In this calculation the axial length of the eye to be made pseudophakic is not taken into account. The two eyes having the same focal length would have the same image size if the corrections were placed at their respective anterior focal points. Since usually the spectacle correction is closer to the eye than the anterior focus and since usually the refraction of the pseudophakic eye will be less hypermetropic or more myopic than the fellow eye, there is still a problem with the image size. The image will usually be slightly larger in the pseudophakic eye than in the fellow eye. To calculate the intraocular lens power, which would compensate for these factors in a given situation, is a very complicated procedure. In general the intraocular lens would have to be 0.25 to 0.5 D stronger. This correction can be added to the calculated intraocular lens power; for intraocular lens implants available in 0.5 D steps, the next step up should be used.

As with the calculations described on p. 132, R. D. Binkhorst has programmed these calculations for the Texas Instruments TI-59 and Hewlett-Packard HP-65 calculators.

Comprehension of these formulas and their derivation may not appeal to most ophthalmologists. Most intraocular lens implant surgeons still use standard power lenses, some select lens powers based on the basic refraction, and only a few resort to sophisticated measurements and utilize the formulas discussed. With the increasing accuracy and simplicity of A-scan ultrasound equipment and with the availability of relatively inexpensive calculators, it is likely that this trend will change.

The implant surgeon must decide when to make a pseudophakic eye emmetropic and when to make it ametropic. It is difficult to set rigid rules for this decision, since implant surgeons use varying guidelines for indications and contraindications for implant surgery.

When should emmetropia be the goal?

1. When bilateral pseudophakia is planned. There is no useful purpose in aiming for myopia if the opposite eye has a visually disturbing cataract. The surgeon may elect to implant a lens in the second eye later. Therefore emmetropia in both eyes would be a more satisfactory goal. If the first eye is made myopic, the second eye should be made the same to avoid aniseikonia. Frequently the cataract in the second eye is sufficiently advanced and binocular vision is so rudimentary that the goal of iseikonia is unrealistic. Another factor to be considered is the possibility of increasing lenticular myopia in the second eye. It is probably wise not to correct this changing refractive error.

2. When there is hypermetropia of 1.5 to 2.5 D in a useful fellow eye. This is a frequent situation, since a small to moderate degree of hypermetropia is near the peak of the curve of refractive errors. It is possible that the fellow eye may not have a cataract, or if it does, that it may not change for many years.

3. When there is known or suspected absence of binocular vision. The indication for emmetropia is particularly valid in high ametropia.

4. When surgery on only one eye is planned. Many elderly patients who have undergone a successful lens implantation find that this is entirely adequate for their needs. Since they have none of the visual handicaps of unilateral aphakia, surgery on the second eye is often unnecessary.

5. When senile macular choroidal degenera-

tion is present in both eyes. There is less demand for iseikonia in these patients.

6. When a contact lens is used in the fellow eye in patients with higher amounts of hypermetropia or myopia. However, it may be argued that if a patient can successfully manage a contact lens in a phakic eye, why bother with an implant in the cataractous eye? A routine cataract extraction with contact lens correction is probably a better choice.

7. When a contact lens is used in an aphakic fellow eye. To achieve iseikonia with an implant in the second eye would necessitate making the pseudophakic eye several diopters hyperopic, a high price to pay. Bilateral contact lens correction would of course achieve iseikonia. If, however, an implant is preferred and that eye is made emmetropic, the aniseikonia is less than in unilateral aphakia corrected with a contact lens and a normal fellow eye. The implant provides some magnification and lessens some of the image size disparity between the two eyes.

When should ametropia be the goal? The only indication to make the pseudophakic eye ametropic exists in unilateral pseudophakia. The rationale for this is the avoidance of aniseikonia, which has been discussed earler. The only important exceptions are when there is hypermetropia of 1.5 to 2.5 D in the fellow eye and when surgery on only one eye is planned in patients with bilateral cataracts or absence of binocular vision.

It was stated on p. 133 that the schematic eye requires 1.7 D myopia to restore the original image size if the spectacle correction is worn at the anterior focal point (about 17 mm). Thus an acceptable method would be to change the refraction of the pseudophakic eye 2.25 D for the iris-clip lens, 2.1 D for the iridocapsular lens, and 2 D for the Copeland iris-plane lens. The discrepancy is because of the vertex distance of the spectacle correction (about 12 mm), which is always within the anterior focal point.

TECHNIQUE

A full description of the techniques of implantation of all currently available intraocular lenses could easily fill a complete volume. Therefore general features common to all will be emphasized.

Intracapsular methods

Surgeons should perform their standard procedures for intracapsular cataract extraction, except that a greater emphasis should be placed on the reduction of vitreous and orbital volume. Although a flat or slightly convex anterior vitreous face is satisfactory for routine lens extraction, it is less than optimum for lens implantation. It is comforting to find a deep concavity in the anterior surface of the vitreous immediately after delivery of the lens. I have been able to achieve this in a high percentage of cases by applying digital pressure for a longer period than I customarily use for an intracapsular lens extraction without lens implantation. Most surgeons have little experience with 7 to 10 minutes of digital pressure. The globe appears well sunken into the orbit, on palpation the cornea feels mushy soft, and the Schiøtz tonometric reading is between 15 scale units and off the scale. In my experience, it is easier to achieve profound hypotonia in elderly patients, in whom vitreous degeneration is common and in whom scleral rigidity permits the vitreous to fall back after lens extraction. In recent years I have tended to rely more on digital pressure than on hyperosmotic agents. The latter must be used with caution because of their cardiovascular side effects in elderly patients. I consider the rapidity of the fall in intraocular pressure with digital pressure a fairly reliable indicator of vitreous decompression.

If all goes according to plan, the anterior hyaloid membrane will be markedly concave immediately after lens extraction. Balanced salt solution is irrigated into the anterior chamber to float the iris up from the vitreous. If the pupil is excessively dilated, acetylcholine solution is placed in the anterior chamber. It is also helpful to keep the anterior chamber free of blood during the procedure, since clotted blood on the surface of the iris and in the angle of the anterior chamber may prevent the pupil from constricting around the implant.

If after the delivery of the lens the vitreous face does not fall back but instead shows an anterior convexity, I proceed as follows. The 12 o'clock 7-0 silk suture is secured with a slip knot. The anterior chamber is repressurized with air. This pushes the vitreous posteriorly. An intravenous injection of 50 ml of 25% mannitol may be rapidly

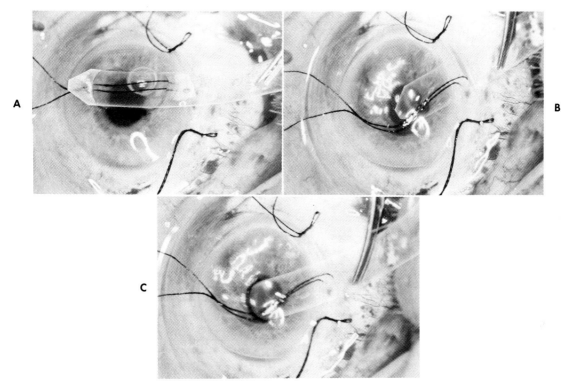

Fig. 5-26. Use of Sheets glide to permit insertion of pseudophakos under air. **A,** Appearance of glide prior to insertion. **B,** Glide being advanced into anterior chamber. **C,** Glide in situ with tip under pupillary margin. (From Jaffe, N. S., et al.: Pseudophakos, St. Louis, 1978, The C. V. Mosby Co.)

given. This is optional. Two additional corneoscleral 7-0 silk sutures are placed at 10 and 2 o'clock, approximately 7 to 9 mm from each other. They are tied with triple knots. The 12 o'clock slip knot is opened and the suture is looped out of the incision. The anterior chamber must remain filled with air. A lens glide (Fig. 5-26) as recommended by Sheets is then made available. The glide most commonly is made of Silastic and may be fashioned from the plastic tear-off strip (0.3 mm thick) of the sterile eye drape. The usual lens glide dimensions are 2 cm in length and 4.5 mm in width. A lens glide punch is manufactured by the Storz Instrument Company (St. Louis, Catalogue No. E 2973 S). Several dozen strips can be punched out at one time from the plastic tear-off strip. They may be individually packaged in sterile containers and made available when needed. (In this way the jaws of the punch will not be dulled by excessive autoclaving.) Sheets

prefers to pass the glide into the eye under the air bubble, over the iris and pupil, and over the inferior iris leaf. I prefer to pass the glide under the inferior iris leaf. If the pupil has remained quite large, acetylcholine solution is injected into the anterior chamber. The Binkhorst 4-loop iris-clip lens is held in the right hand, and the anterior lip of the wound is retracted slightly to allow passage of the lens into the anterior chamber. With moderate pressure against the lens glide and against the posterior lip of the wound, the lens is slid down the glide into the anterior chamber, displacing the iris and the vitreous face posteriorly. This results in a relative negative pressure within the anterior chamber, and hence further air will pass into the anterior chamber as the lens reaches its position. If the lens glide has been passed over the inferior iris leaf, it is slowly withdrawn as the inferior loop of the lens reaches the inferior margin of the iris, thus allowing the posterior loop to fall behind the iris below. If the glide has been passed under the iris leaf, the posterior loop of the lens is passed behind the inferior iris but over the lens glide. The glide is slowly withdrawn. With either method, the superior margin of the iris is retracted slightly as the glide is withdrawn toward 12 o'clock, thus allowing the superior posterior loop to pass behind the iris. The intraocular lens cannot be held with the larger forceps described later because of the relatively small open portion of the incision. It may be held with tying, Shepard, or Hirschman forceps.

The Worst 2-loop Medallion suture lens is introduced in the same way. However, instead of inserting the lens in the usual manner with the loops in the horizontal position, it is introduced with the loops in the vertical position so that it will slide down the glide easily. It can also be inserted through a smaller incision. After the lens is in position, the pupil is constricted, and the loops are well behind the iris, the lens is rotated to the normal position by a combination of maneuvering with a Hirschman notched spatula and gentle traction on the iris suture. It is important to avoid tangling the suture during insertion of the lens.

The lens glide is also useful for a Choyce anterior chamber angle-supported lens. The wound is closed to 6 to 7 mm, and an air bubble is injected into the anterior chamber. The pupil is constricted with acetylcholine solution. The lens glide is passed over the iris, the pupil, and the inferior iris leaf, thus blocking the pupil and allowing insertion of the lens. In addition to keeping back the vitreous, the glide can prevent incarceration of the iris in the angle by the haptic of the lens. The glide is not withdrawn until the lens reaches the inferior angle.

The lens glide cannot be used as easily with the Copeland iris-plane lens or the Binkhorst-Fyodorov (type 1) lens. However, if one haptic is placed in the anterior chamber first, the other three can be nudged in one at a time by patiently rotating the lens counterclockwise.

If air tends to escape during these maneuvers, it is useful to have an assistant refill the anterior chamber with a fine air cannula through the side extremity of the incision.

The lens-glide method is a highly practical

way to avoid damage to the corneal endothelium and the face of the vitreous in eyes with a vitreous bulge following removal of the cataract. It should be learned by all implant surgeons.

A less satisfactory, but alternate, method is an aspiration of retrovitreal fluid through the peripheral iridectomy (Fig. 5-27). A 22-gauge needle attached to a 2 ml syringe is used. If this procedure is successful, the vitreous face will fall well posteriorly. Vitreous strands in the iridectomy opening are excised. The implant is then inserted.

Another alternate method being investigated at this time is the use of Healon (Pharmacaea, Inc.), a 1% solution of sodium hyaluronate. This viscous material is injected into the anterior chamber. It pushes back the vitreous and allows insertion of the lens with less danger of damage to the cornea of the vitreous. When in doubt, the surgeon should not hesitate to close the incision permanently and omit the intraocular implant lens. This possibility should have been discussed with the patient prior to surgery, and it should have been agreed between patient and surgeon that the decision would be left to the surgeon during the surgery.

The technique of iridectomy usually varies with the type of implant being inserted. For a Binkhorst 4-loop iris-clip pseudophakos with a transiridectomy suture and a Worst Medallion lens with a platinum "safety pin" device, a fairly large peripheral iridectomy at 12 o'clock is performed. For all other implants, smaller peripheral iridectomies or iridotomies are placed at 10 and 2 o'clock, since a central peripheral iridotomy plays no role in the fixation of these lenses.

The management of the iris is important in other situations. If the pupil is extremely miotic due to long-term miotic therapy, cataract extraction should not be attempted through this small opening because multiple sphincter tears are likely. Such tears make it difficult to achieve adequate constriction of the iris around the optic portion of the implant. A peripheral iridectomy is performed at 12 o'clock. The iris is then incised from the apex of the iridectomy through the sphincter.

A 10-0 polypropylene suture swaged onto a special needle without cutting edges (Ethicon

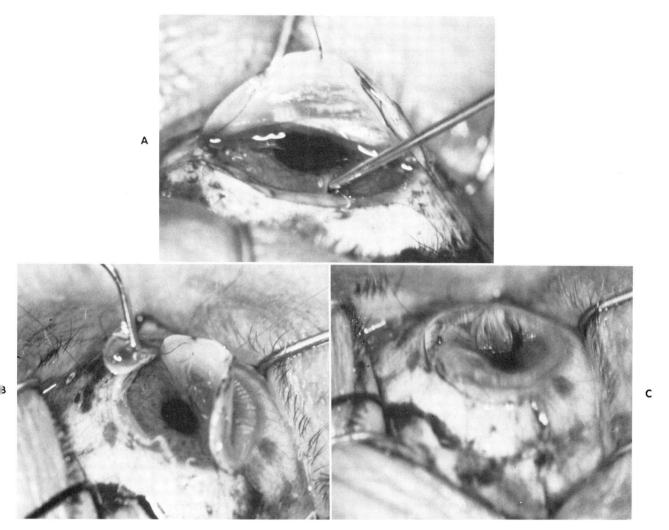

Fig. 5-27. Retrovitreal aspiration of fluid via peripheral iridectomy. **A,** Needle inserted into retrovitreal space through peripheral iridectomy. **B,** Posterior displacement of iris as fluid is aspirated. **C,** Collapsed globe resulting from aspiration of retrovitreal fluid.

2794G) is placed through the margins of the incised iris close to the sphincter. The needle of this suture is particularly useful because it does not tear the delicate iris tissue. The suture is looped out of the eye. The lens is extracted, and the margins of the incised iris are brought together by the nylon suture. The implant is then inserted (Fig. 5-28).

Management of the iris is also important if an iris coloboma is present because of a previous sector iridectomy, previous ocular trauma, or a congenital defect. The coloboma is closed in the same manner, and the remainder of the procedure is as just described.

If vitreous loss occurs during cataract extraction, the surgeon must decide whether or not to implant the pseudophakos. Following a partial anterior vitrectomy, the wound may be sutured and the plan for pseudophakia abandoned. However, if the vitrectomy proceeds well, and there is no obvious intravitreal hemorrhage, the implant may be inserted. However, the surgeon must expect a greater likelihood of postoperative complications. These may occur even if the implant is not inserted, but the patient is more likely to place the blame on the implant. Vitreous loss increases the possibility of retinal detachment, cystoid macular edema, macular pucker, persistent iritis, and so on. Whether the presence of the implant increases the possibility of these sequelae or makes them more severe is not known.

The scope of this book makes it impossible to describe the technique of implantation of all available pseudophakos. Therefore, I will discuss some types that I hope will provide a general understanding of other methods.

1. Copeland iris-plane implant with an intracapsular cataract extraction (Fig. 5-29). Techni-

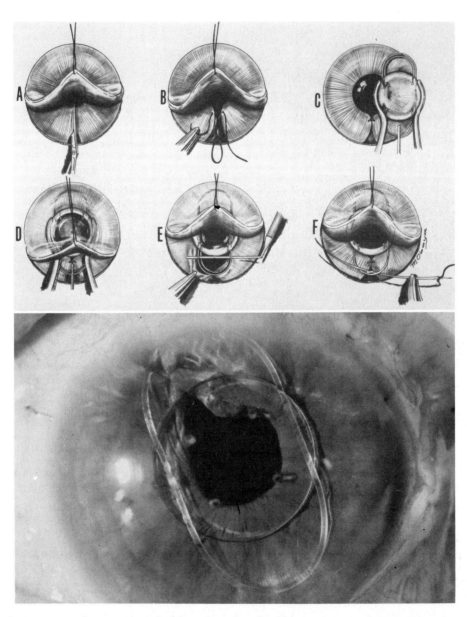

Fig. 5-28. A, Iridotomy extended from peripheral iridectomy to pupil. **B,** Preplaced nylon suture. **C,** Binkhorst 4-loop iris-clip implant held in forceps. **D,** Implant clipped onto iris at 6 o'clock. **E,** Iris placed between loops at 12 o'clock. Optic portion of implant is stabilized with fine spatula. **F,** Transiridectomy suture is placed. *Below,* Postoperative appearance of patient.

cally this is the easiest implant to insert. One of the four solid, flat haptic supports is grasped with a needle holder without a lock or Shepard or Clayman forceps. If it is held in the 12 o'clock position, one of the supports is slid under the iris either temporally or nasally. The opposite support is then slid under the iris in the other horizontal meridian. To facilitate these maneuvers, the iris may be gently lifted with fine forceps. As an alternative, a horizontal support may be grasped by the needle holder, and the two hap-

tics 90 degrees away are placed behind the iris in the vertical position. The inferior haptic is placed first and then the superior haptic. The implant may also be placed in an oblique position (Figs. 5-30 and 5-31). The requirement is that two haptics rest posterior to the iris in one meridian and the other two haptics lie anterior to the iris in the opposite meridian. Since all four haptics lie in the exact plane of the optic portion of the lens, the posterior supports tend to push the iris forward in that meridian while the anteriorly placed

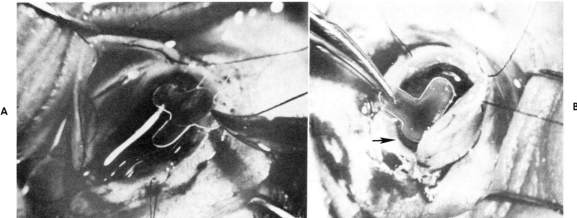

Fig. 5-29. A, Iris-plane lens held by needle holder without lock. **B,** Haptic portion placed behind nasal portion of iris *(arrow)* prior to insertion of temporal haptic portion behind temporal part of iris. Opposite feet of implant rest anterior to superior and inferior portions of iris.

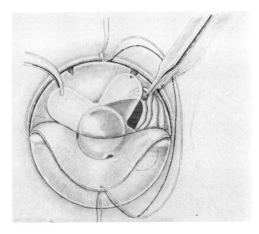

Fig. 5-30. Insertion of Copeland lens implant. Inferior arm is placed under iris at 7 o'clock. Iris is grasped at 1 o'clock and pulled over superior arm. (From Jaffe, N. S., et al.: Pseudophakos, St. Louis, 1978, The C. V. Mosby Co.)

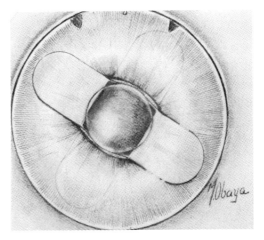

Fig. 5-31. Implant in situ in oblique axis (7-0 suture tied). (From Jaffe, N. S., et al.: Pseudophakos, St. Louis, 1978, The C. V. Mosby Co.)

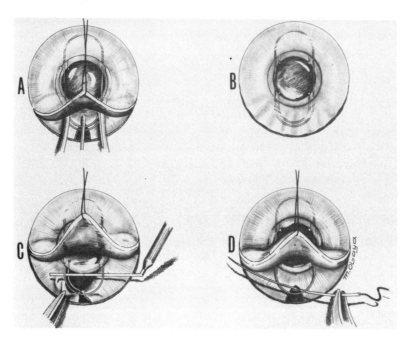

Fig. 5-32. Technique of implantation of Binkhorst 4-loop iris-clip implant (Jaffe modification). **A,** Implant held in Binkhorst implantation forceps (note end of irrigating cannula). Implant clipped to iris at 6 o'clock. **B,** Forceps removed, leaving implant in correct position at 6 o'clock but with both loops anterior to iris at 12 o'clock. **C,** Iris placed between anterior and posterior loops with Hoskins No. 19 forceps. Fine spatula placed between anterior and posterior loops stabilizes implant during this maneuver. **D,** Transiridectomy suture passed around posterior and anterior loops through peripheral iridectomy.

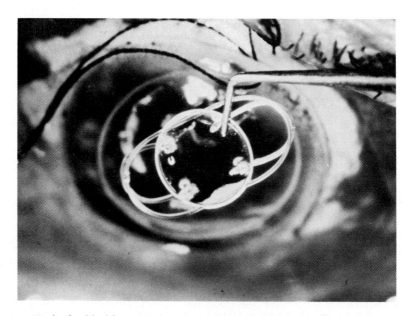

Fig. 5-33. Method of holding implant with Clayman forceps. (From Clayman, H. M.: Ophthalmology [Rochester] **83:**147-148, 1977.)

haptics tend to indent the iris. The pupil has the appearance of a square.

2. Binkhorst 4-loop iris-clip implant with an intracapsular cataract extraction. The iris-clip lens is grasped with a special cross-action forceps. The latter comes with an attached cannula through which the anterior chamber can be irrigated during implantation. This protects against corneal damage and rupture of the anterior face of the vitreous. There are various techniques for inserting this implant. The forceps hold the optic portion of the lens with the four loops in the vertical position (Fig. 5-32). The two inferior loops are clipped onto the iris at 6 o'clock. The forceps is disengaged and removed from the eye. A fine spatula is inserted between the two upper loops, and the optic portion of the implant is gently pushed toward 6 o'clock. The iris is grasped at 12 o'clock by a fine, blunt iris hook. It is threaded between the two upper loops. I find it easier to grasp the iris in its middle portion at 12 o'clock with smooth forceps (Hoskins No. 19) and thread it between the loops. It is better if the entire procedure is accomplished in a single maneuver by using Clayman (Fig. 5-33), Shepard, or Hirschman forceps. These are manufactured with, and

without, an attached irrigating cannula. The inferior loops are clipped to the iris below, and by displacing the implant further toward 6 o'clock, the superior loops are engaged. With this method the cornea does not have to be retracted (Figs. 5-34 and 5-35). These maneuvers are best accomplished with a small pupil. If the iris does not completely lie in contact with the optic portion of the implant, acetylcholine solution is irrigated into the anterior chamber. The superior loops are lined up so that they overlay and underlay the peripheral iridectomy at 12 o'clock. The superior anterior loop is grasped with the fine forceps and elevated so that the corresponding posterior loop appears in the iridectomy opening. A monofilament 10-0 polypropylene suture swaged onto a special 10 mm blunt tapered needle is passed through the two loops from a posterior to anterior direction so that the loops may be loosely tied together. This transiridectomy suture minimizes the possibility of dislocation. Since it is not sutured to the iris, pupillary dilatation is possible without the lens being displaced to 12 o'clock (Fig. 5-36). The 12 o'clock suture is tied, and air is placed in the anterior chamber so that the incision may be sutured without the optic portion of

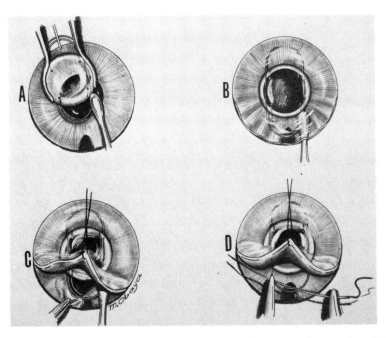

Fig. 5-34. Technique of implantation of Binkhorst 4-loop iris-clip implant (Clayman modification). **A,** Implant transferred from Binkhorst to Shepard forceps. Shepard forceps grasp anterior loop close to its attachment to optic portion if implant. **B,** Implant clipped to iris at 6 o'clock. **C,** Iris placed between anterior and posterior loops at 12 o'clock while implant is still in Shepard forceps. **D,** Transiridectomy suture placed.

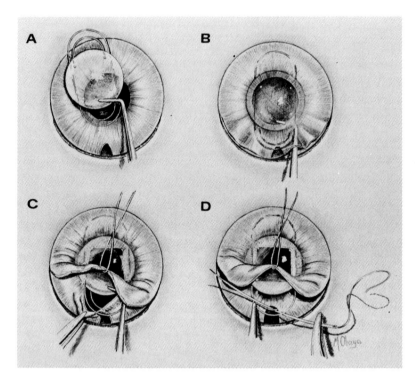

Fig. 5-35. Clayman technique of Binkhorst 4-loop iris-clip implant insertion. **A,** Implant grasped at optic where right arm of superior loop originates. **B,** Implant inserted into anterior chamber with inferior loops straddling iris. **C,** Implant is *still* held while iris is placed between superior loops with forceps. **D,** Transiridectomy suture is passed. (From Jaffe, N. S., et al.: Pseudophakos, St. Louis, 1978, The C. V. Mosby Co.)

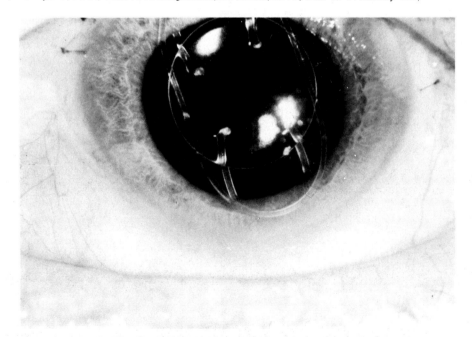

Fig. 5-36. Dilatation of pupil of eye in Fig. 5-13, A.

the lens touching the cornea. A portion of the air bubble is replaced with balanced salt solution after completion of the suturing.

There are many other methods of employing a suture for fixation of the implant to the iris. The simplest technique, and the one I prefer, is to take a small bite in the iris at 12 o'clock midway between the sphincter and the base with the special 10-0 polypropylene suture described on p. 138. Both ends of the suture are laid aside outside the eye. The cataract is extracted. The needle of the suture is then threaded through the superior anterior loop of the implant from bottom up. The slack is taken up and the implant is inserted. The suture is then tied under air. This attaches the superior anterior loop to the anterior surface of the superior iris leaf. To keep air in the anterior chamber while tying the suture, a preplaced 7-0 silk suture is placed at 2 o'clock after the incision is made. This is in addition to the 12 o'clock suture. When the implant is in position, the 2 o'clock suture is tied with a slip knot. Air is then placed in the anterior chamber, and the implant suture is tied. The ends are cut with the aid of slight corneal retraction by the 12 o'clock suture. The air tends to remain in the anterior chamber, thus preventing the optic portion of the implant from making contact with the cornea during these maneuvers.

3. Worst Medallion lens with an intracapsular cataract extraction (Figs. 5-37 to 5-41). Before the lens extraction, a 9-0 or 10-0 monofilament polypropylene suture is passed through the iris just peripheral to its sphincter at 12 o'clock. A special ski-shaped needle (Ethicon) is useful. The width of the bite corresponds to the two holes in the extension of the optic portion of the implant. The suture ends are left long. The cataract is extracted. The ends of the iris suture are passed through the corresponding holes in the Medallion lens so that the knot will be behind the lens. This prevents contact of the free suture ends with the corneal endothelium. The lens is held by a Clayman, Hirschman, or Shepard forceps. One loop is passed behind the iris to the surgeon's right; the other is then passed behind the iris in the opposite horizontal meridian. The pupil is constricted with acetylcholine solution. The iris suture is tied under air behind the haptic portion, and the suture ends are cut short. Because of oc-

casional chafing and disintegration of the suture, a modified design of implant in which the two loops lie in the vertical position has been in use. A small platinum or polypropylene rod extends from the haptic at 12 o'clock. After the implant is inserted, the rod is bent so that it enters the peripheral iridectomy and curves posteriorly under the superior loop of the implant. This is known as the safety pin principle. A suture is not used with this technique. When the pupil is dilated with both of these variations of the Medallion lens, the

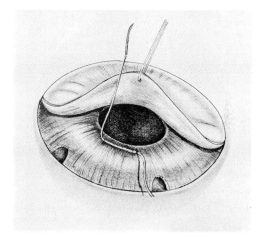

Fig. 5-37. Placement of iris suture in Worst Medallion implant technique. (From Jaffe, N. S., et al.: Pseudophakos, St. Louis, 1978, The C. V. Mosby Co.)

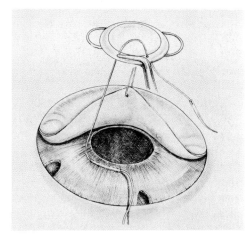

Fig. 5-38. Iris suture threaded through holes in Worst Medallion implant. (From Jaffe, N. S., et al.: Pseudophakos, St. Louis, 1978, The C. V. Mosby Co.)

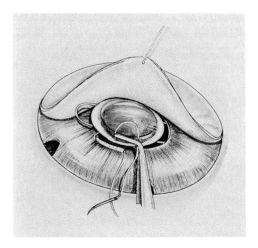

Fig. 5-39. Worst Medallion lens implant inserted with right loop under iris. (From Jaffe, N. S., et al.: Pseudophakos, St. Louis, 1978, The C. V. Mosby Co.)

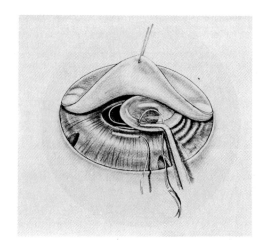

Fig. 5-40. Pupil is displaced slightly to right so left loop can clear pupillary margin. (From Jaffe, N. S., et al.: Pseudophakos, St. Louis, 1978, The C. V. Mosby Co.)

lens rides up toward 12 o'clock because of its fixation to the iris.

Extracapsular methods

The surgeon should perform an extracapsular cataract extraction by the technique described on p. 73 or by phacoemulsification described on p. 191. Many surgeons add their own variation of these methods. In a planned extracapsular extraction, the incision is closed to 7 to 9 mm before the implant is inserted. In phacoemulsification, the incision is enlarged to 7 to 9 mm. If there is positive vitreous pressure, the lens glide should be used. It is passed under the inferior iris and the inferior capsular flap.

1. Binkhorst 2-loop iridocapsular implant with an extracapsular cataract extraction. The optic portion of the implant is grasped in the same manner as the 4-loop iris-clip implant. The vertical loops are passed behind the iris. The loops rest in the capsular bag. Binkhorst recommends that a sufficient amount of lenticular debris should remain behind the iris to ensure adhesion of the loops to the capsule. The pupil is constricted with acetylcholine solution. It is important not to perform too large an anterior capsulectomy, to avoid removal of the posterior capsule. To test for capsular fixation, the pupil is carefully dilated on the fourth postoperative day with 0.5% mydriacyl (Fig. 5-42). If the implant is fixated, it will

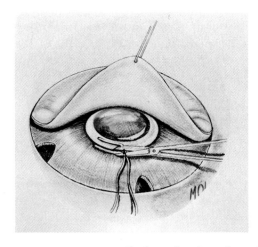

Fig. 5-41. Iris suture cut flush with edge of implant. (From Jaffe, N. S., et al.: Pseudophakos, St. Louis, 1978, The C. V. Mosby Co.)

remain centric in the pupillary aperture. If not, it will displace inferiorly. If this occurs, the pupil is constricted, and 2% pilocarpine solution is placed in the eye three times daily for 1 week. Dilatation is again attempted. With this method the implant is intended to be independent of the iris. Therefore it represents capsular, rather than iridocapsular, fixation.

Most surgeons who use microscopes leave little or no residual cortex in the capsular bag. Ante-

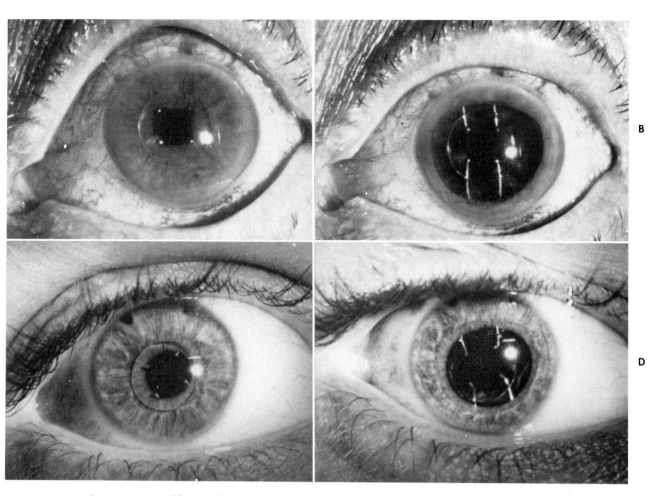

B

D

Fig. 5-42. A, Binkhorst 2-loop iridocapsular implant in situ 4 days postoperatively. **B,** Same eye as **A,** after dilatation of pupil. Note centric fixation. **C,** Binkhorst 2-loop iridocapsular implant in situ 4 weeks postoperatively. **D,** Same eye as **C,** after dilatation of pupil. Note centric fixation.

rior capsular flaps are created, which are used to fold over the inferior and superior loops of the implant. This lessens the possibility of dislocation. Some surgeons also suture the superior capsular flap and the iris to the superior loop.

2. Shearing posterior chamber implant with an extracapsular cataract extraction (Figs. 5-43 and 5-44). After the cataract extraction has been completed, two previously placed 7-0 silk sutures are tied, leaving a 7 mm corneal opening. The anterior chamber is filled with air. The polypropylene loop that emerges from the optic on the surgeon's left is grasped with Kelman-McPherson forceps 2 mm from the optic. The inferior loop

and the optic are passed into the anterior chamber under the air bubble. The inferior loop passes under the inferior iris leaf. When the upper edge of the optic reaches the corneoscleral incision, the forceps then grasps the loop near its end. The loop is bent inferiorly into the anterior chamber until the convexity of the upper loop can be passed under the superior iris leaf. The forceps is then released. To avoid excessive bending of the superior loop and also to avoid an inferior zonular dialysis, the superior iris may be retracted as the superior loop is passed beneath it. The loops should pass under the iris and over the anterior capsular flaps and reach the vicinity

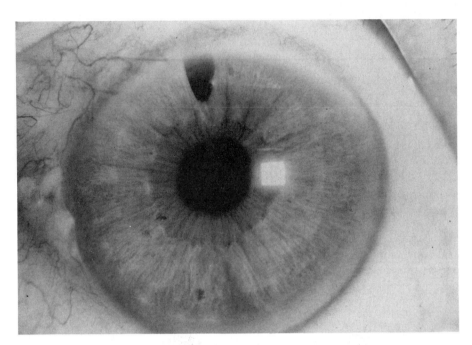

Fig. 5-43. Shearing posterior chamber lens implant before dilation.

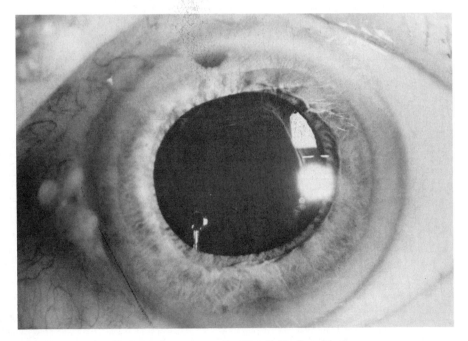

Fig. 5-44. Same eye as in Fig. 5-43 after dilation.

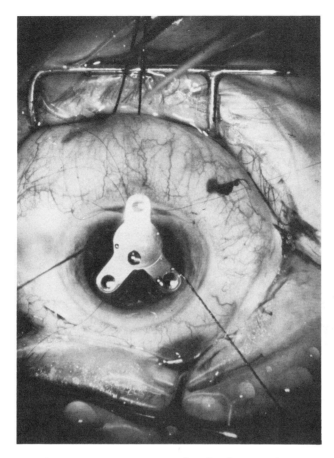

Fig. 5-45. Pearce posterior chamber lens implant.

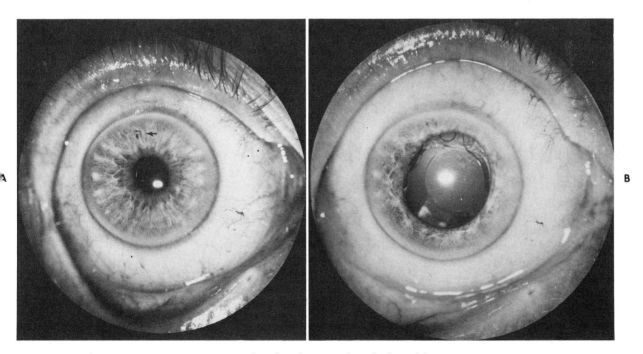

Fig. 5-46. A, Pearce posterior chamber lens implant before dilation. Note iris suture *(arrow).* **B,** Same eye after dilation.

of the ciliary sulcus. This is done with the pupil dilated. When the implant is properly positioned, the pupil is constricted with acetylcholine solution. A peripheral iridectomy is performed at 12 o'clock. The posterior capsule may be left intact, or a capsulotomy may be performed through the iridectomy. The incision is then closed.

3. Pearce posterior chamber implant with an extracapsular cataract extraction (Figs. 5-45 and 5-46). A 10-0 polypropylene suture (Ethicon 2794G) is passed through the pupil behind the superior iris. The point of the needle emerges at 12 o'clock about 2 mm from the limbus and is then laid aside. The loose ends of the iris suture are passed through the haptic foot of the lens and tied, and the free ends are cut. The anterior chamber is filled with air, and the lens is placed within the capsular bag. The iris at 12 o'clock is placed over the superior limb of the implant, and another bite of the iris is taken circumferentially just behind or in front of where the suture emerges from behind the iris, leaving a small loop; the suture is tied and the ends are cut. Pearce considers a peripheral iridectomy unnecessary. If done, it may be placed at 10:30 o'clock, 1:30 o'clock, or in both locations.

Implants used with intracapsular or extracapsular cataract extraction

Any implant that can be used with an intracapsular cataract extraction can be used with an extracapsular cataract extraction. However, the posterior chamber lenses and the Binkhorst iridocapsular lens can be used only with an extracapsular cataract extraction. Four additional common implants that can be used with either technique of cataract extraction will now be described.

1. Choyce Mark VIII implant. Two peripheral iridectomies are performed at 10 and 2 o'clock, at last 8 mm apart, space sufficient for the implant to be slid between them. The correct length of the implant is crucial to the success of the surgery. It is determined by adhering to the "horizontal corneal diameter plus 1 mm rule," regardless of the axis of insertion of the implant (Figs. 5-47 and 5-48). If the implant "falls" into the anterior chamber at the time of operation, it is very likely too short. If the proximal feet protrude more than 1.5 mm over the scleral edge of a properly cut

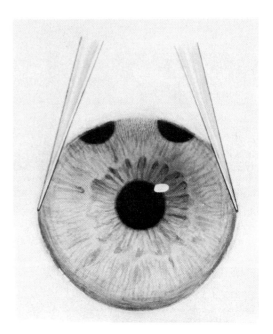

Fig. 5-47. Horizontal corneal diameter, limbal white to limbal white, measured with calipers. (From Jaffe, N. S., et al.: Pseudophakos, St. Louis, 1978, The C. V. Mosby Co.)

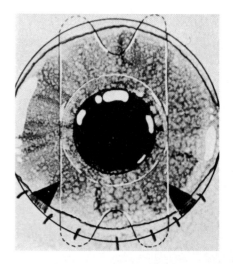

Fig. 5-48. Vertical insertion of Mark VIII implant. Implant length still equals *horizontal* corneal diameter + 1 mm. (Courtesy Dr. Jerald L. Tennant; from Jaffe, N. S., et al.: Pseudophakos, St. Louis, 1978, The C. V. Mosby Co.)

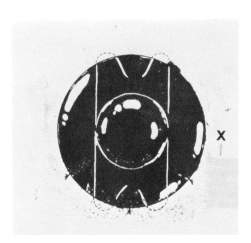

Fig. 5-49. Tap test to detect too short an implant at end of operation. Sclera is tapped at *x*. Iris moves under lens, but lens itself is stable. (Courtesy Dr. Jerald L. Tennant; from Jaffe, N. S., et al.: Pseudophakos, St. Louis, 1978, The C. V. Mosby Co.)

section, it is probably too long. If in doubt, the surgeon should err on the side of too long rather than too short an implant. Tennant[39] has devised two useful tests to determine the correctness of the length of the implant. The "nudge" test is used after the implant has been inserted but before the incision has been sutured. Gentle downward movement with a spatula placed in the crotch of the haptic should not bring the upper feet completely into view if the implant is the right length. If they are clearly seen, the implant is too short. The "tap" test is used at the conclusion of the operation, after reinflation of the anterior chamber. A tap is applied to the sclera in the region of the pars plana at a right angle to the long axis of the inserted implant. It should cause iridodonesis but not pseudophakodonesis unless the implant is too short (Fig. 5-49). The implant is inserted after the corneal opening has been reduced (increased with phacoemulsification) by sutures to 8 mm. The implant is usually inserted under air along the 12 to 6 o'clock axis. After the distal feet have reached the inferior angle, the

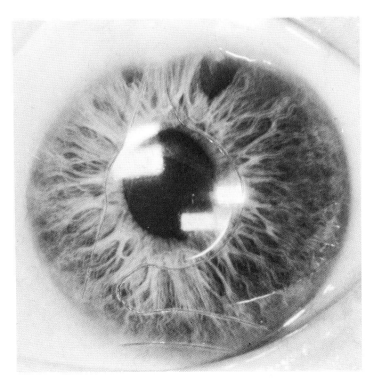

Fig. 5-50. Kelman anterior chamber lens. (Courtesy Dr. Charles Kelman; from Jaffe, N. S., et al.: Pseudophakos, St. Louis, 1978, The C. V. Mosby Co.)

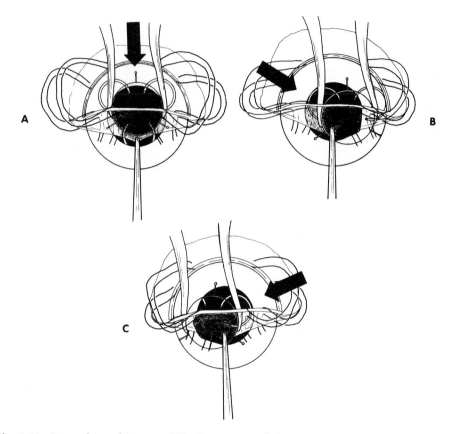

Fig. 5-51. Open-sky technique of Fyodorov sputnik lens insertion. **A,** Implant is held with special forceps. Straight forceps below retracts cornea. Inferior loop is inserted under iris. **B,** Right loop is passed under iris. **C,** Left loop is passed under iris. (From Jaffe, N. S., et al: Pseudophakos, St. Louis, 1978, The C. V. Mosby Co.)

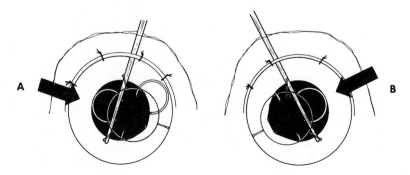

Fig. 5-52. Closed-eye technique of Fyodorov sputnik lens insertion. Fine spatula is inserted through incision to position horizontal loops behind iris. (From Jaffe, N. S., et al.: Pseudophakos, St. Louis, 1978, The C. V. Mosby Co.)

proximal feet are implanted in the superior angle by retracting the scleral lip of the incision. It is not implanted by displacing the implant further toward 6 o'clock because iridodialysis and hemorrhage may occur. If the iris bulges in front of the lower margin of the implant, it should be relieved by piercing the root of the iris around the 6 o'clock position with a single blade of curved Vannas scissors and then snipping through the iris stroma in the direction of its root.

2. Kelman implant (Fig. 5-50). This is a 3-point anterior chamber angle implant that can be inserted through a very small corneal opening. It is ideally suited for implantation with phacoemulsification. The length of the implant is determined by a "dipstick," which measures the diameter of the anterior chamber. This is usually done after the lens nucleus has been emulsified but before the lens cortex is irrigated and aspirated from the eye.

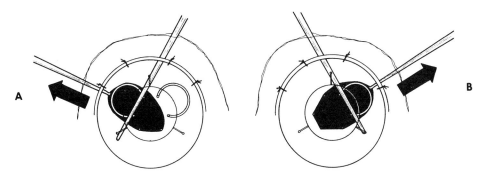

Fig. 5-53. Closed-eye technique of Fyodorov sputnik lens insertion with small pupil. Fine hook is used with spatula. (From Jaffe, N. S., et al.: Pseudophakos, St. Louis, 1978, The C. V. Mosby Co.)

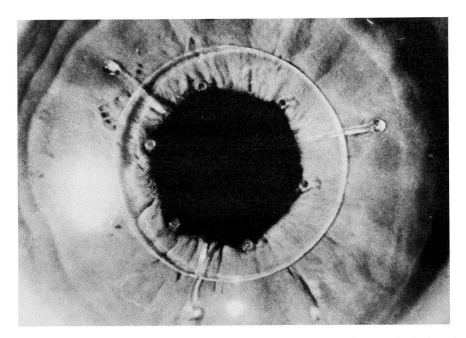

Fig. 5-54. Fyodorov sputnik lens in situ. (From Jaffe, N. S., et al.: Pseudophakos, St. Louis, 1978, The C. V. Mosby Co.)

3. Fyodorov-Binkhorst implant (Fig. 5-9). This implant is similar to the Copeland iris-plane lens in that the four haptics are separated from each other by 90 degrees. However, the haptics are loops rather than solid, and those in one meridian are offset from those in the opposite meridian. The Binkhorst cross-action, Clayman, Shepard, or Hirschman forceps may be used during implantation. The anterior haptics may be placed vertically, horizontally, or at any oblique angle, according to the surgeon's preference. It is difficult to insert this implant through a small incision.

4. Fyodorov sputnik implant (Fig. 5-10). This lens can be inserted in an open-sky (Fig. 5-51) or closed-system (Figs. 5-52 and 5-53) method. The implant is held by an edge holder and inserted into the anterior chamber in its intended iris relationship. The inferior loop is positioned behind the iris. The edge holder is removed, and the wound is made watertight by drawing up the preplaced sutures and adding additional sutures. The anterior chamber is deepened with fluid or air. The two remaining posterior loops are positioned with a fine spatula placed against the vertical portion of the loops where they emerge from the back of the optic. The implant is moved in the opposite direction until the loop pops under the iris. This maneuver is repeated with the remaining loop. A 5 to 6 mm pupil is ideal for these maneuvers. Once the implant is correctly positioned, the pupil assumes a hexagonal shape (Fig. 5-54). If the pupil becomes too small, it is necessary to employ a small blunt hook like a shepherd's crook as well as a spatula. The hook should first be tried in the iris stroma to pull the iris to one side as the lens is slid toward the other side with the spatula. This will usually cause an oblique pupillary opening sufficient to permit the loop to pop into position. If the pupil is too small to allow this, it is necessary to grasp the iris sphincter with the crook of the hook and lift the iris over the posterior loop as the lens is again moved away from the direction of the hook with a spatula.

Postoperative care

I have not used postoperative miotics with the Binkhorst 4-loop or Worst lenses because these involve methods designed to prevent dislocation.

I have used miotics for about 2 weeks with the Copeland iris-plane lens to ensure some adhesion of the iris to the implant. Pilocarpine solution (2%) is used three times daily. Some implant surgeons consider this unnecessary. Steroid therapy administered either systemically or subconjunctivally at surgery, or both, is probably beneficial when using the Copeland lens because of the greater tendency to postoperative iritis. It may or may not be used with Binkhorst or Worst lenses. Except for the test dilation at 4 days with the Binkhorst 2-loop lens, my postoperative regimen does not differ from that used after a routine intracapsular lens extraction.

SURGICAL INDICATIONS AND CONTRAINDICATIONS*

A successful implantation of an intraocular implant lens is pleasing to the patient but even more so to the surgeon who is accustomed to the complaints of patients attempting to adjust to the optic handicaps of aphakia. This satisfaction could lead to an overly liberal attitude in planning the management of the patient with cataracts. Therefore the anticipated advantages must be weighed against the slightly greater risk of lens implant surgery.

Some of the problems related to lens implant surgery are due less to the intraocular lens implant itself than to the poor selection of patients and to inadequately trained surgeons. Therefore it would appear reasonable to establish a set of guidelines for intraocular lens implant surgery for those surgeons with average technical skill and those with less experience. As skill and experience grow, these guidelines can and should be altered.

At this time a wide variance among implant surgeons exists as to surgical indications for the procedure. This variance is underscored by the fact that some surgeons implant intraocular lenses in nearly 90% of their cataract patient population while others reserve the procedure for 10% to 20%.

My personal experience dates back to 1967. My approach has been conservative. Because of

---

*Sections of this discussion have been modified from Jaffe, N. S., et al.: Pseudophakos, St. Louis, 1978, The C. V. Mosby Co.

the greater surgical risks and because of few available statistics on the long-term tolerance of intraocular lenses, I have favored their use in the elderly. I have found the following indications to include nearly all of my implantations. It is emphasized that this is not intended to reflect unfavorably on indications used by other surgeons. However, pending long-term clinical experience, the approach is designed to emphasize caution.

Indications

I have classified indications into three categories: general, special, and specific.

General indications

1. Intraocular lens implants are most easily inserted and are most successful in older patients and initially should be restricted to the elderly.

2. Intraocular lenses are implanted in eyes of those younger patients who are not likely to succeed with a contact lens.

3. Intraocular lens implants are initially restricted to one eye unless the needs of the patient indicate otherwise.

The reasons for restricting implants to the elderly should be apparent. Older people adapt poorly to spectacles for aphakia and to contact lenses. In addition, more hard data need to be obtained about the long-term safety of polymethylmethacrylate, polyamide, polypropylene, platinum-iridium alloy, titanium, and the additives that an implant comprises. If a young patient can be reasonably expected to manage the wearing of a contact lens, an implant is generally not performed by many surgeons. The surgery for routine cataract surgery without an implant is far less burdensome, and certain postoperative complications such as dislocation of the implant or development of an intraocular lens membrane are not encountered.

Surgery on one eye is often sufficient. Many patients who achieve good vision with a pseudophakos can manage well with one eye even if the opposite eye is nearly blind. They do not have to cope with the problem of spatial disorientation, pincushion distortion, and the ring scotoma inherent in cataract spectacle lenses, and they do not require the dexterity and central vision necessary to manage contact lens wear. It should be obvious that these statements do not apply to all patients. Any ophthalmologist knows patients who manage extremely well after routine cataract surgery in only one eye where a contact lens is used, in spite of poor vision in the second eye. Ophthalmologists also know many patients who complain bitterly about the loss of binocularity. The same applies to the use of an implant in one eye. Some patients find unilateral surgery adequate for their needs, others do not.

Special indications

1. There are certain occupational drawbacks to contact lens wear, for example, in ranchers, miners, and divers. In addition, contact lenses may disqualify some people for certain occupations, for example, pilots. Ophthalmologists who treat such patients are familiar with the difficulties of contact lens wear. Opththalmologists who do not treat persons in these categories may not be overly sympathetic to the occupational handicaps of a contact lens.

2. It is well known that we usually have been unsuccessful in preventing amblyopia in children ages 3 to 8 years who sustain a traumatic cataract. In spite of successful cataract removal and diligent contact lens wear, these eyes usually become amblyopic. The use of an intraocular lens in this situation has been studied widely in the Netherlands. American ophthalmologists have only limited experience in this situation.

Specific indications

1. An elderly patient who has an advanced cataract in one eye and visual acuity of 20/40 to 20/60 in the other eye basically has a unilateral cataract. The patient may perform poorly in bright sunlight and may have lost his license to drive an automobile. The same indication might also include those patients who have even better vision than this in the other eye but who have an advanced cataract that interferes with their activities.

2. The same indication exists in slightly younger people with infirmities such as rheumatoid arthritis, parkinsonism, hemiplegia, or mental retardation. These patients are poor candidates for contact lenses, although there may be a poor, but partially satisfactory, solution in bilateral cataract surgery corrected with spectacles.

3. An elderly patient who has disabling cataracts in both eyes, with a visual acuity of, for example, 20/100 in each eye, appears to manage

satisfactorily if implant surgery is performed in one eye. They manage well because they are not confronted with the obstacles of the spectacle correction of aphakia. There is some controversy in this indication. Some ophthalmologists prefer to do surgery in both eyes while others favor surgery in one eye only. If surgery is undertaken in both eyes, it would appear prudent to leave a reasonable period between the two operations. Certainly one should be more conservative in this case than in the management of bilateral cataracts where routine cataract surgery is performed. The trend in the United States in the latter situation appears to be toward cataract surgery within a brief period, for example, 1 week. There are still enough uncertainties in implant surgery so that a longer interval between operations would be in the best interest of the patient. This interval should be longer for younger patients. In patients over 80, the interval can be shortened. However, in patients of this age range, it is questionable whether bilateral surgery is indicated in all cases. Again, this is a judgment decision.

4. It is well known that patients who have extensive bilateral macular degeneration and later develop advanced cataracts in both eyes perform poorly with spectacles after cataract extraction. The loss of peripheral field represents a severe obstacle to these patients, since this is the only field of vision they possess. In addition, they have insufficient central vision to manage a contact lens. When such patients undergo lens implant surgery successfully, they are some of the happiest patients one might encounter. In spite of the absence of a central visual field, they are delighted by the improvement of vision after implant surgery.

5. An elderly patient has worn a contact lens for unilateral aphakia for many years but is faced with a nearly mature cataract in the second eye. This prevents him from managing the contact lens in the first eye. Most patients who wear a contact lens successfully after a cataract extraction in one eye do just about as well as patients who have a successful lens implantation in one eye. However, the management of the contact lens requires a certain amount of vision in the opposite eye. If the cataract in the opposite eye advances sufficiently, the patient may have some difficulty with the contact lens in the aphakic eye. Therefore a lens implant in the second eye is usually a very satisfactory solution for this problem.

It is repeated that these indications cannot be imposed on all surgeons. In the end surgeons are expected to exercise their own judgment in the best interest of the patient. There is a marked difference in the surgical abilities of different surgeons and a marked difference in their attitudes toward indications and contraindications. Therefore what has just been said can only be called a set of guidelines and not a strict list of indications.

To illustrate some of these indications, consider the following actual situations.

Situation: An elderly patient has aphakia in the first eye and wears a contact lens.

Treatment: An implant may be used in the second eye if the cataract in the second eye interferes with the patient's ability to manage the contact lens in the first eye. If the patient is doing well with the contact lens, no surgery need be done in the second eye no matter what the status of the cataract.

Situation: A patient has aphakia in the first eye, has adapted well to spectacles, and likes them.

Treatment: Routine intracapsular cataract extraction is indicated in the second eye; spectacles are prescribed for both eyes.

Situation: A successful implant has been performed in the first eye of a patient under 70.

Treatment: No implant is indicated for the second eye unless the cataract disturbs the patient. The surgeon may then choose between an implant in the second eye or a routine cataract extraction with contact lens correction.

Situation: A successful implant has been performed in the first eye of a patient over 70.

Treatment: No implant is indicated for the second eye in many cases. Alternate choices could be an implant for the second eye in a patient over 70 with a reasonable follow-up period for the first eye or a shorter postoperative period if the patient is over 80.

Situation: The patient has aphakia in the first eye and has not successfully adapted to spectacles or to a contact lens.

Treatment: Routine cataract extraction is preferred for the second eye with spectacles prescribed for both eyes. A secondary implant in the first eye is still considered risky because the risks are greater than with primary implantation. This problem really gets to the heart of the problem of secondary implantation. Since so many patients who wear a spectacle for the first eye after cataract extraction are unhappy with this method of optic correction of aphakia, there is a great danger of an epidemic of secondary implantations. It has been demonstrated that there is a significant risk of complications in secondarily implanted iris-supported pseudophakoi. The most reasonable solution might be a Choyce Mark VIII implant. However, the surgeon must weigh the possibility that even though the patient cannot tolerate the method of optic correction of aphakia in the first eye, there is danger of reducing the vision in this eye by secondary implantation. Again this is a judgment decision to be made by the surgeon. Some patients appear to benefit when the cataract is removed from the second eye and spectacles are used for both eyes. However, this is not a satisfactory solution for all patients. If secondary implantation is performed in the first eye, the patient must be fully informed about the risk of reducing the functional status of that eye even though he had not been able to use the first eye with either a spectacle or a contact lens. If the patient is fully informed and is really intolerant of the spectacle or contact lens, a secondary implantation may prove to be the procedure of choice. However, this situation has not been followed for long in the United States. Therefore the procedure is still in a period of clinical evaluation.

Another important judgment decision is whether an extracapsular cataract extraction lowers the incidence of cystoid macular edema and retinal detachment seen after a routine intracapsular cataract extraction. To date, there are no extensive age-matched series that support this view. Proponents of planned extracapsular extraction, whether by phacoemulsification or by the conventional method, usually reserve this technique for younger cataract patients. However, according to the criteria used by most implant surgeons, these patients would not qualify for an implant, since they could reasonably be expected to manage contact lens wear.

Contraindications

Indications for pseudophakos implantation having been enumerated, contraindications may now be considered. In a controversial area such as lens implant surgery, it is not surprising that there would be more contraindications than indications. Some of these contraindications appear to be well defined. Others are questionable at this time.

1. The patient does not want an implant or expresses anxiety over the procedure.

2. Axial myopia is greater than 7 D. The advantages of an implant are minimal in this situation, since the residual refractive error is small.

3. A poor result was obtained with an implant in the first eye.

4. The patient has only one eye with potentially good vision. It is hoped that contraindications 3 and 4 would be universally accepted by implant surgeons.

5. The patient is young. The definition of young is a judgment decision to be made by the surgeon. Most significant is the surgeon's impression as to whether the patient could be reasonably expected to manage a contact lens.

6. Postoperative follow-up is impossible. The patient who lives far from the nearest implant surgeon may receive inadequate management of late complications from ophthalmologists inexperienced in implant surgery.

7. Severe senile macular choroidal degeneration is present without a nearly mature cataract in both eyes. Such a patient will derive little benefit from implant surgery.

8. Endothelial corneal dystrophy is present. Implant surgery requires greater intraocular manipulation than a routine cataract extraction. Therefore there is a much greater likelihood of postoperative corneal edema.

9. Proliferative diabetic retinopathy is present. Cystoid macular edema and other postoperative complications are more likely in these eyes.

10. Uncontrolled glaucoma is present. Postoperative inflammation with its effects on the anterior chamber angles may be disastrous for such eyes.

11. There has been previous retinal detachment. Since vitreous problems are more likely in implant surgery than in routine cataract surgery, there is a greater risk of redetachment. In addition, if extensive synechiae of the iris to a pseudophakos occur or if a membrane develops over the surface of the implant, visualization of small breaks in the retinal periphery is more difficult.

12. Congenital cataracts, especially of the rubelliform type, are present. With the exception of postnatal zonular cataracts, many of these eyes could not be expected to tolerate or benefit from an intraocular lens implant.

13. The cataract is associated with other abnormalities such as recurrent iritis, essential iris atrophy, or atopic dermatitis.

Although it is conceded that the technical abilities of some intraocular implant surgeons may make some of these contraindications appear unusually conservative, the human eye should not be an arena for surgical heroics. Since it is likely that more surgeons will engage in intraocular implant surgery, and therefore more eyes will be subjected to the procedure, the conservative approach to indications and contraindications should reasonably be expected to be in the best interests of our patients.

In these days of increasing peer review, it is becoming mandatory to formulate a reasonable set of guidelines that would be universally accepted. Greater permissiveness in selection of patients should be guided only by additional favorable experience. It should be apparent that a less conservative approach to lens implant surgery should only be undertaken after surgical education and patient experience has significantly increased.

COMPLICATIONS AND MANAGEMENT
Operative complications

1. Inadequate incision. An incision of 165 to 180 degrees is ideal for intraocular lens implantation with an intracapsular cataract extraction. A smaller incision increases the likelihood of damaging the corneal endothelium during the process of inserting the pseudophakos. It also increases the risk of rupture of the lens capsule, operative loss of vitreous, and detachment of Descemet's membrane. When the lens is implanted under air, the incision is closed with sutures, leaving a 7 to 9 mm opening.

2. Excessive bleeding (p. 45). This must be controlled, since it not only reduces visibility, but clotted blood in the angle and on the surface of the iris may prevent the pupil from constricting around the optic portion of the implant. Bleeding is usually controlled by irrigation, but if this should fail, a bubble of air in the anterior chamber will tamponade the bleeding vessels and prevent access of blood into the anterior chamber. In addition, it is better to approach the cornea at the horizontal extremities of the incision to avoid the larger vessels.

3. Iridodialysis. An inadvertent iridodialysis occurring during enlargement of the incision or during the performance of the iridotomies or iridectomies is usually not serious. If excessive, it should be sutured with a 10-0 monofilament nylon suture. On a rare occasion the iridodialysis appears much larger postoperatively than it does at surgery. This may result in a markedly displaced pupil and bring the optic portion of the pseudophakos and its haptic supports dangerously close to the cornea. The iridodialysis may be repaired postoperatively by the McCannel method.[40]

4. Excessive pupillary dilatation. This may prevent suitable implantation and favor dislocation. It may be avoided by refraining from excessive preoperative use of cycloplegics or mydriatics. If the pupil does not contract after acetylcholine solution is placed in the eye, gentle stroking of the anterior surface of the iris may irritate the iris sufficiently to produce miosis. If the pupil still fails to constrict, there may have been some iris sphincter damage. In such a case, it is probably wise to abandon the implantation.

5. Inadequate pupillary dilatation. These are eyes with small pupils due to long-term miotic therapy. If cataract extraction is attempted through too small a pupil, it usually causes one or more ruptures of the iris sphincter. The resulting atonic pupil precludes lens implantation. The procedure to be followed in this situation has already been described (Fig. 5-28). Another such case is illustrated in Fig. 5-55. Epinephrine bisulfite solution should not be used to promote mydriasis because of the possible deleterious effect of the bisulfite on the corneal endothelium. In addition, epinephrine bisulfite is usually ineffective in those eyes whose pupils fail to dilate adequately with conventional cycloplegics or mydriatics. Occasionally the pupil will constrict during an extracapsular cataract extraction as a result of iris irritation. This makes it very difficult to visualize residual cortex. I have used intracardiac epinephrine containing no preservative (Ephinephrine HCL Solution, CSD, IMS Ltd., South El Monte, Calif). This contains 0.1 mg/ml. Using a 1 ml tuberculin syringe, 0.1 ml of the epinephrine is diluted with 0.9 ml of balanced solution. This will be effective only in those

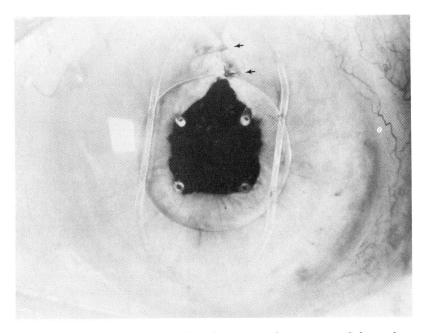

Fig. 5-55. Binkhorst iris-clip implant placed in eye with miotic pupil due to long-term miotic therapy. Iris incision is closed with two 10-0 nylon sutures *(arrows)*. (From Jaffe, N. S., et al.: Pseudophakos, St. Louis, 1978, The C. V. Mosby Co.)

eyes whose pupils dilate preoperatively but constrict during the surgery.

6. Iris sphincter damage. This may occur as a result of inadvertent freezing of the iris sphincter with the cryoprobe. It may also occur accidentally while performing a partial anterior vitrectomy. If inadequate pupillary constriction results, it may be useful to perform a small radial iridotomy through the damaged sphincter and place a suture as described earlier.

7. Dislocation. If the implant should dislocate after its insertion, it may be corrected by grasping the optic portion with smooth tying forceps and repositing the loops. The Binkhorst cross-action forceps should not be used for this maneuver. If the dislocation is observed after the wound is sutured, one or two sutures should be removed so that a smooth (Jaffe) or notched (Hirschman) spatula may enter the anterior chamber to reposition the lens.

8. Rupture of posterior capsule. This may occur during the performance of an extracapsular cataract extraction. If the rent in the posterior capsule is small and vitreous loss has not occurred, the procedure need not be altered. If the rupture is large and vitreous has not escaped, it is best to use an implant designed for an intracapsular cataract extraction. If vitreous loss has occurred, a partial anterior vitrectomy should be performed as well as removal of all retained lens material. The implantation may be abandoned, or an intracapsular type of implant may be used.

9. Vitreous bulge. It is possible to implant a lens in the presence of a mild vitreous bulge without losing vitreous. The maneuvers should be performed without corneal retraction. The management of a more serious bulge has already been described in the section on technique.

10. Vitreous loss. In spite of all the prophylactic measures described earlier, vitreous loss is inevitable in a small percentage of cases. Its management has already been discussed.

11. Choyce implant complications. Some complications seen with this implant are related directly to the surgery itself. Bulging of the iris in front of the margins of the implant may occur, suggesting that adequate apertures were not made in the iris or that wound closure is imperfect so that leakage of aqueous is occurring. If the iris bulge persists for more than a few days and there is no wound leakage, an additional ab externo peripheral iridectomy over the apex of the

bulging iris should be performed and the anterior chamber reinflated with balanced salt solution. The implant may reveal itself to be too short by tending to revolve around the anterior chamber like a propeller. Pseudophakodonesis may also be present, as is not the case if the implant is a snug fit. It most instances the implant actually takes a constant position, and the eye gradually settles down and can be left alone, so there is no immediate urgency to intervene. If after 3 to 6 months it is clear that the too-short implant is acting like a loose foreign body in the anterior chamber, it must be removed and replaced with a longer one. Slight deformation of the pupil sometimes occurs; it usually becomes oval in the long axis of the implant. This suggests, however, that the implant used was a little on the long side or that, when it was inserted, a portion of the peripheral iris was trapped by one of the feet. This is usually not a serious complication.

12. Shearing implant complications. The main operative complication seen here is related to faulty insertion of the implant into the posterior chamber. The upper loop of the implant may lodge itself in the iris rather than in the ciliary sulcus. This results in retraction of the iris superiorly. This is easily corrected during surgery by moving the implant inferiorly with a Sinskey or Jaffe hook (Katena). The tip of the hook is placed in the superior hole of the optic of the implant. As the implant is moved toward 6 o'clock, it may be necessary to push it slightly posteriorly. The superior iris will usually correct its position as the incarcerated loop is freed. The loop of the implant may also get caught in the capsular bag during insertion. This usually causes a decentration of the implant. The maneuver just described should be tried first. If this fails, the implant can be rotated 90 degrees by engaging both holes of the optic with bent-tipped needles.

As stated on p. 147, excessive bending of the superior loop of the implant during the second part of the insertion may cause an inferior zonular dialysis. This is prevented by retracting the superior iris as the superior loop is passed into position.

Another complication may arise during the posterior capsulotomy. It is possible to pass the bent needle through the peripheral iridectomy but behind the posterior capsule. The needle will than pass into the vitreous. This must be avoided!

Early complications

1. Pupillary block. This is an uncommon complication. It may occur if the openings in the iris are made too peripherally and the cataract incision too anteriorly. It may also occur if the iris opening is not patent. Air pupillary block is also a possibility. If miotics are being used, they should be discontinued, and careful mydriasis should be attempted along with the systemic administration of a hyperosmotic agent. If this fails, one or more of the following should be tried: peripheral iridectomy, reopening of a closed iridectomy, transfixion of the iris, or vitreous aspiration through a peripheral iridectomy. If the pupillary block is due to air, repositioning the patient's head may correct the situation. If not, the air should be aspirated.

2. Flat or shallow anterior chamber due to wound fistula. With a pseudophakos in situ, this is a surgical emergency, since irreversible corneal damage may result. The wound should be resutured and a partial bubble of air left in the anterior chamber.

3. Shallow anterior chamber associated with a ciliochoroidal detachment. This should be managed the same way as after a routine cataract extraction with the following exception. If the chamber is sufficiently shallow so that there is danger of the optic portion of the implant touching the cornea, the condition should be remedied in the usual manner.

4. Striate keratopathy and corneal edema. These conditions are usually more marked than after a routine cataract extraction because of the greater manipulation of the tissues that occurs in lens implantation. The conditions are usually transient but in some cases may persist for a long time (Fig. 5-56). There is no effective treatment.

5. Vitreous in the anterior chamber. This may be due to unrecognized rupture of the anterior face of the vitreous during the surgery or to residual formed vitreous after a partial anterior vitrectomy. It usually is of no consequence.

6. Lens precipitates. There are three types. One consists of pigment deposits on both surfaces of the implant (Fig. 5-57). They arise from the pigment epithelium of the iris because of

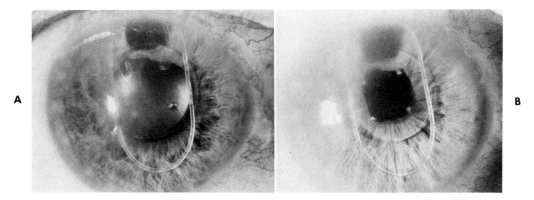

Fig. 5-56. A, Corneal edema, resulting from surgical trauma, seen 8 weeks postoperatively. (Visual acuity = 20/800.) **B,** Same eye 6 months later. (Visual acuity = 20/20.) (From Jaffe, N. S., et al.: Pseudophakos, St. Louis, 1978, The C. V. Mosby Co.)

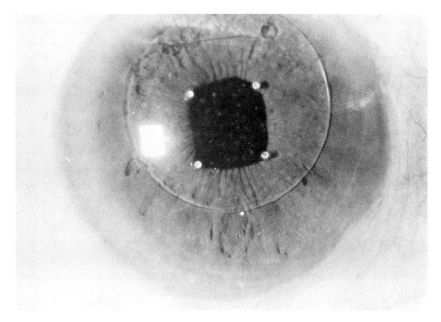

Fig. 5-57. Pigment deposits on posterior surface of Worst Medallion implant. (From Jaffe, N. S., et al.: Pseudophakos, St. Louis, 1978, The C. V. Mosby Co.)

dispersion by the loop supports behind the iris. The other consists of grayish white precipitates that are the residues of lens material after an extracapsular cataract extraction. Similar deposits may be seen after recurrent bouts of uveitis. They resemble K.P. on the back of the cornea. (Fig. 5-58). Lens precipitates tend to lessen with time. If the deposits on the implant are heavy, they occasionally lessen with steroid therapy given topically, by sub-Tenon's route, or both.

7. Endophthalmitis. This rare postoperative complication does not appear to be more frequent than after routine cataract extraction. However, there are theoretical reasons why it should be greater. They involve the numerous variabilities associated with sterilizing and packaging a plastic implant. There have been two serious epidemics of septic endophthalmitis due to contamination of the neutralizing solution when the Ridley caustic soda method was used. One

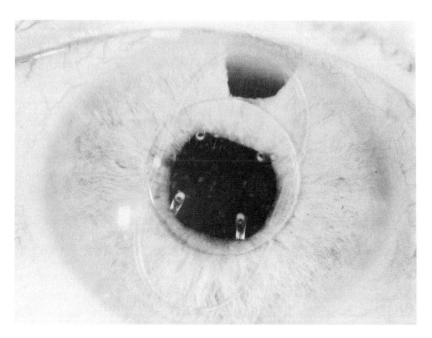

Fig. 5-58. Deposits, resulting from inflammation, on posterior surface of Binkhorst iris-clip implant. (From Jaffe, N. S., et al.: Pseudophakos, St. Louis, 1978, The C. V. Mosby Co.)

was bacterial *(Pseudomonas aeruginosa)* and one fungal *(Paecilomyces lilalicum)*. Ethylene oxide sterilization has replaced the wet-pack method in the United States. There appears to be a higher incidence of sterile endophthalmitis with Ethylene oxide sterilization, for as yet undetermined reasons, than with the Ridley caustic soda method. Gamma radiation was also used for a short time in 1976. This was discontinued because of a high incidence of inflammation. The management of septic endophthalmitis is discussed on p. 457; the treatment of sterile endophthalmitis is discussed on p. 461.

Early or late complications

1. Dislocation. This may be due to the following:
   a. Too much air in the anterior chamber
   b. Too wide a pupil as a result of rupture of the sphincter of a miotic pupil during cataract extraction or sphincter damage by the cryoprobe
   c. Premature discontinuation of pilocarpine in those implants not secured by a fixation suture or device
   d. Accidental use of mydriatics
   e. Pupillary dilatation at night
   f. Pupillary dilatation due to excitement
   g. Loop length of implant too short
   h. Ocular trauma

Reposition is initially attempted pharmacologically (Figs. 5-59 and 5-60). A short-acting mydriatic that is easily reversible such as 10% phenylephrine solution or 1% tropicamide (Mydriacyl) is instilled. The patient's head is placed in an optimum position, which is determined by the portion that has dislocated. As soon as the pupil dilates sufficiently so that the distal portion of the dislocated haptic is cleared by the iris, the patient's head is placed securely in the proper position, and a miotic such as echothiophate iodide 0.12% solution is placed in the eye. If this fails (Fig. 5-60), instrumental repositioning must be used. There are a number of fine instruments available. Disposable needles are very sharp and very useful for this purpose. I have used a 25- or 27-gauge needle attached to a 2 ml syringe filled with balanced salt solution. The needle enters the anterior chamber through the limbus and maneuvers the implant into proper

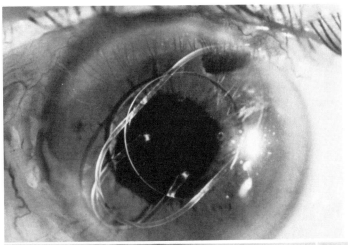

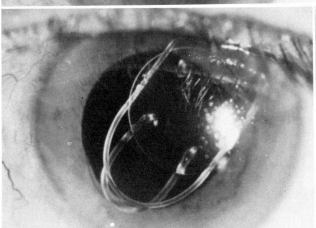

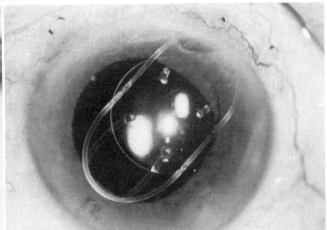

Fig. 5-59. **A,** Spontaneous dislocation of Binkhorst 4-loop iris-clip implant. Both loops are anterior to iris at 6 o'clock. Condition of eye at diagnosis of dislocation. **B,** Pupil dilated with 10% phenylephrine solution. **C,** Pupil sufficiently dilated for repositioning with echothiophate iodide 0.12% solution. **D,** Implant properly positioned. (**D** from Jaffe, N. S.: Pseudophakos, St. Louis, 1978, The C. V. Mosby Co.)

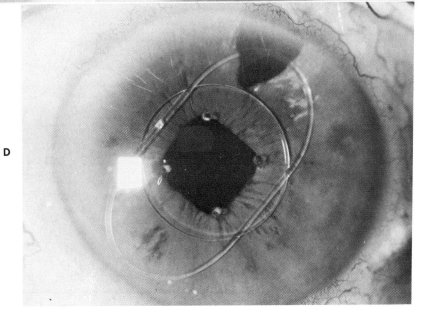

position. If aqueous escapes, it should be replaced with the balanced salt solution. If dislocation of a capsule-supported lens occurs, it may be possible to reposition it with eye drops, as just described. Pilocarpine solution should be used indefinitely. It may be possible to suture one of the loop supports to the iris. In some instances it may be wise to remove the implant and replace it with an iris-supported lens such as a Binkhorst 4-loop iris-clip pseudophakos. If the optic portion of a capsule-supported implant dislocates behind the iris, it can usually be left in this position as a posterior chamber lens (Fig. 5-61).

If repeated dislocations of an implant with loops occur, in spite of daily miotic medication, a more permanent method of securing fixation must be undertaken. McCannel has suggested a method that has become popular (Fig. 5-62). A stab wound is made just within the limbus through a clear cornea closest to the position where the suture will end up being tied to the iris below. A double-arm 9-0 nylon or polypropylene (Prolene, Ethicon, Inc., Somerville, N.J.) (a half-curve needle is best for this purpose) suture is passed through this incision, through the iris, around the loop that may be anterior or posterior

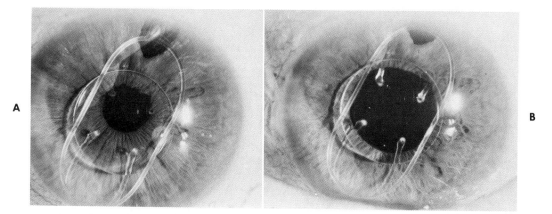

Fig. 5-60. A, Dislocation of Binkhorst iris-clip implant. **B,** Maximal mydriasis obtained in this eye is insufficient for repositioning by pharmacologic means. (From Jaffe, N. S.: Pseudophakos, St. Louis, 1978, The C. V. Mosby Co.)

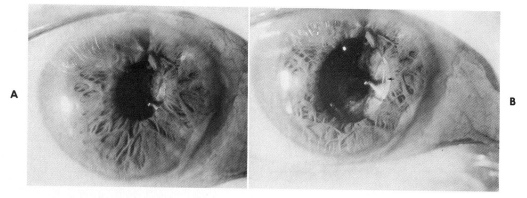

Fig. 5-61. A, Extracapsular cataract extraction has been performed in eye with miotic pupil. Superior iris was incised and sutured. Optic portion of Binkhorst iridocapsular implant has dislocated into posterior chamber. **B,** After mydriasis, edge of optic portion *(arrow)* is seen. Capsular fixation is adequate. (Visual acuity 2 years postoperatively = 20/20.) (From Jaffe, N. S.: Pseudophakos, St. Louis, 1978, The C. V. Mosby Co.)

to the iris (according to the implant type), back out through the iris, and finally out through the cornea at any point where the needle ends up. At this point we have a suture that is passing through the stab wound, through the iris, around a loop, through the iris again, and out through another area of the cornea. The needle is cut off from the leading end of the suture that has emerged from the cornea. Five to 7.5 cm of suture is left outside the cornea after the needle is cut off. A small iris hook is introduced through the stab wound, and the free end of the suture is grasped and withdrawn from the eye through the stab wound. Both ends of the suture are now emerging from the stab wound. These two ends are then tied together with four knots. This brings the loop and iris up to the stab wound. The suture is cut close to the knot. The iris and the sutured loop will then retract into the anterior chamber.

2. Decentration. When this occurs, it nearly always does so within the first 6 postoperative months. It may be caused by asymmetric adhesion of the loop supports to residual capsulolenticular material after an extracapsular cataract extraction. It may also be caused by iris incarcera-

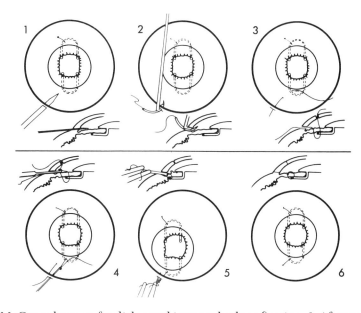

Fig. 5-62. McCannel suture for dislocated intraocular lens fixation. *1,* After small limbal incision at 8 o'clock, long narrow spatula used to reposition loop of intraocular lens into its proper place behind iris. *2,* Small, short, grooved 2.5 mm spatula introduced into incision guides 10-0 monofilament nylon suture on half-circle needle, which is directed into anterior chamber under spatula. This prevents needle point from catching on corneoscleral tissues as it enters anterior chamber. *3,* Needle point is then directed down posteriorly through iris and under now properly positioned loop of intraocular lens. Without releasing needle holder grip, needle point is brought up again through iris and vertically across anterior chamber to exit through cornea. *4,* Anterior chamber suture segment is then pulled out in a loop through same corneoscleral stab wound with delicate, blunt iris hook or 25-gauge needle with its point bent into small hook. *5,* Corneal suture is then cut flush on epithelial surface, allowing end to be brought out in single strand at limbus. Triple throw suture tie is placed, using two ends of suture. As knot is drawn down firmly, shift is seen in anterior chamber, intraocular lens, and pupil toward corneal incision. *6,* When knot is fully tied, ends are cut flush at knot, releasing suture tension so iris can then resume normal shape with intraocular lens and pupil centering again. This results in a tied fixation suture around iris and intraocular lens loop within anterior chamber. Miotic solution may be injected into anterior chamber. (From McCannel, M. A.: Ophthalmic Surg. **7:**98-103, 1976.)

Table 5-1. Incidence of angiographic-proven cystoid macular edema (812 angiograms)

	4 months	8 months	16-24 months
ICCE — implant	24/140° (17%)	14/114 (12%)	18/117 (15%)
ECCE — implant	4/48° (8%)	3/51 (6%)	2/48 (4%)
ICCE — no implant	16/113† (14%)	13/87 (15%)	8/94 (9%)

°Although there were 210 implant (ICCE + ECCE) eyes in the study, only 188 had a 4-month angiogram.
†Although there were 133 control eyes in the study, only 113 had a 4-month angiogram.

tion, peripheral anterior synechiae, an atonic pupil, too tight a suture used for fixation to the iris, and vitreous strands in the anterior chamber. The implant may not only decenter; it may tilt. This usually does not require treatment since vision is not at all altered, or only minimally so. This may be because the optic portion of the lens rests close to the first principal plane of the eye.

The most frequent cause of decentration is fibroplasia of vitreous left in the anterior chamber when operative loss of vitreous has occurred. If there is extensive incarceration of vitreous in the wound, the implant may be decentered so that the optic portion or an anterior loop (iris-clip lens) may touch the cornea or be dangerously close to it. This must be surgically corrected by removing the offending vitreous and repositioning the implant.

3. Uveitis. This may be a reaction to surgical trauma. It may be sufficiently exaggerated to be considered a sterile endophthalmitis. It may be a response to retained lens material (phaco-anaphylaxis). When due to the first two causes the condition responds well to steroid therapy. The third cause is much more difficult to treat. Evacuation of all lenticular remains may be necessary. I am somewhat surprised that the renewed popularity of the extracapsular cataract extraction has not yet brought forth a reappearance of phacoanaphylactic uveitis as a significant postoperative problem. Occasionally a dense anterior vitreous membrane and posterior synechiae result from intraocular inflammation. In such cases, vision may be restored by a trans pars plana anterior vitrectomy (p. 490).

4. Cystoid macular edema. The cause of this complication is still speculative. It occurs between 1 and 4 months after surgery but in some instances does not appear until years later. There still remains some question about the influence

Table 5-2. Visual acuity in eyes with angiographic-proven cystoid macular edema

	Total no. of eyes	No. of eyes with visual acuity less than 20/40	Percent
ICCE — implant	28	6	21
ECCE — implant	8	1	13
ICCE — no implant	29	6	21

of an intraocular lens or the presence of an intact posterior capsule on the incidence of cystoid macular edema. Jaffe and co-workers[41] performed a fluorescein angiographic study of patients undergoing the following surgical procedures: an intracapsular cataract extraction with a Binkhorst 4-loop implant (153 eyes), an extracapsular cataract extraction with a Binkhorst 2- or 4-loop implant (57 eyes), and an intracapsular cataract extraction without an implant (133 eyes). The posterior capsule was left intact in 53 of the 57 extracapsular cases. Angiograms were performed 4, 8, and 16 to 24 months postoperatively. All three groups were age matched (67 years or older) and ocular status matched. The results are shown in Table 5-1.

The visual acuity in eyes with angiographic-proven cystoid macular edema is shown in Table 5-2.

The following conclusions were reached:

a. Standard intracapsular cataract extractions and intracapsular cataract extractions with a Binkhorst lens implant have a comparable incidence of cystoid macular edema as determined by fluorescein angiography 4, 8, and 16 to 24 months postoperatively.

b. Extracapsular cataract extractions with a Binkhorst lens implant and an intact posterior capsule have a significantly lower incidence of angiographic-proven cystoid macular edema than intracapsular cataract extractions with a Binkhorst lens implant 16 to 24 months postoperatively. The differences were less significant at 4 and 8 months. There was a lower incidence of angiographic-proven cystoid macular edema in the extracapsular-implant group than in the intracapsular – no implant group at all three periods.

c. Visual function, as measured by visual acuity, was 20/40 or better in approximately 80% of eyes with angiographic-proven cystoid macular edema in all groups. The study did not consider the problem of distortion.

The role of an intact posterior capsule in preventing cystoid macular edema is discussed on p. 368. The treatment of cystoid macular edema is difficult to assess because of the tendency to spontaneous resolution. A trial of steroids or some other anti-inflammatory drugs might be tried. I prefer three injections of 40 units (1 ml) of triamcinolone by sub-Tenon's route at weekly intervals. Indomethacin, 25 mg, three times a day, after meals, might be tried for 2 weeks. I am still unconvinced of the efficacy of these agents.

5. Secondary membranes. After a planned extracapsular cataract extraction, an excess of unevacuated lens material may migrate into the pupillary space. With the implant in situ, the passage of this material into the anterior chamber where absorption is more likely is retarded. This slowing of absorption encourages dense secondary cataracts that occasionally vascularize due to migration of iris vessels. In most of these cases, one need not be concerned about dislocation due to attempted dilatation of the pupil. The pupil should be kept dilated as much as possible with hyoscine or atropine solution. Dilatation helps prevent pupillary block and aids in absorption of the retained lens material. If the secondary cataract membrane shows no tendency to absorb or becomes severely involved in adherence to the iris, surgical intervention is indicated.

Surgery designed to create an adequate pupillary aperture in a secondary membrane must be carefully planned. It is easy to underestimate the difficulties one might encounter with a very thick capsulolenticular membrane. A relatively thin secondary membrane lends itself easily to surgery. If the membrane has disturbed the patient's vision and appears to be getting progressively more dense, surgery should not be delayed. Early surgery is more effective and less complex. The surgeon should be assured that the decline in vision is in accord with the view of the fundus (direct ophthalmoscope or Hruby lens). For most thin secondary membranes the following procedure has been found useful (Fig. 5-63). A stab wound is made just inside the limbus with a Beaver No. 75 disposable razor blade fragment or a similar instrument. This location for the initial entry into the anterior chamber is selected to avoid bleeding from a more peripheral location. It is mandatory to maintain clear visibility for this procedure. A tiny hook is made at the tip of a disposable 25-gauge needle by bending it with a needle holder so that the opening is at the inside of the bent tip. The angle of the bend may be from 45 to 90 degrees. The needle is attached to an irrigating handle such as the Cavitron irrigation-aspiration handle. The handle is attached to the plastic tubing of a container of irrigating solution. The irrigating container is elevated sufficiently for free flow through the needle. All air should be evacuated from the tubing. The needle is passed through the stab wound, under the optic portion of the implant, until the opposite edge of the pupil is reached. The continuous flow of fluid pushes the posterior capsule posteriorly. When the hook of the needle is in the correct position, the plastic tubing is pinched closed by the surgeon or an assistant. This permits the posterior capsule to float foward against the tip of the needle. A tiny tear is made in the posterior capsule, and the irrigation flow is permitted to resume. The fluid passes through the hole and pushes the vitreous posteriorly. The tear in the posterior capsule is than completed across the entire pupil. The needle is withdrawn from the eye. The stab wound may be left unsutured, or a single 10-0 nylon suture may be used to close the small opening.

This procedure works very well for thin secondary membranes and for thin membranes that develop on the surface of the vitreous after an intracapsular cataract extraction. Thick membranes are much more difficult and often impossible to manage by this technique. These membranes may be so extensive as to adhere to the ciliary processes. It would be dangerous to pull on such a membrane. Another approach is recom-

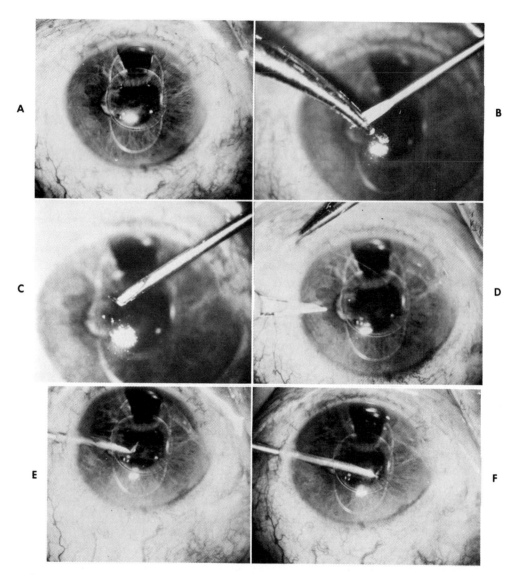

Fig. 5-63. A, Secondary membrane after extracapsular cataract extraction (12 weeks) with implantation of Binkhorst iris-clip lens. Maximum mydriasis shown. (Visual acuity = 20/400.) **B,** Hook created at tip of 25-gauge disposable needle using needle holder. **C,** Bent tip shown. **D,** Limbal stab wound made with No. 75 Beaver blade. **E,** Needle is attached to irrigating solution and enters anterior chamber, passing behind implant. **F,** Tip of needle engages membrane as irrigating flow is stopped.

mended in this situation. One of the various types of vitrectomy instruments may be used, for example, Douvas Roto-Extractor, Machemer Vitreous Infusion Suction Cutter, Girard ultrasonic fragmentor, or Berkeley Ocutome. In these cases the iris on all sides of the pupil is often pulled centrally except at the origin posts of the poste-

rior loops or at the apices of the Copeland implant. The pupil may have the shape of a vertical or horizontal hourglass. The cutting instrument is usually passed through a pars plana incision until it appears in the pupillary space. If the membrane is confined to the posterior capsule or the anterior vitreous, fiber optics illumination is

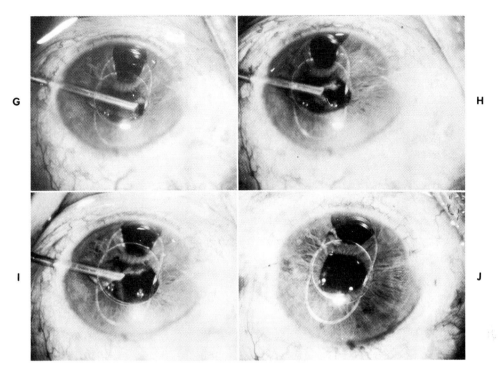

Fig. 5-63, cont'd. G, Hole in membrane is created as irrigating flow resumes. **H,** Membrane is drawn toward limbal wound. **I,** Opening in membrane is enlarged still further. **J,** Final result. Visual acuity improved to 20/25 3 months later. (From Jaffe, N. S.: Pseudophakos, St. Louis, 1978, The C. V. Mosby Co.)

not required. The dense membrane is removed. The pulled-in portions of iris may also be resected. This will usually not result in undue mydriasis. The iris is resected until a square-shaped pupil is fashioned (Fig. 5-64). The surgeon may elect to create a V-shaped notch in the inferior border of the pupil. The surgery is concluded when a clear fundus reflex is visible through the surgical microscope. Some surgeons prefer to perform the surgery through the anterior chamber via a limbal incision. The advantage of avoiding an incision through the pars plana is somewhat offset by the increased possibility of dislocating the implant and the lessened freedom of maneuvers behind the implant. When properly performed, this technique rarely damages or dislocates the implant.

In summary, a discission is recommended for thin, postlental membranes and a membranectomy with a vitrectomy instrument for thick membranes.

Another satisfactory procedure is to use a scalp vein infusion needle connected to a bottle of Ringer's lactate to keep the anterior chamber inflated. A stab wound with a knife needle is made at the limbus. A fine spatula is inserted into the anterior chamber, passed beneath the optic portion of the implant, and used to gently separate iris-capsular adhesions. The secondary membrane may then be handled in one of two ways. A 27-gauge disposable needle with a bent tip enters the limbal incision and tears an opening in the membrane. This may be facilitated by passing a knife needle into the anterior chamber from the opposite limbus and gently lifting the membrane so that is may be split more easily with the first instrument. This can also be accomplished with two knife needles (p. 487). These procedures are best performed with all the prepupillary implants but with great difficulty with the Copeland iris-plane implant.

6. Retinal detachment. Fortunately, with im-

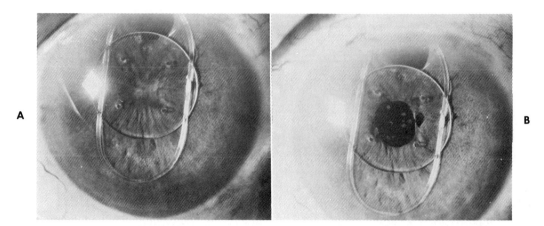

Fig. 5-64. A, Dense retrolental membrane in patient who suffered hypopyon uveitis 3 days after intracapsular cataract extraction and implantation of Binkhorst iris-clip lens. (Visual acuity = hand motion at 1 foot.) **B,** Membrane and anterior vitreous removed with Douvas Roto-Extractor. Pupil reshaped. Visual acuity 4 months later was 20/40. (From Jaffe, N. S.: Psuedophakos, St. Louis, 1978, The C. V. Mosby Co.)

proved methods of examining the fundus, a satisfactory examination is usually possible. However, reattachment of the retina may be more difficult with than without an implant because of an undilatable pupil, optic distortion from metal loops, and optic discontinuity between the implant and the aphakic portion of the dilated pupil. Moreover, a dense intraocular lens membrane or a dense secondary membrane is a serious obstacle to satisfactory localization of retinal breaks. These obstacles may be eliminated at the time of retinal surgery by the methods just discussed. In spite of these obstacles, most recent reports indicate that there is little difference in the reattachment rates between aphakic and pseudophakic retinal detachments. However, these same reports show poorer visual acuity after surgery for pseudophakic detachments. This is probably due to the higher incidence of massive preretinal proliferation (MPP) in pseudophakic eyes.

Late complications

1. Secondary cataract. This has been described.

2. Intraocular lens membrane (Figs. 5-65 and 5-66). This appears to be more common with the iris-plane lens, since this implant lies closer to the vitreous face. Vitreous may contact the posterior surface of the optic portion of the implant and proliferate on the surface. The iris may migrate over the back or front of the implant. Recurrent iritis may also cause such a membrane. Retained lens remnants may do likewise, but this possibility tends to lessen with time.

3. Opacification of the anterior face of the vitreous. This usually results from a severe hyphema or recurrent iritis. If it interferes with vision, it can be incised as in performing a discission of a secondary membrane. It may also be managed by a trans pars plana anterior vitrectomy, as previously mentioned.

4. Cystoid macular edema. This may appear some years after implantation for no apparent reason.

5. Corneal edema. This complication has become far less frequent than in the days of anterior chamber angle implants. It may occur due to intermittent contact between the anterior loops of the implant or the optic portion and the cornea (Fig. 5-67). It is theoretically possible for this condition to result from degradation of the plastic implant, although this has never been proven. It is more likely to result from senescent corneal degeneration, especially in eyes with endothelial abnormalities. It may follow repeated attacks of iritis, especially with secondary glaucoma. If mild, localized corneal edema results from a defective or malformed loop support touching

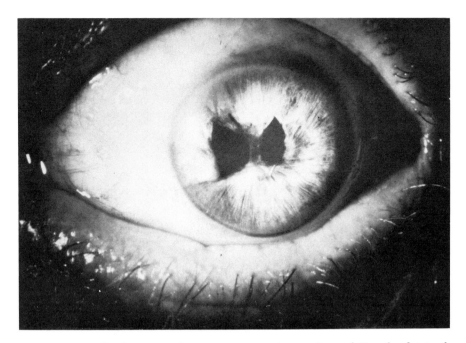

Fig. 5-65. Intraocular lens membrane over posterior surface of Copeland iris-plane implant.

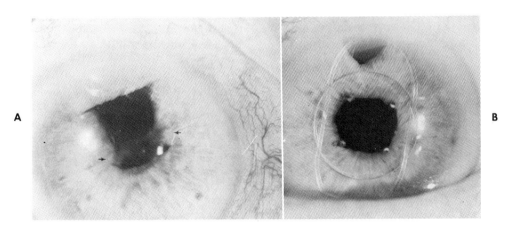

Fig. 5-66. A, Right eye of patient 6.5 years after implantation of Copeland lens. Note membrane *(arrows).* (Visual acuity = 20/25.) **B,** Left eye of same patient 6 months after implantation of Binkhorst iris-clip lens. Pupil is dilatable. (Visual acuity = 20/25.) (From Jaffe, N. S.: Pseudophakos, St. Louis, 1978, The C. V. Mosby Co.)

the cornea, the situation should be corrected immediately. Procrastination in this situation usually leads to total corneal edema. The defective loop may be excised (Fig. 5-68). In irreversible corneal edema, the only treatment for visual restoration is a penetrating keratoplasty. This usually has a favorable prognosis, since the im-plant prevents the vitreous from contacting the cornea.

Postoperative corneal edema is not restricted to implant surgery; it has also been a significant complication of both intracapsular and extracapsular cataract extraction without lens implanta-tion. Nevertheless, from the inception of lens

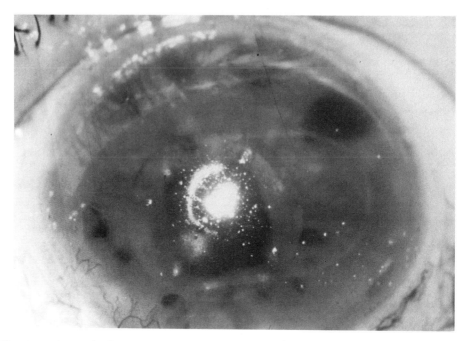

Fig. 5-67. Corneal edema in old style Binkhorst 4-loop iris-clip implant. There was intermittent contact between periphery of haptic loop and cornea.

implant surgery, corneal edema has been the most dreaded complication related to the surgery and the one most responsible for the seemingly endless number of changes in implant design and techniques of surgery.

It would be illogical to assume that corneal edema is merely a sign of senescence and that the surgery is just a minimal cause. If one were to compare a large population of patients with clinically normal corneas who have never had cataract surgery with an equal number of patients with normal corneas who have had cataract surgery, one would expect to find a higher incidence of corneal edema in the latter group at a particular age level. One relates this directly to the trauma of surgery and the alteration in the intraocular morphology. For example, some patients have unusually traumatic surgery and some have problems related to a particular postoperative occurrence such as vitreocorneal adherence. The eye that has never had surgery has not been exposed to these events. Carrying this logic further, it would appear justified to anticipate a higher incidence of corneal edema after lens implant surgery than after routine cataract extraction. The reason for this is simple. Implant surgery begins

where routine cataract surgery ends. Even the most skillful insertion of an intraocular lens involves an additional number of surgical manipulations not required in a routine cataract extraction. In addition, there are a number of postoperative complications related specifically to the implant, and these probably outweigh those that are not seen after implant surgery, for example, corneal edema due to vitreocorneal adherence.

In general, one might expect lens implant surgery rather than conventional cataract surgery more likely to be followed by corneal edema for the following reasons:

1. Improper selection of cases (for example, preexisting corneal disease, severe diabetes)
2. Greater risk of operative and postoperative endothelial damage
3. Use of a badly designed implant that can make contact with the cornea (Fig. 5-68)
4. Toxic influence of degenerative products of the implant, although this has never been demonstrated

Probably the single most important factor causing corneal edema after lens implant surgery (or after any intraocular surgery) is a lowered en-

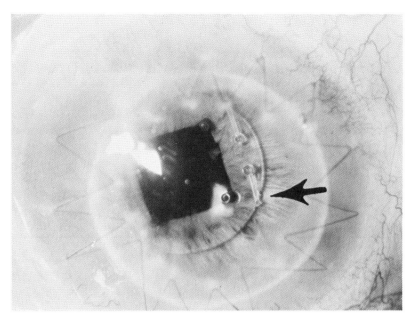

Fig. 5-68. Corneal edema, resulting from contact of lower loop of Fyodorov-Binkhorst implant with cornea. Penetrating keratoplasty and amputation of loop *(arrow)* performed. (From Jaffe, N. S.: Pseudophakos, St. Louis, 1978, The C. V. Mosby Co.)

dothelial vitality. This term appears nebulous only because we do not yet possess reliable clinical means of grading corneal endothelial health. The slit lamp is of some help in pointing out certain degenerative changes such as cornea guttata, but is of little help when the cornea appears normal. It has been shown that endothelial cell population decreases with age, but until recently there have been no reliable clinical indicators of this. Pachymetry is occasionally useful but is probably not yet a significant tool. Specular microscopy of the endothelial cells holds far greater promise (discussed later), but its widespread use will certainly require some time.

Endothelial vitality varies greatly among individuals, which leads one to suspect that it might be inborn. Note how susceptible some eyes are to corneal edema after minor trauma such as a simple needling or during an attack of iritis. Some eyes show a strong tendency to striate keratopathy or edema of the wound margins. In this there is a strong tendency to bilaterality. This is a warning that endothelial vitality has exceeded its critical level of decompensation. On the other hand, some corneas fare remarkably well after the most difficult surgical procedures. That there

are individual differences in endothelial vitality is certain, on the basis of clinical experience. This probably explains why some eyes develop persistent corneal edema immediately after surgery, whereas others do not develop it for many years, although its origin is the surgery itself. There is no such thing as atraumatic surgery; trauma is merely a matter of degree. Every eye subjected to a cataract extraction suffers some damage from instruments, retraction of the cornea, inflammation, toxic and mechanical effects of intraocular solutions and medications, alterations of intraocular pressure (high and low), and so on. Conditions occur immediately following the surgery that favor decreased endothelial vitality. A certain amount of iritis is inevitable. The intraocular pressure may be elevated for several days. This may be due to the use of alpha-chymotrypsin or to the current tendency to tight wound closure. Epithelial corneal edema is frequent and may be due to these factors as well as to others. A wound leak or pupillary block associated with a flat or shallow anterior chamber may cause vitreocorneal or iridocorneal contact, which damages corneal endothelium. As stated previously, the response of the eyes of different individuals to these surgical and postoperative traumas vary. Even among those eyes that appear to make a complete clinical recovery, there will be marked differences in the residual endothelial cell population. It would be naive to consider that these corneas have resumed their preoperative health. That they have not is to be seen in eyes that develop an unexplained iritis months or years after surgery. In some there is an associated corneal edema, indicating endothelial decompensation, while in others there is no clinical evidence of corneal edema.

Binkhorst listed the following three causes as the most frequent etiologic factors (in nearly equal frequency) in a survey of intracapsular cataract extractions with a 4-loop implant: (1) low endothelial vitality before surgery, (2) surgical and postoperative complications, and (3) late contact of implant with cornea.

It is not difficult to accept that corneal edema may result from surgical trauma or postoperative problems. However, late corneal edema remains a problem in etiology, especially when there are no postoperative problems such as recurrent iritis, secondary glaucoma, or corneal contact. Such an example is illustrated in Fig. 5-69. Corneal edema occurred in this eye 6½ years after an uneventful intracapsular cataract extraction with implantation of a Copeland iris-plane lens. The postoperative course was entirely normal. Of interest is that pachymetry revealed a corneal thickness of 0.74 mm in this eye and 0.54 mm in the fellow eye. The latter showed no slitlamp evidence of corneal abnormality, although pachymetry suggested the possibility of lowered corneal vitality. Occurrences such as this have been observed after routine cataract extraction without implantation. However, when it occurs after lens implant surgery, the cause is usually related to poor behavior of the implant, in spite of no evidence to support this.

A recent attempt was made to explain the apparent higher incidence of late corneal edema after lens implant surgery as compared to routine cataract surgery. This was done with the aid of the specular microscope, which was used in 1968 for observing corneal endothelium in vitro and modified later for clinical examination of the human corneal endothelium in vivo. Using this technique, an extensive evaluation of the effect of cataract extraction and lens implantation on the central endothelial cell density is possible.

Forstot and co-workers[42] studied a series of patients operated on by one surgeon, Norman Jaffe

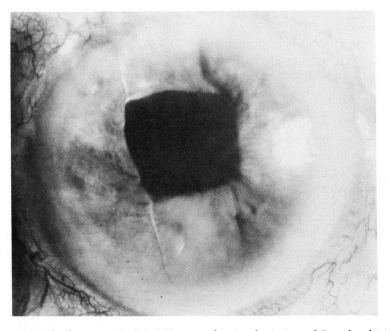

Fig. 5-69. Corneal edema, occurring 6.5 years after implantation of Copeland iris-plane lens. (From Jaffe, N. S.: Pseudophakos, St. Louis, 1978, The C. V. Mosby Co.)

(Fig. 5-70). All patients examined had clear corneas without edema or scarring. The 76 patients included in the study were divided into four groups.

Group I included 12 consecutive patients, studied prospectively, who had lens implantation after intracapsular cataract extractions. Preoperative and postoperative cell counts (measured 7 to 15 days postoperatively) were compared. Ten of these were uncomplicated. The average decrease in cell density preoperatively to postoperatively was 28.6%. One patient had a sterile hypopyon postoperatively that cleared; cell density was 57.6% less postoperatively (Fig. 5-71). A second patient had vitreous loss at surgery requiring an extensive sponge vitrectomy; cell density was 84.1% less postoperatively. Overall the decrease in cell density in this prospective group was 35.7%. Group IA was a similar prospective study of five additional consecutive patients undergoing intracapsular cataract extraction without lens implantation; the average decrease in cell density was only 8%.

Group II consisted of 38 monocular pseudophakic patients studied retrospectively. All cell counts of pseudophakic eyes were compared to those of the unoperated phakic fellow eye. These patients were subdivided into groups by lens type. There were five patients with a Copeland iris-plane lens inserted following intracapsular cataract extraction. The time from surgery varied from 3 to 7 years. The average cell density was 47.9% less in the implant eye. Nine patients had a Binkhorst 2-loop implant inserted following planned, conventional extracapsular cataract extraction. The time from surgery varied from 7 months to 4 years. The average cell density was 47.5% less in the implant eye. Twenty-one patients with Binkhorst 4-loop implants inserted after an intracapsular cataract extraction, the time from surgery varying from 1 week to 15 months, had a cell density in the implant eye averaging 43.5% less than in the fellow eye. One patient had a Fyodorov-Binkhorst lens implanted after an intracapsular cataract extraction 2.5 years previously; the difference in cell count was 84.1%. Two unilaterally pseudophakic patients with Binkhorst 4-loop lenses had postoperative dislocations. One patient's lens was repositioned pharmacologically. The difference in cell count between his unoperated and implant eye was 54.5%. The second patient required surgical repositioning and had 72.2% less cells in the implant eye than in the unoperated eye. An analy-

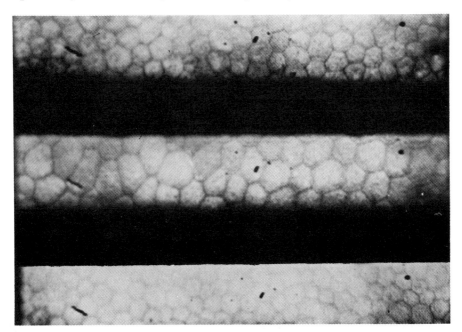

Fig. 5-70. Specular microphotograph. *Upper*, Endothelial cells in eye of 21-year-old woman. *Middle*, Endothelial cells in eye of 79-year-old woman 4 years after uneventful intracapsular cataract extraction. *Lower*, Endotheilal cells in opposite, unoperated eye of same 79-year-old woman. (From Jaffe, N. S.: Pseudophakos, St. Louis, 1978, The C. V. Mosby Co.)

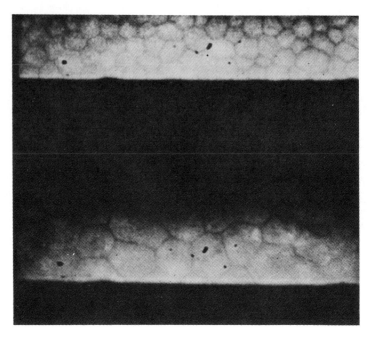

Fig. 5-71. *Upper,* Endothelial cells in 81-year-old man preoperatively. *Lower,* Same eye 11 days after implantation of Binkhorst iris-clip lens. Hypopyon uveitis occurred on second postoperative day. This cleared with aid of steroid therapy. (From Jaffe, N. S.: Pseudophakos, St. Louis, 1978, The C. V. Mosby Co.)

sis was performed to determine any correlation between the percent differences in cell density (unoperated eye and implant eye) and the time from surgery (1 week to 7 years) in the 36 uneventful implant procedures. There was no correlation to indicate progressive endothelial damage.

Group III was a study of eight patients, comparing a standard uneventful cataract extraction in one eye with an uneventful intracapsular cataract extraction with an implant in the fellow eye. There were six patients with Copeland iris-plane lenses and two with Binkhorst 4-loop lenses. All implant eyes had less cells (six of eight had significantly less cells). The average difference in cell density was 41.4%.

Group IV retrospectively compared the eyes of seven bilaterally aphakic patients to those of eight bilaterally pseudophakic patients. Of the bilaterally pseudophakic patients, two had an iris-plane lens in one eye and a Binkhorst 4-loop lens in the fellow eye, and one had an iris-plane lens in one eye and a Binkhorst 2-loop lens in the fellow eye. The average cell count for aphakic eyes was 1882 cells per square millimeter. The

average cell count in the pseudophakic eyes was 1078 cells per square millimeter. The difference between these average cell counts was 42.7%.

This study is not represented as a statistical analysis, but the trend of the results is overwhelming. The most obvious conclusion is that an intraocular lens implantation procedure is more traumatic to the corneal endothelium than an uneventful cataract extraction. A striking similarity was observed in the monocular pseudophakic series. Comparing three lenses (iris-plane, Binkhorst 2-loop, and Binkhorst 4-loop), the average difference in cell count between phakic unoperated and pseudophakic eyes was 47.9%, 47.5%, and 43.5%.

The cell loss associated with lens implantation is probably related to several factors. The first, and probably most obvious, is contact between the intraocular lens and the cornea, however brief this contact might be. A second factor is the increased manipulation required by this procedure. Folding of the cornea occurs with routine cataract extraction but is greater with lens implantation. In the case of the Binkhorst 4-loop lens the cornea must be retracted for placement of the transiridectomy suture. In addition, there is more drug use. In this series, alpha-chymotrypsin was always used with the intraocular lens implantations (except in extracapsular extraction), and acetylcholine was used to constrict the pupil. There was also more use of irrigating solutions, greater with extracapsular extractions. It is by no means clear at this time which of these factors may be the most significant contributor to cell loss, but the endothelial microscope should make it possible to define the roles of these separate maneuvers.

The data also suggest that the lens itself appears to cause no further endothelial damage or cell loss with time once it is implanted. Analysis of cell loss versus time from surgery (1 week to 7 years) in the monocular pseudophakic patient group showed no greater comparative loss with time. This evidence is not as conclusive as consecutive measurements on the same patient over many years, but it does provide evidence for good tolerance of the lens by the eye following the surgical procedure. Further cell loss probably does occur with intraocular inflammation or mechanical trauma (lens dislocation).

Cell counts in the implant eyes varied from 2900 to 380 cells per square millimeter. In all eyes the corneas were clear and without edema. This clearly indicates that eyes can tolerate the procedure well and corneas can remain clear with significant reductions in endothelial cell numbers. As yet the minimum number of central endothelial cells per square millimeter required to maintain corneal dehydration cannot be determined. Eyes with less cells, however, may be more susceptible to corneal edema due to inflammation or trauma; the possible effect of further cell death with age is unknown.

This study should not serve as an incrimination of the intraocular lens implant procedure. At the outset, it was stated that it is only logical to anticipate a higher incidence of corneal edema after lens implant surgery than after routine cataract surgery simply because there are greater manipulations required in the former. The study tends to point to endothelial cell damage at the time of surgery, rather than to toxic degradation of the implant, as the principal cause of late corneal edema. However, the study serves as a challenge

to all implant surgeons. Every step of the operation must be guided by the most fundamental principle of surgery, minimal trauma. Assiduous attention to details such as avoidance of corneal endothelial contact, minimal folding back of the cornea, less irrigation, better irrigating solutions, less intracameral drugs, and so on will protect the cornea against undue trauma. In the meantime, it appears justified to assume a conservative approach to surgical indications, since, as shown, the cornea may not show clinical evidence of degeneration in spite of lowered endothelial vitality. It is possible that as the patients age, any further loss of cells may be enough to result in corneal edema.

Returning to Binkhorst's three most frequent causes of corneal edema (p. 174) — low endothelial vitality, surgical and postoperative complications, and late contact of implant with cornea — only the last requires further comment. Contact between the optic portion of the implant and the cornea can only result from some abnormality in anterior chamber depth such as wound leak, pupillary block, and so on. If this is not corrected rapidly, corneal edema will inevitably result. More insidious is intermittent contact between the haptic supports of the implant and the cornea. Since the contact is usually made with the periphery of the cornea and is intermittent, the edema may not appear until quite late in the postoperative course. A portion of the blame rests directly with improper implant design and a portion with improper methods of implantation.

A good illustration of this is seen if one follows the evolution of the Binkhorst implant. Both the implant design and the method of implantation were occasionally at fault. Early designs of the 4-loop iris-clip lens included anterior loops that measured only 7.5 to 8.0 mm. Suture fixation was unknown at that time. The result was a high incidence of dislocations. Therefore the length of the anterior loops was increased to 8.5 to 9.0 mm. This caused fewer dislocations but increased the incidence of corneal edema because of loop contact with the periphery of the cornea. Another unfavorable element appeared to be that the loops were placed in a horizontal position. Since horizontal ocular rotations predominate over movements in other directions, the possibility of intermittent corneal contact became more than theoretical. To lessen the chance of corneal edema due to loop contact, the length of the anterior loops was shortened again to 7.5 to 8.0 mm, the anterior and posterior loops were angled posteriorly 10 to 15 degrees, and the implant was inserted in a vertical position. To prevent dislocation, a method of secure fixation was adopted. The transiridectomy suture is discussed on p. 143. The current implant design and method of insertion are likely to result in a far lessened tendency to corneal contact.

It was further reasoned that an implant without loops in the anterior chamber would lessen the possibility of corneal edema due to corneal contact. This is partly (not wholly) responsible for the genesis of the Binkhorst 2-loop iridocapsular implant and the Worst 2-loop Medallion implant. Support for this concept usually cites the research of Nordlohne, who ingeniously measured the depth of the anterior chamber with the patient prone and supine. Comparing the Binkhorst 4-loop and 2-loop implants, he observed that the anterior chamber was shallower by only 0.12 mm with the former when the patient lay flat on his face. The validity of these findings in incriminating loop contact remains speculative with cur-

rently designed implants. No one would argue with this thesis if the loops are too long or if they are defective in manufacture so that they bend anteriorly.

One might safely conclude from this discussion that the most important causes of corneal edema resulting from implant surgery are lowered endothelial vitality and surgical trauma to the endothelial cells of the cornea. Because of greater manipulation than during routine cataract extraction without an implant, a decreased endothelial cell population may result. The cornea may decompensate much later due to age senescence or other intraocular complications. In irreversible corneal edema the only treatment for visual restoration is a penetrating keratoplasty (Fig. 5-72). This usually has a favorable prognosis, since the implant prevents the vitreous from contacting the cornea.

6. Retinal detachment. This may occur as a late complication and is managed in the same manner as after routine cataract extraction.

7. Hyphema. A minihyphema is occasionally seen and is easily confused with an iritis. I have seen it most often with the iris-plane implant. The dense adhesions that form at the apices of

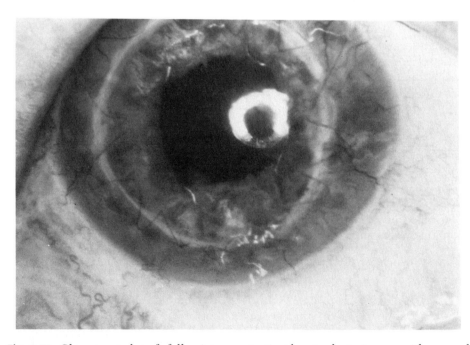

Fig. 5-72. Clear corneal graft following penetrating keratoplasty in eye with corneal edema following implantation of Copeland iris-plane implant.

the square pupil may vascularize. The action of strong light on the pupil may cause a rupture of one of these vessels. The patient complains of blurred vision that may persist for hours or days. There is no effective treatment. Hyphema, occasionally seen with anterior chamber angle-supported implants, is usually associated with uveitis and secondary glaucoma. Ellingson[43] was the first to describe it. The cause of it appears to be defective manufacture of the implant; warpage of the feet of the implant and sharp edges of the implant have been implicated.

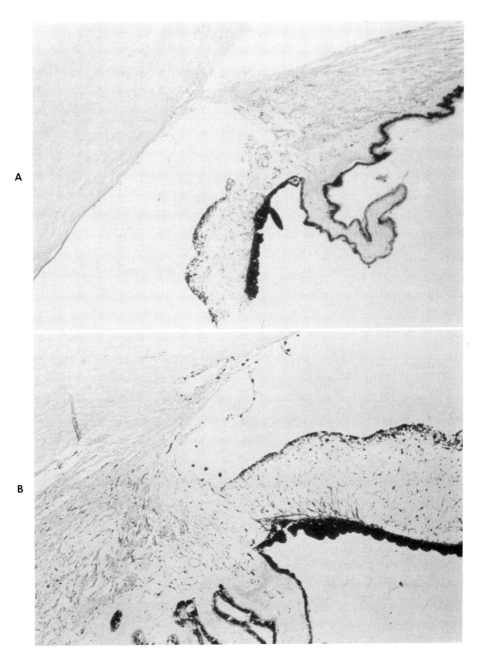

Fig. 5-73. A, Postmortem eye of 81-year-old woman who died 1 year after insertion of Copeland iris-plane implant. Note lack of inflammation in upper angle. **B,** Lower angle of same eye.

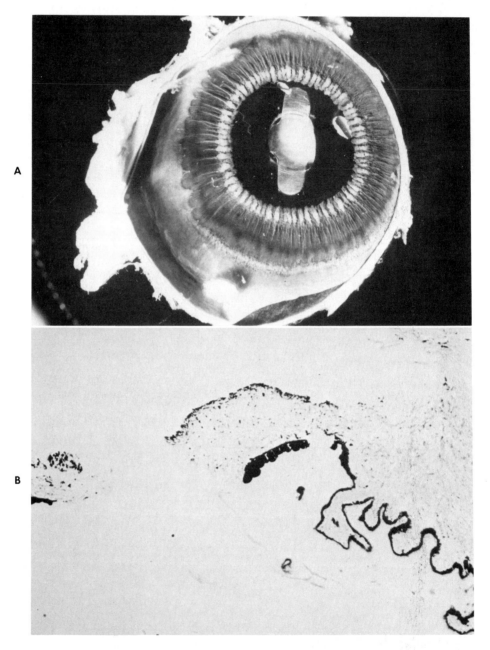

Fig. 5-74. A, Postmortem eye of 63-year-old man who died 7 months after insertion of Copeland iris-plane implant. Note optic portion of implant in pupillary space and two solid haptic supports behind iris in vertical position. **B,** Upper angle in area of iridectomy in same eye. **C,** Lower angle of same eye. Note remarkable lack of inflammation. **D,** Note flattening of pigment epithelium of iris in same eye where haptic support made contact behind iris.

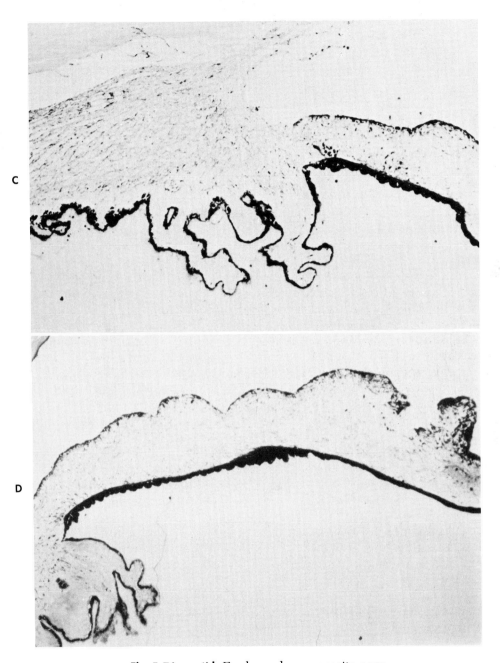

Fig. 5-74, cont'd. For legend see opposite page.

Postmortem findings

It would be useful to obtain postmortem specimens of eyes containing intraocular lenses. At
this time, I have two such specimens (Figs. 5-73
and 5-74) with Copeland iris-plane implants.
They show a remarkable lack of inflammation.
The only pathologic finding is a flattening of the
pigment epithelium of the iris where contact is
made with the haptic portion of the pseudophakos. Atrophy of the iris sphincter also occurs
where the pupillary margin makes contact with
the supporting loops of the Binkhorst, Worst, and
Federov implants.

CURRENT STATUS*

Thirty-one years have passed since Ridley
implanted his first intraocular lens. Thirteen
years have passed since I implanted my first intraocular lens, an experience initiating more than
4000 lens implantations. Nonetheless, even the
most enthusiastic advocate of this procedure
would agree that it has polarized the American
ophthalmic community like nothing else in recent memory. The intraocular implant lens was
born in controversy, has been controversial, and
remains controversial.

An attempt is made here to depolarize current
positions by presenting a reasonable list of advantages and disadvantages of the intraocular
implant lens and by presenting a current position
on the subject. This is done with the full realization that no single person can speak authoritatively for a huge community of ophthalmologists
and with the further understanding that progress
is so dynamic that today's vogue may be tomor-
row's obsolescence. However, it may be possible
to place the intraocular implant lens in reasonable perspective and gain acceptance for it in the
broad spectrum of American ophthalmology.
Objectivity based on experience should guide
future positions on lens implantation.

The following statements are those of one
ophthalmologist and are not intended to reflect
unfavorably on the positions of others.

Advantages of the intraocular implant lens

1. In uncomplicated cases, the quality of vision far exceeds that of a routine cataract extraction corrected with spectacles.

---

*This discussion is modified from Jaffe, N. S.: Ophthalmology
(Rochester) **85**:52-58, 1978.

Image-size magnification is virtually eliminated, spatial disorientation is nonexistent, pincushion distortion is absent, and there is no restriction of the peripheral visual fields. The vision of
the pseudophakic eye resembles that of the normal phakic eye more closely than vision with any
other method of optic correction of aphakia. In
addition, constant adjustment of aphakic spectacles is eliminated. None of the adverse effects of
aphakic spectacles on the patient's coordination
in simple manual tasks and mobility are apparent
in pseudophakia.

2. For those unable to manage a contact lens
(the elderly, arthritics, those with parkinsonism,
hemiplegics, the mentally retarded), intraocular
implant lens surgery is often the procedure of
choice.

When cataract extraction is indicated in patients with a unilateral cataract, an intraocular
lens is the best solution for those who are unlikely to succeed with a contact lens. This applies
particularly to elderly, infirm, and mentally incompetent patients. The younger, healthy patient is a suitable candidate for a contact lens.

3. In an elderly patient with bilateral cataracts,
unilateral intraocular implant lens surgery may
be adequate for the patient's needs.

Elderly and infirm patients often manage well
with an intraocular lens in one eye. This is far
superior to a unilateral aphakic spectacle after
routine cataract surgery in one eye. Some patients require binocular vision. This may be accomplished with a contact lens in one eye and an
intraocular lens in the other. A reasonable alternative is bilateral routine cataract extraction with
spectacles for both eyes. Only time will tell if
bilateral lens implantation in the younger,
healthy patient, even with a suitable interval between operations, is justified. However, if a single operation with an intraocular lens can meet
the needs of an elderly patient, that is a definite
argument for the procedure.

4. The patient with a successfully implanted
intraocular lens in one eye usually is more mobile than a patient who is bilaterally aphakic and
wears spectacles.

This is an advantage attested to by thousands
of patients who have undergone intraocular lens
implantation. Contact lenses became popular for
aphakic patients because of the disadvantages of
spectacles. Intraocular lenses became popular

because of disadvantages with both contact lens and spectacle lens correction of aphakia. In retirement communities where a high number of aphakic patients live close together, it is readily apparent that the patients with intraocular lenses and contact lenses (when they can be successfully managed) are more mobile than those wearing aphakic spectacles. The psychologic adjustment to aphakia has been considerably eased by the intraocular implant lens.

5. Long-wear contact lenses are still unproved.

Although claims have been made for several years that long-wear contact lenses will replace the intraocular lens, we are no closer to this realization than we were 5 years ago. Long-wear contact lenses are successful in a significant number of patients, but problems still arise in an unacceptably high number of patients. Unfortunately, if cataract extraction is performed with the expectation that a contact lens will be worn, failure to manage a contact lens is highly disappointing. The options facing the patient—no correction for the aphakic eye, a cataract spectacle with a balance lens for the opposite eye, or a secondary implantation of an intraocular lens—are less satisfactory than the primary implantation of an intraocular lens.

Disadvantages of the intraocular implant lens

1. The operation is technically more difficult than a routine cataract extraction.

This should be readily apparent, since the process of lens implantation commences where the routine cataract extraction ends. It requires a high degree of skill and judgment. Whether one prefers an intracapsular or an extracapsular cataract extraction, a bulging vitreous without actual vitreous loss is not a serious problem so long as lens implantation is not planned. However, one can imagine the danger to the corneal endothelium and the anterior hyaloid membrane if an implant is inserted. Techniques are available to safely implant a lens in such a situation, but they require intense training and extraordinary skill.

2. The rate of complications is therefore greater, although only slightly greater, with our present knowledge. This varies with the skill of the surgeon.

The additional intraocular maneuvers required in the implantation of an intraocular lens after the cataract is removed expose the corneal endothelium and anterior hyaloid membrane to greater risk of injury. The incidence of postoperative corneal edema and operative loss of vitreous is higher than after a routine cataract extraction. Skillful surgery can restrict this difference to a minimum. However, most reports indicate that endothelial cell population is reduced to a greater degree after lens implantation than after routine cataract operation and that, if vitreous loss occurs, there is a higher rate of cystoid macular edema and retinal detachment.

3. Some postoperative complications associated with both intraocular implant lens surgery and routine cataract extraction are more serious with the former, for example, flat or shallow anterior chamber and retinal detachment.

A flat or shallow anterior chamber after a routine cataract extraction, while not to be taken lightly, usually does not require urgent therapy. If this complication does not respond to observation or medical therapy over a period of days, minor surgical intervention usually corrects the problem. However, when an intraocular implant lens is in situ, this is a surgical emergency. Contact with the back of the cornea can easily result in permanent corneal decompensation. Immediate treatment of the cause of the anterior chamber depth abnormality is mandatory.

Some reports indicate that the rate of reattachment of the retina is the same whether or not an implant is present. Others contend that the rate of reattachment is lower in pseudophakia. However, there is little contention with the observation that visualizaton of the retina is more difficult with an implant in situ, since pupillary dilatation may be inadequate. It is made even more difficult if a posterior capsule or other lens remnants are present.

4. Closer follow-up care, both short and long term, is required, especially if we are to assess the risks and advantages of intraocular lenses.

Since a relatively large foreign body remains inside the eye, it becomes necessary to give the patient closer follow-up care than that given for a routine cataract extraction. This is both for the short and long term. The eye may show more early or late recurrent iritis. There may be evidence of intermittent contact between the cornea and a haptic support or even the optic portion of the implant. A subluxation of the implant may go unrecognized. Equally important from the point of view of close observation is the information that becomes available. These data are useful in assessing the risks and advantages of intraocular lenses both for short and long periods.

5. Colleague resistance. Complications are more severely criticized.

Because the intraocular implant lens is still controversial, criticism is often emotionally stimulated. Colleagues who elect not to perform lens implantation because they feel insecure with the surgery or unconvinced of its advantages tend to be more critical of the procedure. Complications that occur after lens implantation and routine cataract extraction such as retinal detachment, hyphema, and cystoid macular edema are often not judged impartially.

6. Dependence on quality manufacturing.

This is a significant disadvantage. An implant lens is placed inside the eye where it is intended to remain for a lifetime. The quality of the optics, the quality of the design, and the absolute assurance of the sterility of the implant are crucial. Breakdowns in quality have occurred in the past and will probably occur in the future. The eagerness of manufacturers to enter what they consider to be a lucrative market makes it difficult to police the traffic. This is a definite disadvantage of the intraocular implant lens.

Current position

1. Intraocular implant lens surgery should be performed only after adequate training.

The curriculum of every residency program in ophthalmology should include lens implant surgery and careful supervision of the resident ophthalmologist by an experienced lens implant surgeon. Supervisory personnel must accept this obligation with the realization that a great responsibility rests with them. It would be a disservice to permit less skilled surgeons to progress to lens implantation during their period of training. They should be discouraged from attempting this surgery. Courses for the graduate ophthalmologist must be upgraded. These courses must place the intraocular implant lens in perspective. Minimally, they should include instruction in the materials that constitute an implant, indications and contraindications for the surgery, surgical technique including animal laboratory experience, management of complications, and information concerning manufacturers and their products.

2. For less experienced surgeons, the initial indications should be extremely conservative.

The beginning implant surgeon will never regret a conservative start in lens implant surgery. Extremely elderly patients should be selected because of their shorter life expectancy and lesser tendency toward vitreous bulge after the cataract is extracted. Where extracapsular cataract surgery is planned, the procedures should not be overly complex. Difficult phacoemulsification procedures should be converted to a standard extracapsular method with a larger incision. Miotic pupils and eyes with anterior segment abnormalities should be avoided. There should be a logical progression to more complex procedures and cases, based on the surgeon's personal experience.

3. Surgery should be restricted to those patients not likely to manage a contact lens or those who refuse a contact lens.

Examples of such individuals have been cited earlier. Although the rate of complications is only slightly greater with lens implantation than with routine cataract surgery, it is the majority opinion that lens implantation is less safe. There are patients who would obviously be poor candidates for a contact lens and others who could reasonably be expected to manage a contact lens. Extended-wear contact lenses are an alternative to intraocular lenses, but their long-term safety is still unproved. In the final analysis, the decision whether the patient is a reasonably good candidate for a contact lens rests with the surgeon.

4. Intraocular lens surgery on both eyes within a short time is unacceptable.

Opinion is nearly equally divided about the acceptability of routine cataract extraction in both eyes within a week. Good arguments can be presented to support both points of view. The situation is different with intraocular lenses. Serious complications in both eyes of the patient are more difficult to correct in the case of intraocular lenses. It is difficult to define what one means by operating on two eyes close in time. In general, the time between operations in an elderly patient can be shorter than that for a younger patient. Once again, the standard for a reasonable interval between operations on both eyes must be established by the surgeon. However, most ophthalmologists would agree that operations close in time are unacceptable, based on present knowledge.

5. The patient's decision to undergo intraocular implant lens surgery should be based on a reasonably informed consent that includes the advantages and disadvantages of the procedure as well as alternatives.

The requirement for an informed consent by the patient is currently mandatory. However, even if this were not the case, the patient's decision to undergo lens implant surgery should not be based on unscientific information disseminated by the news media. The decision should be made only after a careful explanation of the advantages and disadvantages of the procedure as well as the advantages and disadvantages of alternative procedures. The surgeon must present this to the patient as objectively as possible in language the patient or his family can understand.

6. A surgeon who performs an adequate cataract extraction but feels insecure with the demands of intraocular implant lens surgery or is unconvinced of its benefits should not perform lens implantation.

It is ironic that it is now possible for a surgeon to be criticized for not implanting a lens in instances considered acceptable by a lens implant surgeon. It is certainly not in the patient's best interest for surgeons who consider lens implantation beyond their expertise to perform the surgery. Many ophthalmologists are unconvinced of its benefits. It would be improper for them not to be guided by their own experience and judgment. In fact, since lens implantation is still a controversial procedure, surgeons on both sides of the issue should respect each other's opinion and not confuse the patient by making unscientific remarks about the surgery. Implant surgeons must be especially respectful of their colleagues who do not do the operation, since the latter are often under pressure from patients who want the procedure. It would be unrealistic to expect full objectivity on both sides, but one can expect the advice afforded the patient to be based on an honest assessment of the procedure by a consulting surgeon.

7. There are still too many breakdowns in good manufacturing processes.

This has been discussed earlier. The implant surgeon must assume the role of watchdog over industry and should expect quality optics, quality design, and absolute assurance of sterility from the manufacturer. Breakdowns in quality should be reported to the American Intra-Ocular Implant Society, which has played a valuable role in the past in rapidly apprising its members of problems. The section on Medical Devices and Diagnostic Products of the Food and Drug Administration should be expected to monitor the manufacturer and his products. The lens implant surgeon should cooperate fully with this federal agency, whose role it is to protect the patient as well as the surgeon.

8. The long-range results are still uncertain. There is a need for well-documented retrospective studies.

The existing uncertainty about the long-range safety of the intraocular implant lens is a result of a paucity in the medical literature of well-documented retrospective studies of a particular implant procedure with a specific implant. Techniques and implants have changed frequently, making it difficult to assess the long-range safety and efficacy of a particular implant technique with a particular implant. Implant surgeons must be encouraged to collect data and report their long-term results. Patients cannot be promised what is not known.

9. The short-term safety is still controversial. There is a need for well-controlled prospective studies.

Most lens implant surgeons are convinced of the short-term safety and consider that the risk is only slightly greater than with a routine cataract extraction. Some lens implant surgeons and many nonimplant surgeons consider the risks to be significantly greater. This difference can be best resolved by well-controlled prospective studies. The National Eye Institute of the National Institutes of Health is ideally suited to conduct such studies.

10. It is inevitable that the current position will change in the future.

Progress is dynamic. The current position expressed here and the current position of others must be expected to change in the future. This change will be based on continued accumulation of experience in the field of lens implant surgery.

It is hoped that proponents of opposing points

of view can place the intraocular implant lens in reasonable perspective. This will help defuse the sometimes heated controversy over the procedure and insure an orderly and sequential growth of intraocular lens implantation.

REFERENCES

1. Ridley, H.: Intra-ocular acrylic lenses, Trans. Ophthalmol. Soc. U.K. **71**:617-621, 1951.
2. Baron, A.: Tolérance de l'oeil à la matière plastique. Prothèses optique cornéennes. Prothèses optique cristalliniennes, Bull. Soc. Ophthalmol. Paris **9**:982-988, 1953.
3. Strampelli, B.: Sopportabilità di lenti acriliche in camera anteriore nella afachia e nei vizi di refrazione, Ann. Ottal. **80**:75-82, 1954.
4. Strampelli, B.: Due anni di esperienza con le lenti camerulari, Atti Soc. Oftal. Ital. **15**:427-433, 1955.
5. Dannheim, H.: Vorderkamerlinse mit elastischen Halteschlingen, Ber. Dtsch. Ophthalmol. Ges. Heidelberg **60**:267-268, 1956.
6. Strampelli, B.: Fissazione di lenti camerulari mediante filo di supramid, Atti Soc. Oftal. Ital. **17**:669-682, 1957.
7. Strampelli, B.: Anterior chamber lenses, Arch. Ophthalmol. **66**:12-17, 1961.
8. Strampelli, B.: Anterior chamber lenses. In Fasanella, R. M., editor: Modern advances in cataract surgery, Philadelphia, 1963, J. B. Lippincott Co.
9. Strampelli, B., Marchi, W., and Valvo, A.: Lentine in camera anteriore con fissazione esterna (10 anni di esperienza clinica), Ann. Ottal. **94**:9-42, 1968.
10. Barraquer, J.: In Strampelli, B.: Complications de l'opération de Strampelli, L'Année Thérap. Clin. Ophthalmol. **9**:349-370, 1958.
11. Epstein, E.: Modified Ridley lenses, Br. J. Ophthalmol. **43**:29-33, 1959.
12. Binkhorst, C. D.: Iris-supported artificial pseudophakia. A new development in artificial intraocular lens surgery (iris clip lens), Trans. Ophthalmol. Soc. U.K. **79**:569-584, 1959.
13. Federov, S. N.: Application of intraocular pupillary lenses for aphakia correction (translation), Vestn. Oftalmol. **78**:76-83, 1965.
14. Federov, S. N. (in an interview): Scientific research in behalf of the medical practice (translation), Nauka i zjiznj (Science and Life) **8**:93-95, 1972.
15. Jaffe, N. S.: Current status of intraocular lenses, EENT Monthly **52**:290-296, 1972.
16. Jaffe, N. S., and Duffner, L. S.: The iris-plane (Copeland) pseudophakos, Arch. Ophthalmol. **94**:420-424, 1976.
17. Worst, J. G. F.: Over fixatie van de "Binkhorst-lens," Ned. Tijdschr. Geneeskd. **114**:489, 1970.
18. Binkhorst, C. D.: Praxis und Theorie der "iris klipp Linse" und der "irido-kapsular Linse." Sitzungsber. 125. Vers. Ver. Rhein.-WestfaL. Augenärzte Bonn. Balve/Sauerland, 1972, Grafischer Betr. Gebr. Zimmermann.
19. Binkhorst, C. D.: Perspektiven der Iris-Klipp-Linse und der Irido-Kapsularlinse, Klin. Monatsbl. Augenheilk. **161**:477-481, 1972.
20. Binkhorst, C. D.: The iridocapsular (two loop) lens and the iris clip (four loop) lens in pseudophakia, Ophthalmology (Rochester) **77**:589-617, 1973.
21. Nordlohne, M. E.: The intraocular implant lens, The Hague, 1975, Dr. W. Junk, p. 34.
22. Binkhorst, C. D., and Gobin, M. H. M. A.: Pseudophakia after lens injury in children, Ophthalmologica **154**:81-87, 1967.
23. Woods, A. C.: The adjustment to aphakia, Am. J. Ophthalmol. **35**:118-122, 1952.
24. McLemore, C. S.: Cadillacs, Volkswagens and aphakic corrections, Arch. Ophthalmol. **70**:734-735, 1963.
25. Welsh, R. C.: The roving ring scotoma with its Jack-in-the-box phenomenon of strong-plus (aphakic) spectacle lenses, Am. J. Ophthalmol. **51**:1277-1281, 1961.
26. Linksz, A.: Optical complications of aphakia. In Theodore, F. H., editor: Complications after cataract surgery, Boston, 1964, Little, Brown, and Co., pp. 597-534.
27. Welsh, R. C.: Experimental simulation of aphakia, Br. J. Ophthalmol. **49**:84-86, 1965.
28. Girard, L. J., et al.: Intraocular implants and contact lenses, Arch. Ophthalmol. **68**:762-775, 1962.
29. Binkhorst, C. D., and Gobin, M. H. M. A.: Injuries to the eye with lens opacity in young children, Ophthalmologica **148**:169-183, 1964.
30. van Balen, A. T. M.: Binkhorst's method of implantation of pseudophakoi in unilateral traumatic cataract, Ophthalmologica **165**:490-494, 1972.
31. Bierlaagh, J. J. M., et al.: Techniques and perspectives of lens implants (pseudophakoi) in children, Proceeding of Second International Orthoptics Congress Amsterdam (Int. Cong. Series No. 245), Amsterdam, 1971, Excerpta Medica Foundation.
32. Stenström, S.: Untersuchungen über die Variation und Kovariation der optischen Elemente des Menschlichen Auges, Acta Ophthalmol. (Suppl.) (Copenh.) **26**: 1946.
33. Sorsby, A.: Epidemiology of refraction, Int. Ophthalmol. Clin. **11**:1-18, 1971.
34. Binkhorst, R. D.: The optical design of intra-ocular lens implants, Ophthalmic Surg. **6**:17-31, 1975.
35. Colenbrander, M. C.: Calculation of the power of an iris clip lens for distance vision, Br. J. Ophthalmol. **57**:735-740, 1973.
36. Fyodorov, S. N., Galin, M. A., and Linksz, A.: Calculation of the optical power of intraocular lenses, Invest. Ophthalmol. **14**:625-628, Aug. 1975.
37. Binkhorst, C. D.: Power of the prepupillary pseudophakos, Br. J. Ophthalmol. **56**:332-337, 1972.
38. Duke-Elder, S.: System of ophthalmology. Vol. V. Ophthalmic optics and refraction, St. Louis, 1970, The C. V. Mosby Co., p. 119.
39. Jaffe, N. S., et al.: Pseudophakos, St. Louis, 1979, The C. V. Mosby Co., p. 122.
40. McCannel, M. A.: A retrievable suture idea for anterior uveal problems, Ophthalmic Surg. **7**:98-103, 1976.
41. The Miami Study Group: Cystoid macular edema in aphakic and pseudophakic eyes, Am. J. Ophthalmol. **88**:45-48, 1979.
42. Forstot, S. L., et al.: Effect of intraocular lens implantation on corneal endothelium, Ophtholmology (Rochester) **83**:OP195-203, 1977.
43. Ellingson, F. T.: Complications with the Choyce Mark VIII anterior chamber implant, J. Am. Intraocul. Implant Soc. **3**:199-201, 1977.

CHAPTER 6

Phacoemulsification

CHARLES D. KELMAN

Ophthalmologists the world over have worked on surgical techniques in cataract surgery until the procedure is probably the most refined, precise, safe, and successful surgical operation performed. The decades just past have produced tremendous advances in ophthalmology such as improved illumination and magnification with the use of the operating microscope, better anesthesia and akinesia, osmotic agents, enzymes, sharper needles, better sutures, and the use of cryoextraction.[1] With these advances the recuperation period for the patient has shortened from the almost total immobilization endured many years ago to a hospitalization of from 2 to 4 days followed by a 2- to 4-week recuperation period at home. The concern about wound dehiscence with its multiplicity of complications has prompted adherence to such a regimen. Variations of the size and plane of the corneal incision have been employed with varying success. In general the basic premise has been that a significantly smaller incision makes recuperation much shorter. I felt that a 1 to 2 mm incision could dramatically reduce the recuperative period, with all the attendant advantages to the patient.

Aspiration of cataracts in young people has been done for centuries. Scheie popularized the technique for congenital cataracts.[2] Others have done extensive work with congenital and traumatic cataracts.[3] The size of the incision fit the criterion for minimal incapacity, but the aspiration technique could not be applied to most adult and senile cataracts because the nucleus is a hard, insoluble protein.[4] Initial needling would not soften the nucleus sufficiently to make aspiration possible.

In 1963, with these problems in mind, I began to work on the possibility of transforming a mature cataract into a solution or an emulsion, thus making aspiration possible.[5]

Various methods were attempted in the earliest experiments. An encapsulating membrane was used to enclose the entire lens after dislocation with enzyme, with subsequent fragmentation by microdissectors within the membrane. The procedure proved too traumatic and often resulted in displacement of vitreous. Following this, rotary devices such as drills and microblenders were tried. It was soon discovered that with these devices the lens only rotated and was not emulsified, the iris was entrapped and disinserted, and eddy currents with lens particles in the anterior chamber denuded the corneal endothelium.

Slow-turning drills were designed to circumvent the rapidity of lens rotation, with little success. Sharp prongs were used in counterpuncture to impale the lens. However, manipulation was cumbersome, and the sharp points further endangered both the corneal endothelium and the posterior capsule of the lens. Low-frequency vibrators were tried. The iris was not disinserted, the lens, rather than being emulsified, merely vibrated with the tip, and the corneal endothelium was still damaged. Each of these devices was tried experimentally but was discarded as dangerous and ineffective. Through this trial and error method it became increasingly clear that, for the lens to remain stationary, the acceleration of the moving tip must be high enough not to overcome the standing inertia of the lens and that this could only be accomplished with an ultrasonic frequency. A dental ultrasonic unit with irrigation and a nonlongitudinal motion was used but was unsuccessful because of the high energy radiated. Additionally, iron filings were shed into the animal eyes. To correct these problems, a longitudinal movement was introduced, and the tip construction was changed from iron to titanium. Then, in addition to the irrigation and emulsification, suction was added, thus allowing fixation of the lens and withdrawal of the emulsate.[4]

After a step-by-step solution to each problem a workable prototype machine was used in 1966 in animal trials of phacoemulsification. The first operations on patients were performed in 1967. Further refinements in the handpiece, a silicone sleeve for the titanium needle, and a prototype flowmeter were developed during the following 2 years. Modifications in the equipment continued with the addition of an improved flowmeter and a nonultrasonic aspirator. The lastest Cavitron/Kelman phacoemulsifier embodies all the elements developed through the years, making possible the performance of this surgical procedure.

Three specific innovations constitute the originality of this work. First, the concept of using high-frequency vibrations to fragment and emulsify the lens; second, a highly refined logic system for aspiration and prevention of anterior chamber collapse; and third, the concept and technique of prolapsing the lens nucleus into the anterior chamber.[4]

INSTRUMENTATION

The present Cavitron/Kelman phacoemulsifier console is, then, the end result of years of trial and development. The console, in use since 1969, embodies all the necessary instrumentation for an effective procedure. The handpiece consists of a magneto-strictive ultrasonic mechanism that activates a hollow, 1 mm titanium needle covered with a soft silicone sleeve, which vibrates 40,000 times per second longitudinally in the axis of the needle. The stroke amplitude is 1/3000 of an inch in air and 1/1500 of an inch in fluid and develops an acceleration of 240,000 G

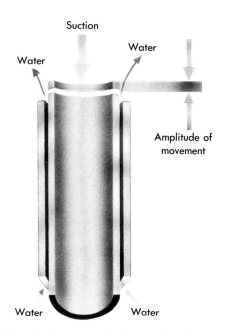

Fig. 6-1. Phacoemulsification handpiece.

at the tip. The mechanical vibration transforms the lens into an emulsion, hence the name phacoemulsification. Actually, while emulsification is occurring, other phenomena are also taking place. The soluble protein portion of the lens is dissolved in the irrigating fluid, which enters between the needle and the silicone sleeve at a given rate and pressure not to exceed 25 mm Hg (Fig. 6-1). Thus part of the lens is fragmented, part is suspended, and part is unaffected.[6] Excessive heat buildup is circumvented by the constant flow of the irrigating solution. Ultrasonic waves are not significantly transmitted to affect any other part of the eye.

The suction control system is extremely important. Irrigation and aspiration must be balanced. This has been accomplished by the introduction of a highly refined logic system with a constant-volume pump. Irrigating solution passes between the sleeve and the outer wall of the needle while suction is applied through the central, hollow portion, which emulsifies through its longitudinal action. Thus as the lens is held against the needle point by suction, irrigation and emulsification also occur at this point, producing all three functions necessary in the procedure. The logic system with its peristaltic pump, vent

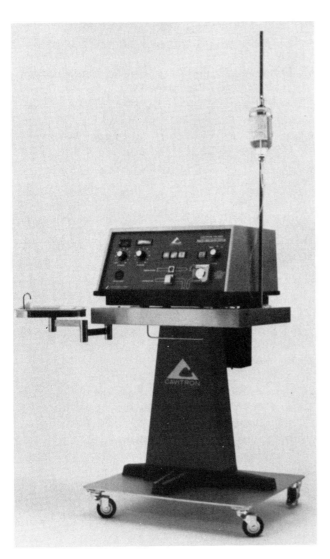

Fig. 6-2. Phaco-Emulsifier Aspirator. (Courtesy Cavitron Surgical Systems, Irvine, Calif.)

valves, and bypass valve prevents a collapse of the anterior chamber. The use of the older model machine required the constant assistance of a trained technician. The new console embodies all the essential elements refined to such a degree that a circulating nurse in the operating room can handle the necessary adjustments (Fig. 6-2).

A foot pedal activates each level of machine operation. Initial depression activates level I, which is for irrigation only; further depression of the pedal activates level II, which is for both irri-

gation and aspiration; total depression of the pedal activates level III, which adds ultrasonic emulsification to the existing irrigation and aspiration.

Three basic handpieces are now used: the first is an air cystotome, used to deepen the anterior chamber while at the same time performing an anterior capsulotomy and prolapsing the nucleus; the second is the basic unit for phacoemulsification; and the third is a special nonultrasonic aspirator and tip designed for cortical remnants.

TRAINING

By its very nature, ophthalmic surgery is a delicate, precise, and carefully learned discipline. As in every field, there are those whose natural dexterity gives them a facility in operating techniques that comes more slowly to others. However the training programs with their emphasis on patient, step-by-step learning procedures have produced in the ophthalmic community a large number of competent surgeons. Over the years, some decide to limit their activities to certain procedures. Surgery is an acquired art, honed to a fine edge through constant attention to detail and an appreciation of the delicate nature of the tissue involved. The ethical integrity of the individual ophthalmologist combined with the level of training often determines the nature of procedures. Cataract surgery in particular has developed dramatically. The addition of the cryo technique for intracapsular extractions has produced a high level of competence with a minimum of complications. However, it must be remembered that training is the key. Even those who feel highly skilled must continue to apply themselves. Phacoemulsification, with its proven efficacy and its advantages for the patient, is not an easy procedure, and it is for this reason that I insist on an intensive training program to learn the basic technique and continued practice on animal and eye bank eyes.

The procedure is difficult, and several factors contribute to this difficulty. First, the margin of error is small. Surgical judgment allowing for this margin of error is extremely important. One must develop a new set of rules, since what applies to cryoextraction will not necessarily apply here. Second, surgeons must develop a sixth sense about the equipment—they must learn to "hear" what the machine is doing. It is possible to determine, by feeling the vibrations of the tubing at the handpiece, whether there is an adequate stroke. An awareness of the technician's activities may give an indication of a properly or improperly functioning machine. Third, it is imperative that one develop a facility with the operating microscope, and some surgeons find this a drawback. Finally, the level of difficulty is often enhanced because this technique has been controversial and thus places added pressure on the surgeon.

Additionally, this procedure is a demanding one. Things do not always go the way they should, and the surgeon must learn to be in control of the situation. A tremor that may not interfere with an intracapsular extraction may be unacceptable. Certain precautions should be taken such as the avoidance of coffee, tea, or alcohol for at least 12 hours prior to performing surgery. Even a long drive just prior to surgery may increase the tremor.

The compounding of errors is one of the most serious problems. It is important to know the contraindications to the beginning or continuation of the procedure.

The surgeon must have excellent depth perception, good stereopsis, and perfect development of visual proprioceptive reflexes. Considerable patience is required, especially near the end of the procedure.

In spite of the problems, there are definite reasons for learning this technique. It is personally rewarding to know that one has mastered a difficult procedure. The patient emerges with a quiet eye and has complete mobilization, which is extremely important to a large number of patients. It is the easiest, most effective aspiration technique for children. In competent, well-trained hands there are now minimal complications. Finally, it is gratifying to the surgeon to have the approval of peers for having acquired this expertise.

My training course, which is 5 days in length, consists of a thorough indoctrination in the mechanics and use of the machine, didactic lectures on the history and development of the technique, and intensive instruction on the performance of the surgical procedure. Videotapes of interesting and difficult cases are shown, and open discussions are held to answer any questions concerning technique, pitfalls, and possible complications.

Each ophthalmologist has the opportunity to perform surgery on several cat eyes under basic operating room conditions. During the week, surgery on nine patients is observed, and careful postoperative evaluations are made. Further cat surgery is performed, and surgeons have the opportunity to see their surgical results. Lectures are also given on anesthesia, postoperative care, and the management of complicatons. It is an intensive course, designed to incorporate as much as possible into the 5-day period.

CASE SELECTION

There are many patients who are ideally suited for phacoemulsification.
1. A young patient with a capsular-hyaloid adhesion
2. Patients in whose eyes the anterior capsule is already ruptured
3. Active patients, young and old, who cannot afford to be away from their occupations
4. Elderly patients who must care for themselves

When surgeons, after their training course and subsequent repeated animal procedures or practice on eye bank eyes, feel confident in their ability to handle phacoemulsification, they should be keenly aware of the type of patient who is the ideal candidate for this procedure. Many factors are involved.

1. *Lens followability.* The direct ophthalmoscope or slit lamp may be used to evaluate the lens. The red reflex will give a definite indication as to the followability, or ability of the lens to be aspirated. This may be graded on a scale of +4 to 0 based on the density of the lens, with +4 having the greatest followability.

Congenital or traumatic cataracts may be gray with no red reflex, yet be quite followable. A hypermature lens in the older patient does not have a highly followable nucleus, and the capsule is so delicate that the posterior capsule may be easily ruptured.

2. *Pupillary dilatation.* This is one of the most important factors in patient selection. If the pupil will not dilate to at least 7 mm, do not attempt the procedure.

3. *State of the cornea.* Surgery on patients with endothelial problems should not be attempted until the surgeon has had at least 100 cases. As I have gained experience, I no longer consider cornea guttata a contraindication, since many patients with advanced cornea guttata have had successful operations without complications. However, phacoemulsification of these eyes should not be attempted until one has gained considerable expertise.

4. *Depth of the anterior chamber.* Again, at the outset of a surgeon's experience, patients with shallow anterior chambers and narrow angles should be avoided.

5. *Age of the patient.* As with other surgical or medical problems, the younger patient generally tolerates the procedure much better than does the older patient. Of course, in cataract surgery the older patient has the hard, brunescent lens, which is much more difficult. I have successfully emulsified brunescent lenses, but these cases should be avoided early in the surgeon's experience.

6. *Subluxated or dislocated lenses.* Although these lenses may be operated on successfully, they should be avoided at first.

7. *Emotional status of the patient.* In the use of a new technique the surgeon has enough to think about without adding to the pressure by having a nervous, highly emotional patient. These pa-tients tend to relate any complication to the technique employed. Do not compound the problem.

The first operation should be done under general anesthesia. Later the surgeon may choose to use local anesthesia in most cases. Caution must be exercised in early case selection. As one develops facility in the procedure, case selection may be expanded. Good surgical judgment must always be exercised. Perhaps the surgeon should even plan to convert the first 10 to 12 cases to a planned extracapsular extraction.

This is not to discourage the ophthalmologist from using this procedure, for its advantages outweigh the initial disadvantages, but to encourage the ophthalmologists to approach each case with a logical plan and to choose the ideal cases first. The greatest temptation, and the greatest threat, is to persist in phacoemulsification when the procedure should be converted. Learning the procedure well is worth the effort, since for many patients this may be the procedure of choice.

Technique

The patient is given mannitol, 1 g/kg of body weight, intravenously 1 hour prior to surgery. Dilatation is achieved by the following regimen:

Neo-Synephrine 10% is administered topically: 2 drops 2 hours before surgery, 2 drops 1 hour before surgery, and then at 5-minute inter-

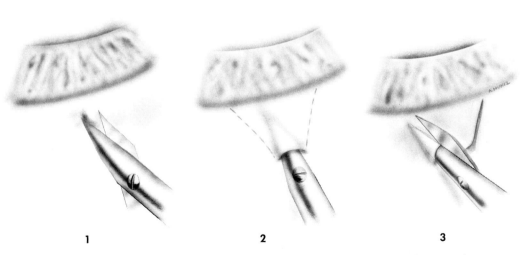

1   2   3

Fig. 6-3. Preparation of triangular limbus-based conjunctival flap, which serves for retraction and as valve to help keep air in anterior chamber.

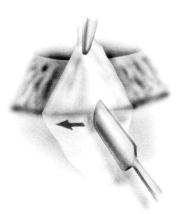

Fig. 6-4. Tooke knife being used to clean limbus.

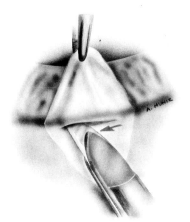

Fig. 6-5. Razor blade incision (3 mm) made at limbus.

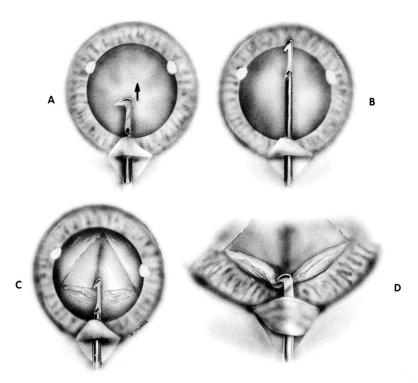

Fig. 6-6. A, Air cystotome is introduced into anterior chamber, and large air bubble is instilled. **B,** Cystotome extended to 6 o'clock position. **C,** Point of cystotome engages anterior capsule and is withdrawn superiorly, forming Christmas tree–shaped wedge of capsule. **D,** Apex of torn capsule being withdrawn to limbal wound.

vals until full mydriasis is achieved. Cyclopento-late hydrochloride (Cyclogyl, Alcon, Ft. Worth, Texas) is given in the same manner. Hyoscine 0.25%, 1 drop, is given on call to surgery.

A wire speculum is used for lid retraction. Soap is not used to prepare the patient, since it may cloud the cornea. Iodine is applied to the brows and lids. No intraocular infections have occurred in 1600 cases.

Use of the operating microscope with coaxial illumination is imperative, since without the microscope proper control of the procedure is impossible.

The superior rectus muscle is grasped with forceps, and a bridle suture is inserted 3 to 4 mm posterior to the muscle insertion. A triangular, limbus-based conjunctival flap is developed for retraction and as a valve to help keep air in the chamber (Fig. 6-3). A Tooke knife is helpful in cleaning the lumbus (Fig. 6-4). Light cautery achieves hemostasis. A 3 mm razor blade incision is made at the limbus with the sharp edge of the blade rather than the point (Fig. 6-5). The incision must be smooth to prevent the silicone sleeve from catching. If the incision is too near the cornea, instruments may touch the endothelium; if too far posterior, the sleeve will irritate the iris, and the root of the iris may ballon out during surgery, thus obstructing the flow of fluid. Further, if the incision is too large, fluid may leak out, making maintenance of the anterior chamber difficult. A small opening may compress the silicone sleeve and prohibit the inflow of irrigating solution.

The air cystotome is then introduced, and a large air bubble is instilled into the anterior chamber. The cystotome is extended to the 6 o'clock position; the point engages the anterior capsule and is withdrawn superiorly, forming a Christmas tree-shaped wedge of capsule (Fig. 6-6). The apex of the capsule is excised outside the globe, as shown in Fig. 6-7. The next procedure is perhaps the most important of the entire operation. The point of the cystotome engages the nucleus and through a vertical seesaw maneuver or, if necessary, a lateral seesaw, the nucleus is prolapsed into the anterior chamber (Fig. 6-8). At this point a definite decision must be made. If the pupil begins to constrict and if the nucleus cannot be prolapsed, the procedure must be converted.

The ultrasonic tip is then placed in the anterior chamber, and for the next 1 to 2 minutes the lens is emulsified and aspirated. Emulsification is performed either with a cartwheel approach, in which the tip is placed almost tangentially to the lens, or with the croissant technique, in which

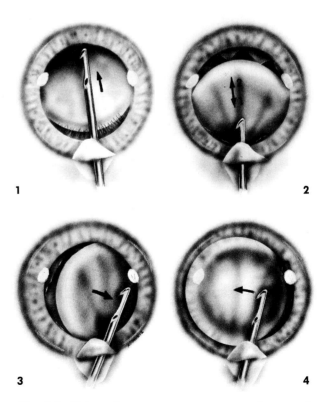

Fig. 6-8. Point of cystotome engages nucleus, and through vertical seesaw maneuver (or, if necessary, lateral seesaw), nucleus is prolapsed into anterior chamber.

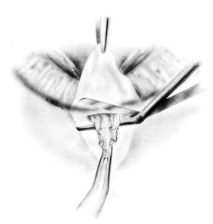

Fig. 6-7. Apex of capsule is excised outside globe.

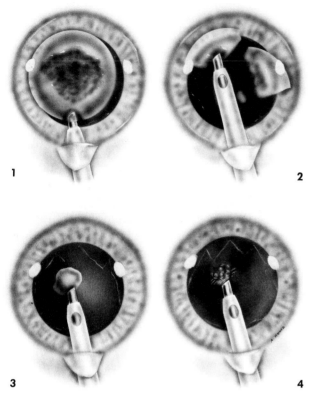

Fig. 6-9. Ultrasonic tip performing emulsification and aspiration.

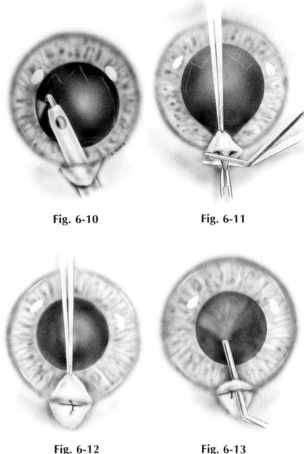

Fig. 6-10. Nonultrasonic tip is used with only irrigation and aspiration to clear out cortical remnants.
Fig. 6-11. Peripheral iridectomy.
Fig. 6-12. Incision closed with one suture.
Fig. 6-13. Air bubble instilled into anterior chamber after capsulotomy.

the central core is hollowed out (Fig. 6-9). The ultrasonic tip should be kept above the 3 to 9 o'clock position to prevent tumbling of the lens.

The nonultrasonic tip is then used with only irrigation and aspiration to clear out the cortical remnants (Fig. 6-10). In the last portion of the procedure the power should be cut down by at least 50% to prevent rupture of the posterior capsule.

A peripheral iridectomy is performed after acetylcholine solution is instilled into the anterior chamber (Fig. 6-11). The incision is then closed with one suture (Fig. 6-12).

A Zeigler knife is used to do a posterior capsulotomy in all patients under 65 years of age. The capsulotomy is performed by passing the knife through the incision. The knife, held flat, touches the posterior capsule, is turned 45 degrees, engages the capsule, is then turned to 90 degrees, and is swept from the 3 to the 9 o'clock position.

The capsule is actually ripped rather than cut. The knife is removed from the eye, and an air bubble is instilled into the anterior chamber (Fig. 6-13). Methylprednisolone sodium succinate (Solu-Medrol, Upjohn) is inserted under the conjunctiva, which is not sutured.

The following important surgical principles must be observed:

1. Any instrument in the anterior chamber should be supported by two hands.
2. The emulsifier tip should remain parallel to

the iris plane; if it must move, the tip should be pointed only slightly toward the cornea, not toward the posterior capsule.

3. If the procedure must be converted, the incision should be slightly more than 180 degrees.

4. The safest place to have the tip inside the eye is in the pupillary center—farther away from the cornea, the iris, and the posterior capsule.

It must be appreciated that this procedure is performed between two of the most delicate tissues in the body, the endothelium and the posterior capsule.

The possibility of converting the procedure must always be kept in mind. The following are specific indications:

1. The pupil does not dilate well.

2. Air cannot be kept in the anterior chamber.

3. The pupil constricts before the lens is in the anterior chamber.

4. The zonules are ruptured, and the lens is seen to be subluxed.

Phacoemulsification in the posterior chamber

The original phacoemulsifications, performed between 1967 and 1970, were all done in the posterior chamber. The difficulties with emulsification in the posterior chamber are as follows:

1. If the pupil constricts during the emulsification, as it often does, visibility of the lens is greatly reduced and the surgeon must perform a sector iridectomy, abandon emulsification in favor of a larger incision and a planned extracapsular extraction, try to redilate the pupil, or engage in the risky business of emulsifying a lens "blind," behind the small pupil.

2. The further the lens is from the cornea, the less acute the visualization is, especially if the cornea develops any stria or loss of epithelium during the surgery.

3. With the lens in the posterior chamber, the emulsifier is of necessity pointing down toward the lens and therefore toward the posterior capsule. As the emulsifier breaks through the lens, it can, and often will, engage and open the posterior capsule. With the lens in the anterior chamber, the emul-

sifier tip is pointing either parallel to the posterior capsule or slightly up toward the cornea, with much less danger of rupturing the capsule.

For these reasons, I abandoned emulsification in the posterior chamber except in young adults, in children, and in unusual circumstances. Techniques were developed for bringing the lens into the anterior chamber where it was more visible, less dependent on iris dilatation, and safer for the posterior capsule.

At this time, my feelings remain unchanged, especially regarding the surgeon who is a novice with the technique. For the surgeon who has done fewer than 100 phacoemulsifications in the anterior chamber, my advice is: When the lens cannot be brought into the anterior chamber for emulsification, open the incision 180 degrees and do a planned extracapsular extraction, with a sector iridectomy if necessary.

For the experienced surgeon, emulsification in the posterior chamber offers one theoretical advantage: the lens is brought less in contact with the corneal endothelium, and there is less chance of losing important endothelial cells. In theory, in careful endothelial cell counts, the experienced surgeon will find only about 10% or less of endothelial cell loss with emulsification in the anterior chamber, and this compares favorably to the percentage of cell loss in any other type of cataract extraction, including emulsification in the posterior chamber.

For those who are experienced and wish to perform posterior chamber emulsification, the technique is as follows:

1. After the anterior capsulotomy is performed, the phacoemulsifier rides along the anterior surface of the lens, forming deep grooves. Since the lens is held in place at this point by the zonules, this portion of the emulsification is quite easy. The surgeon leaves an inferior ridge of lens (Fig. 6-14) close to the 6 o'clock margin of the iris.

2. When the lens has been sculptured down to approximately half thickness, a spatula is introduced through a small lateral incision to press against the ridge of lens material, in effect prolapsing the upper border of the lens and exposing it to the emulsifier (Fig. 6-15).

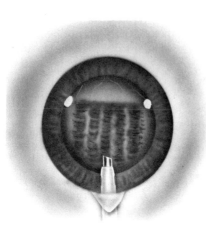

Fig. 6-14. Deep grooves formed along anterior surface of lens with phacoemulsifier. Inferior ridge of lens left close to 6 o'clock margin or iris.

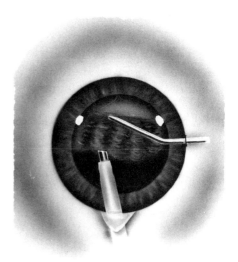

Fig. 6-15. Spatula introduced through small lateral incision to assist in prolapsing upper border of lens nucleus and exposing it to emulsifier.

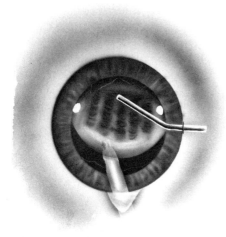

Fig. 6-16. Upper portion of nucleus is totally emulsified; lower portion is still held in place by inferior capsule.

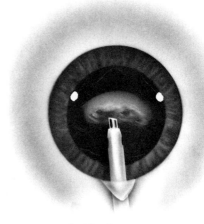

Fig. 6-17. Lower half of nucleus is spontaneously pulled out of capsule and engaged by phacoemulsifier.

3. With the spatula holding the lens in place, the upper portion of the lens is totally emulsified while the lower portion is still held in place by the inferior capsule (Fig. 6-16).
4. When the upper half of the lens is removed, the lower half of the lens will spontaneously be pulled out of the capsule and will come toward the phacoemulsifier. At this point the surgeon can remove the second instrument or use it to tap the lens gently toward the phacoemulsifier tip (Fig. 6-17).

Some surgeons prefer not to use a second instrument in the eye with posterior chamber emulsification; their technique is similar except that somewhat more of the lens is sculptured away (Fig. 6-18) until enough has been removed so that the lens will tumble into the chamber (Fig. 6-19).

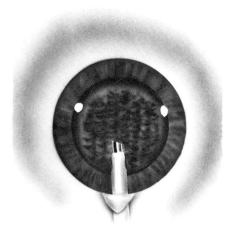

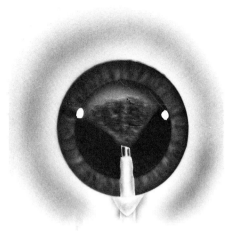

Fig. 6-18. Alternate technique not using spatula. More of nucleus is sculptured away than in spatula technique.

Fig. 6-19. Remaining nucleus tumbles into anterior chamber.

POSTOPERATIVE CARE

Postoperative care is always an important facet of surgery; however, in phacoemulsification the patient has a great advantage in that minimal postoperative care is needed. Postoperatively the eye is quiet, there is usually no photophobia, and there is little or no tearing or discomfort. The patient is allowed to return to full activity the day following surgery. This includes all types of work and physical activity.[6]

The patient is discharged on a regimen of Hyoscine 0.25% solution twice a day and Chloromycetin hydrocortisone four times a day. No patch is used, but a shield is worn at night for approximately 2 weeks to protect the eye.

The patient is examined the day of discharge and again in 1 week. If minimal striate keratitis is present, hypertonic sodium chloride (Murocoll No. 4, Muro) is added four times a day. If plaque edema or confluent areas of striate keratitis are present, hypertonic sodium chloride, topical steroids, and glycerine are added to detergesce the cornea. The eye need not be patched.

A contact lens, hard or soft, is usually prescribed in 3 weeks. Induced astigmatism is extremely low.[6]

COMPLICATIONS

Since the first phacoemulsification in 1967, the rate and severity of complications have decreased. With refinement of the instrumentation and the surgical technique, the contraindications and the complications have been minimized.

Cornea

Early in my experience, prolonged ultrasonic time and excessive manipulation produced 12 cases of striate keratitis that lasted from 2 to 3 weeks. At present, striate keratitis is rare and quite transient when it does occur. Permanent keratitis occurred in three of the early cases and in one of the latest. One, in a 76-year-old, was probably due to excessive intraocular manipulation. A severe preoperative case of cornea guttata progressed postoperatively, and in one case vitreous adhered to the cornea.

Vitreous adhesion to the wound

Along with the other advantages of a small incision, it is relatively simple to insert a spatula through a counterpuncture and sweep any vitreous strands that may touch the wound. Vitreous adhesions have been noted to occur in approximately 16% of uneventful intracapsular extractions, with a 7% incidence of peaked pupils.[7] Since the first 100 cases, the incidence of peaked pupils has been less than 1%.[8]

Glaucoma

Aphakic glaucoma has not been a problem except in one instance. In the last 400 patients followed for 6 months, glaucoma has not occurred.[6] A transient rise in intraocular pressure has occurred in approximately 5% of patients but has rarely lasted beyond 2 to 3 days.

Uveitis

Only one patient had a severe postoperative uveitis. This was followed by a retinal detachment. The retina was surgically reattached, and after detachment surgery the vision returned to 20/40. There have been no additional instances in the last 100 cases.

Opacification of the posterior capsule

It has been found that in patients over 65 years, opacities of the posterior capsule rarely occur. In patients under 25 years, almost 100% of the capsules opacity to some degree. In patients between 25 and 65 years, 20% of the eyes required discission. With these statistics in mind, a posterior capsulotomy is performed now on all patients under 65.

Retinal detachment

Retinal detachment has not been a significant problem in phacoemulsification. In the first 500 cases only five cases occurred, three of which were simple aphakic detachments. One patient had Marfan's syndrome, and another detachment occurred secondary to trauma.[8] In a series of 100 patients who have been followed for at least 6 months postoperatively, 12 cases of maculopathy occurred. One patient was diagnosed as having hypertension and leukemia and had a final visual acuity of 20/200. Myopic degeneration was present in two patients, both with final visual acuity of 20/40. Six cases of cystoid macular edema were recorded. Four patients had a final visual acuity of 20/20, one had 20/25, and one had 20/30.[6]

CONCLUSION

Since 1963 when phacoemulsification was an experimental project, it has progressed to the point that in experienced hands the results are better than the results of comparable intracapsular extractions. It is now possible to state that in the hands of a well-trained ophthalmic surgeon, the results are as good or better than the results of intracapsular extractions, although this of course would not be true if the technique were performed by a novice.

With its well-recognized advantages for the patient of a brief recuperative period and no physical restrictions, phacoemulsification has achieved its place in the ophthalmic armamentarium.

REFERENCES

1. Kelman, C. D.: Cataract emulsification and aspiration, Trans. Ophthalmol. Soc. U.K. **90:**13-22, 1970.
2. Scheie, H. G.: Aspiration of congenital or soft cataracts, Am. J. Ophthalmol. **50:**1048-1056, 1960.
3. Girard, L. J.: Aspiration-irrigation of congenital and traumatic cataracts, Arch. Ophthalmol. **77:**387-391, 1967.
4. Kelman, C. D.: Phaco-emulsification and aspiration of senile cataracts, Can. J. Ophthalmol. **8:**24-32, 1973.
5. Kelman, C. D.: Phaco-emulsification and aspiration, Am. J. Ophthalmol. **64:**23-35, 1967.
6. Kelman, C. D.: Symposium: Phaco-emulsification. Summary of personal experience, Ophthalmology (Rochester) **78:**OP 35-38, 1974.
7. Ruiz, R. S.: Personal communication, Jan. 1972.
8. Kelman, C. D.: Phaco-Emulsification and aspiration. A report of 500 consecutive cases. Am. J. Ophthalmol. **75:** 764-768, 1973.

CHAPTER 7

Keratomileusis and keratophakia in the surgical correction of aphakia

JOSÉ I. BARRAQUER

The cataract extraction has restored vision to more patients than any other surgery. However, even with good vision, persons with aphakia are still liable to certain visual limitations, not to mention the handicap imposed by absolute dependence on optic correction, without which they are semi-invalids. Any surgical method, then, that will eliminate, or significantly decrease, these aftereffects of the surgery is justified, as long as it does not cause an extremely high additional risk.

Intraocular lenses are a good optic solution. Nevertheless, since they are intraocular foreign bodies, they must be regarded with a certain reservation in relation to long-term results. Extended use of the new intraocular lenses has demonstrated to the surgeons of this generation the benefits and the drawbacks of the surgical correction of ametropia. The drawbacks, in turn, have motivated surgeons to develop alternate methods such as refractive keratoplasty in their search for other procedures to extend the field and the indi-

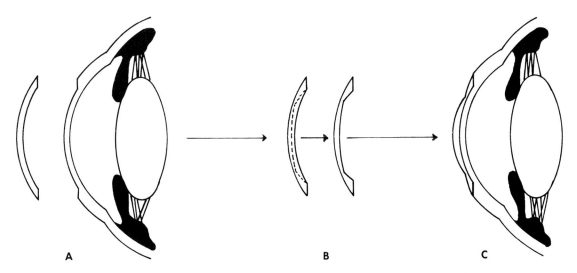

Fig. 7-1. Sketch of keratomileusis for correction of hypermetropia and aphakia. **A,** Corneal disc of parallel faces separated by microkeratome. **B,** Frozen disc, cut on its parenchymal face, becomes lenticule. **C,** Lenticule repositioned in bed of operated eye.

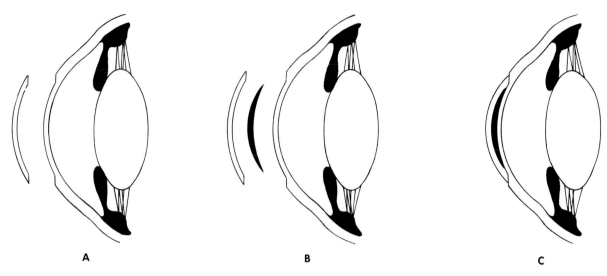

Fig. 7-2. Sketch of keratophakia. **A,** Disc of parallel faces resected by microkeratome. **B,** Lenticule, made from parenchyma of donor eye, is placed into inferface. **C,** Cornea is reconstructed.

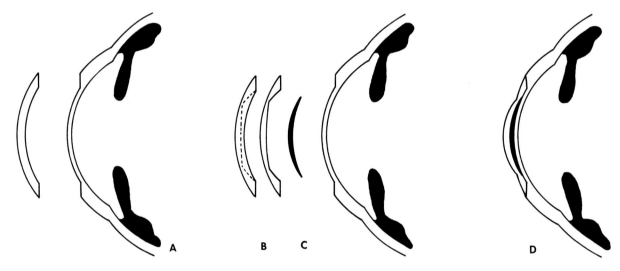

Fig. 7-3. Sketch showing combination of hypermetropic keratomileusis and keratophakia. In this operation, both corneal disc *(A)* obtained by microkeratome *(B)* and lenticule from parenchyma of donor eye *(C)* are cut in lathe. When reconstructing cornea *(D)*, care must be taken to leave central thickness of not more than 0.70 mm.

cations of the surgical correction of ametropia.

By modifying the radius of the corneal curvature, refractive keratoplasty aims to correct or decrease an ametropia, including aphakia, to abolish or diminish dependence on prosthetic devices. Keratomileusis and keratophakia are extraocular surgical techniques to modify the curvature of the anterior surface of the cornea by modifying its thickness. The former is an autoplastic operation, in which the periaxial thickness in the zone of the optic axis is decreased (Fig. 7-1); the latter is homoplastic and results in an increase of the corneal thickness in its optic vertex (Fig. 7-2). If necessary, both techniques may be combined (Fig. 7-3). The satisfactory long-term results obtained with lamellar and penetrating keratoplasties in different diseases and 16 years' experience in refractive keratoplasty have led me to believe that this corneal surgery is a good method for the permanent correction of ametropias, including aphakia. At present the greatest handicap of this surgery is the great precision required in each of its steps, especially in the optic cut, and in the use of instruments and equipment unfamiliar to the surgeon, which call for a long learning period.

Because of the complexity and scope of the subject, this chapter will necessarily be general.

BACKGROUND

Until the mid-1940s, attention in corneal grafts was directed mainly to the fixation of the graft and its transparency. Once success at this stage was achieved, attention was turned to the refractive errors secondary to corneal graft surgery. This led me to consider utilizing this quality of the cornea, which caused great ametropias, in an opposite way, that is, to correct them. Thus in 1949 the concept of refractive keratoplasty was born, with different experimental techniques, some of which resemble those used at present.

These techniques confirmed the hypothesis but were difficult to perform and did not add great precision to the corrections obtained. When in 1950 I became acquainted with Ridley's discovery and performed my first intraocular lens implantations in the posterior and then in the anterior chamber, with lenses of the Strampelli and Dannheim types, I thought the problem of the surgical correction of aphakia had been solved. Unfortunately experience soon showed that this was not the path to follow in all cases. As a result I began experimenting again to determine the factors that influence the radius of the corneal curvature, ways to control them, and the possibility of influencing these factors by surgical means with the precision required by optic laws.

As a result, both the keratophakia and keratomileusis techniques were developed, the former based on my first operations with intracorneal glass lenticules, and the latter based on the law of thicknesses. In 1963 the technique, instruments, and equipment were sufficiently developed for me to perform my first operations in humans. The

results obtained confirmed my experimental work. Since then the techniques, instruments, and calculation programs have been developed further to make the corrections more accurate and to facilitate performance of the procedures.

TERMINOLOGY AND TECHNICAL POINTS

The word keratomileusis is derived from the Greek, and means "sculptured cornea." To perform this surgery a round corneal disc of parallel faces and predetermined thickness is resected from the anterior layers of the operated eye. Hardened by freezing, this tissue disc is cut on its parenchymal face to give it the necessary dioptric power, as if it were a contact lens. Next this disc (now called lenticule) is replaced in the globe, and the cornea is reconstructed (Fig. 7-1). Keratomileusis was the first surgery in which an organ (the cornea) was separated from the human body, modified in its function (refraction), and replaced in its original location.

In keratophakia, from the Greek words for cornea and lens, an adequately shaped lenticule is obtained from the parenchymal tissue of the cornea of a donor eye. This lenticule is placed interlamellarly within the operated cornea to modify the radius of its anterior surface (Fig. 7-2).

In both the optic cut must be performed with great precision — beyond that attainable by manual technique alone — and, since corneal tissue is not inert, the necessary calculations must be performed quickly. In this technique a computer was first used in surgery to determine the degree of surgical action necessary to correct an anomaly.

INSTRUMENTATION

For this surgery, it was necessary to develop or adapt instruments and equipment appropriate for each specific surgical step. To obtain the anterior lamellar disc a microkeratome was designed; to make the optic cut a cryolathe was created; to reconstruct the globe a surgical ophthalmometer was developed; and to perform the calculations a programmable electronic calculator or computer was introduced.

Microkeratome

The microkeratome is based on the principle of the carpenter's plane. Its cutting blade, powered

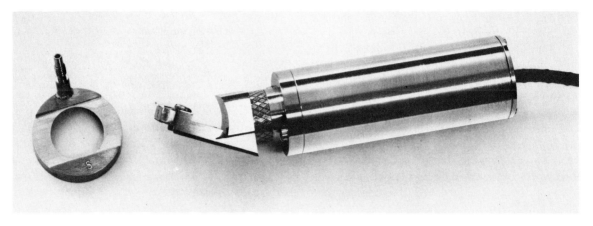

Fig. 7-4. Microkeratome. (Courtesy Steinway Instruments.)

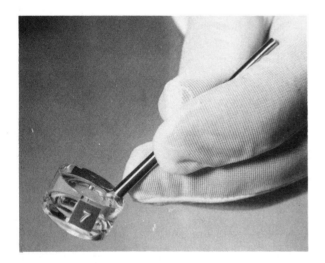

Fig. 7-5. Sclerometer.

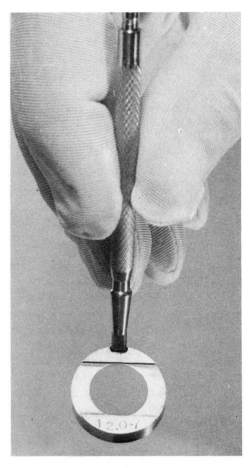

Fig. 7-6. Pneumatic fixation ring, from above.

by a small electric motor, has an oscillating motion to obtain round corneal resections 7.00 to 8.75 mm in diameter and 0.200 to 0.450 mm in thickness (Fig. 7-4).

For use in refractive surgery the microkeratome has been provided with the following special devices:

1. *Sclerometers.* To determine the scleral radius to select the radius of the pneumatic ring (Fig. 7-5).
2. *Pneumatic fixation rings.* To fix the ocular globe, regulate the intraocular pressure, and guide the sliding of the microkeratome (Fig. 7-6).
3. *Applanation lenses.* To select the adequate height of the fixation ring, according to the required diameter of resection (Fig. 7-7).
4. *Surgical tonometer.* To measure the intraocular pressure at the time of the keratectomy (Fig. 7-8).
5. *Denuded-surface protector.* To prevent dust, cotton fibers, and other foreign bodies from falling on the raw corneal surface.

Cryolathe

A Levin Radius Turning Machine for contact lenses, to which several elements for cutting corneal tissue lenses have been added, is transformed into a cryolathe. The added elements are as follows:

1. *Freezing circuits.* To harden the corneal tissue by freezing and make it firm enough for cutting. The equipment uses CO_2 as the freezing agent, and is provided with two circuits controlled by solenoid valves. One circuit freezes the tissue, and the other cools the cutting tool to prevent the tissue from thawing with its friction, especially in the center where the cutting speed is low.
2. *Thickness measuring device.* To measure the thickness of the corneal disc obtained with the microkeratome.
3. *Increment measuring device.* To measure the increase in the thickness of the tissue as a result of freezing.
4. *Digital displacement indicator.* To increase accuracy in measuring the thickness of the resected tissue.
5. *Sphere comparator.* To increase precision in selecting the cutting radius.

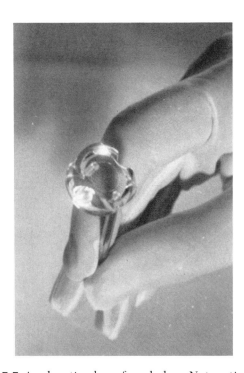

Fig. 7-7. Applanation lens, from below. Note reticule.

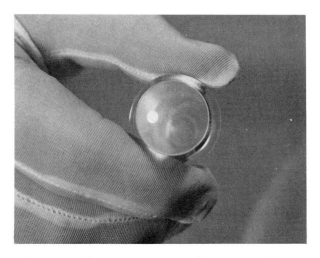

Fig. 7-8. Applanation tonometer, for presurgical use.

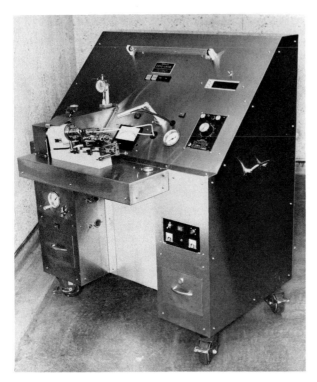

Fig. 7-9. Cryolathe. (Courtesy Steinway Instruments.)

6. *Comparator of angle turning.* To increase the precision in measuring the diameter of the optic zones, with an accuracy of up to 0.01 degree.
7. *Micrometric stops for angles alpha and beta.* To preselect the dimension of the carved zone.

The cryolathe is mounted in a console (Fig. 7-9) provided also with a chronometer, suction equipment, a power source for the microkeratome, cold light, ultraviolet tubes, and a heater (to evaporate the paraformaldehyde used to sterilize the equipment).

Surgical ophthalmometer

The models we use at present (Fig. 7-10) are still prototypes. However, commercially available models such as those of Troutman and Terry and the Zeiss Op-Keratoscope are excellent for our purpose.

CALCULATIONS

The basic calculations for keratomileusis are simple. The corneal disc is adapted to the radius

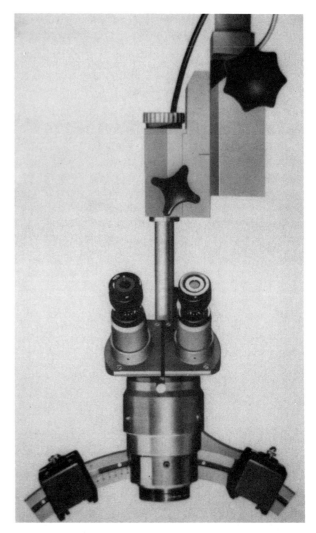

Fig. 7-10. Barraquer surgical ophthalmometer.

it must acquire to correct the ametropia, by cutting it on its parenchymal side to the radius of the corneal surface left exposed when it was resected and over which it must be adapted again (Fig. 7-11).

In keratophakia, the corneal tissue disc is adapted to the final radius that corrects the ametropia, by determining the characteristics of the void space created inside the cornea. The lenticule that will fill this void must have these same characteristics (Fig. 7-12).

These calculations would be simple if corneal tissue were inert. The cornea modifies its thickness, however, contracting its diameter when

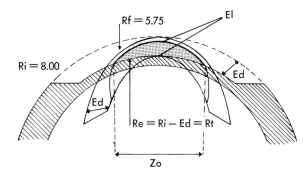

Fig. 7-11. Sketch of calculations for keratomileusis. Adapting disc resected to final radius in interface. By substracting thickness of intersection zone, thickness and diameter of optic available can be calculated.

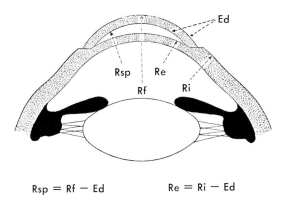

Fig. 7-12. Sketch of calculations for keratophakia. Adapting disc resected to final radius in interface of operated eye. Empty space that must be filled by lenticule of stromal tissue of same characteristics can be seen.

frozen. Also, donor corneas are always more or less hydrated. Therefore, all of these factors must be taken into account because they cause a considerable deviation from the preliminary simple calculations.

In addition, the location of the edge of the cutting tip of the tool is not the same when a small radius is cut as when a large radius is cut. Consequently a modification of this location must be considered in the calculations to determine the dimension of the corresponding optic zones.

Between 300 and 1000 mathematical operations must be performed during each surgery when the characteristics of the tissue disc are known, both before and after freezing. These calculations must be performed within a few seconds so that the conditions do not change; they are possible only with the aid of a programmable electronic calculator or a computer. We use the TI-59 Texas Instruments calculator, but the programs developed may easily be translated into the language of other machines.

Finally it is necessary to establish comparisons with preset limits of minimum or maximum measurements compatible with good vision, such as diameter of the optic zone, remaining thickness, thickness of the lenticule. The programs must include these considerations and provide the best possible data for each given case, limiting the correction, if necessary, to give the closest correction compatible with the preestablished limits.

The programs are previously made and easy to operate, but the surgeon who wishes to introduce modifications, as a result of personal experience, must know the principles of programming, conditional jumps, loops, subroutines, and so on.

To facilitate the performance of these techniques, new models of equipment, which will require only the initial data to perform the calculations and the optic cut, automatically, are being manufactured. However, for a good understanding of the procedure, it is important to be able to perform the surgery with manual equipment alone, such as that presently available.

CASE SELECTION

Keratomileusis and keratophakia for the correction of aphakia are not indicated in the following cases:
1. Those in which corneal surgery is contraindicated
2. Irritated eyes
3. Decentered pupils
4. Pathologic corneas
5. Corneas thinner than 0.45 mm
6. Corneas steeper than 7.30 mm
7. Corneas flatter than 9.00 mm
8. Glaucoma
9. Marked lacrimal hyposecretion

Among highly favorable cases are unilateral aphakia with poor tolerance for contact lenses or inability to wear them (unless this is because of lacrimal hyposecretion).

Among potential cases are those of uncomplicated cataracts, since the operation may be performed as primary surgery, simultaneous with the cataract extraction, or secondary surgery, on a previously aphakic eye. In the first case the diopters of correction are determined by the ultrasonic axial method; in the second case they must be determined by the more accurate refraction method.

The operation is also indicated in surgery on the second eye when the first eye has been operated on with refractive keratoplasty or an intraocular lens.

At present, hypermetropic keratomileusis is the surgery of choice because it does not require a donor eye and has only one interface, which permits a faster recuperation of visual acuity. But if during surgery the resected corneal disc does not have the adequate thickness to permit a satisfactory correcting cut, a combined operation or keratophakia may be performed. Whenever justified, the latter may also be used as a complementary procedure in the correction of a residual ametropia (Fig. 7-3).

LIMITS OF CORRECTION

The possibility of correcting an ametropia is limited by the initial radius of the cornea and the thickness of the tissue.

Initial radius of the cornea

At the present we have set 5.75 mm as the steepest radius of the optic zone of the cornea compatible with good visual acuity. This radius corresponds to 57.74 D of corneal power; therefore, the possibilities of correction may be estimated as the difference between this figure and the dioptric power of the cornea before surgery. Thus, for example, a cornea with a radius of 7.70 mm and a power of 43.05 D will allow correcting 14.68 D of hypermetropia; a cornea with a radius of 8.30 mm and a power of 40 D will allow correcting 17.74 D of hypermetropia; and one with 7.30 mm will only allow correcting 12.25 D of hypermetropia.

Thickness of the tissue

Limiting the thickness. Experience has shown that to obtain high visual acuity corneal thickness must not exceed 0.72 mm. As a consequence, we have set 0.20 mm as the maximum thickness of a lenticule for keratophakia. In theory, this thickness allows a correction of up to 17.00 D; in practice, it is limited by other variables.

In hypermetropic keratomileusis the correction may be limited by the thickness of the tissue disc available. A disc of 0.420 theoretically allows a correction of 20.00 D, but one of 0.320 only allows 13.00 D of correction. In both cases the correction may also be limited by an exceedingly low value of the final radius or the diameter of the optic zone.

Limiting the optic zone. In theory, any power may be corrected with a given thickness of tissue. However, if this thickness is low, the diameter of the lens will be too small and therefore inadequate for the ocular optic apparatus. We have set 5.45 mm as the minimum useful diameter of the optic zone in these operations.

When both techniques are combined, however, there is no limitation other than the final radius, since an excessively curved cornea distorts the images. The interrelations of these factors must be well understood to determine a correct surgical indication.

TECHNIQUE

These operations may be performed under general or local anesthesia, although I prefer the former. Ocular hypotensive agents must not be used before performing the keratectomy, but if they are necessary, as in the case of surgery combined with an intraocular maneuver or operation, these agents must be administered after the corneal disc is resected.

Besides being aseptic, the surgery must be amoric (from the Greek, a = without and morion = particle). Consequently in the operating room, filtered air must be used at positive pressure, all sources of foreign bodies (talcum powder, textile fibers, common powder, etc.) must be avoided, and gowns and materials adequate for this purpose must be used. In addition, all containers in which solutions are kept must be washed repeatedly with a filtered saline solution before the solutions used in the surgery are introduced. These in turn must also be filtered immediately before use; the Millipore filters recommended by Jaffe are very useful for this purpose.

Both the corneal tissue disc and the lenticules

must be handled with extreme caution to prevent unnecessary trauma as well as the seeding of epithelial cells or foreign bodies in the interface.

The operating field is prepared in the usual way. The surgery does not require a particular condition of the pupil. Use of the microscope is mandatory.

The operation begins with a superior rectus bridle suture. A reference mark is then made (Fig. 7-13). This is a small radial erosion of the corneal epithelium, beginning 3 mm from the optic center of the cornea and ending 1 mm from the limbus. It is placed in an appropriate meridian. This erosion, performed with a small spherical diamond burr or a small cutting spoon, is designed to allow replacing the resected corneal tissue disc exactly in its original position.

Keratectomy

The pneumatic ring, selected previously, on the basis of experience, is adapted and centered on the optic axis of the cornea (Fig. 7-14). When the vacuum is opened, the ring remains firmly adherent to the ocular globe. This ring serves three functions: it fixes the globe, it increases the intraocular pressure, and it provides a plane and guides for the sliding of the microkeratome. The surgeon must check that the ring selected performs these functions satisfactorily; if not it must be changed. The fixation is checked by moving the globe slightly with the ring, the intraocular pressure is checked with the surgical tonometer (Fig. 7-15), and the location of the plane is checked with the applanation lenses.

The applanation lenses make possible preselecting the diameter of the proposed resection by means of a reticule engraved in the lower surface. If when adapting the lenses to the ring the contact zone of the cornea and the lenses is smaller than the reticule, then the ring must be changed for one of less height to allow greater corneal protrusion; if the applanation is larger than the reticule, the ring must be changed for one of greater height (Fig. 7-16).

The microkeratome (with the adequate plate to regulate its cutting thickness) is placed between the guides of the ring (Fig. 7-17). Then after the motor is started, the microkeratome is passed

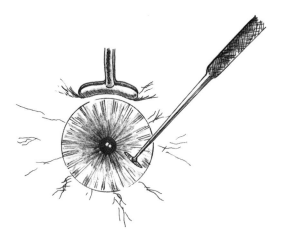

Fig. 7-13. Reference mark is made, by performing slight epithelial abrasion with small diamond burr without hurting Bowman's membrane.

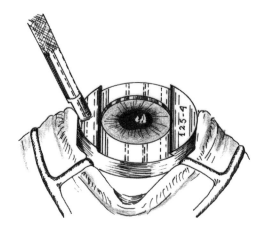

Fig. 7-14. Adapting pneumatic ring to anterior segment of ocular globe to be operated on.

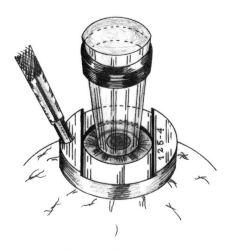

Fig. 7-15. Tonometry.

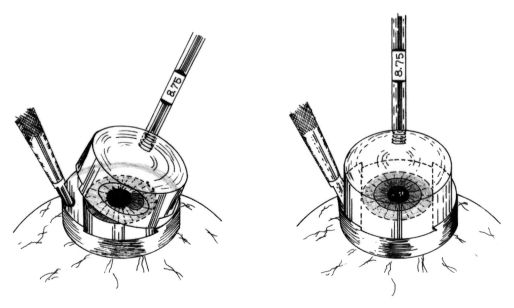

Fig. 7-16. Adapting applanation lenses to guide of pneumatic ring to predetermine diameter of keratectomy.

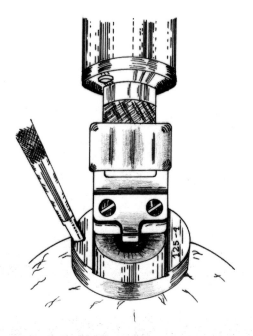

Fig. 7-17. Keratectomy with microkeratome.

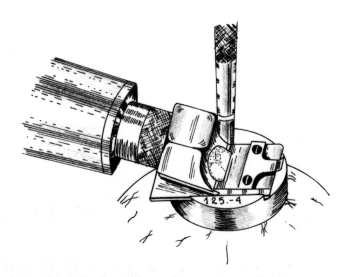

Fig. 7-18. End of keratectomy with microkeratome.

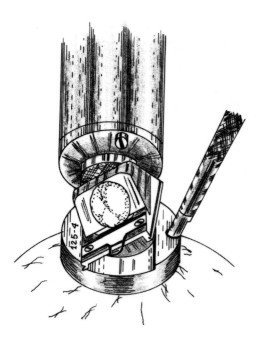

Fig. 7-19. Microkeratome is removed by turning it slightly sideways. (Rings have dovetail in one side only.)

through the guides of the ring with a slow and even motion until the keratectomy is completed (Fig. 7-18). The motor is then turned off, the suction is stopped, and the ring and microkeratome are removed from the globe. To avoid having to cut off the suction, however, single-guide rings were designed to allow withdrawing the microkeratome by inclining it to one side (Fig. 7-19). The corneal tissue disc is withdrawn from the microkeratome and placed on the applanation lens for inspection. It must not be washed because it would become hydrated. Next the thickness of the corneal disc is measured, and the data are given to the operator of the computer.

In keratophakia the disc is replaced in its bed; in keratomileusis it is frozen and carved. In both cases the reconstruction of the globe is identical. The reconstruction begins by replacing the disc in its bed, orienting it to its original position with the reference mark (Fig. 7-20), and placing two previous Perlon stitches, one at 12 o'clock and the other at 6 o'clock, to center and distribute it evenly (Fig. 7-21).

The disc is fixed with an antitorque 10-0 Perlon suture in eight steps, as shown in Figs. 7-22 to 7-24. Once the suture is secured, the knot is buried in the peripheral cornea, and the suture is adjusted under keratometric control (Fig. 7-25). In hypermetropic keratomileusis a second suture must be placed between the stitches of the first for better closure of the coaptation edge to pre-

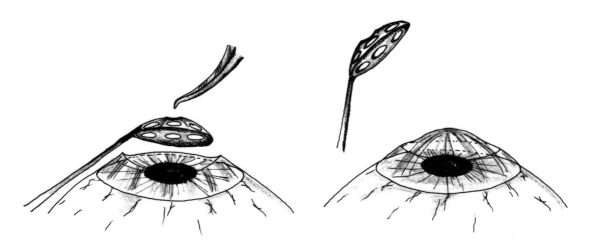

Fig. 7-20. Lenticule, placed in spatula, is placed in its bed by pushing it with forceps through central perforation of spatula.

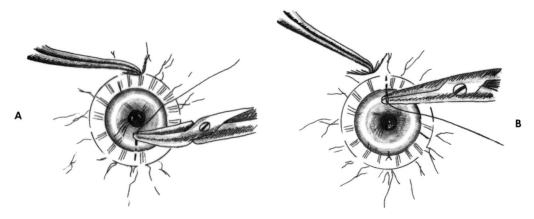

Fig. 7-21. Placing two previous stitches—one at 12 o'clock *(A)*, the other at 6 o'clock *(B)*—to distribute tissue evenly without fixing lenticule with forceps.

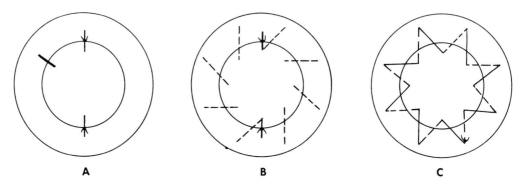

Fig. 7-22. A, Two previous stitches are placed, matching reference mark perfectly. **B,** Interlamellar path of antitorque running suture. **C,** Finished antitorque suture.

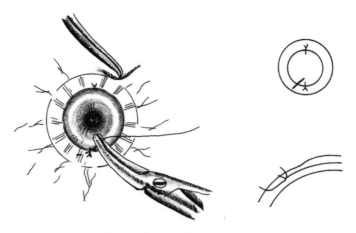

Fig. 7-23. Placing first stitch of antitorque suture.

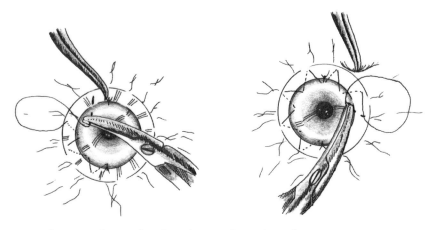

Fig. 7-24. Placing fourth and seventh stitches of antitorque suture.

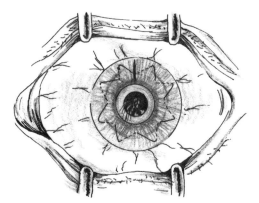

Fig. 7-25. Finished suture.

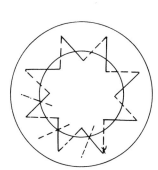

Fig. 7-26. Double antitorque suture.

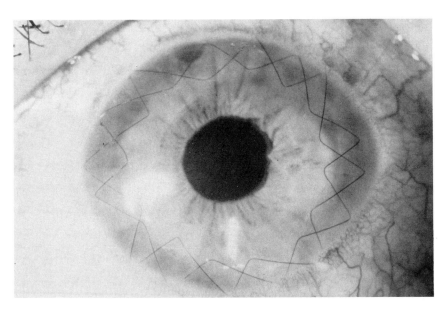

Fig. 7-27. Photograph of antitorque suture at end of surgery.

vent migration of epithelial cells into the interface (Figs. 7-26 and 7-27).

The operation ends with a subconjunctival injection of gentamicin 10 mg and instillation of 1 drop of undiluted glycerin, in the center of the cornea to dehydrate it. A cutaneous tarsorrhaphy stitch is placed in the outer third of the palpebral fissure, and the eye is dressed with a protective shield.

Keratomileusis

For the correction of aphakia, or in corrections of ± 15 D of corneal vertex, a tissue disc 8.50 to 8.75 mm in diameter and 0.400 mm in thickness is required. These dimensions have a tolerance of 8.35 to 8.85 and 0.375 to 0.420 and are obtained by using the 8.50 applanation lens and the 0.35 mm plate in the microkeratome. (In this instrument, individual gauging is important.)

Once the disc is obtained, it is placed on a concave base, where it is left to desiccate at room temperature for 2 or 3 minutes. Next it is submerged in a dyeing and cryopreserving solution for 1 minute. Meanwhile, the cryolathe, already preregulated with its base at a radius of 7.0 mm and its initial point fixed at 20, is checked.

The preserved tissue disc is placed with its epithelial face on the base of the lathe, and excess liquid is removed from its anterior and posterior surfaces. It is then centered with the edge of a spatula as the lathe revolves slowly. The disc is protected from atmospheric moisture by a special protective cap. It is then frozen by opening the corresponding solenoid valve to let the gas through. Freezing takes place in 20 to 30 seconds. Fifteen seconds later the protective cap is removed, and another 15 seconds later the thickness of the frozen disc is measured with a device installed in the cryolathe for this purpose. The new data are fed into the computer, which then performs all operations and comparisons in a few seconds, providing the best possible data to regulate the lathe for the optic cut.

With a cutting tool that has a tip 0.1 mm in radius, the cut begins in the periphery, is always performed with a radius of 5.00 mm, and ends exactly at the outer limit of the optic zone where it will leave a tissue only 0.12 mm thick. Next the lathe is regulated to cut the optic zone so that the tissue in its center is left untouched, and in the periphery a remnant tissue is left, also 0.12 mm thick. This creates a perfect coincidence between the level of the optic zone and the peripheral zone or wing.

For good cell survival and minimal postoperative edema, these maneuvers should be performed in less than 8 minutes. Lately, however, I have been using a tool 1.5 mm in radius (Fig. 7-28), which allows cutting both the optic zone and the peripheral zone (wing) in a single stroke, starting at the center, to obtain an even coincidence between the optic zone and the wing, thereby reducing the freezing period to 3 minutes. Once the corneal disc (lenticule) is cut, it is removed from the lathe along with its plastic base and submerged in a solution of 10% glycerin at room temperature for thawing and examination. It is then removed from the solution with a concave fenestrated spatula, replaced in its bed, and set into place by the technique already described (Fig. 7-20). The sutures must run through the lenticule at the coaptation edge of the wing and not through the intersection zone because it is very thin (0.12 mm) and might easily be torn. The suture must be tightened until there is ±0.10 mm between the epithelium of the lenticule and the peripheral epithelium. Astigmatism is minimized by using the ophthalmometer during suturing.

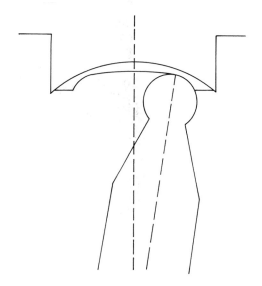

Fig. 7-28. With round-tipped tool 1.5 mm in radius, optic zone and wing can be cut in a single stroke.

Keratophakia

As in keratomileusis the corneal disc of the eye operated on must also be 8.50 mm in diameter, but its thickness may be 0.250 to 0.300 mm; the 0.30 plate is applicable in most cases. The donor eye should be fresh, so that corneal edema is minimal and the viability of its stromal cells high.

With the same technique as in keratomileusis, a corneal tissue disc from the donor eye is resected, preferably 7.50 to 8.00 mm in diameter and 0.30 to 0.35 mm in thickness.

While the donor disc is being measured, desiccated, and preserved (as in keratomileusis), the remaining posterior layer of the central part of the cornea of the donor globe is resected with a 5.0 mm trephine. The thickness of this disc is also measured, and the data are passed on to the computer operator to ascertain the degree of hydration of the whole donor cornea.

The preserved donor disc, which has been cut with a radius of 7.00 mm, is placed with its parenchymal face on the base of the freezing chamber. When it is frozen the thickness of the disc is measured, and the data are fed into the computer. The properly programmed computer will provide the radius to be used in cutting the lenticule, the angle necessary for its proper diameter, and the tool displacement, so that its thickness is not above 0.20 mm. As a rule, thicker lenticules do not allow good visual acuity. It is important to note that the anterior membrane structure has been carved away, so that the final lenticule consists only of stroma.

After the lenticule is thawed, it is kept in a closed container (with the fenestrated spatula with which it was removed from the solution) to prevent its desiccation and contamination with foreign bodies before it is implanted. Once the proper lenticule is obtained, the eye is operated on with the technique already described.

After the antitorque suture is placed, its superior loops are moved aside, and after the upper half of the corneal disc is raised, the lenticule is introduced into the interface with its convex side

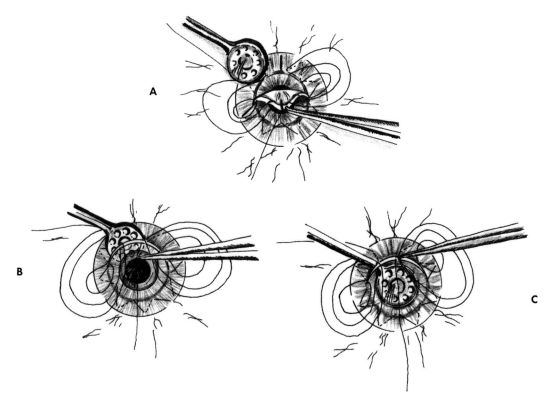

Fig. 7-29. Keratophakia. **A,** Interface is opened. **B,** Lenticule is inserted with spatula. **C,** Spatula is removed.

facing forward (Fig. 7-29). When the lenticule is centered on the optic axis of the globe, care must be taken to leave it well extended with a perfectly circular shape. A lenticule that is incorrectly extended or decentered will lead to high degrees of astigmatism.

The suture is tightened, and a narrow gap is left at the edge of the whole perimeter. The gap required is approximately 0.2 mm, but it varies from eye to eye according to the degree of the correction, the diameter of the corneal disc, and the diameter of the lenticule. The traction of the sutures must be distributed evenly to leave 2 to 3 D of astigmatism against the rule. This astigmatism is compensated for in the postoperative period, and any final astigmatism is usually with the rule. The medication, dressing, and so forth are as in keratomileusis.

In both procedures, when the operation is finished, slit lamp examination is necessary to observe the change in thickness of the cornea and, most of all, to detect foreign bodies that may have gone unnoticed during surgery. These may be removed with fine toothless forceps.

POSTOPERATIVE COURSE

In keratophakia the dressing may be removed 24 to 48 hours after surgery. Corticosteroids are instilled two or three times daily, and a mydriatic as well if there is spasm of the pupillary sphincter. If there is edema of the lenticule, the instillation of undiluted glycerin two or three times daily speeds its reabsorption.

After the first week the corticosteroid is discontinued or reduced. The sutures are removed 15 to 20 days postoperatively. In the examination performed 30 days after the surgery, the patient is given complementary optic correction for distant vision and addition for close vision. Visual acuity improves progressively. The second optic correction is given 3 months later, and the last 1 year postoperatively.

In keratomileusis, since the epithelium was frozen, it is best to keep the tarsorrhaphy suture and the occlusive patch for 5 or 6 days. The corticosteroid is instilled every third day, and a mydriatic and glycerin, or a 5% sodium chloride solution, is added whenever necessary. The administration of vitamin A parenterally favors epithelialization.

The occlusive dressing must not be removed until epithelialization is complete. Corticosteroids in small doses and moisturizers three times daily may be instilled.

The sutures are removed 20 to 25 days postoperatively. The first refraction is performed 30 days after surgery, and the remainder of the postoperative period is as in keratophakia.

In both operations the patient must avoid rubbing the eye to prevent epithelial erosions in the unsensitive cornea. For the first month protective glasses must be worn during the day, and a protective shield, fixed with surgical tape, during sleep.

COMBINED OPERATIONS

Refractive keratoplasty may be performed as a primary procedure, that is, simultaneously with the cataract extraction, or as a secondary operation in aphakia.

As a primary procedure, the order of the surgical steps is different in a classic cataract extraction from that in a lens aspiration or phacoemulsification. In the classic cataract extraction, the refractive surgery is performed first, then the cataract extraction, where care is taken not to alter the traction of the running suture that fixates the lenticule. In lens aspiration or phacoemulsification, once the keratectomy is performed but before the lenticule is replaced, the lens is aspirated to provide a better view of the anterior chamber. This visibility improves even more when a few drops of an aqueous solution of 10% glycerin is instilled into the interface. Once the lens is extracted the paracentesis must be closed with one or several sutures to allow resumption of a normal intraocular pressure and facilitate suturing the lenticule. It is better to use liquid than air because air produces reflexes that make suturing visibility difficult and is not ideal for use with the keratometer.

Finally if a keratomileusis does not provide enough correction or if a keratophakia requires an excessively thick lenticule to accomplish the correction, both operations may be combined to achieve a correction nearer to emmetropia.

RESULTS

Both operations give good and stable results (Figs. 7-30 and 7-31). Thirty days postoperatively,

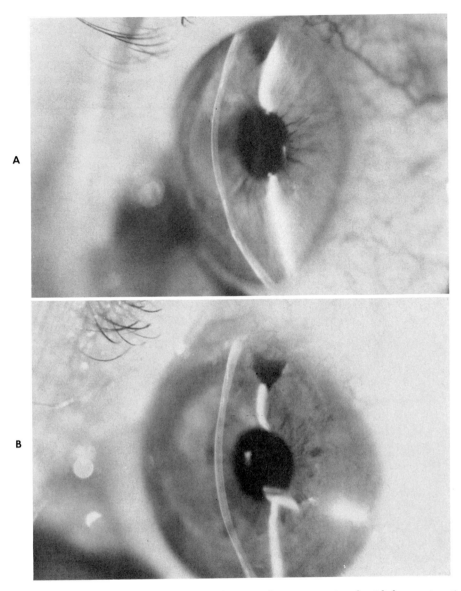

Fig. 7-30. Two cases of hypermetropic keratomileusis associated with lens extraction. **A,** One month postoperatively. **B,** One year postoperatively.

one may expect an acuity of 20/40 or more in eyes without other pathologic conditions. With keratomileusis, 20/30 vision 30 days postoperatively is not exceptional. Because of the double interface in keratophakia, recovery is somewhat slower, requiring 6 months or more, but the architecture of the anterior surface of the cornea is more uniform. Astigmatism with keratomileusis is minimal or nil; in keratophakia, on the average, it is

1.00 to 2.00 D greater than what it was preoperatively (Tables 7-1 to 7-7).

Since patients function without difficulty and do not complain of ring scotomas of any kind, it would seem that the zone of negative curve encircling the optic zone in keratomileusis does not cause any visual problem. Those who drive a vehicle do not complain of lateral visual difficulties either. In addition, binocular vision is satis-

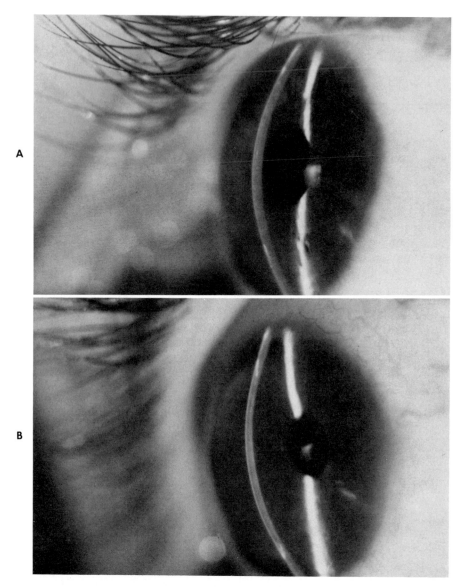

Fig. 7-31. Two cases of keratophakia associated with lens extraction. **A,** Eighteen months postoperatively. **B,** Eight years postoperatively.

factory if the resulting anisometropia is lower than 4 D. Some patients can tolerate 6 D, but they are exceptions. Whenever 6 D of anisometropia persists, the diplopia without optic correction becomes more evident than diplopia with an anisometropia of 12 or 13 because with the latter the acuity of the anisometropic eye is very low. Contrary to the practice with intraocular lenses, it is not convenient to make the eye myopic, since this would require a very small radius of curvature. As a rule, patients close to emmetropia read at a distance of 40 cm without the aid of glasses.

The examination of the fundus does not present any difficulties, and the periphery is easily seen with an indirect ophthalmoscope or a three-mirror lens.

If the surgery has been atraumatic and amoric, there should not be any dark shadows in the skiascopic reflex. Interfaces are scarcely visible

Table 7-1. Average results of keratophakia in 32 cases of aphakia in 1976

	Preoperative	1 year	Late*
Ametropia (D)	+12.38	+1.52	+1.11
Ametropia correction		87.7%	91.0%
Visual acuity	0.45	0.49	0.64
Astigmatism (D)	1.07	1.78	1.97
Anisometropia (D)	12.61	2.33	2.89
Stereopsis			253″
Ametropia variation (D)		0.10 D per year	

*The average time for eyes examined more than 1 year postoperatively is 4.8 years.

Table 7-2. Average of late results with keratophakia in aphakia in 1974 to 1976

	1974	1975	1976
Preoperative			
Ametropia (D)	+11.56	+10.61	+12.38
Acuity	0.50	0.34	0.45
Postoperative			
Ametropia (D)	+1.35	+1.22	+1.11
Acuity	0.62	0.53	0.64
Correction	88.21%	86.34%	91.00%
Astigmatism (D)	1.56	1.93	1.97
Stereopsis		180″	253″
Annual change (D)		0.06	0.10
Follow-up (years)	3.5	3	4.8
Cases	50	49	32

Table 7-3. Late visual acuity in keratophakia

Acuity	Cases	Percentage
1.00-0.67	21	65.6
0.60-0.35	5	15.6
0.33-0.10	5	15.6
Less than 0.10	1	3.1

Table 7-4. Hypermetropic keratomileusis in 100 cases of aphakia at 1-year follow-up*

	Preoperative	3 months	1 year
Ametropia (D)	+12.23	+4.26	+4.26
Acuity		0.62	0.65
Astigmatism (D)	1.00	1.56	1.50

*Contraction factor 1.05.

Table 7-5. Hypermetropic keratomileusis in 12 cases of aphakic eyes in 1979*

		Postoperative	
	Preoperative	1 month	3 months
Ametropia (D)	+12.35	+1.12	+0.92
Astigmatism (D)	−1.10	−1.52	−1.58
Vision			
Without correction	0.06	0.24	0.31
With correction	0.70	0.50	0.70

*Program 1; contraction factor (Fcc) = 1.09.

Table 7-6. Visual acuity in hypermetropic keratomileusis in 100 cases of aphakia*

Acuity	1 month (%)	3 months (%)	6 months (%)
1.00-0.60	28	61	76
0.60-0.40	50	31	20
0.40-0.05	22	8	4

*Causes of vision under 0.40: macular edema, two cases; epitelitis, one case; opaque posterior capsule, one case.

Table 7-7. Hypermetropic keratomileusis plus cataract extraction in 50 cases in 1979*

	Preoperative	Postoperative 1 month	Postoperative 3 months
Ametropia (D)	Cataract	+1.33	+1.18
Vision (average)	Cataract		
Without correction		0.20	0.20
With correction		0.41	0.51
Vision (1.00-0.60)		24%	30%
Vision (0.60-0.40)		30%	56.67%
Vision (0.40-0.20)		34%	13.33%
Vision (0.20)		12%	0%

*Program 1; contraction factor (Fcc) = 1.09.

in the optic zone, even with the slit lamp. They become more visible in the peripheral zone, especially in the coaptation edge, which very often is the only place where they may be noticed.

In the first days of the postoperative period, some patients complain of monocular diplopia, due to the existence of the interface. This phenomenon is more frequent in keratophakia, but it usually disappears spontaneously once the corneal structure becomes uniform.

COMPLICATIONS

Because of the complexity of the surgery, most complications are caused by the omission of a checkpoint or an operating step. That is why use of a checklist or a prerecorded tape is highly recommended.

Keratectomy

If a small irregularity of the resection with the microkeratome results, the operation may be continued; if it is significant, the resected disc must be replaced in its bed and the surgery postponed.

A disc thinner than the one programmed will not provide the necessary correction in keratomileusis. A certain hypocorrection must then be accepted; otherwise a keratophakia will have to be performed, if a donor eye is available.

Calculations. When a computer is used, errors may result from wrong feeding of the data or incorrect placement of a decimal point. Before regulating the lathe according to the data provided by the computer, the surgeon must check the accuracy of the input and the values of the output.

Optic cut. If the data are in error or the regulation of the lathe is deficient, the cut will not be correct. The lenticule may be perforated and destroyed. In keratophakia, another lenticule may be obtained, but in keratomileusis, a homoplastic procedure must be performed with a lenticule from a donor eye.

Reconstruction. Both the repositioning and suturing must be precise. Otherwise the apposition of the edges will be faulty, leaving openings for epithelial cells or inducing astigmatism. If the surgery is not amoric, there will be a large number of particles and foreign bodies in the interface or interfaces that will produce a cellular reaction and low transparency of the interface.

In keratophakia the lenticules may become decentered or herniated during the postoperative period because of a suture that is either too loose or too tight. In such case the pressure of the corneal disc pushes the lenticule outward. However, in general the lenticule may be replaced easily.

It is improbable, but possible, that the suture may break or the knot become untied. To prevent this complication, care must be taken not to cause trauma to the suture during surgery. The knots must be made in the right direction and buried well. A double suture makes this accident more improbable.

A postoperative complication related to this type of surgery is epithelialization of the interface (Fig. 7-32). Epithelial cells may reach the interface by seeding during surgery, by a faulty coaptation of the edges of the wound, or by mi-

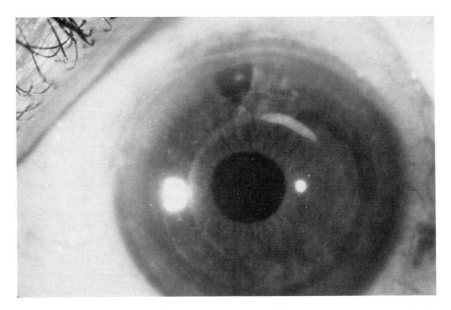

Fig. 7-32. Epithelialization of intersection zone in hypermetropic keratomileusis.

gration by attraction through an empty space, caused by a defective optic cut or irregular tightening of the suture, inside the cornea. As a rule, if these epithelializations are marsupialized, they stop growing. Only if they are left to grow or if they multiply and reach the optic zone will it be necessary to perform a homoplastic procedure.

Cases of immune reaction have not been observed in keratophakia, but it is possible that some cases of delayed recovery of visual acuity because of edema of the lenticule may be due to this.

In keratomileusis, where the epithelium of the lenticule is frozen, normalization of the epithelium may be delayed. If this condition persists, it may be followed by necrosis of Bowman's membrane and scar formation. In those cases in which this condition was reported, it was of traumatic origin. It is wise to advise the patient to be careful when drying the eye and to use a protective shield at night during the first month.

To summarize, the complications inherent in refractive keratoplasty show themselves early, are not very serious (since they are extraocular), and are few, once the surgical technique is mastered. Up to the present, with 16 years' experience, I have not found any special late complication resulting from these techniques.

I consider refractive keratoplasty to be a phys-

iologic method for the correction or decrease of aphakic ametropia that will find its place within the ophthalmologic armamentarium in the near future.

APPRENTICESHIP

Learning the techniques of refractive keratoplasty is difficult, even for experienced ophthalmologists, because they require the assimilation of new concepts and the handling of new mechanical and electronic instruments with which the ocular surgeon, even a specialist in anterior segment and corneal surgery, is not familiar.

The greatest difficulties are encountered in using the microkeratome and the cryolathe and in understanding the various mathematic and physical relationships.

Learning to handle programmable calculators is easy enough, although it takes time to learn how they function and what their possibilities are. Yet this is a good way to enter the field of the more sophisticated computers, which have increased capacity and speed. Without this knowledge the surgeon will have to depend on a program technician to introduce modifications into a program.

After learning the functions of each element that makes up the machinery, the surgeon must become familiar with them. This can be achieved only by spending many hours in the laboratory, cutting bases, centering and decentering the lathe, and becoming aware of the alterations (and their consequences) introduced into the cut surfaces by erroneous handling of each of its parts.

Learning to cut lenticules in wax is the next step, beginning with myopic keratomileusis (the simplest operation), continuing with keratophakia, and ending with hypermetropic keratomileusis (the most difficult). Errors in technique may be corrected during this laboratory training.

Once the control and alignment of the parts of the lathe and the ability to perform the cut quickly and confidently are mastered, the surgeon may begin to measure the contraction of the base and of the tool and to make a contraction table adequate for the equipment for a given time and gas pressure.

Once this is accomplished, optic cuts on animal corneas may be performed, with presumptive data in the absence of real data and actual figures when these may be measured.

Following this, eye bank eyes may be used for practicing with the microkeratome. Practice must continue until all the accidents and incidents described (and perhaps new ones) have been faced and the surgeon has firsthand experience of their causes and understands their intrinsic nature. At the same time the ever scarce globes can be used in performing the whole surgical procedure, from the reference mark to the final suturing, concentrating on those steps found most difficult. Some of these corneal discs should be used to check the value of the contraction in individual working conditions.

Keratophakia should be used as an introduction to refractive keratoplasty in humans because the most difficult step—the optical cut—is performed on a donor eye and may be repeated as often as wished or as many times as necessary.

Finally, or better, simultaneously, it is wise to watch experienced surgeons perform surgery of this type and whenever possible to collaborate with them in a specialized center for a few months.

REFERENCES

1. Barraquer, J. I.: Refractive keratoplasty, vol. I, Bogotá, 1970, Instituto Barraquer de América.
2. Barraquer, J. I.: Refractive keratoplasty, vol. II, Bogotá, 1975, Instituto Barraquer de América.
3. Barraquer, J. I.: Keratomileusis and keratophakia, Bogotá, 1980, Litografía Arco.

CHAPTER 8

Subluxation and dislocation of the lens

Until recently the subject of subluxation and luxation of the lens has been confusing and its proper management one of the most controversial in all of ophthalmology.

When the lens is displaced from its normal position, it is considered subluxated if it remains in the pupillary area and luxated, or dislocated, if it is completely displaced from the pupil. The latter implies separation of all zonular attachments.

ETIOLOGY

Lens displacements may be divided into three types: traumatic, heritable, and spontaneous.

Traumatic ectopia lentis

The incidence of these types varies somewhat in the literature, but trauma is the main factor in slightly more than 50% of all lens displacements. It may vary from a slight blow to the eye to a major contusion. A peculiar relationship appears to exist between syphilis and traumatic dislocation of the lens.[1] Nevertheless, it is still unknown whether the spirochete weakens the zonule so that minimal trauma can cause a displacement of the lens or whether patients who acquire syphilis are more prone to ocular trauma.

Subluxation is relatively common after a blow to the eye. After a contusion, with or without resulting hyphema, the eye is usually soft with a deep anterior chamber. As the eye recovers, with the return of the lens to its normal position the depth of the anterior chamber gradually becomes normal. In a severe injury in which the zonular attachments are ruptured, the lens may not be displaced because of its attachment to the vitreous. In such a case the lens may float on the vitreous surface in the manner of a compass, with obvious iridodonesis. The vitreous may herniate through the pupil, and the anterior chamber may become of unequal depth.

The subluxated lens may remain in the pupillary aperture indefinitely, giving rise to variable optic disability. In cases of complete traumatic luxation the lens may be displaced into the anterior chamber, into the vitreous, beneath the retina, or if the globe is ruptured, even subconjunctivally.

Heritable ectopia lentis

Heritable forms of ectopia lentis may be associated with other systemic anomalies, with other ocular anomalies, or appear as an isolated anomaly.

Associated systemic anomalies

1. *Marfan's syndrome* is characterized by ectopia lentis, slender development of bones, poorly developed musculature, absence of subcutaneous fat, and cardiopathy. Thus, a triad of skeletal, cardiovascular, and ocular anomalies is found. The skeletal anomalies are expressed as general thinness and elongation of the limbs, sternal deformities, kyphoscoliosis, joint hyperextensibility, and a low ratio of upper segment to lower segment. Arachnodactyly is found at birth. The cardiovascular anomalies include cardiopathy, aortic dilatation, dissecting aneurysm, and mitral regurgitation. Mental retardation is rare.

The most characteristic ocular anomaly is ectopia lentis, which is found in 70% to 80% of cases, is nearly always bilateral, is usually partial, is rarely progressive, and is characteristically displaced superiorly and temporally. The lens displacement is usually seen early in life — at 5 years in 50% of patients. The pupils are usually miotic and dilate poorly due to hypoplasia of the dilator muscle of the iris. Myopia is common and is associated with a lenticular, as well as an axial, component.[2] Gonioscopic examination of the iridocorneal angle reveals the presence of mesodermal abnormalities of varying degrees.[3] These include pectinate ligaments, iris processes, peripheral mounds of iris tissue, and vascular anomalies. A recent series[4] described similar findings, including an inconspicuous Schwalbe's line and a broad trabecular meshwork in 75% of patients examined by gonioscopy. Strabismus, retinal detachment, and glaucoma are found in a much smaller number of patients.

The heredity is autosomal dominant with a variable expressivity. The molecular defect remains unknown, although there is apparently a faulty formation of collagen. There is no specific amino acid abnormality. No specific therapy is available.

2. *Homocystinuria* is also characterized by a triad of skeletal, cardiovascular, and ocular anomalies. This unfortunate enzymopathy may resemble Marfan's syndrome, with at least 50% of patients showing a similar clinical appearance. Some differences are subtle, others emphatic. Many patients with homocystinuria are tall and slender with an abnormal upper segment to lower segment ratio. However, the arachnodactyly is usually less marked. Other skeletal anomalies are genu valgum (knock-knee), flat feet, kyphoscoliosis, joint laxity, deformed sternum, generalized osteoporosis with vertebral collapse, and high arched palate. Anomalies of the skin are also characteristic. These consist of malar flush, light, fair, and dry skin, and hair that is fair, coarse, and sparse. Some patients have hernias and hepatomegaly. Mental retardation, not seen in patients with Marfan's syndrome, is not uncommon. The cardiovascular problems are more serious than those in Marfan's syndrome. Thromboembolic phenomena in the veins and middle-sized arteries occur in at least 50% of cases. These are due to blood coagulation disorders or increased blood viscosity due to platelet stickiness. Cerebrovascular thromboses, myocardial infarctions, pulmonary emboli, and intermittent claudication may occur at a relatively early age. Premature death occurs in about 40% of patients. The ophthalmologist must be alerted to these possibilities, since the thromboembolic phenomena

are more likely to occur after vessel puncture or general anesthesia.

Ectopia lentis is a characteristic finding in 90% of eyes of patients with homocystinuria. Unlike with Marfan's syndrome, the lens displacement is usually inferior and is often toward the nasal side. Ectopia lentis, however, is also found early in life. Complications associated with ectopia lentis are more frequent, probably because the lens is much more mobile. Thus the incidence of pupillary block glaucoma and total dislocation is much higher. In a recent series[4] one third of the lenses in homocystinuria became totally dislocated into the anterior chamber or the vitreous. Unlike with Marfan's syndrome, anterior chamber angle anomalies do not occur. However, glaucoma and retinal detachment are associated ocular anomalies, the former higher in incidence and the latter about equal in incidence to the eyes of patients with Marfan's syndrome.

The heredity is autosomal recessive. It is caused by the lack of cystathionine synthetase. Homocystine, an amino acid, is found in the urine. The sodium nitroprusside test of the urine is a simple diagnostic screening test (Brand reaction). Attempted dietary therapy has consisted of foods poor in methionine and rich in cystine in early cases. Pyridoxine has also been advocated. Although some patients have benefited from this dietary regimen, the therapeutic results are far from encouraging. Cases of homocystinuria are being reported with increasing frequency. It is possible that this disorder may even surpass phenylketonuria as the commonest inborn error of metabolism.

3. *The Weill-Marchesani syndrome* is much more rare than Marfan's syndrome. Although this is also a mesodermal dystrophy, especially of the anterior segment, there is a marked contrast in the appearance of these patients. The skeletal anomalies consist of brachymorphy, short stature, and spadelike hands and feet. These patients have large thoraces and reduced joint motility. There are no vascular, cutaneous, mental, or urinary abnormalities.

Microspherophakia is occasionally seen in this syndrome and, when present, is frequently associated with ectopia lentis. The lens displacement tends to occur later in life.

Both dominant and recessive inheritance have

been reported, with partial expressivity in the heterozygote.[5]

4. *Other heritable conditions* associated with ectopia lentis include hyperlysinemia, a rare, recessively transmitted disorder of lysine metabolism, and a variety of disorders in which the ectopia lentis may be nothing more than a random association. These include the Ehlers-Danlos syndrome, the Sturge-Weber syndrome, the Crouzon syndrome, dwarfism, oxycephaly, polydactyly, mandibulofacial dysostosis, sulfite oxidase deficiency, and Sprengel's deformity.

Associated ocular anomalies

1. *Ectopia lentis et pupillae* is a disorder in which lens and pupillary anomalies are associated. The pupils are oval or slit-shaped and are usually ectopic. As a rule, the pupillary displacement is in a direction opposite that of the ectopic lens. The condition is often bilateral and symmetrical.[6] Cataract, glaucoma, and retinal detachment may be associated.[6] The inheritance is recessive.

2. *Aniridia* may be complicated by ectopia lentis. However, the ectopia lentis is only a minor constituent of the clinical picture.

The isolated anomaly. Ectopia lentis may occur as an isolated anomaly. In this event it may occur either congenitally or spontaneously later in life. The congenital type (presumed to be congenital) of ectopia lentis resembles that of Marfan's syndrome in that it is seen early in life, is bilateral and symmetrical, is usually upward and temporal, and is usually transmitted in an autosomal dominant fashion.

The spontaneous, late ectopia lentis is more puzzling. It may occur at any time during adulthood. There is a downward direction to the dislocation. Like the congenital type, this form may show a tendency toward cataract formation, glaucoma, and retinal detachment.

Spontaneous ectopia lentis

Spontaneous displacements of the lens are slightly more frequent than the heritable varieties and are related to mechanical stretching of the zonule. In certain middle-aged or older individuals the lens gradually tilts backward as the upper zonules give way and eventually becomes dislocated into the vitreous cavity.

However, spontaneous displacement is probably more often related to some other ocular pathology. It may be seen in high myopia when enlargement of the eyeball results in stretching of the zonule to the breaking point. It is seen in endophthalmitis where inflammation may soften the zonule to the point of rupture. The lens may be displaced by the resulting cyclitic inflammatory adhesions. Similar adhesions may cause ectopia lentis after treatment of retinal detachment by diathermy, in Eales' disease, chalcosis, and so on. It may be associated with other ocular disorders such as buphthalmos, megalocornea, and coloboma of the iris and choroid. An acute dislocation may follow perforation of a corneal ulcer when the lens-iris diaphragm is suddenly thrust forward. The lens may also be pushed out of position by the growth of an intraocular tumor.

DIAGNOSIS AND CLINICAL FINDINGS

The diagnosis of ectopia lentis in a minor subluxation may be difficult. This is especially true in infants. The greater the lens displacement, the more apparent the diagnosis. Both phakodonesis and iridodonesis are observed with ocular movements. The anterior chamber is deep, usually of aphakic depth, except in cases of pupillary block where it may be very shallow. It is also not unusual to observe an uneven anterior chamber depth, the depth being greater where the lens and iris are dislocated posteriorly. When the edge of the dislocated lens appears in the pupillary spaces, it shines brightly in focal illumination. The edge of the lens may have a scalloped appearance, which results from a local deficiency of the zonule rather than a loss of lens substance. On ophthalmoscopy the edge of the lens may appear as a dark, curved line in the fundus reflex. This is due to internally reflected light. There may be two ophthalmoscopic images, one through the phakic portion of the pupil and the other through the aphakic portion. In most instances the zonules appear intact, although they may be stretched or thickened. It is rare to see torn edges of the zonular fibers attached to the lens capsule, since they usually retract to the ciliary processes. Vitreous may protrude between the lens and iris and be present in the anterior chamber.

Visual disturbance

The patient usually has a visual disturbance related directly to the displacement of the lens. If the lens is only minimally displaced, lenticular myopia may occur because of increased curvature as a result of relaxation of the suspensory ligament. Anterior displacement also causes myopia. Tilting of the lens may cause a marked irregular astigmatism that is not entirely correctable with glasses or contact lenses. Monocular diplopia may be caused by the lens being partly in and partly out of the pupil. If the lens is luxated posteriorly, out of the visual axis, the optic condition of aphakia results. The visual disturbance may be variable if the lens moves freely in the visual path with movements of the head. The visual impairment will also depend on whether the lens is clear or cataractous. Traumatic dislocations of the lens are occasionally associated with chorioretinal degeneration, which may also affect vision.

Glaucoma

There has been some confusion in the past concerning the cause of glaucoma in displacements of the lens. It is now known that the etiology of the glaucoma is varied. The following four causes may exist alone or in various combinations.

Pupillary block by vitreous or the lens is particularly important in those cases in which the lens enters the anterior chamber. It is the pupillary block mechanism that pushes the lens forward. This is demonstrated by the fact that the lens tends to recede behind the iris if a peripheral iridectomy is performed. In Marfan's syndrome, and especially in spherophakia (Weill-Marchesani syndrome), the zonules are characteristically longer and looser than normal. If miotics are used, the further relaxation of the zonules permits the lens to move forward and block the pupil. Vitreous gel may wedge itself between the pupillary margin and the ectopic lens and cause pupillary block, or it may block aqueous flow without the lens being present in the pupillary space. In these cases, relief of the pupillary block by peripheral iridectomy or discission of the vitreous will relieve the glaucoma, except in neglected cases. Pupillary block glaucoma and lens touching the corneal endothelium are less frequent with Marfan's syndrome than with homocystinuria or the Weill-Marchesani syndrome.

Peripheral anterior synechias are usually the result of a prolonged attack or repeated episodes of pupillary block. However, the congenital anterior chamber angle deformities seen with some of the heritable forms of ectopia lentis, as in the syndromes of Marfan and Weill-Marchesani, may be associated with glaucoma.

Postcontusion angle deformity is the third cause. In eyes with lens displacement and glaucoma with wide open angles, the most likely cause of the glaucoma is the syndrome of postcontusion glaucoma described by Wolff and Zimmerman.[7] In these eyes the glaucoma shows an insidious onset but a protracted course, as demonstrated by a median interval of 15 years between trauma and enucleation in one series[8] and 17 years in another.[7] Contusion angle deformity is characterized by an increased depth of the anterior chamber, which is often measurable by slit lamp examination. Gonioscopy reveals a marked deepening of the anterior chamber angle in which the exposed face of the ciliary body appears unusually wide and the iris root is found posteriorly displaced. The defect may occupy one or more quadrants of the globe. This picture is caused by a tear in the face of the ciliary body and is observed after an ocular contusion in which the lens may or may not be displaced. In some of these eyes, after a lapse of years a mother-of-pearl, grayish white hyaline membrane may be observed covering the entire angle recess.

It is this peculiar angle deformity that is responsible for much of the early confusion regarding the incidence and mechanism of glaucoma after traumatic lens displacement. Rodman[8] has pointed out that the incidence of glaucoma in eyes with a subluxated or luxated lens is difficult to determine because the glaucoma may not appear for a long time. Therefore the incidence reported by different investigators depends on the length of the follow-up interval. In his series, 97% of enucleated eyes with open-angle glaucoma had postcontusion angle deformities. The latter were found in 74% of cases with anterior dislocations and in 66% of cases of posteriorly dislocated and subluxated lenses with closed angles. In the latter two groups the glaucoma was caused by the closed anterior chamber angle, and the postcontusion deformity was only of secondary interest.

In those eyes with open-angle glaucoma associated with postcontusion angle deformity, there is no evidence of hypersecretion of aqueous resulting from irritation of the ciliary body by a freely moving lens. Tonography reveals instead that a decreased facility of outflow is the cause of the elevated intraocular pressure. It should be obvious that removal of the lens in these eyes is not likely to influence the course of the glaucoma, since the errant position of the lens is not related to the deformity of the angle. Both are caused by the ocular contusion. Therapy should be directed toward the medical treatment of the glaucoma, and if this fails, some type of filtration procedure should be performed.

In phacolytic glaucoma, the fourth cause, the glaucoma is directly related to the lens, since the trabecular meshwork becomes blocked by macrophages laden with lens debris. The diagnosis may be made by passing anterior chamber fluid through a Millipore filter and demonstrating the characteristic cytology. In this instance, lens extraction is definitely indicated.

Retinal detachment

The association of ectopia lentis and retinal detachment after ocular trauma is due to widespread ocular damage. The displacement of the lens by cyclitic membranes resulting from diathermy treatment of retinal detachment has been mentioned previously.

Retinal detachments are relatively common in eyes with heritable ectopia lentis. They occur in about 10% of eyes with Marfan's syndrome (Fig. 8-1) and homocystinuria. The relationship between the lens displacement and the retinal detachment is unclear. There may be no significant difference in the incidence of retinal detachment between the eyes that have undergone surgery for the displaced lens and those that have not.[4] It would appear logical to ascribe the complication of a retinal detachment to the motion of the dis-

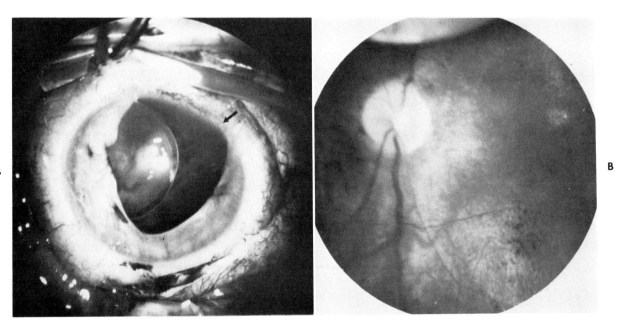

Fig. 8-1. A, Eye of 15-year-old boy with Marfan's syndrome who had optic iridectomy (*arrow*) 8 years before photograph was taken. Three retinal detachment procedures were performed in past 2 years. He had subluxed lens and total retinal detachment with massive periretinal proliferation. Following procedures were performed: pars plana lensectomy, vitrectomy, scleral buckling, and intraocular gas. B, Postoperative photograph shows clear view to fundus. Preoperative fundus photograph was not possible because of subluxed lens and vitreous opacities. (Courtesy Dr. Robert Machemer.)

placed lens and the subsequent trauma to the vitreous. However, the retinal detachment may be primarily due to abnormalities such as lattice degeneration in the retina itself.[2,9] The presence of a retinal detachment may require removal of a dislocated lens if the lens prevents adequate visualization of the retina.

Uveitis

There are two likely mechanisms for the complication of uveitis. The first is phacolytic. A totally opaque lens may be hypermature, which results in leakage of lens material. This has been discussed with the glaucoma mechanisms. In some patients, no specific etiology can be found. These cases are characterized by recurrent iritis, and it is assumed that the abnormal motility of the lens with its associated traction on the zonule and ciliary body may be the cause.

Corneal edema

Corneal edema may be due to contact between the dislocated lens and the corneal endothelium, peripheral anterior synechias as a result of the iris being pushed forward, or elevated intraocular pressure.

Strabismus and amblyopia

There is a high incidence of strabismus and amblyopia in ectopia lentis. In traumatic cases the injury occurs in early childhood. In the heritable types of ectopia lentis the dislocations occur early in life and are frequently asymmetrical. Therefore, amblyopia may result from the associated anisometropia. The amblyopia may explain why some patients may fail to show an improvement in vision after lens extraction. This was presumed to be the case in 14 out of 84 eyes that had undergone lens surgery as a result of ectopia lentis at the Wilmer Institute.[10]

MANAGEMENT

When surgery for displacement of the lens has been considered, the pendulum has swung from a liberal attitude toward removal of the lens to one of pessimism and caution. A rational approach would be to regard these eyes as sick, and the first consideration should be preservation of the globe. There have been numerous reports of long-term tolerance of a posteriorly dislocated lens; and the results of surgery have not been impressive.

A study[1] from the Wilmer Institute reported that less than 50% of 94 eyes had better vision after removal of a dislocated lens. The results of lens removal are poorer in traumatic dislocations than in Marfan's syndrome, probably because trauma causes other ocular problems such as contusion deformity of the anterior chamber angle, commotio retinae, macular scarring, and retinal detachment. In most eyes with glaucoma associated with dislocation of the lens, the usual cause of both is trauma. Only rarely (as outlined later) does lens extraction cure the glaucoma.

The least controversial indications for removal of the subluxated or dislocated lens are phacolytic glaucoma and the necessity for optic improvement in a one-eyed individual. The most controversial is the removal of a posteriorly dislocated lens in an eye with open-angle glaucoma to cure the glaucoma.

Principles of management

Because of the unusual positions a displaced lens may find and because of its frequent association with other ocular pathology, it is not surprising that the approach to management of the lens is multivarious. Each situation should be carefully analyzed and undertaken with a rational goal in mind. It is impossible to outline an approach that would gain the approval of all surgeons. For many years I have managed these situations in much the same fashion as that outlined several years ago by Iliff and Kramar.[11]

Traumatically dislocated lenses

The likelihood of associated ocular damage must be kept in mind. There may be recession of the anterior chamber angle, iris laceration, injury to the ciliary body, choroid, and retina, retinal detachment, rupture of the lens capsule, intraocular hemorrhage, rupture of the globe, and so on. In most instances the removal of the ectopic lens will not benefit these conditions. There are certain complications directly related to the lens displacement, such as pupillary block glaucoma, that will improve by removing the lens. Other complications such as retinal detachment might be aggravated. If the globe is ruptured or the retina detached, these conditions should be treated first. If angle-recession glaucoma has occurred, it should first be treated medically. If this is unsuccessful, surgery for the glaucoma should be performed. If vision is relatively good, a filtering procedure such as a trabeculectomy is a reasonable choice. If the lens is sufficiently opaque to reduce vision significantly, I would favor a combined lens extraction and trabeculectomy. A partial anterior vitrectomy is recommended if vitreous is in the anterior chamber. There are certain recommended approaches to management of the displaced lens, according to its position.

Subluxated lens still in pupillary space. If the lens is subluxated in the pupillary space, I tend to leave it in situ even if it becomes cataractous. This, of course, is if the opposite eye has adequate vision for the patient's needs. If binocular vision is required for occupational reasons, a cataractous lens is removed. These patients should be followed closely for evidence of progressive dislocation of the lens. If this occurs, the lens should be removed before it luxates completely into the vitreous. A lens aspiration is recommended for patients under 35 years of age. If the lens capsule is ruptured, aspiration is more effectively performed if one waits for the lens to become nearly totally opaque. This usually occurs rapidly. For older patients a routine cryoextraction may be possible if the rent in the lens capsule is not too large. If the subluxation has resulted in pupillary block glaucoma and visual acuity is relatively good, a peripheral iridectomy is usually curative. If vision is poor due to cataract, the lens is extracted and a peripheral iridectomy is performed. A partial anterior vitrectomy is usually necessary in these cases.

Subluxated lens in anterior chamber. The lens should be extracted in these cases. The pupil is constricted to trap the lens in the anterior chamber. A Flieringa ring is useful. Hyperosmotic agents are used in older patients. The incision should be large enough to prevent corneal endothelial damage that occurs as a result of molding the lens through an inadequate opening.

Subluxated lens in vitreous. The lens may be fixed to the retina or may be floating freely in the vitreous. If the eye appears to be tolerating the dislocated lens without undue inflammation, as is often the case, no surgery need be done. If the lens is fixed to the retina, surgery is contraindi-

cated. However, if the free-floating lens produces lens-induced uveitis or glaucoma or if it seriously interferes with vision in a one-eyed individual, the dislocated lens should be removed.

Heritable ectopia lentis

Whether or not lens surgery is performed probably makes no difference in the incidence of retinal detachment associated with heritable ectopia lentis. Although long-term follow-up series are not yet available, a lens aspiration, if indicated, should not be delayed because of fear of a late retinal detachment. However, the removal of the lens in an eye with a preexisting retinal detachment may worsen the prognosis.

Subluxated lens still in pupillary space. Surgery should be performed only if vision appears decreased. The problem is that although we are seeing these children at an early age, it is usually too early to assess the vision of the eye. As mentioned earlier, amblyopia may be present. If the zonular fibers are so relaxed that pupillary block occurs or if because of absent zonular fibers the lens and vitreous cause pupillary block, surgery is indicated. A conservative approach would be a peripheral iridectomy, which would relieve the pupillary block. However, if the lens appears responsible for decreased vision, it may be aspirated at the same time.

Subluxated lens in anterior chamber. The lens should be removed in this case. If it is still partially held by relaxed zonular fibers, it should be aspirated. Phacoemulsification is ideally suited for this situation. If the lens is completely free in the anterior chamber, it can be trapped by constricting the pupil. The surgeon may choose between a lens aspiration, phacoemulsification, or removing the entire lens through a larger incision.

Subluxated lens in vitreous. A freely floating lens in the vitreous is best left alone unless it is producing uveitis, phacolytic glaucoma, or obscuring vision. If the lens is fixed to the retina, it should be left alone. Any associated iritis or glaucoma should be treated separately. This is not easy if the complications are lens-induced.

SURGICAL PROCEDURES

A lens aspiration is indicated in patients under 35 years of age. Maximum mydriasis is obtained.

A soft eye is achieved by the usual techniques discussed on p. 257. Although not considered essential by many surgeons, I use a Flieringa ring in these cases. A 14, 16, 18, or 20 mm ring is employed, depending on the size of the eye. A small limbus-based conjunctival flap is prepared at 12 o'clock. A peritomy may be performed, if preferred. Since most of these lenses are poorly supported in the pupillary space, I prefer a two-knife discission of the anterior capsule. A knife needle is passed through an oblique incision in clear cornea just inside the limbus in the inferior temporal quadrant. The second knife passes through the limbus at 12 o'clock. One knife is used to fixate or support the lens while the other incises the anterior capsule and stirs up the lens cortex. The posterior capsule should be left intact. The knife at the lower incision site should be removed. The 12 o'clock incision site is enlarged to at least 3 mm as the knife is being withdrawn. At this juncture the surgeon has several choices of procedure, depending on personal experience. Aspiration may be performed with an inflated anterior chamber by passing a dull-tipped 25-gauge needle through the lower knife incision. This needle is attached to sterile intravenous tubing and balanced salt solution or Ringer's lactate solution passes into the anterior chamber at a sufficient rate to keep the chamber full. A scalp vein needle set may also be used for this purpose. A lens aspiration needle (I prefer the Gass needle) is passed through the 12 o'clock incision, and the lens material is carefully aspirated so that the corneal endothelium and posterior capsule are avoided. The surgeon may perform the aspiration part of this technique entirely through the 12 o'clock incision by using a combination aspiration-irrigation needle such as that of O'Gawa (Storz) (Fig. 3-60) or Thomas (Karl Ilg). I find the tips of the Fuchs or Fink-Weinstein double-barreled syringes too large in these eyes. The surgeon may elect to use the irrigation-aspiration element of the phacoemulsifier for this purpose. The 12 o'clock incision is closed with a single 7-0 chromic catgut suture. If the posterior capsule has been broken or if vitreous is present in the anterior chamber, it is swept free of the 12 o'clock site across the anterior chamber through the lower incision site. The pupil is kept dilated, and air is placed in the anterior chamber. If adequate pupillary dilatation cannot be obtained, a sector iridectomy is performed through the 12 o'clock incision. One should not hesitate to do this, if necessary.

There have been numerous other approaches to the surgical removal of a dislocated lens. An attempt may be made to trap the lens in the anterior chamber by placing the patient in the prone position and then constricting the pupil. This is rarely successful. If the lens is situated in the posterior vitreous, it may be floated into the pupillary space where it may be grasped by directing a stream of saline into the vitreous cavity. This procedure, originally recommended by Verhoeff[12] is best suited for those eyes in which the vitreous is mostly fluid. Breinin[13] recommended the use of a straight toilet-plunger type of erisiphake to extract a lens from the posterior part of the eye after vitreous is first aspirated.

The following two approaches have also been effective in the removal of a dislocated lens.

The first is probably best exemplified by a procedure recently recommended by Douvas.[14] The intraocular pressure is lowered by using an orally or intravenously administered hyperosmotic agent and applying digital pressure to the globe. A Flieringa ring is used in young patients. The incision is placed in a location that makes it unnecessary to traverse the area where formed vitreous has herniated into the anterior chamber around the edge of a dislocated lens. A limbus-based conjunctival flap and a grooved incision with preplaced sutures is desirable. Hemostasis is mandatory to avoid irrigating the anterior chamber. This is achieved by lightly searing a saline-moistened limbus with the Scheie cautery before making the groove. The superficial scleral tissue only is to be whitened; charring is avoided. Air is placed in the anterior chamber to serve as a tampon until the incision is completed. If there are residual attached zonules, alpha-chymotrypsin is used after the lens is grasped by a cryoextractor, since they may be very resistant. If an erisiphake is used, the bulb is filled with the enzyme instead of saline solution. This prevents the lens from going completely into the vitreous. If the vitreous must be traversed by the cryoextractor, it must be done by an instrument that can be applied with a warm tip with the probe shaft insulated by a silicone sleeve. Freezing is initiated once the capsule is contacted. Visualization is aided by the binocular indirect ophthalmoscope and the Wood ultraviolet light in the case of posteriorly dislocated lenses. The Amoils self-illuminating intravitreous cryoprobe[15] may be used. Miotics and acetazolamide (Diamox) are used to combat secondary glaucoma and iris prolapse.

Douvas[14] has modified Breinin's technique[13] by using a Silastic aspirating tube, a clamping hemostat, intravenous tubing with a collecting bottle, and a Stedman vacuum pump. On command by the surgeon, the hemostat is clamped on the aspirating tube by the assistant. The surgeon can position the gentle aspiration of the transparent Silastic tube with one hand while the other is free for placement of the cryoextractor.

The second approach is exemplified by a procedure popularized by Barraquer.[16] A double-pronged needle is inserted 6 mm behind the

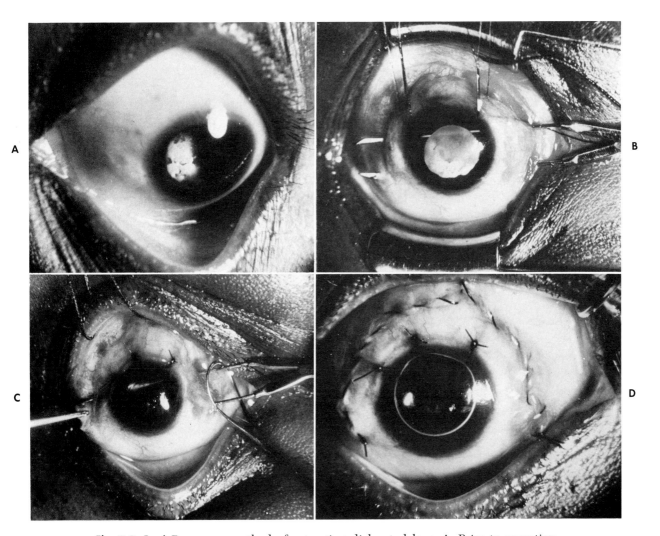

Fig. 8-2. José Barraquer method of extracting dislocated lens. **A,** Prior to operation. Note cataractous dislocated lens at nasal margin of pupil of left eye. **B,** Lens (6.5 mm in diameter) has been trapped in pupillary area by Calhoun needle, with patient in prone position. **C,** After cataract is removed and sutures are tied, sclera is fixed at needle exit sites, and slight counterpressure is applied around exit sites with lens loop prior to withdrawal of needle. **D,** At completion of operation, air bubble in anterior chamber. (From Calhoun, F. P., Jr., and Hagler, W. S.: Am. J. Ophthalmol. **50:**701-715, 1960.)

limbus through the pars plana and emerges from the globe on the opposite side 6 mm behind the limbus. The needles come in two sizes, 20 and 25 mm. Calhoun and Hagler[17] have modified this needle. They use a 27-gauge steel needle with 25 mm shafts and cutting edge tips that face outward. The shafts are spaced 4.5 mm apart. A small, lightweight handle is placed on one end to facilitate insertion. In the case of a posteriorly dislocated lens the patient is placed prone on a neurosurgical table. When the lens appears in the anterior chamber, the surgeon, working from beneath the patient's head, inserts the needle. A Flieringa ring is not used because the needle provides good scleral support. The patient is rolled over into the supine position on an adjacent table as soon as the lens is held in the anterior chamber by the needle. The surgery can then proceed by opening the anterior chamber and removing the lens by any convenient technique (Fig. 8-2). In removing the needles, good scleral fixation should be made on both sides, since there is a strong tendency for the globe to collapse with resultant vitreous loss.

In the case of a subluxated lens the patient is kept in the supine position. The needle should be inserted in the meridian in which the zonular attachment remains so that its points can be passed behind the lens and the lens can simply be lifted forward by the needle. For a small lens a triple needle may be used.

One should not leave this subject without repeating that many eyes tolerate posteriorly dislocated lenses very well and that the results of surgical removal of the lens are often poor.

REFERENCES

1. Jarrett, W. H., II: Dislocation of the lens; a study of 166 hospitalized cases, Arch. Ophthalmol. **78:**289-296, 1967.
2. Allen, R. A., Straatsma, B. R., Apt, L., and Hall, M. O.: Ocular manifestations of the Marfan's syndrome, Ophthalmology (Rochester) **71:**18-38, 1967.
3. von Noorden, G. K., and Schultz, R. O.: A gonioscopic study of the chamber angle in Marfan's syndrome, Arch. Ophthalmol. **64:**929-934, 1960.
4. Cross, H. E., and Jensen, A. D.: Ocular manifestations in the Marfan syndrome and homocystinuria, Am. J. Ophthalmol. **75:**405-420, 1973.
5. Marchesani, O.: Brachydaktylie und angeborene Kugellinse als Systemerkrankung, Klin. Mbl. Augenheilk. **103:**392-406, 1939.
6. Francois, J.: Heredity in ophthalmology, St. Louis, 1961, The C. V. Mosby Co.
7. Wolff, S. M., and Zimmerman, L. E.: Chronic secondary glaucoma associated with retrodisplacement of iris root and deepening of the anterior chamber angle secondary to contusion, Am. J. Ophthalmol. **54:**547-563, 1962.
8. Rodman, H. I.: Chronic open-angle glaucoma associated with traumatic dislocation of the lens; a new pathogenic concept, Arch. Ophthalmol. **69:**445-454, 1963.
9. Probert, L. A.: Spherophakia with brachydactyly, Am. J. Ophthalmol. **36:**1571-1574, 1953.
10. Jensen, A. D.: Heritable ectopia lentis. In Goldberg, M. F., editor: Genetic and metabolic eye disease, Boston, 1974, Little, Brown and Co., pp. 325-336.
11. Iliff, C. E., and Kramar, P.: A working guide for the management of dislocated lenses, Ophthalmol. Surg. **2:**251-257, 1971.
12. Verhoeff, F. H.: A simple and safe method for removing a cataract dislocated into fluid vitreous, Am. J. Ophthalmol. **25:**725, 1942.
13. Breinin, G. M.: Removal of the dislocated lens (a motion picture), Ophthalmology (Rochester) **66:**544, 1962.
14. Douvas, N. G.: Management of luxated and subluxated lenses, including a new surgical technique utilizing mechanical fluid vitreous: aspiration and cryoextraction, Ophthalmology (Rochester) **73:**100-106, 1969.
15. Amoils, S. P.: A self-illuminating intravenous cryoprobe, Arch. Ophthalmol. **80:**484-487, 1968.
16. Barraquer, J. I.: Surgical treatment of lens displacements, Arch. Soc. Am. Oftal. Optom. **1:**30-38, 1958.
17. Calhoun, F. P., Jr., and Hagler, W. S.: Experience with the José Barraquer method of extracting a dislocated lens, Am. J. Ophthalmol. **50:**701-715, 1960.

CHAPTER 9

Cataract surgery combined with glaucoma surgery or keratoplasty

SIMULTANEOUS GLAUCOMA AND CATARACT SURGERY

Senile cataract and open-angle glaucoma are common eye disorders arising independently in the same age group, yet the problem of how to manage these eyes when vision is sufficiently reduced to require a cataract extraction is controversial. This question arises frequently, since the treatment of the glaucoma in an eye with a lens opacity is usually done at the expense of the patient's vision. For example, miotic therapy for glaucoma often reduces visual acuity in proportion to the density of the cataract and its axial position. In addition, stronger miotics, such as echothiophate iodide, may accelerate progression of the lens opacity. If an antiglaucomatous filtering operation is performed in an eye with a lens opacity, it often hastens the development of the cataract, especially if prolonged hypotonia occurs or if the lens is accidentally traumatized. Conversely a cataract extraction performed subsequent to a filtering procedure may cause closure of a previously functioning bleb. In addition, if cataract extraction alone fails to control intraocular pressure despite maximum medical therapy, subsequent surgery for the glaucoma is definitely more unpredictable.

Thus, in a patient with senile cataract and open-angle glaucoma, the ophthalmologist is faced with four choices:

1. Cataract surgery alone
2. Filtering procedure followed by cataract extraction at a later date
3. Cataract surgery followed by a cyclodialysis or a trabeculectomy at a later date
4. Simultaneous cataract and glaucoma surgery

It is becoming increasingly apparent that cataract extraction has a favorable influence on the therapy of open-angle glaucoma in a high percentage of eyes. This is discussed on p. 318. Many patients require no glaucoma medication for a considerable time after the cataract extraction. However, they must be examined periodically because there is a tendency for the intraocular pressure to rise again in most of these eyes, since the lens extraction itself probably exerts little influence on the course of the open-angle glaucoma. I have found that it is extremely rare for these patients to require stronger medical therapy after the cataract extraction than preoperatively. It is not unusual to find that some patients require no medication permanently, although it is possible that in some of these the original diagnosis of open-angle glaucoma was in error. However, the medical therapy for the glaucoma appears to be more effective after the cataract has been removed. This has been my impression in patients requiring mild, moderate, or strong glaucoma medication preoperatively. For example, echothiophate iodide works very effectively in these eyes. Most of the contraindications and side effects of this agent disappear once the lens is removed. Obviously, we are not concerned with its cataractogenic tendency. Even more important, we are less concerned about its ability to produce edema in the uveal tract. This edema can secondarily narrow the angle and produce angle-closure glaucoma in the phakic eye. Most phakic eyes with marginal glaucoma control respond well to this drug after lens extraction. Of course, other agents such as epinephrine, timolol, and acetazolamide are available to be used in combination with the echothiophate iodide.

Therefore, if the intraocular pressure is controlled by mild, moderate, or strong medical therapy, one should not hesitate to perform a lens extraction alone, if indicated, since it is highly probable that the glaucoma will be easily managed postoperatively. The problem may arise of what to do if the intraocular pressure fails to respond to medical therapy after the lens extraction. I have found this to occur very rarely. In the past it has usually been associated with a postoperative abnormality of anterior chamber depth that resulted in peripheral anterior synechias. Cyclodialysis has proven disappointing in a high percentage of these patients. However, cyclocryothermy has proven useful here, since it is a safe and simple procedure. Although its benefit is rarely permanent or even of long duration, it may be repeated. Therefore, it is more ideally suited for the elderly patient. The younger patient with a greater life expectancy may respond better to other procedures. Trabeculectomy has been successful in some of these eyes, although its success rate does not approach that seen in phakic eyes with open-angle glaucoma. It is less likely to succeed if vitreous is present in the anterior chamber. It is better suited for aphakic eyes with an intact, posteriorly displaced anterior hyaloid membrane and even better if a posterior capsule is present.

The older procedure of initially performing a filtering operation and then a lens extraction 6 months to a year later has little to recommend it, since the frequent failure of the filtering bleb after the lens extraction may place the eye in jeopardy. In elderly patients in whom the lens opacity is advanced in both eyes there is an unduly long delay in restoring vision.

Performing a lens extraction in poorly controlled eyes, to be followed at a later date by a cyclodialysis or a trabeculectomy is probably also unsafe. As stated earlier, if the glaucoma control is marginal, there may be adequate justification in first attempting the lens extraction, since the glaucoma is often more easily controlled. However, poorly controlled cases are usually not benefited by lens extraction alone. Glaucoma surgery must then be performed under less favorable circumstances.

In my opinion, if an eye requires strong medical therapy in combination such as the stronger anticholinesterases, epinephrine derivatives, and carbonic anhydrase inhibitors, and if the level of intraocular pressure is frequently abnormal, and especially if visual field loss has progressed, the surgical procedure should be a simultaneous cataract and filtering operation. This is a difficult decision. In the end, the surgeon comes to rely on personal experience or that of a consultant in planning the surgery. Unfortunately, some reports of the benefits derived from simultaneous cataract and glaucoma surgery are based on cases in which the urgency for the glaucoma surgery is not well established. I have found simultaneous surgery to be rarely indicated. Admittedly, however, there will be patients in whom such a procedure is justified.

Although a simultaneous cataract extraction and filtering operation was recommended[1] nearly 40 years ago, enthusiasm for such procedures did not materialize until recently. The ophthalmologist who labors meticulously to seal the cataract incision finds it difficult to generate support for a procedure that intentionally creates a wound leak. Several ophthalmologists[2-8] have advocated combining a cataract extraction with filtering procedures such as iridencleisis, sclerectomy, or trephination. Stocker[9] was the first to recommend cautery sclerostomy and buried sutures combined with cataract extraction. His was followed by other reports[10-13] that favored this procedure. More recently, cataract extraction combined with trabeculectomy has been advocated.[14] A simultaneous cyclodialysis and cataract extraction has also received favorable attention.[15-18] Proponents of this procedure claim that the disadvantages of a wound fistula and shallowing of the anterior chamber are avoided.

Simultaneous cautery sclerostomy and cataract extraction

After eyelid akinesia and retrobulbar injection composed of a combination of lidocaine (Xylocaine), hyaluronidase, and epinephrine, digital pressure is applied to lower intraocular pressure, as for a routine cataract extraction. A superior rectus suture is placed. After the anesthetic solution is injected subconjunctivally, an arcuate incision is then made through conjunctiva and Tenon's capsule from 9 to 3 o'clock, approximately 8 mm posterior to the limbus. The flap is then dissected down to the limbus. A scalpel with a No. 15 Bard-Parker blade is used to brush the remaining fascia toward the limbus. The rounded surface of the blade—not its tip—is used to avoid perforating the flap. Bleeding vessels are cauterized. A razor blade groove approximately two thirds the thickness of the sclera is made at an angle ranging from 70 to 90 degrees to the surface of the sclera, from 9:30 to 2:30 o'clock. The groove is placed about 0.5 mm posterior to the blue and white junction of the limbus (p. 47) or midway between Schwalbe's line and the iris root. A single 10-0 nylon or 9-0 black silk suture is preplaced at 12 o'clock. The lips of the wound are cauterized at points on both sides of the central suture by use of the Hildreth cautery (Fig. 9-1). The retraction is limited to the outer half of the sclera. The anterior chamber is entered at one end of the grooved incision with a keratome, a razor blade, or some other suitable instrument. The incision is enlarged with Barraquer scissors with the stop device, which prevents the tips from closing completely, to avoid uneven edges. Peripheral iridotomies or iridectomies are placed at 10:30 and 1:30 o'clock. The lens is removed by cryoextraction. The central suture is tied. An additional suture is placed on each side midway between the point of cautery and the periphery of the incision. The knots are pulled to the scleral side, and the sutures are cut flush with the knot. The knots should be pulled into the suture track. This is more important with 10-0 nylon than with 9-0 silk, since the ends of the former show a greater tendency to erode through the flap. The anterior chamber is filled with balanced salt solution. Air is avoided, since it may cause sufficient compression to prevent filtration. The conjunctival flap is then sutured in only two places with the same material. No attempt is made to make this wound watertight.

The blebs usually appear on the second or third postoperative day and progressively assume a flat succulent appearance. The anterior chamber is usually well formed on the first day. The patient should be followed closely for several months, and if the bleb appears to diminish, ocular massage should be initiated in an attempt to maintain filtration. Acetazolamide should be avoided because it diminishes aqueous flow.

The procedure is simple to perform, and I have been satisfied with its results. Maumenee and Wilkinson[12] performed this procedure in 20 eyes and reported that 12 had filtering blebs 6 months to 3 years later with satisfactory pressures and no medication. Seven eyes required medication for adequate control of the glaucoma, and one eye had a normal pressure without medication but no evidence of filtration. For 3 years Boyd[13] followed up 370 eyes in which he had performed a simultaneous filtering cautery sclerostomy and cataract extraction. He divided the eyes into four groups.

Group 1 (125 eyes). Moderately strong medical therapy was required to control intraocular pressure to a level of 19 mm or less. Seventy-five percent were controlled without medication after 3 years; no eyes required stronger medication than preoperatively, and no eyes were uncontrolled medically.

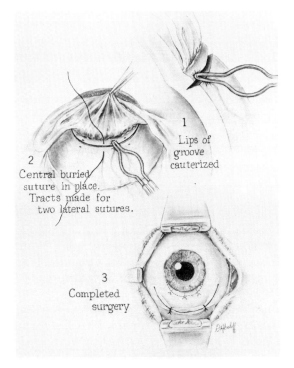

1
Lips of groove cauterized

2
Central buried suture in place. Tracts made for two lateral sutures.

3
Completed surgery

Fig. 9-1. Simultaneous cautery sclerostomy and cataract extraction. (From Maumenee, A. E., and Wilkinson, C. P.: Am. J. Ophthalmol. **69:**360-367, 1970.)

Group 2 (125 eyes). Strong to maximum medical therapy was required to control intraocular pressure to a level of 19 mm or less. Sixty percent were controlled without medication after 3 years, no eyes required stronger medication than preoperatively, and no eyes were uncontrolled medically.

Group 3 (80 eyes). Maximum medical therapy without control of intraocular pressure was followed; preoperative range of pressure was 21 to 36 mm. Forty-five percent were controlled without medication after 3 years, the remainder required medication less strong than preoperatively for control of pressure, but 10% required cyclodialysis because of intolerance to medications.

Group 4 (40 eyes). Maximum medical therapy in addition to a previous filtering operation was followed. In 24 eyes the preoperative intraocular pressure was 19 mm or less. Forty-two percent were controlled without medication after 3 years, 48% were controlled on less strong medication than preoperatively, and 10% required cyclodialysis. In 16 eyes the preoperative intraocular pressure ranged from 21 to 34 mm. Thirty-five percent of these were controlled without medication after 3 years, 40% were controlled on less strong medication than preoperatively, and 25% required cyclodialysis.

Simultaneous trabeculectomy and cataract extraction

Since Cairns'[19] modification in 1968 of a trabeculectomy procedure introduced by Sugar[20] in 1961, there has been widespread interest in this surgical method for the control of open-angle glaucoma. The operation is based on the proposition that the obstruction to outflow of aqueous in this disease is situated in the trabecular meshwork. Objections have been raised to the term trabeculectomy as applied to this procedure. Since the block of tissue removed contains not only trabeculum but also canal of Schlemm, cornea, and sclera, such objections are reasonable. However, the term is in general usage, and no attempt will be made to modify it.

Trabeculectomy was originally designed to allow aqueous to gain entry into the cut open ends of Schlemm's canal, thus bypassing the impermeable trabecula. Considerable evidence has accumulated against this hypothesis. Histopathologic studies by Spencer[21] revealed that the cut ends of Schlemm's canal had fibrosed closed. Ridgway and co-workers[22] reported that histological examination of a specimen of the sclerocorneal excision demonstrated the presence of trabecular meshwork in only one third of the specimens. In addition, it has been shown that, with rare exceptions, blood cannot be refluxed into the anterior chamber from Schlemm's canal after trabeculectomy. Finally, a most significant point is the appearance of a filtering bleb in nearly all successfully treated cases. Thus the originally intended mechanism, egress of aqueous into Schlemm's canal, has changed to the extent that trabeculectomy permits filtration of aqueous from beneath a scleral flap into the subconjunctival space. This would indicate that it is just another filtering operation except that it is performed under a scleral flap. Cairns[23] has enumerated three other possible mechanisms: that it bypasses Schlemm's canal, not into the subconjunctival space directly but into the collector channels and aqueous veins; that it acts by virtue of a localized cyclodialysis (the negligible effect of even large cyclodialysis procedures on intraocular pressure suggests that this explanation is unlikely to be correct); or that the effect is purely one of hyposecretion (the duration of control in many cases makes this unlikely). However, as just stated, the currently accepted view is that the mode of action is by filtration of aqueous into the subconjunctival space.

It is now apparent that trabeculectomy has about the same success rate as other filtering operations. It shares with other filtering operations a tendency to fail in young patients, in black patients, and patients with secondary glaucoma.[24] Some[25] ophthalmic surgeons feel that the pressure is not as low and is of shorter duration than after other filtering operations, but that is not definitely known. The main advantage of trabeculectomy may be that it causes fewer complications than other filtering procedures. Two advantages that may make it ideally suited for a simultaneous glaucoma and cataract procedure is that there is a decidedly lower incidence of postoperative flat anterior chamber and that the bleb is thick-walled and diffuse. The former is a definite advantage after cataract extraction, and the latter

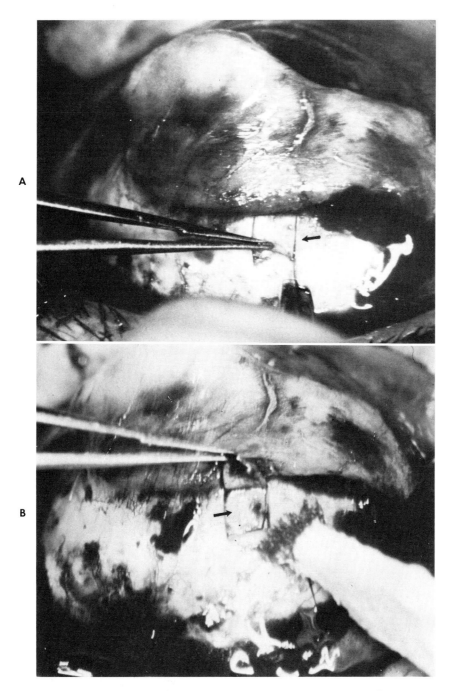

Fig. 9-2. A, Half-thickness lamellar scleral flap 4 mm wide and extending 4 mm posterior to limbus is raised at 12 o'clock *(arrow)* with razor blade. **B,** Lamellar scleral flap is retracted, exposing bed of flap *(arrow).*

(still unproven) reduces the risk of late bleb infections and may even allow contact lens wear in some patients. The bleb is definitely less cystic and more posteriorly situated. There is less tendency for migration of the bleb over the cornea.

The preliminary steps in the technique are identical to those enumerated for a simultaneous cautery sclerostomy and cataract extraction regarding eyelid akinesia, retrobulbar injection, digital pressure, superior rectus suture, and the preparation of the conjunctival flap. A half-thickness lamellar scleral flap 4 mm wide and extending 4 mm posterior to the limbus is raised at 12 o'clock (Fig. 9-2). The flap is hinged in the cornea. The outline of the flap is made with a razor blade section. The undermining is completed with a Beaver No. 66 lamellar blade. A 7-0 silk or catgut suture is used to retract the scleral flap. The surgical landmarks are easily visualized. A dark blue zone designates the usually transparent cornea. This is sharply demarcated from a white zone. This division overlies Schlemm's canal. A rectangular block of tissue containing cornea, trabecula, Schlemm's canal, and sclera is excised (Fig. 9-3). This is done by entering the anterior chamber with a perpendicular razor blade incision, which is made posteriorly for a distance of 2 mm. This creates an inner flap that can be everted, allowing the surgeon to observe directly the trabecular meshwork and the base of the iris. The everted block of tissue is dissected posteriorly to a point of firm attachment at the base of the iris. This marks the attachment of the scleral spur and provides the posterior limit of the trabecular block dissection. The 4 by 2 mm inner flap is excised with the razor blade tip or fine-tipped scissors (Vannas or Westcott). If the iris should prolapse during the preparation of the inner flap, it may be punctured to allow it to fall back. After the excision of the inner flap, a peripheral iridectomy is performed through this opening (Fig. 9-4). Since this is an extremely basal iridectomy, care must be taken to avoid the ciliary body. A corneoscleral incision is then made as for a routine cataract extraction with right and left scissors (Fig. 9-5). Care must be exercised to avoid the iridectomy opening at the beginning of the right and left portions of the incision. At this juncture, some form of iris manipu-

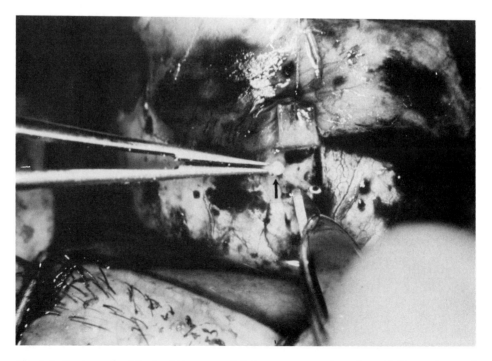

Fig. 9-3. Rectangular block of tissue containing cornea, trabeculum, Schlemm's canal and sclera *(arrow)* is excised.

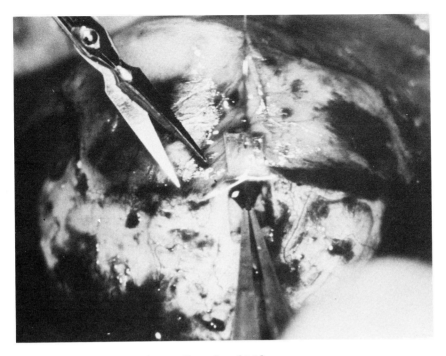

Fig. 9-4. Peripheral iridectomy.

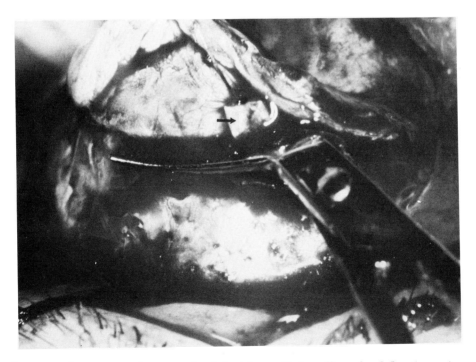

Fig. 9-5. Enlargement of corneoscleral incision with lamellar scleral flap *(arrow)* retracted.

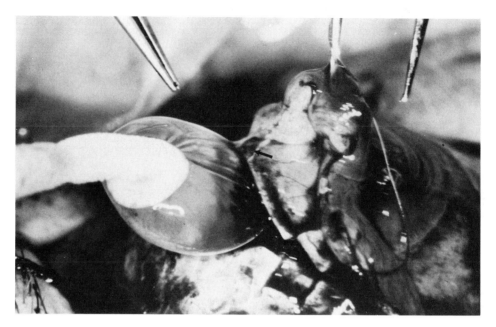

Fig. 9-6. Cryoextraction of lens. Note bed of lamellar scleral flap *(arrow).*

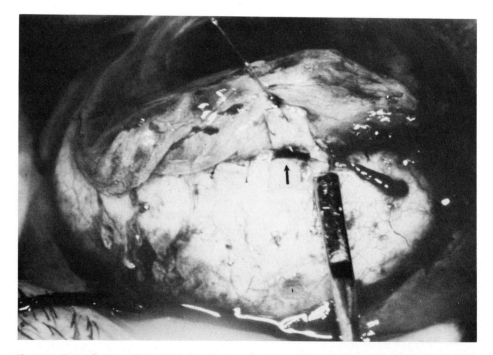

Fig. 9-7. Completion of corneoscleral wound suturing. Lamellar scleral flap is still retracted. Note defect *(arrow)* from excision of rectangular block of tissue.

lation is required. These patients have usually been on a regimen of long-term miotic therapy, resulting in a fixed small pupil due to fibrosis of the iris sphincter. Posterior synechias may also be present. An iris spatula is placed under the iris through the pupil and gently separates any posterior synechias. Small sphincterotomies may be made at 12, 4:30, and 7:30 o'clock. This greatly facilitates lens extraction. Alpha-chymotrypsin is instilled. A 10-0 monofilament nylon corneoscleral suture is placed at each side of the lamellar trap door. The sutures are looped out of the wound. Additional preextraction corneoscleral sutures may be placed, if desired. After the anterior chamber is irrigated, the cataract is extracted (Fig. 9-6). The preplaced sutures are tied, and additional sutures are placed as needed (Fig. 9-7). The lamellar scleral flap is closed with two interrupted 10-0 monofilament nylon sutures, one at each posterior corner of the flap. Recognizing that subconjunctival filtration is now accepted as the mechanism of pressure lowering in trabeculectomy, I have encouraged filtration by using very light thermal cautery of the sclera adjacent to each vertical arm of the scleral flap. The anterior chamber is filled with balanced salt solution. The limbus-based conjunctival flap is closed with a continuous 7-0 or 8-0 plain catgut suture.

The anterior chamber is usually fully formed on the first day. The bleb may not be apparent at first and is usually less bullous than that seen after other filtering procedures. It has the appearance of conjunctival edema. It is my impression that there is a greater number of bleb failures with this combined procedure than with trabeculectomies without lens extraction. The success rate for glaucoma control is apparently high even in those eyes where a bleb is not seen. However, this may be the effect of the lens extraction. Longer follow-up will determine the permanence of the control. Since filtration is the apparent mechanism, the precise localization and excision of the trabecular meshwork and Schlemm's canal may not be necessary to achieve success. Therefore, the technique need not be overelaborate. However, to avoid ciliary body damage, the entry into the anterior chamber should not be made too posteriorly.

The advantage of a combined trabeculectomy and cataract extraction, as stated previously, appears to be its avoidance of early (anterior chamber depth abnormalities) and late (bleb infection) complications. More cases must be accumulated before this assumption is considered valid.

Simultaneous cyclodialysis and cataract extraction

Adequate akinesia, anesthesia, and hypotonia of the globe are obtained as for a routine cataract extraction. Galin and co-workers[18] advocate the following simple procedure (Fig. 9-8): A 2 to 3 mm limbus-based conjunctival flap is dissected superiorly for 180 degrees. A shallow limbal groove is made over the upper half of the globe, and corneoscleral sutures are preplaced. A cyclodialysis site is prepared approximately 5 mm

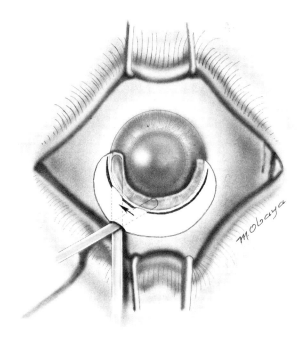

Fig. 9-8. Simultaneous cyclodialysis and cataract extraction. A 2 to 3 mm limbus-based conjunctival flap is dissected. Shallow 180-degree limbal groove is prepared. A 2 to 3 mm scleral incision down to ciliary body is made, parallel to and 5 mm from limbus. Cyclodialysis spatula is then inserted into supraciliary space, and single sweep of approximately 90 to 120 degrees is carried out. Anterior chamber is then reformed and entered through limbal groove. Cataract is then extracted according to surgeon's preferred technique.

superior to the corneoscleral limbus at the 2 or 10 o'clock meridians. With a cautery or knife a 2 to 3 mm groove is created parallel to the limbus until the choroid is reached. A cyclodialysis spatula is then inserted into the supraciliary space, and a single sweep of approximately 90 to 120 degrees is carried out. Saline or balanced salt solution is

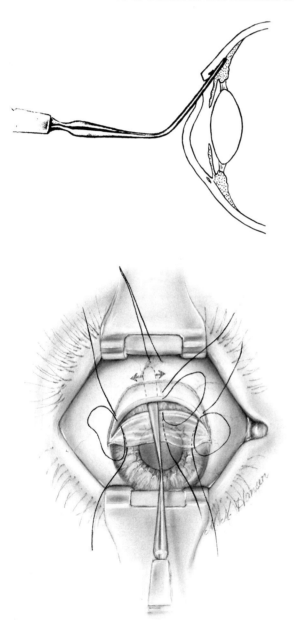

Fig. 9-9. Combined operation of intracapsular lens extraction and reverse type of cyclodialysis. (From Harrington, D. O.: Am. J. Ophthalmol. **61:**1134-1140, 1966.)

injected through the cyclodialysis cleft to reconstitute the chamber. The anterior chamber is then entered through the preplaced groove, and the lens is extracted according to the surgeon's preferred technique. The procedure is safe and, according to the authors, has resulted in normalizing the intraocular pressure without medication in more than 60% of patients. It is still unknown whether the pressure-lowering effect is caused by the suprachoroidal drainage of aqueous through the cleft or by hyposecretion hypotonia related to ciliochoroidal detachment.

A variation of this procedure was reported earlier by Harrington[17] (Fig. 9-9). A beveled limbal groove, starting 1 mm on the scleral side, is prepared over the upper half of the globe. Preplaced sutures are inserted across the groove. The anterior chamber is entered perpendicularly, and scissors enlargement proceeds at a right angle to the surface of the globe. Thus a beveled-perpendicular incision is made. The corneal lip of the wound is retracted, and the scleral lip is grasped at about the 11 o'clock position with fine-toothed forceps and is slightly elevated. A round-ended, smooth spatula is then gently pushed up into the angle of the anterior chamber beneath the forceps, fixating the scleral wound lip until it encounters slight resistance in the angle recess. The upper surface of the spatula hugs the sclera as it is pushed past the trabecula between the sclera and ciliary body for a distance of 6 to 7 mm from the cut edge of the corneoscleral wound. The cyclodialysis cleft is widened over a portion of a quadrant by sweeping the spatula to the left as it is withdrawn. The procedure is then repeated in the other upper quadrant from the 1 to 2 o'clock position. Thus a "reverse" cyclodialysis is accomplished. Lens extraction then proceeds in the usual manner.

SIMULTANEOUS CATARACT EXTRACTION AND PENETRATING KERATOPLASTY

Until recently it has been considered an essential requirement that an eye with both a corneal leukoma and a cataract should undergo a penetrating keratoplasty first and a cataract extraction 6 months to 1 year or more later. When one considers that the first procedure has a definite failure rate and the second causes opacification of the graft in a significant number of cases, the failure rate after the two procedures is fairly high. It is not surprising, therefore, that the simultaneous performance of penetrating keratoplasty and cataract extraction has become increasingly attractive.

The presence of a corneal opacity is certainly not an absolute indication for a penetrating keratoplasty. A cataract extraction combined with an optic iridectomy will often result in satisfactory vision. It is only in those eyes where a cataract extraction is likely to cause a worsening of the corneal pathology or where the corneal opacification is sufficiently extensive that both procedures become necessary. The most frequent indication for simultaneous surgery is the presence of a cataract in an eye with Fuchs' dystrophy. The final result is probably equal to or better than that obtained when the procedures are done consecutively with an interval of 6 months to 1 year or longer allowed between them. Moreover, the prolonged convalescence and prolonged interval without usable vision with the latter are serious drawbacks. In addition, a recent analysis[26] of 300 consecutive keratoplasties indicates that combined keratoplasty and cataract extraction have approximately the same success rate as keratoplasty alone. This success rate of 70% to 80% in patients[27,28] with advanced bullous keratopathy appears superior to what might be expected from keratoplasty and cataract extraction as separate procedures.[29]

The improved rate of success of the combined operation may be attributed to several factors: better suture material and wound closure techniques, prevention of pupillary block, and the realization that the most frequent cause of failure is adherence of vitreous to the back of the grafted cornea.

The following are suggestions for the prevention of vitreocorneal adherence:

1. Measures to prevent operative loss of vitreous, such as preoperative systemically administered hyperosmotic agents, posterior sclerotomy through the pars plana, Flieringa ring, general anesthesia, and others discussed on p. 256

2. Artificial devices to prevent vitreocorneal adherence, such as the spatula of Filatov[30] or an anterior chamber lens[31]

3. Round pupil, preferably miotic

4. Extracapsular cataract extraction with preservation of the posterior capsule of the lens

5. Partial anterior vitrectomy in the event of operative loss of vitreous

One of the most important predisposing factors in vitreous loss is scleral collapse (Fig. 9-10). When the eye is open, the scleral shell tends to collapse, and if the sclera can be reinforced, vitreous loss can be minimized. This factor is especially important in young people, keratoconus patients, and those with high myopia. The use of a ring tends to lessen scleral collapse while serving other useful purposes. It aids in suture placement by maintaining the regular circumference of the remaining host cornea after excision of the corneal button. It prevents distortion of the shape of the eye during the suturing. It maintains the integrity of the global wall during the extraction of the cataract. Since the lens is often larger than the opening in the cornea, it tends to press against the side of the corneal opening, distorting the globe as well as collapsing the sclera. The use of the ring minimizes these problems.

Kaufman[26] has offered a reasonable argument for the advantage of a double (Legrand) ring over a single ring. Although a single ring can be used to support the anterior segment, it may cause

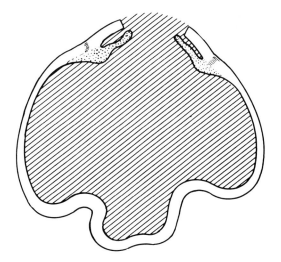

Fig. 9-10. Common cause of vitreous loss is collapse of scleral shell. This is especially likely to happen in myopic patients, patients with keratoconus, and young children in whom scleral shell lacks rigidity. (From Kaufman, H. E.: Am. J. Ophthalmol. **77:**824-829, 1974.)

what one is trying to prevent. If the same sutures are used to attach the sclera to the ring and to provide traction, any nonradial pull on the sutures slides the sutures along the ring causing the sclera to fold in and actually cause vitreous loss (Fig. 9-11). For proper use of a ring, therefore, one set of sutures should be applied for fixation and others to provide traction on the ring. The double ring, on the other hand, provides a more effective technique of scleral support. In most eyes, four sutures can be placed just central to the posts connecting the anterior and posterior ring. These four supports generally provide sufficient support for the globe and can also be used for superior and inferior traction, since they cannot slide around the ring and are held stationary by the post connecting the anterior and posterior ring (Fig. 9-12). In very myopic eyes or eyes particularly prone to scleral collapse, one may elect to place two to four additional sutures to fix the posterior ring to the sclera. This is usually unnecessary, since the posterior ring simply serves to help lift away the eyelids and adnexal tissue from the globe. The ring is simple to fixate, is effective, and provides excellent fixation for trephining while it is held by forceps (Fig. 9-12).

Technique. The technique of the simultaneous cataract extraction and penetrating keratoplasty is as follows:

1. Local anesthesia including retrobulbar injection.
2. Digital pressure for at least 7 minutes.
3. Aspiration of 0.25 to 0.5 ml of retrovitreal fluid by pars planotomy with a 25-gauge needle (Fig. 17-9). This is optional and is usually reserved for eyes with increased orbital pressure as with endocrine exophthalmos.
4. Double ring of Legrand sutured to sclera, as just described.
5. Beveled knife-needle limbal incision with injection of air.[32]
6. Donor button of 7.5 to 8 mm prepared.
7. Trephination of 7.5 to 8 mm in recipient eye (Fig. 9-12).
8. Three peripheral iridotomies at 10, 12, and 2 o'clock (Fig. 9-13). These are difficult to perform through a central corneal opening

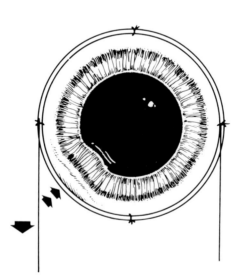

Fig. 9-11. Nonradial pull on Flieringa ring with suture attached to sclera can slide suture along ring and cause infolding and collapse of sclera with consequent vitreous loss. (From Kaufman, H. E.: Am. J. Ophthalmol. **77:**824-829, 1974.)

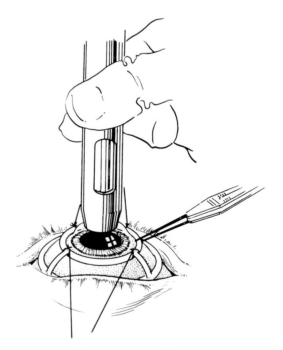

Fig. 9-12. Double ring (Legrand) with traction above and below. Traction sutures also anchor sclera and cannot slide around ring because of posts connecting two rings. Sutures are attached just central to posts connecting anterior and posterior ring. (From Kaufman, H. E.: Am. J. Ophthalmol. **77:**824-829, 1974.)

without causing iridodialysis and hemorrhage. They are performed by grasping the iris with forceps near the pupillary border, slightly depressing it, and sliding sharp-tipped, slightly curved scissors (Wescott or Vannas) between the cornea and iris to make small, transverse, full-thickness incisions in the iris near its base.

9. Injection of 1.5 ml of alpha-chymotrypsin 1:5000 under the iris.
10. Irrigation of anterior chamber with balanced salt solution after 90 seconds.
11. Cryoextraction of the lens. The usual technique is modified because the lens cannot usually be held at its superior or inferior pole but generally is held slightly below the middle. As the ice ball forms, the lens is elevated and moved slightly superiorly. The iris and corneal tissue are then milked around the border of the lens, usually beginning with the inferior border, and are pushed off the lens rather than simply lifting out the lens. This procedure, as pointed out by Kaufman,[26] reduces the resistance to lens movement but also mechanically breaks the zonules, in the inferior

portion first and later elsewhere, and facilitates removal of the lens (Fig. 9-14). A variety of spatula-like instruments may be used for this maneuver.

12. If vitreous loss occurs, a partial anterior vitrectomy should be performed (p. 268). This is important. One should aim at leaving no vitreous in the anterior chamber.
13. Donor graft anchored in place using four equally spaced, interrupted 10-0 nylon sutures.
14. Air injection into anterior chamber.
15. A continuous 10-0 monofilament nylon suture is placed and tied to itself in one location. After the suture is placed and before it is tied, each loop is pulled up, one at a time, until the wound is tightly closed. After the suture is tied, the wound is tested for areas of poor closure. Interrupted sutures are placed in these locations. An attempt is made to bring the suture knot of the continuous suture into the suture track. One may substitute 15-0 (13 μm) monofilament nylon for the continuous suture.
16. Aspiration of a portion of the air bubble and replacement with balanced salt solution.
17. Postoperatively, 6 ounces of 50% glycerin are given orally twice daily for 4 days to prevent adherence to the cornea. This is optional. The interrupted sutures are removed in about 1 to 3 months. The continuous suture is left in for at least 6 months.

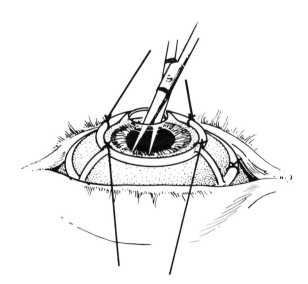

Fig. 9-13. Small pointed scissors inserted under cornea and above iris makes contact with iris at its base, so that when scissors is closed, peripheral iridotomy is produced. (From Kaufman, H. E.: Am. J. Ophthalmol. 77:824-829, 1974.)

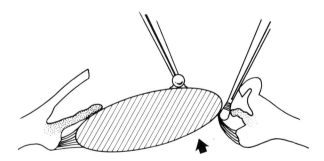

Fig. 9-14. In extracting cataract through keratoplasty incision, lens is grasped with cryophake slightly below middle. Lens is elevated and moved slightly superiorly with cryoprobe as cornea and iris are pushed over its inferior margin with spatula, and zonules are mechanically ruptured. (From Kaufman, H. E.: Am. J. Ophthalmol. 77:824-829, 1974.)

To remove it, one must cut through the corneal epithelium. It may have to be removed one loop at a time and at different sessions. It may be left in permanently in some cases.

Because of the advantage of an intact posterior lens capsule in preventing vitreous contact with the grafted cornea, a simultaneous phacoemulsification cataract extraction and penetrating keratoplasty has been recommended.[33] However, these cases must be chosen carefully, since corneal opacification can limit the surgeon's ability to visualize the lens during its emulsification.

The postoperative management differs little from that of a routine cataract extraction with the following exception: These patients are likely to run high intraocular pressures. The pressure may be checked with a Mackay-Marg electronic applanation tonometer. If there is elevation of intraocular pressure, it usually can be controlled with medication. If after a few weeks the pressure cannot be lowered by medical means alone, cryotherapy of the ciliary body may be very useful and does not cause clouding of the corneal graft.

REFERENCES

1. Wright, R. E.: Lectures on cataract. IV. Posterior-segment complications in the postoperative period; some difficult extractions, Am. J. Ophthalmol. **20:**376-387, 1937.
2. O'Brien, C. S.: Ocular surgery: random observations, Arch. Ophthalmol. **37:**1-7, 1947.
3. MacMillan, J. A.: In discussion of Ramsay, G. A. S.: Glaucoma and cataract, Arch. Ophthalmol. **43:**195, 1950.
4. Birge, H. L.: Glaucoma with cataract surgically cured with a single operation, Trans. Am. Ophthalmol. Soc. **50:**241-263, 1952.
5. MacLean, A. L.: In discussion of Birge, H. L.: Glaucoma with cataract surgically cured with a single operation, Trans. Am. Ophthalmol. Soc. **50:**259-260, 1952.
6. Wenaas, E. J., and Stertzbach, C. W.: Cataract extraction with iris inclusion, Am. J. Ophthalmol. **39:**71-75, 1955.
7. Hughes, W. L.: Report on a combination operation for cataract with glaucoma, Am. J. Ophthalmol. **48:**1-14, 1959.
8. Sugar, H. S.: Extraction of cataract in glaucomatous eyes, An. Inst. Barraquer **3:**494-502, 1962.
9. Stocker, F. W.: Combined cataract extraction and scleral cauterization, Arch. Ophthalmol. **72:**503-504, 1964.
10. McLean, J. M.: Personal interview between the editor and Dr. J. M. McLean: Cataract surgery, Highlights Ophthalmol. **7:**125-149, 1964.
11. MacLean, A. L.: Limbal lip cautery for glaucoma, Arch. Ophthalmol. **71:**653-661, 1964.
12. Maumenee, A. E., and Wilkinson, C. P.: A combined operation for glaucoma and cataract, Am. J. Ophthalmol. **69:**360-367, 1970.
13. Boyd, B. F.: Cataract extraction in eyes with open angle glaucoma, Highlights Ophthalmol. **12:**259-302, 1969.
14. Dellaporta, A., and Fahrenbruch, R. L.: Trepano-trabeculectomy, Ophthalmology (Rochester) **75:**283-295, 1971.
15. Guyton, J. S.: In discussion of Birge, H. L.: Glaucoma with cataract surgically cured by a single operation, Trans. Am. Ophthalmol. Soc. **50:**261-262, 1952.
16. Boberg-Ans, J.: Simultaneous operation for cataract and glaucoma: report on 30 cases, Trans. Ophthalmol. Soc. U.K. **84:**113-125, 1964.
17. Harrington, D. O.: Cataract and glaucoma: management of the coexistent conditions and a description of a new operation combining lens extraction with reverse cyclodialysis, Am. J. Ophthalmol. **61:**1134-1140, 1966.
18. Galin, M. A., Baras, I., and Sambursky, J.: Glaucoma and cataract: A study of cyclodialysis-lens extraction, Am. J. Ophthalmol. **67:**552-526, 1969.
19. Cairns, J. E.: Trabeculectomy: Preliminary report of a new method, Am. J. Ophthalmol. **66:**673-679, 1968.
20. Sugar, H. S.: Experimental trabeculectomy in glaucoma, Am. J. Ophthalmol. **51:**623-627, 1961.
21. Spencer, W. H.: Histologic evaluation of microsurgical glaucoma, Ophthalmology (Rochester) **76:**389-397, 1972.
22. Ridgway, A. E., Rubinstein, K., and Smith, V. H.: Trabeculectomy, Br. J. Ophthalmol. **56:**511-516, 1972.
23. Cairns, J. E.: Trabeculectomy, Ophthalmology (Rochester) **76:**384-388, 1972.
24. Schwartz, A. L., and Anderson, D. R.: Trabecular surgery, Arch. Ophthalmol. **92:**134-138, 1974.
25. Spaeth, G. L., Joseph, N. H., and Fernades, E.: Trabeculectomy: a re-evaluation after three years and a comparison with Scheie's procedure, Ophthalmic Surg. **6:**27-38, 1975.
26. Kaufman, H. E.: Combined keratoplasty and cataract extraction, Am. J. Ophthalmol. **77:**824-829, 1974.
27. Fine, M.: Corneal grafts and aphakia. In Rycroft, D. V., editor: Corneo-plastic Surgery, proceedings, International Corneo-Plastic Conference, 2nd, Royal College of Surgeons of England, 1967, New York, 1969, Pergamon Press Inc., p. 289.
28. Capella, J. A., Kaufman, H. E., and Polack, F. M.: Prognosis of keratoplasty in phakic and aphakic patients and use of cryopreserved donor tissue, **76:**1275-1285, 1972.
29. Lemp, M. A., Pfister, R. R., and Dohlman, C. H.: The effect of intraocular surgery on clear corneal grafts, Am. J. Ophthalmol. **70:**719-721, 1970.
30. Filatov, V. P.: Transplantation of the cornea, Arch. Ophthalmol. **13:**321-347, 1935.
31. Casey, T. A.: Penetrating keratoplasty in aphakia, Int. Ophthalmol. Clin. **2:**801-808, 1962.
32. Girard, L. J.: Combined cataract extraction and penetrating keratoplasty. In Welsh, R. C., and Welsh, J.: The new report on cataract surgery, Miami, 1969, Miami Educational Press, pp. 194-195.
33. Praeger, D. L., and Schneider, H. A.: Combined Kelman procedure (phaco-emulsification cataract extraction) and simultaneous aphakic penetration keratoplasty, Ophthalmol. Surg. **6:**56-59, 1975.

CHAPTER 10

Postoperative care

Reciting a routine for postoperative management suitable for every patient or for every surgeon is impossible. Although there are principles of intelligent postoperative care that can be listed, personal variations are unavoidable. Each surgeon must establish a course of management for patients that best suits their needs. The following takes heed of this, but my personal opinions will be apparent.

Postoperative care commences immediately after the conclusion of the cataract extraction. If local anesthesia has been used, the surgeon may inform the patient that the operation is over, that all has gone well, and that he has been very cooperative. Every patient enjoys hearing this. If general anesthesia has been used, the surgeon must forego direct communication until the patient is awake.

The patient is given instructions for the day. Increasing permissiveness has been apparent in recent years. Formerly, patients were hospitalized for 10 days to 2 weeks, kept at bed rest for 2 to 3 days, had binocular occlusion for 2 days, had sandbags placed at the sides of the head to discourage head movements, and had both wrists bound with restraints while in bed. Some hospitals, because of legal suits involving patients falling while attempting to climb over the side rails of the bed at night, required the patient to wear a body restraint. This resulted in a high incidence of mental disorientation, prostatic obstruction, and pulmonary problems. In some patients the enforced immobility produced the opposite effect from that desired—thrashing about in bed, bronchial asthma, marked disorientation, accidental falls from the bed, and numerous other accidents upsetting to the patient, the family, and the surgeon. As a result of marked improvements in methods of wound closure, these rigid restraints are no longer considered necessary.

If the patient has been given local anesthesia, if premedication has been light and has worn off, and if a systemic preoperative hyperosmotic agent has not been given, the patient may safely be transferred to a wheelchair, returned to his room, and placed in a comfortable chair. If a hyperosmotic agent has been administered preoperatively, the patient should be returned to his room on a stretcher and instructed to lie flat in bed for 3 to 4 hours. This will usually prevent a lumbar puncture type of headache and permit the effects of other premedication to wear off. The patient may then sit in an upright chair and watch television or listen to music to pass the time.

On the first postoperative day the patient should leave or enter the bed only with assistance. The location of the nurse's signal should be made clear. It can be pinned to his gown while he is in bed. The patient may walk to the bathroom unaided once out of bed. Side rails should be mandatory while he is in bed. Mild analgesics, tranquilizers, and sedatives may be prescribed when needed. Visitors should be few on the first day. A regular diet is prescribed (except where medically contraindicated), and he is permitted to feed himself. This routine must be varied for feeble, crippled, or otherwise disabled patients. Special nursing care and the cooperation of the patient's personal physician are required for these patients.

My personal routine is to make an effort to visit each patient in his room before leaving the hospital on the day of surgery. Questions asked by the patient or the family can be answered. Reassuring words from the surgeon are highly therapeutic. The surgeon must never lose sight of the fact that this is one of the most important events in the patient's life and must try to avoid impatience with what seems like an unending barrage of trivial questions and requests. Some of the physician-patient dialogue can occur in the operating room immediately after completion of the surgery if local anesthesia has been used. Additional instructions and responses to questions can be postponed until the first postoperative visit (discussed later).

The operated eye is examined on the morning following surgery. The eye pad (if one is used) and the plastic eye shield are removed. In cleansing the eye, an individual, sterile dressing package is used. It contains wet absorbent cotton balls, gauze pads, an eye pad, and tape. A combination antibiotic-steroid solution is given to the patient with the dressing kit. This is far superior to the older method of using a single eye dressing tray for all patients. The surgeon then had to rely on nursing personnel to maintain sterile ophthalmic solutions, ointments, and dressings. It is much simpler and safer to order individual dressing packages and medication for each patient. The examination at this time consists of an external examination, a slit lamp examination, and applanation tonometry. The ability to count fingers with a +12.00 D lens or other appropriate lens is tested. This is good for the morale of the patient. However, this part of the examination is postponed if the media are not sufficiently clear because of hyphema, striate keratopathy, and so on. Following the examination the patient is given instructions for home care, since I currently discharge my patients the morning after surgery. Some surgeons discharge their patients 2 or more days after surgery. There are probably significant advantages to both early and late hospital discharge.

A short hospital stay and a quick return to familiar food and surroundings is best for the patient psychologically, in my opinion. Early discharge from the hospital frees beds for more seriously ill patients. This endears the ophthalmologist to colleagues in other fields of medicine and saves the patient and governmental health insurance programs a considerable amount of money. However, early hospital discharge should never be ordered if a patient has special need for a longer hospital stay.

Longer hospital confinement is advantageous for patients who are alone and for those accustomed to living in institutional surroundings. It is easier to control early postoperative discomfort in the hospital, and medication is more likely to be given as ordered. However, in these days of crowded hospitals and overworked nursing personnel, this observation is not always valid.

I have no experience with outpatient cataract surgery. However, I think that it is probably safe, provided that there are convenient facilities nearby where the patient can be made comfortable and be observed by a family member, a friend, or a trained attendant. It is likely that the trend toward outpatient cataract surgery will continue, and more experience will be gained. In the meantime, if in the judgment of the surgeon there is no added risk to the patient, outpatient surgery is a valid alternative. However, the surgeon should be satisfied that the surgical and immediate postoperative facilities are suitable for cataract surgery.

Outlining a routine for all surgeons and all patients is obviously very difficult. Surgeons practicing in rural areas see patients who often must travel long distances. Then a longer hospital stay is probably justified. Some hospitals do not have a slit lamp. Therefore, it is better in such cases to get the patient to the office sooner. The patient who must travel a long distance might find it more convenient to take up residence near the office for 7 to 14 days.

Before leaving the hospital the patient, or a member of the family, is instructed about cleansing the eye and using eye drops. I prefer a combination antibiotic-steroid solution used three times daily initially. The value of this is open to question. A printed list of instructions for postoperative care is given to the patient. For those who require it a careful explanation of the instructions is given. I instruct the patient to lead a sedentary life for 2 weeks. Daily baths are permitted, but no showers for 2 weeks. The hair may be washed after 2 weeks. Bending and lifting weighted objects are prohibited during this period. If the patient wears no distance glasses, the eye shield is used for about 12 days. The patient sleeps with the shield for 3 weeks. If aphakic spectacles are worn for the opposite eye, I remove the shield on the first office visit and permit the patient to wear the glasses until bedtime when the shield is placed over the operated eye. If the patient wears distance spectacles for the opposite phakic eye, the glasses are worn over the eye shield for a few days. If an aphakic contact lens is used for the opposite eye, its use is resumed on the first office visit. In the hospital, the patient's aphakic spectacles, or temporary loaner aphakic spectacles, may be worn. The patient is asked to report to the office 3 days after hospital discharge.

During the first office visit, visual acuity is estimated with a pinhole disc. Tonometry is again performed.

No matter which routine is used, it is important to follow the patient very closely during the early postoperative period. This can be done with the patient in or out of the hospital. For example, an eye with an aseptic uveitis may show few external signs but, if ignored or missed, will soon suffer serious exudation into the anterior chamber as well as into the vitreous. Early therapy makes this complication much easier to control. Wound disruptions, shallowness of the anterior chamber, infections, and corneal edema from vitreocorneal adherence must all be diagnosed as early as possible.

After the first office visit, weekly visits are made. Glasses are ordered as soon as the keratometry reading or refraction stabilizes. This usually occurs at the sixth to eighth week after surgery. However, I have ordered aphakic spectacles after only 4 weeks and sometimes after 8 weeks. Such prescription depends partly on the technique of making the incision (Chapter 4). I seldom permit contact lenses to be worn before 8 weeks.

If the cellular response in the anterior chamber is moderate to severe, atropine solution is added to the antibiotic-steroid solution. I seldom prescribe systemic steroids because I have found an injection of 1 ml (40 mg) of triamcinolone (Kenalog) beneath Tenon's capsule to be most effective in combatting iritis. It may be repeated after 7 days, if necessary. Anterior chamber cells may be of four types: inflammatory cells from surgical trauma, red blood cells, pigment cells (especially in diabetics and patients with dark

irides), and macrophages laden with blood-breakdown products or lens material in a case of an extracapsular extraction.

Some patients show a mild-to-moderate corneal edema during the first 72 hours after surgery. This may be associated with a slight elevation of intraocular pressure. It is occasionally related to the use of alpha-chymotrypsin during surgery. Only rarely does it give rise to serious complications. I prefer to treat this with timolol, having found acetazolamide to be of limited benefit. Descemet's membrane folds are usually present to some degree, especially with corneal or anterior limbal incisions and with poor wound closure. Whether corneal edema or folds are present, the surgeon must be satisfied that vitreous is not adherent to the back of the cornea. Corneal edema can be temporarily minimized by a drop of a hyperosmotic solution. As discussed in Chapter 17, this requires early treatment.

Visual acuity is again determined through a +12.00 D lens with a multiple pinhole disc on the second postoperative office visit (approximately 4 to 5 days after surgery). If visual acuity drops on a later examination, it is probably caused by cystoid macular edema (Chapter 18). Keratometry is performed at 3 weeks, and the eye is refracted at this time and on subsequent office visits.

The one-eyed patient is a special problem. I remove the eye shield after 24 hours and permit the patient to wear one of the several tinted, plastic, temporary cataract spectacles. The eye shield is worn at bedtime. The partial sight is a great morale booster. However, extra precautions are taken in nursing care and physical activity.

When a person may resume an occupation varies and must be established for each patient individually. I permit a female patient who lives alone to do light cooking and perform light house chores after 14 days. At this time, I also permit schoolteachers and other people in sedentary occupations to resume activities on an escalating scale. This assumes, of course, that the opposite eye has relatively useful vision.

The ingenuity of the surgeon is severely tested in introducing the patient to aphakic spectacles for the first time. The patient must be adequately prepared for this experience. I place the prescription in a trial frame and ask the patient to shake my hand. Invariably, he will underestimate the distance and miss the hand because of the 25% to 30% image-size magnification. Pains must be taken to explain to the unilaterally aphakic patient that both eyes cannot be coordinated through spectacles. As any ophthalmologist knows, the unhappiest patients are those with visual acuity of 20/60 or better in the unoperated eye. These patients are instructed to use their new glasses for activities performed in a chair such as reading or watching television for the first 2 weeks. They are then to walk carefully around the house and in the street. They are not to drive an automobile until they are fully adjusted. If the visual acuity in the opposite eye is very poor, the patient adjusts more readily to the new situation, is elated with the restored vision, and complains very little.

Those patients who do not adjust well to unilateral aphakia are encouraged to try a contact lens, provided that they are not too elderly or infirm. Some elderly patients are very happy and their needs fully satisfied after surgery on one eye. In these individuals, surgery on the second eye may be postponed indefinitely. All younger patients are encouraged to try a contact lens.

Although there is much to be said in favor of surgery on the second eye within 1 to 2 weeks of the first operation, I usually wait 2 to 6 months unless there is an urgent reason not to wait. In practice I have found such reasons uncommon. I like to approach surgery on the second eye only after evaluating the long-term result of surgery on the first eye (p. 4). This is a personal preference and is stated with the full realization that many surgeons prefer to operate on the second eye within a week of the first eye and justify this by their favorable results.

PART TWO

COMPLICATIONS
OF CATARACT SURGERY

CHAPTER 11

Major operative complications

Most complications that may occur during cataract extraction have been considered in Chapter 3 in the discussion of the various portions of operative techniques. Three of the most serious complications that occur during the surgery are rupture of the lens capsule, expulsive hemorrhage, and loss of vitreous.

RUPTURE OF THE LENS CAPSULE

The lens capsule may rupture at any stage during intracapsular cataract extraction from the moment of application of the capsule forceps or erisiphake to any time during the delivery. This operative complication has been reduced considerably but not eliminated by the introduction of the cryoextraction technique.

Causes of capsule rupture

1. Resistant zonules
2. Fragile lens capsule
3. Intumescent cataract
4. Capsule rupture from trauma or hypermature cataract
5. Capsulohyaloid adhesion
6. Inadequate incision
7. Inadequate pupillary opening
8. Unsuspected posterior synechias
9. Faulty application of capsule forceps: too large a bite of lens capsule, grasping lens capsule too close to anterior pole where capsule is thinnest
10. Excessive vacuum pressure of the erisiphake
11. Defective capsule forceps or erisiphake cup
12. Precipitate extraction

Prevention of capsule rupture

Cryoextraction technique. Cryoextraction should virtually eliminate capsular rupture. However, it may still occur in eyes with a swollen, liquefied cataract. If a fragile lens capsule is suspected, it is the procedure of choice.

Enzymatic zonulysis. Zonulysis is particularly applicable to patients under 50 years of age in whom the zonules are likely to be tough and the capsulohyaloid ligament tenacious.

Adequate incision. Unless a cryoextraction technique is employed a small incision invites capsule rupture and other complications. This is particularly applicable to corneal incisions made anterior to a filtering bleb. A large lens may mold with difficulty through a small incision if the grasp of the capsule is made with forceps or an erisiphake. The incidence of capsule rupture with a small incision has been reduced with the cryoextraction technique, but it still occurs.

Adequate pupillary aperture. The pupillary aperture must be adequate as determined by previous mydriasis. If the pupil constricts during the surgery, it is not a serious problem. If the pupil did not dilate adequately with mydriatic drops or the retrobulbar injection, the iris sphincter is probably rigid. It is poor judgment to attempt a lens extraction through such a pupil. A sector iridectomy or one or more sphincterotomies should be done.

Instrument inspection. Instruments such as capsule forceps and an erisiphake should be inspected for defects before use.

Close attention to technique. The forceps or erisiphake should be applied properly to the lens capsule, and the delivery of the lens should be slow.

Management of lens capsule rupture

If the capsule ruptures in a mature or nearly mature lens, it is of little consequence. Capsule forceps with teeth are used to remove a wide portion of the anterior lens capsule, and an extracapsular extraction is performed (p. 72). Frequently if the rent in the anterior lens capsule is small, an intracapsular extraction may still be salvaged. The cornea is retracted by an assistant. The margins of the torn capsule are grasped by two smooth capsule forceps (such as Arruga forceps), and an attempt is made to lift the lens from the eye solely by traction. In this same situation a cryoprobe may be applied to an area of intact capsule and left in contact for as long as 10 seconds until a solid ice ball is formed. A satisfactory lens extraction may then be possible. It is usually impossible to apply the cryoprobe to the region of the capsule rupture because of the soft cortex. If alpha-chymotrypsin was not instilled in the eye beforehand, it should be used at this time, before either of these two techniques are attempted. If the capsule rupture enlarges during these maneuvers, as much of the anterior capsule as possible should be removed and the nucleus expressed by applying pressure from without at 6 o'clock and intermittent depression of the posterior lip of the wound above as in a routine extracapsular extraction.

Retained cortical material is less serious than retained lens capsule material because the former will absorb, whereas the latter usually does not. If the eye is soft and the vitreous pressure low, pieces of lens capsule may be removed by a hand-over-hand maneuver, with two capsule forceps. As the piece of capsule is grasped and pulled up with one forceps, the second forceps is applied close to its base, creating further traction on the capsule. In this way, large pieces of capsule may be removed. It may be difficult to visualize capsule remnants unless a surgical microscope or an ultraviolet lamp (Hague lamp) is used. Occasionally, filling the anterior chamber with air helps distinguish lens material from vitreous. Irrigation of the anterior chamber with balanced salt solution will usually remove most of the lens cortex.

The nucleus of the lens must be removed because it will not absorb and may cause serious intraocular inflammation. If the eye is so soft that the nucleus is impossible to deliver safely by the techniques just described, one may spear the nucleus with a fine sharp needle while the tip of a muscle hook applies counterpressure from without at 6 o'clock.

The two most serious complications of these attempts to remove retained lens material are damage to the corneal endothelium and loss of vitreous. The surgeon must always bear in mind the delicacy of the corneal endothelium. The instruments must not come in contact with it. The maneuvers should be performed with the preplaced sutures slightly closed and the anterior chamber filled with balanced salt solution. Rupture of the anterior hyaloid membrane is always serious but especially so when formed vitreous mixes with retained lens material. It is better to leave lens material behind than to damage the cornea or lose vitreous. If formed vitreous escapes, a partial anterior vitrectomy should be performed (p. 268). Another important complication is incarceration of lens capsule material in the wound. Its relationship to epithelial invasion of the anterior chamber and fibrous ingrowth are discussed elsewhere. Before closing the wound, the surgeon should sweep the lips of the incision free with a spatula. A bubble of air should be left in the anterior chamber to prevent postoperative incarceration of lens capsule material in the wound.

The postoperative consequences and treatment of retained lens material are discussed in Chapter 24.

EXPULSIVE HEMORRHAGE

Since expulsive hemorrhage is at least as likely to occur after the cataract extraction as during, it is considered in Chapter 21 in the section on postoperative complications.

OPERATIVE LOSS OF VITREOUS

Aside from expulsive hemorrhage, loss of vitreous is the most serious ocular complication that occurs during cataract surgery. Its importance is underscored by the fact that it is largely preventable.

The past 25 years have been marked by significant progress in reducing the incidence of operative loss of vitreous. Those surgeons whose experience spans this period can bear adequate testimony to the validity of this statement. It is difficult to appreciate this from the literature, which is replete with reports of the incidence of vitreous loss during cataract surgery and measures recommended to prevent its occurrence. When one reads these surveys, which date back to the middle of the last century and arise from centers all over the world, a sense of frustration arises if one attempts to draw meaningful conclusions. The variables that exist are so numerous that these reports educate us very little. Nevertheless, it is clear that the results of cataract surgery have markedly improved and the incidence of operative loss of vitreous has sharply declined. It would be of interest to investigate the reasons for the lessened rate of vitreous loss. However, some of the variables that influence all large statistical surveys of complications of cataract surgery should first be discussed.

The first of these concerns the surgeon, whose surgical ability, era of education, locale, and reputation for accurate and objective reporting of results must all be considered. The second variable involves the predominant type of patient in the survey. Private patients generally are easier to follow up, obey instructions better, and report complicating symptoms more readily than other patients. Patients from countries where poverty and malnutrition predominate are more likely to lower the incidence of surgical success. Another consideration is the institution in which the surgery is performed. Modern facilities supply more and better operating room personnel, equipment, and postoperative care than less well-equipped hospitals. In addition, medical records are likely to be kept orderly. It would be difficult to compare the nursing care in any modern first-rate hospital with that in some of the antiquated facilities in poverty-stricken areas. Considerations such as these, and others too numerous to list, tend to influence the statistics in most surveys.

A further drawback in comparing the results of older authors with those of modern series is that the former usually included planned extracapsular extractions. Some series relate the incidence of operative loss of vitreous in all types of lens extractions, including those in eyes with dislocated lenses.

The experience of Vail[1] and Barraquer[2] probably reflects most accurately the progress made in recent years. Vail reported a 12.7% incidence of loss of vitreous in 1601 cataract extractions from 1925 to 1942. In a subsequent series of 1292 such operations performed by Schoch and Vail between 1946 and 1961, the rate of operative loss of vitreous fell to 3.7%, an almost 350% decline. Barraquer's rate of vitreous loss fell from 7.3% in 1945 to less than 1% at present. It is probably fair to state that an incidence of vitreous loss of not more than 3% should be attained because of the improvements in surgical training, techniques, instrumentation, and facilities. It is likely that this figure will drop still further as more surgeons become aware of and use these improvements.

The importance of preventing operative loss of vitreous has been known for a long time, as evidenced by this 200-year-old statement of A. G. Richter[3] of Germany:

I confess that I have seen this accident (loss of vitreous) happen but very seldom during the operation, and when it does so, there is always some particular cause for it. Either the assistant who supports the eyelids presses unguardedly on the eye itself or the operator performs his part so awkwardly that the eye is violently irritated or injured, or he makes use of a bad method of operating, or his instruments are ill adapted for the intended purposes, or he persists in his endeavors to force out the lens although he has made the incision in the cornea too small, or he presses hard on the eye without having previously punctured the capsule.

These are circumstances which the operator must avoid if he means to prevent the discharge of the vitreous humor.

Commenting on this, Vail[1] observed that this "remarkable statement of two centuries ago leaves us little to add to the subject of prevention. It is particularly to be noted that Richter rightly puts the blame upon the operator and not the patient."

Ironically the serious import of operative loss of vitreous has been emphasized during the past 25 years, during which time the greatest strides toward its prevention have been made. This change is exemplified in statements made by Colonel Smith,[4] in 1910, and by Vail, Sr.,[5] in 1911, that a small or moderate loss of vitreous is of little or no consequence. This view has been refuted by Vail[1] in a Gifford lecture in 1964, wherein he observed that deleterious results are

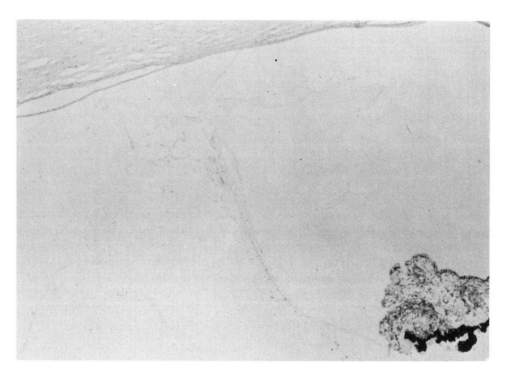

Fig. 11-1. Direct contact of vitreous with back of cornea after cataract extraction.

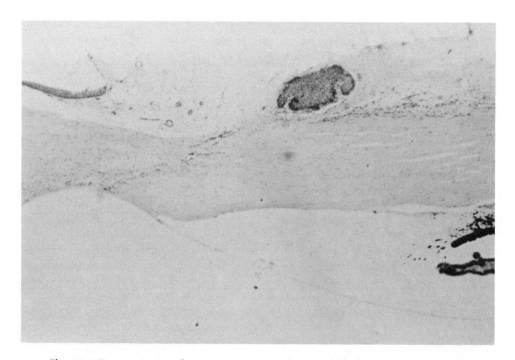

Fig. 11-2. Incarceration of vitreous into operative wound after cataract surgery.

common, and loss of vitreous can indeed have very grave consequences. It also matters little whether a small or a moderate amount of vitreous has been lost.

Consequences of operative loss of vitreous

The complications that result from operative loss of vitreous are not at all related to the loss of vitreous bulk itself but to the morphologic changes in the vitreous body that occur when the anterior hyaloid membrane is ruptured. These complications are thus related to the following mechanisms:

1. Direct contact of vitreous with other structures (such as the cornea) (Fig. 11-1)
2. Incarceration of vitreous into the operative wound (Fig. 11-2)
3. Fibroplasia of the residual vitreous
4. Inflammation

Most consequences of vitreous loss may be explained by one of these mechanisms. A list of the important complications would include the following.

Excessive degree of astigmatism. Excessive astigmatism is undoubtedly related to defects of wound healing when vitreous adheres to the operative site.

Bullous keratopathy. The normal cornea may tolerate apposition of vitreous fibrils to its posterior surface, but if the endothelial cell population is sparse because of dystrophy or surgical trauma, a persistent corneal edema with bullous formation may result (p. 340).

Epithelial invasion of the anterior chamber. As a result of incarceration or prolapse of vitreous into or through the surgical wound, surface epithelium may be encouraged to enter the anterior chamber. If contact with uveal tissue and a plasmoid aqueous humor occurs, an epithelial cyst or a downgrowth of epithelium as a sheet over the cornea and iris may result (p. 506).

Fibrous ingrowth. An ingrowth of stromal elements may result from a similar mechanism (p. 543) or from fibrous metaplasia of endothelial cells due to vitreous adherence to the wound (p. 553).

Wound infection and endophthalmitis. The presence of vitreous fibrils between the lips of the wound delays healing and may provide a portal of entry of pathogenic organisms into the eye.

This is more likely if the conjunctival coverage of the wound is defective, as may occur with a retracted fornix-based flap (p. 441).

Iris prolapse. If vitreous fibrils between the lips of the wound delay healing, external pressure on the globe (squeezing, rubbing, and so on) may favor an iris prolapse.

Updrawn or misshapen pupil. As a result of fibroplasia, the pupil may be severely distorted and result in a hammock pupil, which may interfere with contact lens fitting. It is possible that the pupil in some cases may actually be completely covered by the upper eyelid.

Fibroplastic traction bands. Fibroplastic traction bands that connect the posterior surface of the operative wound to other structures such as the retina and ciliary body may cause a retinal detachment (p. 578) or an intense uveitis.

Secondary glaucoma. Glaucoma may be the result of anterior synechias or chronic irritation and is due to fibroplasia of the damaged vitreous.

Cystoid macular edema and papilledema. The incidence of postoperative cystoid macular edema and papilledema rises sharply when vitreous loss occurs. In addition, it persists for longer periods than when the anterior face of the vitreous is intact. The final result may be a permanent degeneration of the macula with subnormal visual acuity (p. 370).

Vitreous opacities. In addition to whitish, fiberlike membranes in the anterior chamber, vitreous opacities are often found more posteriorly. They may also be associated with hemorrhage or uveitis.

Vitreous hemorrhage. Bleeding into the vitreous is a common accompaniment of operative loss of vitreous. Whether this is caused by separation of angiovitreal adhesions or loss of vascular support is not known (p. 414).

Expulsive hemorrhage. The rare but destructive complication of expulsive hemorrhage may occur more frequently when vitreous is lost at the time of surgery (p. 425).

Fibroplastic condensation of the residual formed vitreous. Fibroplastic condensation may obstruct vision or may cause aphakic pupillary block. The new membrane is occasionally very thick and vascularized. It may prevent passage of water and electrolytes freely through its anterior surface (p. 303).

Retinal detachment. The incidence of retinal detachment after cataract extraction increases greatly in those eyes that suffer operative loss of vitreous.

Chronic ocular irritability. An eye that has lost vitreous at the time of surgery often remains inflamed, tears frequently, and is intensely photophobic. Even a drop of topical anesthetic solution placed in such an eye may cause marked redness.

• • •

This large list of sequelae resulting from a single operative complication should be adequate reason for all ophthalmologists to direct their efforts to the prevention of operative loss of vitreous.

Follow-up of eyes with operative loss of vitreous

Few reports exist in the ophthalmic literature on the long-term follow-up of patients who have suffered operative loss of vitreous. Two carefully documented reports[1,6,7] (Vail and Dunphy) show a striking agreement in the average final visual acuity, 20/56. Most of the complications related to vitreous loss occur during the first year after cataract surgery. Vail showed that 6% of these eyes were totally lost within the first few months after surgery, and about 23% of the surviving eyes had no useful vision at the end of 2 years. Furthermore only 20% of eyes that survived after 3 years had a vision of 20/70 or better.

In a long-term follow-up of these patients, he concluded that if the eye remained quiet for 2 or 3 years after surgery, the chance for the maintenance of useful vision for the rest of the patient's life was very good—as good, perhaps, as if no vitreous had been lost, subject of course to the usual attrition of age.

These series are now obsolete because of significant improvements in the management of operative loss of vitreous (p. 268). Long-term follow-ups of these newer methods are now becoming available.

Recognition of the dangerous eye before surgery

A history of operative loss of vitreous in the opposite eye or, in the absence of a history, clinical signs of loss of vitreous should alert the surgeon to take extra precautions when operating on the second eye. Sometimes, despite every prophylactic measure, the same complication results. The chances of vitreous loss in the second eye is probably much higher if operative loss of vitreous befell the first eye. Such loss may be related to some ocular structural deformity present in both eyes, such as lack of scleral rigidity, which permits the walls of the globe to collapse when the eye is decompressed, or some inherent weakness in the anterior hyaloid membrane, or other unknown causes.

The physical and mental condition of the patient may be such that accidental loss of vitreous may be anticipated, yet surgery should not be postponed if the condition is chronic. One might include such problems as marked obesity, diabetes of long standing, advanced arteriosclerosis with vascular hypertension, a history of infection, a bleeding tendency, malnutrition, bronchial asthma, emphysema, chronic bronchitis, chronic cough, mental agitation, and psychosis. However, there is no real evidence that any of these conditions are related to operative loss of vitreous.

The findings during the examination of the patient may alert the surgeon to the possibility of vitreous loss. They would include proptosis, especially when associated with increased orbital resistance, glaucoma, evidence of previous intraocular surgery, high myopia, subluxated or dislocated lens, eyelid abnormalities such as shortening of the palpebral fissure, conjunctival abnormalities such as essential shrinkage, and a patient with a short thick neck. Theoretically, venous pressure is increased in such a patient when placed in a prone position. This may cause external pressure on the globe.

Measures to prevent loss of vitreous before surgery

Readjustment of preoperative medication and choice of anesthesia. A combination of drugs to produce sedation, analgesia, tranquility, and antiemesis should be selected according to the needs of the patient. A choice of anesthesia—local, general, or a combination of both—should be selected not only to suit the patient but also to suit the temperament of the surgeon under the condition encountered.

Surgery on the soft eye. Soft-eye surgery is in

my opinion the single most important development during the past 30 years to reduce the incidence of vitreous loss. The soft eye may be achieved by three methods — digital pressure, hyperosmotic agents, and a posterior sclerotomy.

Digital pressure. The principal method of achieving the soft eye is the application of 5 or more minutes of digital pressure (relaxed intermittently to prevent vascular occlusion) after a retrobulbar injection of anesthetic solution (Fig. 3-7). Although the ancient Greeks used massage of the eye therapeutically,[8] it is not known whether they realized that the eye softened from the massage. We are certain that the effects of digital pressure in lowering intraocular pressure date back at least to the nineteenth century.[9,10] In more recent times digital pressure has been used for other reasons. Atkinson[11] recommended it to ensure a more thorough diffusion of anesthetic solution within the mascular cone after a retrobulbar injection. It has been used as a tamponade against possible bleeding after the retrobulbar injection. Although the originator of this idea was unknown to me, I used it for this purpose before learning of its hypotensive advantages. Chandler is generally credited with employing digital pressure after the retrobulbar injection to lower the intraocular pressure during cataract surgery. Kirsch and Steinman[12] were primary investigators in popularizing the technique. Kirsch became interested in it after observing its use by Chandler. They lauded its benefits as a result of an excellent study that clearly demonstrated its pressure-lowering qualities, both by tonometric measurement and clinical observation during cataract extraction. They reported a profound decrease in intraocular pressure to an average of 2.3 mm Schiøtz in 100 cases. The average duration of pressure below 10 mm was 14.3 minutes. This short span of hypotension must be kept in mind so that the incision is made during this interval. I have been influenced greatly by them in applying this method during cataract surgery.

It readily became apparent that decreased tonometric readings were accompanied by clinical signs of profound hypotonia such as lessened tendency toward wound gape of spontaneous iris prolapse after the cataract incision, central corneal collapse, marked concavity of the anterior face of the vitreous after the lens is extracted, and the spontaneous filling of the anterior chamber with air as the lens is delivered.

The mechanism for the hypotonia induced by digital massage is not completely clear and has received less attention than that accorded hyperosmotic agents, but the evidence suggests that the escape of fluid from the vitreous is the probable cause.

Hildreth[13] studied the effects of digital ocular compression and considered the induced hypotonia to be mainly caused by loss of fluid from the vitreous and expression of aqueous. Support for this thesis is supplied by the difficulties encountered in softening the eyes of children by digital massage. One speculates that the vitreous in such eyes has undergone little or no liquefaction, as is the case in senile eyes. Further evidence is supplied by Quinn and Porter,[14] who performed experiments in dogs with tritiated water and observed that less water remained in the vitreous of the massaged globes. Using a technique of weighing the vitreous after digital compression, Robbins and co-workers[15] found a reduction in vitreous weight and volume in rabbits sufficient to explain the hypotonia induced. In a more recent report, François and co-workers[16] reported that digital massage caused a decrease in intraocular pressure, especially in adults and elderly patients. They noted that there was no change in the depth of the anterior chamber, which argues in favor of the arrival of fluid from the vitreous to much the same extent as aqueous expelled from the anterior chamber. They noted a decreased concentration of glucose and phosphate in the aqueous, which they attributed to their dilution by water from the vitreous. Using experimental methods, they observed that the sclera, uvea, retina, lens and anterior chamber weighed more after digital massage, but the vitreous weighed less. They concluded that, although the quantity of water chemically linked to the macromolecular structures of the vitreous varies very little, it is the free or nonlinked water that is eliminated. They pointed to Schlemm's canal and the vitreous base as exit sites. Thus they also attributed the hypotensive effect of digital pressure to the elimination of fluid from the eye.

From the practical point of view, we should not lose sight of what we are trying to accomplish with digital pressure. Is it the lowering of intraocular pressure or the reduction of vitreous volume? It has been argued that lowering of pressure is of little benefit, since the intraocular pressure falls to zero as soon as the globe is opened. Thus it is not the intraocular pressure but the volume of vitreous that is important. Would it be safe to perform a cataract extraction on an eye with an intraocular pressure of 80 mm Hg, since the pressure falls to atmospheric as soon as the incision is made? If not, why not? Perform the following experiment on two eye bank eyes. Inject 0.5 ml of water through a 30-gauge needle into the vitreous through the posterior portion of the sclera of one eye. This will make the eye extremely hard. Make an incision into the anterior chamber of both globes. Note the forward propulsion of intraocular contents in the hard eye compared to the that in the soft eye. In clinical practice I have also observed that eyes with hypotonia due to previously performed fistulizing operations may show a tendency to vitreous bulge during cataract surgery if not subjected to digital pressure after the retrobulbar injection. It should also be apparent that it requires a greater force exerted against the globe from without to create a vitreous bulge if vitreous volume is previously decreased.

Although these arguments appear to minimize the factor of lowering intraocular pressure, it is an important monitor of what is going on within the globe during digital pressure. Indeed, I use this in every cataract extraction. Instead of exerting digital pressure for a fixed period and then measuring intraocular pressure, I use a sterile, autoclavable Schiøtz tonometer to make frequent measurements during the massage period. I have occasionally observed that the intraocular pressure may actually rise in some cases during the first minute. Whether this is caused by displacing some of the aqueous into the vitreous is not known. In most eyes the pressure during the second minute of digital pressure will fall precipitously. I have found that those eyes whose intraocular pressure can be massaged to a scale reading of 12 or greater with a 5.5 g weight within 2 minutes or less usually have a markedly dehydrated vitreous. If it requires at least 5 minutes to achieve this hypotonia, a dangerous situation exists. These eyes may not show clinical evidence of hypotonia after the globe is opened. In these the added precaution of a posterior sclerotomy is sometimes taken (as discussed later).

To this point, no mention has been made of the effect of digital pressure on orbital volume, which is probably equal in importance to the reduction of vitreous volume. It should be apparent that if there is less mass exerting external pressure against the open globe, there is less likelihood of operative loss of vitreous. It is difficult to quantify reduction of orbital volume, but there is adequate clinical evidence that this occurs. Note the increasing enophthalmos as digital pressure continues. This is a comforting, as well as a practical, sign of reduction of orbital volume. An interesting observation was made by Curtin,[17] who recommended an alternative to digital pressure. He used a Schiøtz tonometer with a 10 g load and placed it on the cornea to obtain a scale reading of zero (81.7 mm Hg). In 2 minutes the pressures of 70% of the eyes fell to zero, and 50% showed off-the-scale readings in 4 minutes. He attributed this hypotensive effect to the absence of compression of the episcleral veins that occurs to some extent with digital massage. The tonometer also avoids eyelid gland massage. In spite of this, only one half of eyes undergoing cataract extraction showed a concave anterior vitreous face immediately after lens extraction. All patients were operated on under general anesthesia, and no retrobulbar injections were performed. My impression is that this is an effective method of reducing intraocular pressure but less efficient in reducing orbital volume. There are other methods of reducing intraocular and intraorbital pressure that are probably as effective as digital pressure. One of these is called the "super pinkie." Another is the use of a rectal balloon inflated by a sphygmomanometer and placed over the orbit with a Velco strap.

As mentioned earlier, other benefits of digital pressure include a more thorough diffusion of the anesthetic agent within the muscular cone and probably some hemostasis after the retrobulbar injection.

Thus the benefits of digital pressure are:
1. Decreased vitreous volume
2. Decreased orbital volume
3. Better akinesia and anesthesia
4. Hemostasis within the orbit

Hyperosmotic agents. In recent years, hyperosmotic agents, efficacious in reducing intraocular pressure, have been applied to reduce some of the hazards of intraocular surgery. That these agents could be employed effectively to lower intraocular pressure has been known for some time. However, only recently criteria have been established that make certain agents practical in increasing plasma osmolarity. To adequately maintain a significant plasma:aqueous:vitreous osmotic gradient, the following criteria must be met:

1. The agent must have a small molecular weight that provides a greater osmotic effect per unit weight, since it is the number of molecules, not their weight, which is important.
2. The agent must be nontoxic.
3. The agent must show poor ocular penetrance.

Sucrose and sorbitol will maintain an adequate gradient because they penetrate the eye poorly, but because of their large molecular weight, large doses are required that make them impractical. In addition, they may cause renal damage. On the other hand, sodium chloride is nontoxic and of small molecular weight, but it penetrates the eye rapidly.

Although these agents are relatively safe, the ophthalmologist should be familiar with their side effects, which include the following:

1. Cardiovascular side effects associated with rapid expansion of blood volume, angina, arrhythmias, hypertension, congestive heart failure, and pulmonary edema
2. Headache and back pain due to reduced intracranial pressure
3. More serious cerebral complications such as subdural hematoma
4. Diuresis with intravenous agents
5. Nausea and vomiting with oral agents
6. Specific complications related to an agent: slough—urea; hematuria and anuria—intravenous glycerin; gastric disorders and diarrhea—oral vitamin C; hyperglycemia—glycerin

The dosage of these agents has already been discussed (p. 13).

I find oral glycerin (Alcon, Ft. Worth, Texas) and Glyrol (Smith, Miller and Patch, New York City) to be the most convenient of all the agents. It can be given orally, is safe, and does not promote a diffuse diuresis. The incidence of nausea and vomiting is low, which I have attributed to serving the glycerin in cracked ice, not oversedating the patient, and having the patient in the supine position. I have used it in most cataract extractions for more than 11 years. In an experimental study[18] I found that I was able to achieve a lower intraocular pressure by using glycerin preoperatively, along with retrobulbar anesthesia and 5 minutes of digital massage, than I could without the glycerin. Isosorbide (Hydronol, Atlas Chemical Industries, Inc., Wilmington, Delaware) may be substituted for glycerin. With a dose of 1.5 g/kg of body weight its pressure-lowering effect is similar to that of glycerin. It appears to have certain advantages. It has no caloric value and is not metabolized. Therefore it may be safer for diabetics. In addition, side effects such as nausea, vomiting, headache, and backache appear to be less frequent.

If the surgery is performed under general anesthesia, an intravenous preparation such as 20% mannitol (Osmitrol, Travenol Laboratories, Inc., Morton Grove, Illinois) or urea in the form of a 30% lyophilized solution (Urevert, Travenol Laboratories) may be used. The great drawback of urea is the serious consequence of extravasation at the needle site, and therefore mannitol is preferred. An indwelling catheter may be necessary in some cases because the urine flow rate with mannitol is about five times greater than with glycerin. A popular method is the use of 50 ml of 25% mannitol administered rapidly by the intravenous route. If an intravenous solution of 5% glucose in water is administered during surgery, the mannitol may be conveniently injected into the tubing. The total volume is given over a period of 90 seconds. It is not as effective as a full dose of 20% mannitol given over a period of a few hours.

Despite the drawbacks related to all hyperosmotic agents, they are a very useful adjunct to cataract surgery.

The mode of action of these agents is presumed to be removal of fluid from the vitreous, which thus reduces its volume. It is not simple to prove this statement. However, the following data justify this assumption. Bucci and

Neuschüler[19] evaluated with Jaeger's apparatus the depth of the anterior chamber in humans after the oral administration of 50% glycerin in doses of 1 g/kg body weight. The mean deepening of the anterior chambers in normal eyes was 0.004 mm. In glaucomatous and unoperated cataractous eyes it was 0.05 mm, and in operated eyes it was 0.2 mm. From this study, it would appear that the dehydrating effect is exerted on the vitreous, since only in this way can a deepening of the anterior chamber be explained. The same authors[20] previously noted that glycerin administered orally does not inhibit aqueous humor production (unlike acetazolamide) and that on the contrary it facilitates the fluid's passage into the anterior chamber at a given interval after administration. Bucci[21] studied the effect of orally administered glycerin on the weight and volume of the vitreous body in rabbits. He obtained a constant reduction of the weight and volume of the vitreous. It is surprising how a small decrease in volume such as 4% is sufficient to cause a profound drop in intraocular pressure. The removal of 0.12 ml of retrovitreal fluid (slightly greater than 2% of vitreous volume) produces a profound hypotonia. This work was later corroborated by Robbins and Galin,[22] who used a similar technique. Bucci and Virno[23] performed a dramatic experiment wherein they trephined a corneal button from rabbits' eyes and placed a piston attached to a series of levers on the lens. The piston fell as the rabbits were given a hyperosmotic agent. There was no fall in control eyes when a hyperosmotic agent was not given. Presumably the posterior displacement of the lens was due to reduction in vitreous volume.

Posterior sclerotomy. The use of a posterior sclerotomy with drainage of vitreous fluid preparatory to cataract surgery is a seldom used but effective method of preventing operative loss of vitreous. This technique has been recommended by Iliff[24] when medical (hyperosmotic agents) or mechanical (digital massage) means have failed to achieve a tonometric scale reading of 10 units or more with a 5.5 g weight. A pars planotomy is performed in the upper temporal quadrant of the globe in the following manner: A flap of conjunctiva and Tenon's capsule is turned down from the upper fornix, exposing the sclera. A Hildreth or Scheie cautery is applied to the exposed sclera at

6 mm from the limbus and parallel to it until a slight shrinkage of tissue is noted over an area of 1 by 4 mm. A narrow-bladed Graefe knife is then passed through this area of the sclera and pars plana and is directed posteriorly and inferiorly toward the lower temporal quadrant of the globe to a depth of 1 cm, as marked with methylene blue on the blade of the knife. The point enters the temporal vitreous lake, which lies between the central formed vitreous and the temporal retina. The blade is turned, spreading the lips of the wound and creating a channel along which the fluid drains. When the eye is soft, the knife is withdrawn. It is not necessary to suture the scleral incision. Iliff prefers the knife to aspiration with an 18-gauge needle because he considers it less traumatic.

I have modified this technique and find it to be a most useful and simple procedure in the rare instance when it is necessary. At a point 5 mm from the limbus in the superior temporal quadrant, a small conjunctival incision is made to expose the sclera, which is marked at this point. A 25- or 27-gauge Rizzuti-Spirizzi keratome cannula attached to a syringe is passed through the sclera and pars plana at this point and is directed superiorly and posteriorly where the retrovitreal space is usually found. Aspiration pressure is made on the syringe as the cannula is passed through the vitreous. When the retrovitreal space is reached, a sudden gush of aqueous will enter the syringe. The globe will become mushy soft from aspiration of as little as 0.25 ml. These cannulas are perfectly suited for this procedure (Fig. 17-9). They are so sharp they will pass through the sclera without fixation of the globe. No attempt is made to remove formed vitreous, merely retrovitreal aqueous. In fact, formed vitreous will not pass through this needle. A 25- or 27-gauge disposable needle attached to a syringe may be substituted because of its sharpness.

My view is that this technique should be reserved for the very rare patient who cannot be given a hyperosmotic agent or who vomits the preparation, whose intraocular pressure cannot be reduced to hypotonia, or in whom vitreous was lost during surgery on the first eye. In my experience, if a tonometric reading of 10 or more scale units (5.5 g weight) cannot be achieved, a careful search for extraglobal pressure should be conducted. It may be a faulty speculum, an everted upper tarsus by the use of lid sutures, a tight lateral canthus, inadequate akinesia, residual extraocular muscle activity, or a retrobulbar hemorrhage.

The safety of a posterior sclerotomy is open to question. Since it causes a vitreous disturbance, it cannot be considered free of risk. Therefore good surgical judgment is required in its application.

Reduction of external pressure on the vitreous. The advantage of reducing vitreous bulk as just described is obvious, since it will then require a greater force exerted against it to cause a rupture of the anterior hyaloid membrane. Nevertheless, the minimizing of these forces is of critical importance and is clearly the stamp of the skillful surgeon.

Digital pressure. The benefits of digital pressure in reducing orbital volume and thereby decreasing external pressure on the vitreous have been discussed (p. 257).

Technique of separating the eyelids. The technique of separating the eyelids is probably responsible for most of the inadequacies in reducing external pressure on the vitreous. There are probably as many methods of achieving exposure as there are surgeons performing cataract extractions. This is adequate testimony to the inefficacy of most of these methods. Proper exposure of the operative field is essential in all surgery. Several factors alter the degree of exposure in ophthalmic surgery such as a deep-set eye, a short palpebral fissure, microphthalmos, a large globe as in high myopia, and an inadequate orbit as in some cases of exophthalmos.

The most effective method of avoiding pressure on the globe is to use separate upper and lower lid retractors such as those recommended by Desmarres. However, these involve the use of a trained, alert assistant throughout the entire procedure. This inconvenience has detracted from the popularity of the technique.

Exposure must be obtained with the lids well away from the globe and the tarsus in its normal plane. With respect to the tarsus, if its vertical dimension is large, its eversion may press more posteriorly on the globe and in a more perpendicular direction, a situation to be avoided. Lid

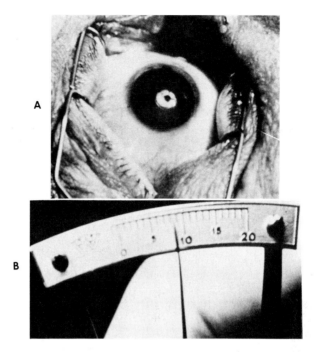

Fig. 11-3. A, One-piece Colybri-Barraquer blepharostat. **B,** Intraocular pressure is 10.2 mm Schiøtz.

sutures and small marginal lid clamps (Castroviejo) provide excellent exposure, but all too often the very dangers they seek to avoid are inherent in this method. The lid speculum is convenient but has limitations. The main source of pressure is from the weight of the central or screw end of the speculum, which is the most dependent part of the instrument; it exerts pressure on the lateral aspect of the globe. This pressure is somewhat minimized by placing a cotton pledget between the screw end of the instrument and the skin surface of the lateral orbital margin. It is surprising that some specula, such as the one-piece Colybri-Barraquer blepharostat, may raise intraocular pressure to a dangerous level before the incision is made (Fig. 11-3). Many of the shortcomings of the speculum have been eliminated by the Guyton-Park or Maumenee-Park versions. However, the latter do not permit different degrees of retraction for the upper and lower eyelids.

I find separate upper and lower eyelid retractors[25] made of stainless steel wire most acceptable (Figs. 3-10, 3-11, and 11-4). The curved end of the retractor fits behind the tarsus. It is

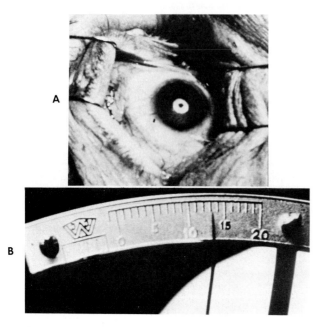

Fig. 11-4. A, Separate upper and lower eyelid Jaffe retractors placed in same eye as in Fig. 9-3 immediately after removing Colybri-Barraquer blepharostat. B, Intraocular pressure is 4.0 mm Schiøtz.

sufficiently broad to eliminate notch type of retraction as with single lid sutures. The curved part is approximately the same length as the tarsus, thereby eliminating any bending or folding of the tarsus. The retraction is in the direct plane of action of the lids. There is no pressure on the globe, and the exposure exceeds that of the speculum and eyelid sutures. A No. 1 nylon suture is tied to the end of the retractor and clamped to the drapes so that no assistance is required for exposure. There are no annoying screws or locks to contend with, and the retractors are easily and readily removed. These retractors permit different degrees of retraction of the upper and lower eyelids. When excessive retraction raises intraocular pressure, the lower eyelid is retracted less so that exposure of the globe above need not be compromised. The use of these retractors was discussed on p. 38.

Satisfactory anesthesia and akinesia. Residual extraoculor or orbicularis muscle activity may exert significant pressure on the globe. If ocular movements persist after the retrobulbar injection, the latter may be repeated or the individual rectus muscles may be injected directly. The technique of performing the retrobulbar injection is important to avoid a retrobulbar hemorrhage. A blunt-tipped needle may be used but is probably not necessary if the fluid is slowly injected as soon as the needle penetrates the skin. Slow injection ensures against perforation of large vessels and the optic nerve. The volume of injected fluid should be small (2 to 3 ml), especially with a shallow orbit, tight lids, or a proptotic globe. A significant retrobulbar hemorrhage is easy to detect, but a smaller one may show few signs. A stainless steel autoclavable tonometer is indispensible in this regard and should be available on the instrument tray. Just as it takes only a small decrease in vitreous volume to cause a profound hypotonia, it requires only a minor extraocular force to displace the vitreous. An elevation of intraocular pressure may be readily detected by using the tonometer. Continued digital massage will often cause a lowering of the pressure to safe levels after minor retrobulbar bleeding, but a significant hemorrhage should result in postponement of surgery.

Serous or hemmorrhagic choroidal detachment. It is probable that serous or hemorrhagic choroidal detachment occurs in every decompression procedure performed on the eye. It appears as a dark, curved, elevated line with the convexity toward the disc. It is peripheral and found mostly in the inferior quadrants. The resulting mass may create a force sufficient to compress the vitreous to a dangerous degree. There are three forces to be considered in its pathogenesis: The first is the intraocular pressure, which tends to prevent transudation from the choroidal vessels. This, of course, falls to zero as soon as the globe is opened. The second is the intravascular pressure. Since transudation occurs chiefly at the capillary level, the blood pressure within the choroidal capillaries is considered. According to Best and Taylor,[26] the blood pressure at the arterial end is about 32 mm and that at the venous end 12 mm. This force favors transudation into the tissue fluids. Offsetting the intravascular pressure is the third force, the oncotic pressure exerted by the protein colloids of the plasma, which tends to draw fluids from the tissues into the vascular tree. This is discussed in detail on p. 294.

A most important consideration may be how long the globe remains open. It is possible that the longer the choroidal vessels are exposed to an intraocular pressure of zero, the greater is the likelihood of choroidal detachment.

One can only speculate on the role played by the transudate in compressing the vitreous at surgery. In considering all the forces that come into play on opening the globe, one wonders if any measures may be adopted to minimize vitreous compression. Theoretically, a sudden, precipitous fall in intraocular pressure favors more massive transudation. The fall may be largely avoided by reducing the intraocular pressure to hypotonia before making the incision.

A rare, but dangerous, phenomenon is the sudden occurrence of a massive serous choroidal detachment. This is illustrated in the following case. A 74-year-old woman had a cataract removed from her right eye without complication. The anterior face of the vitreous appeared concave, and there was not the least sign of a vitreous bulge. Suddenly the vitreous began to push forward. A large choroidal detachment suddenly appeared in the superior temporal quadrant. It was dome shaped and extended more than two thirds the way across the pupil. Formed vitreous escaped from the eye. A hasty diagnosis of expulsive hemorrhage was made. The emergency suture was tied at 12 o'clock. A subchoroidal tap was performed in the region of the choroidal detachment. A clear, slightly yellowish fluid escaped. Finally, a partial anterior vitrectomy was performed when there was no further progression of the choroidal effusion. Ruiz and Salmonsen[27] have described two similar cases. They called this entity "expulsive choroidal effusion."

Collapse of the sclera. Collapse of the sclera may create a force sufficient to compress the vitreous, with subsequent loss of vitreous during cataract surgery. It probably one of the commonest causes of operative loss of vitreous and is usually undiagnosed. Although Flieringa[28] is largely credited with the technique of sleral fixation, van der Hoeve[29] recommended in 1919 the use of four episcleral sutures placed in the sclera between the limbus and the insertion of the rectus muscles. However, if the pull on these sutures by the assistant is too great, the diminution

of the surface will become considerable, and the contents of the globe may be displaced.

Flieringa designed a ring made of stainless steel with a thickness of 0.3 mm and a diameter of 20 mm. He applied this concentric to the cornea. If the eyeball is of normal size, the distance between the ring and the limbus will be 5 mm. In a larger eyeball a ring of 22 mm is used. The ring is fastened in the following manner: In eight places, equally distributed on the total circumference, the conjunctiva is incised and the sclera exposed. Next, at these eight points, the suture is brought through the episclera, and the ring is thus firmly attached to the sclera. Alternate sutures are cut off close to the knot; the others are kept long. By accurate traction on these sutures, it is possible to greatly diminish the tendency to scleral collapse and displacement of intraocular contents.

There have been variations and modifications of the Flieringa ring, notable among which is the double ring of Legrand,[30] which consists of a smaller ring elevated above the level of the larger ring and available in two sizes, 14 × 23 mm and 17 × 24 mm, and those of Neubauer and of Mackensen. Girard[31] has designed a "scleral expander" to prevent scleral collapse during intraocular surgery. It is the most complex and cumbersome of all these instruments but probably the most effective (Fig. 11-5).

Flieringa[28] recommends his perilimbal ring in the following situations: in cataract extraction in eyes with high myopia, in all cataracts in which one suspects a fluid vitreous, in the discission of secondary cataracts as well as inflammatory pupillary membranes, in the extraction of dislocated lenses, in surgery for iris cysts, and in penetrating keratoplasties exceeding 5 mm. However, others consider the indications to be more limited.

Probably its greatest usefulness is in linear extractions, which are usually performed in very young individuals. In these the sclera is highly elastic and collapses easily when the globe is decompressed, producing a marked forward propulsion of the lens-iris diaphragm immediately on entrance into the globe.

Mechanical factors. Mechanical factors that cause pressure on the vitreous include orbital abnormalities such as oxycephaly, orbital masses

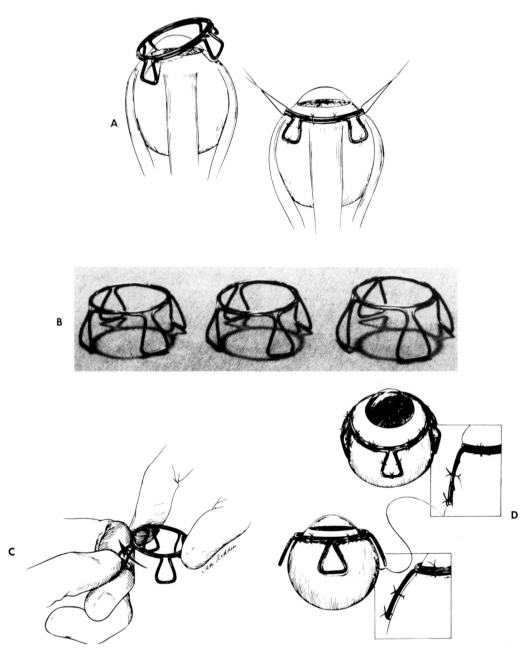

Fig. 11-5. Scleral expander is composed of ring with four malleable wings that can be adjusted to size of globe. **A,** After peritomy and exposure of muscles, expander is best inserted by placing lower wings on either side of inferior rectus, inferiorly, and then inserting upper wings superiorly. **B,** Expanders of different sizes should be available. **C,** Wings of expander should be adjusted so they do not compress globe. **D,** *Upper right,* incorrect size and adjustment of wings illustrating compression of globe. *Lower left,* correct size and adjustment of wings. There should be clearance of 1 to 2 mm. Sclera should be expanded to ring. Expander should not be sutured down on sclera. (From Girard, L. J.: Ann. Ophthalmol. **5:**223-240, 1973.)

such as neoplasms or hyperplasias associated with endocrine exophthalmos, abnormalities of the eyelids such as shortening of the palpebral fissure, and abnormalities of the conjunctiva such as essential shrinkage. There is probably no satisfactory method of managing these problems. It is safe to make use of a liberal lateral canthotomy (Fig. 11-6). In exophthalmos with increased orbital resistance, it may be advisable to eliminate the speculum or lid sutures and merely resort to a superior rectus bridle suture for exposure. If eyelid retraction causes the shrunken conjunctiva to press on the globe, the conjunctiva may be incised. A tonometer is invaluable. If the intraocular pressure cannot be reduced to a safe surgical level, one should consider a preliminary posterior sclerotomy, as previously suggested. It is in these cases that the ingenuity of the surgeon is tested most severely.

The surgeon should be on guard at all times to anticipate vitreous loss during cataract surgery. I have found the following five situations especially dangerous:

1. *Young patients.* Digital pressure and hyperosmotic agents cause little reduction in vitreous volume, probably because there is little free or nonlinked water in the vit-

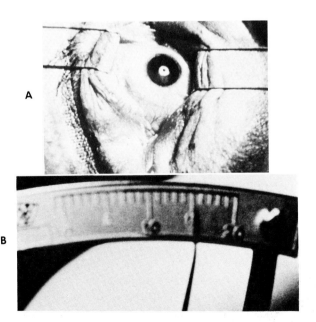

Fig. 11-6. A, Lateral canthotomy performed in same eye as in Fig. 11-3. **B,** Intraocular pressure less than 3.0 mm Schiøtz.

reous. These eyes also show a marked tendency to scleral collapse.

2. *Eyes with a shallow anterior chamber and narrow angle.* Digital pressure may completely occlude the angle and create a misdirected flow of aqueous into the vitreous. The intraocular pressure rises rather than falls as digital pressure is performed; a preliminary posterior sclerotomy is useful in this situation.

3. *Previous peripheral iridectomy.* These eyes often show a forward displacement of the lens-iris-vitreous diaphragm; the iris may prolapse as soon as the incision is made.

4. *Certain anatomic factors — short, thick neck, proptosis, and so on.* The patient's head should be propped up to prevent hyperextension of the neck.

5. *Evidence or positive history of operative loss of vitreous in the opposite eye.* Prolonged digital pressure and a hyperosmotic agent should be used; posterior sclerotomy may be performed if the intraocular pressure does not fall to a safe level.

Recognition of the dangerous eye during surgery

Sometimes despite every precaution just outlined or where the likelihood of vitreous loss was not appreciated beforehand, a dangerous situation will arise immediately after surgical decompression of the globe. Some signs of such impending danger are so obvious that even an inexperienced surgeon will recognize them; other signs are subtle and are appreciated only with experience.

There may be signs of increased vitreous pressure such as forward displacement of the lens and iris with gaping of the wound. This situation may complicate the enlargement of the incision, since it becomes difficult to place the blades of the scissors between the cornea and the bulging iris. The iris may actually prolapse. Another important sign is the appearance of horizontal lines of tension in the cornea. If the vitreous pressure is low, a vertical or a circular indentation of the cornea appears after the incision is made. The presence of horizontal creases, on the other hand, is a dangerous sign. The appearance of conjunctival ecchymosis, increasing in degree, often signals the presence of a retrobulbar hemorrhage or a "retrobulbar" injection outside of Tenon's capsule.

The causes of this critical situation are often not immediately apparent. They are usually related to some form of external pressure being exerted against the vitreous. The method of lid retraction may be faulty. There may be inadequate exposure and pressure against the globe because of a tight lateral canthus. There may be residual ocular movements and some residual orbicularis oculi function. There may be inadequate oxygenation of the patient or a high degree of restlessness. There may be scleral collapse, especially in young patients, although this occurs in older individuals more often than is generally appreciated. A significant retrobulbar hemorrhage may be present. A subchoroidal hemorrhage or serous effusion may also exert pressure on the vitreous.

The surgeon should make every attempt to determine the cause of the situation. The retraction of the lower lid should be terminated by releasing the lower blade of the speculum, loosening the lower lid suture, or removing the independent lower lid retractor. Occasionally this release will cause less wound gape. If it has not already been done, a lateral canthotomy should be performed. The corneoscleral incision may be held closed for several minutes, and mild pressure may be exerted against the cornea from without with a flat instrument such as a scalpel handle. If the wound gapes again when the cornea is retracted, the situation has not been remedied.

The following procedure may be found useful, although it is not always simple to perform: The wound should be closed by drawing up the preplaced sutures. A bubble of air is placed in the anterior chamber. It will often escape if the vitreous is under great pressure. In this case a slipknot is made with each suture. If air still escapes from the anterior chamber, additional sutures should be inserted and a slipknot placed in each. Air will usually be retained at this juncture and the lens-iris diaphragm is forced posteriorly. Once this is accomplished, there is no need to rush. The sclera is exposed in the superior temporal quadrant. A Rizzuti-Spirizzi 25- or 27-gauge cannula needle, attached to a syringe, is inserted through the sclera at a point 5 mm from the limbus. This instrument is so sharp that the pressure exerted against the globe during its insertion is minimal. It is directed superoposteriorly until the retrovitreal space is entered, at which point fluid may be aspirated into the syringe. The cornea will then show a vertical oval fold, indicating lowered intravitreal pressure. The sutures are untied and the wound reopened. The cataract extraction may then proceed in the usual manner. Many times, more often than not, the impending vitreous loss will be averted by this procedure.

If one wishes, a Flieringa ring may be applied after the posterior sclerotomy is performed. This will minimize the effect of scleral collapse if it is a cause of the bulge of vitreous.

If the vitreous has been pushed forward by a subchoroidal hemorrhage, a dark choroidal mass will become evident in the fundus if an indirect ophthalmoscope is used by the surgeon. If a hemorrhage bursts through the choroid and retina, an expulsive hemorrhage has occurred. This is managed in the manner outlined on p. 427.

Management of operative loss of vitreous

No matter how skillful the surgeon or how astute the surgeon's judgment, operative loss of vitreous will occur. There has been a gradual departure from the early tendency to simply close the wound with as little loss of formed vitreous as possible. Numerous methods of managing operative loss of vitreous exist, some of which appear contradictory.

Vitreous replacement. Vitreous replacement has been advocated in case of massive loss of vitreous. When one peruses the literature, one remains perplexed, since some authors extol the benefits of vitreous replacement, whereas others consider it entirely unnecessary. The former are motivated by the fear of an immediate intraocular hemorrhage, a later retinal detachment, or even phthisis bulbi.

As early as 1883, Andrews[32] successfully treated posttraumatic collapse of the globe with injections of sterile saline solution, as did Starr[33] later. Knapp[34] expanded the indications by recommending the injection of lukewarm, sterile saline solution in all cases of profound postoperative hypotonia, in cases of massive loss of fluid vitreous, and especially in those after a bulbar collapse associated with a perforating wound. In the last, he felt that the injected saline solution not only accomplished a refilling of the globe but also served to inhibit inflammation. In 1916 Mayweg[35] stated that vitreous lost in small amount is spontaneously replaced, but in massive vitreous loss, saline replacement is the surest way to avoid phthisis bulbi. However, in the same year, Schreiber[36] performed experiments on rabbits and observed that the removal of vitreous, even in large amounts, was followed by a spontaneous refilling of the vitreous cavity. He related this to his clinical observations that postoperative and posttraumatic massive loss of vitreous is usually followed by a spontaneous refilling. He stated that even if the procedure is well tolerated, it merely adds a supplementary trauma. However, if the collapse persists for 2 or 3 days, a saline injection then may be of value.

There is no valid statistical series relating to the benefits of saline injection as opposed to permitting spontaneous refilling of the globe. Thus there is little to be gained by reviewing the numerous reports on this subject. With the advent of modern cataract surgery, including better methods of wound closure, there is less to be feared from bulbar collapse once the risk of immediate intraocular hemorrhage has passed. Recently a long list of vitreous substitutes has become available.

Ice cold water. Ice cold water poured on the prolapsed vitreous to provoke its retraction has been recommended by Moutinho and Brégeat.[37]

Gas refrigerants. Gas refrigerants such as tetrafluorodichlorethane (Fluogen) have been advocated by Miller and his colleagues[38] to cause vitreous retraction, although Magdalena[39] attributes the benefits obtained to choroidal vasoconstriction.

Reduction of prolapsed vitreous without resection. Castroviejo[40] first closes the wound with an adequate number of corneoscleral sutures. He then engages the prolapsed or incarcerated vitreous by passing a specially designed cyclodialysis spatula (15 mm long and 0.75 mm wide) through the temporal extremity of the wound. The vitreous is drawn inferiorly by a sweep made parallel to the plane of the iris. This is repeated until there is no vitreous in the wound. The anterior chamber is filled with air, and the pupil is

constricted with a miotic. I have been less fortunate than Castroviejo in utilizing this procedure. Too often, I find vitreous regaining access to the wound, with subsequent distortion of the pupil. Maumenee[41] has advocated a similar technique in which he leaves his most temporal suture untied. He inserts a tightly wound cotton stick applicator into the anterior chamber through this opening, engages the prolapsed vitreous, and draws it out of the wound, where it is resected.

Removal of fluid vitreous. Maumenee[42] has advocated an excellent method of reducing prolapsed vitreous that enables one to suture the wound without vitreous between its lips and to place air in the anterior chamber. An 18-gauge needle that has had the tip filed off and is marked 1.5 cm from the tip, is inserted into the vitreous for about a centimeter. Gentle traction is then placed on a 2 ml syringe attached to the needle. As soon as the pocket of fluid vitreous is tapped, 1 to 2 ml may be aspirated. Formed vitreous in the anterior chamber will then retract.

Management of the iris. When the vitreous face ruptures, it is sometimes difficult to sweep all the vitreous back into the pupillary space. The superior portion of the iris is thrown into folds. It may even roll posteriorly and be lost from view. Within a few days these folds become so fibrosed that they cannot be unfolded even with forceps. For this reason a large sector iridectomy has been practiced. This may be combined with an inferior sphincterotomy to avoid an updrawn pupil. However, Castroviejo[43] and Barraquer and co-workers[2] recommend maintenance of the round pupil.

Resection had probably been the most frequently practiced procedure for operative loss of vitreous. Classically, resection has been performed after the wound is closed by pulling up the preplaced corneoscleral sutures. All vitreous that persists between the lips of the wound is resected. A spatula is used to ensure that no residual vitreous remains incarcerated between the lips of the wound. Air is then placed in the anterior chamber. I have used this technique with less than ideal results. The residual vitreous readheres to the wound and causes marked distortion of the iris with displacement of the pupil. Frequently the air penetrates the disrupted vitreous and lodges in the center of the globe.

Partial anterior vitrectomy. The technique of partial anterior vitrectomy has gained popularity in recent years. The term signifies that the entire anterior portion of the vitreous is not resected. That part attached to the pars plana and ora (vitreous base) is not removed. Therefore partial anterior vitrectomy is a more suitable term than anterior vitrectomy. Because of several obvious advantages that make this the management of choice in operative loss of vitreous, the procedure I have followed for the past several years is discussed and outlined in greater detail than the preceding techniques.

Credit for this technique correctly belongs to Kasner,[44] who has employed it since 1961. His first experience involved a boy whose eye was lacerated open from equator to equator along the horizontal axis. Traumatic aniridia and aphakia were present, and most of the vitreous had been avulsed; some vitreous was on the boy's face. He appeared anophthalmic on lid closure. He was taken to the operating room, where the remainder of the vitreous was removed as close down to the retina as possible. The wound was tightly closed with sutures, and the globe was filled with air and saline solution. The eye recovered remarkably, and visual acuity 7 years later was 20/50 with a contact lens. The retina is now normal, and the vitreous cavity appears to be optically empty.

This experience, combined with subsequent examples, teaches us that an eye can survive remarkably well without vitreous. This should come as no surprise, since in the natural course of senescence liquefaction of the vitreous gel occurs, reducing greatly its formed elements. In myopic eyes and in other pathologic and post-traumatic states, it is not unusual to find a vitreous cavity that appears optically empty because of conversion of the gel to a completely fluid state.

Anterior vitrectomy treats the vitreous as if it were a vestigial organ like the appendix. Kasner considers the vitreous the "enemy." When it causes trouble, he gets rid of it. If, as discussed earlier, many of the complications resulting from operative loss of vitreous are due to direct contact of vitreous with other structures, incarceration of vitreous into the operative wound, fibroplasia of the residual vitreous, and inflammation, it would appear prudent to rid the anterior segment of the eye of vitreous before these changes can take place. All previous methods, no matter how expertly applied, usually fail in this regard.

In children, in whom scleral collapse usually occurs, a scleral ring may be applied before the vitrectomy is begun. It is of advantage in adults too for reasons discussed later, although it is not always an absolute necessity. The wound should be closed by drawing up the preplaced sutures

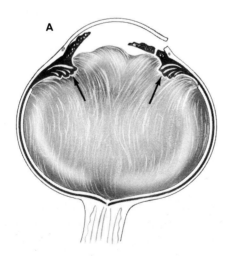
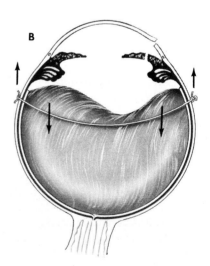

Fig. 11-7. A, Collapse of globe after operative loss of vitreous. Angle of anterior chamber is closed by iris, which is pushed up from below. **B,** Application of Flieringa ring maintains shape of globe. Iris tends to fall back posteriorly as vitreous is removed, thus keeping angle open at all times.

and tying them with a slipknot. This will facilitate the placement of the scleral ring. The beneficial effect of the ring is attributable to the fact that when the globe collapses, the angle is often closed by iris that is pushed up from below (Fig. 11-7). This is caused by the circumferential residuum of vitreous just under the peripheral portion of iris at the vitreous base. It is remarkable how quickly the vitreous over the iris and lips of the wound becomes fibrinous. Its contracture pulls the iris periphery up against the cornea, thus making if difficult to rid the angle of vitreous. The result is usually an angle that becomes permanently closed in many areas. If the ring is applied first, the shape of the globe is maintained. The iris tends to fall back posteriorly as vitreous is removed, thus keeping the angle open at all times.

Once the ring is securely in place (four episcleral sutures instead of the customary eight are usually adequate), the wound is reopened. The incision is enlarged to 180 degrees, or more, to facilitate vitreous removal and avoid damage to the corneal endothelium. The cornea is retracted by the assistant, and the vitrectomy is performed by the open-sky technique.

Chunks of vitreous are picked up by cellulose sponges, such as the Weck-cell sponges (E. Weck and Co., Long Island City, New York). They are cut at the pupillary plane by scissors (Fig. 18-17). These bundles should not be pulled outside the globe to be cut because they may, if stretched to excess, cause a retinal detachment or a vitreous hemorrhage. I prefer to use long-bladed scissors at first and then change to short-bladed scissors such as those of de Wecker or Barraquer when smaller bundles of vitreous are excised from the face of the iris or from the angle. This procedure is tedious, since it must be performed meticulously to be effective. After a moderate amount of vitreous is removed from the pupillary area, the iris will fall posteriorly, exposing the angle. Small triangular bits of the cellulose sponges are then applied to the surface of the iris and the angle to remove the remaining vitreous from the anterior chamber. The sponge will often swell because of absorption of fluid, but it will usually retain its contact with formed vitreous so that it may be cut.

When vitreous can no longer be picked up at the temporal and nasal extremities of the inci-

sion, the anterior chamber is free of vitreous. Additional vitreous should then be removed from the pupillary space. Long, narrow cellulose sponges (2 × 8 mm), presently available, are very useful for picking up vitreous in the pupillary axis behind the level of the iris. This can be done with minimal contact with the iris and will result in much less postoperative iritis. Finally, the pupil is constricted with acetylcholine. If the pupil is round, its shape should be retained, since this aids in preventing later incarceration of vitreous into the wound. The anterior chamber should be filled with air or balanced salt solution to facilitate suturing. It is especially important that wound closure be meticulous. A subconjunctival injection of a long-acting steroid should be made. When properly performed, a partial anterior vitrectomy empties the entire anterior chamber and the anterior one third of the vitreous cavity of formed vitreous (Fig. 11-8). Because of the associated intraocular inflammation—local, as well as systemic—steroids should be prescribed. An injection of 1 ml of a long-acting steroid at weekly intervals under Tenon's capsule may be given, if necessary.

Although I have not found it necessary, Gass[45] prefers to precede the vitrectomy by first performing an aspiration of fluid vitreous according to the technique suggested by Maumenee (p. 267). Such aspiration will cause the formed vit-

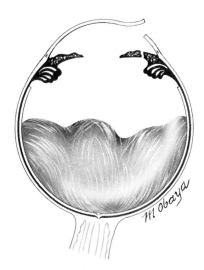

Fig. 11-8. When properly performed, partial anterior vitrectomy empties entire chamber and anterior one third of vitreous cavity of formed vitreous.

reous to retract and perhaps facilitate removal of vitreous from the angle. The tendency, however, is to remove less vitreous. This maneuver may delude the surgeon into thinking that an adequate anterior vitrectomy has been performed, since the iris falls posteriorly when the retrovitreal fluid is aspirated. The pocket may refill after the incision is closed, and formed vitreous may fill the anterior chamber. However, if one keeps this possibility in mind, a combination of the two procedures may be useful because they may shorten the time required for the surgery and perhaps facilitate its performance.

Cerasoli[46] studied a series of partial anterior vitrectomies according to the technique of Kasner performed for operative loss of vitreous at the Bascom Palmer Eye Institute. In the Bascom Palmer series, 17 of the 18 eyes were white, quiet eyes, and only one had cells in the anterior chamber. Twenty-eight percent showed macular lesions; 6% had corneal complications. There were nine peaked pupils and nine unpeaked pupils. Nine eyes had vitreous attached to the surgical wound, three in the form of a sheet, two with thick strands, and four with thin strands. Seven eyes had vitreous at or posterior to the plane of the iris, 11 had vitreous in the anterior chamber. The fundus was normal in 12 eyes, abnormal in 6 eyes. Of the latter, two had cystoid macular edema, one had cystoid macular edema with macular pucker, one had macular pucker, one had atrophy of the pigment epithelium at the posterior pole, and one had a pigmented scar temporal to the macula.

Kasner[47] has kindly informed me about a follow-up of 105 partial anterior vitrectomies performed during the course of cataract extraction by former residents at the Bascom Palmer Eye Institute who were in private practice from 1966 to 1972. The resulting visual acuities were as follows:

Visual acuity	No. of eyes	Percent
20/20-20/30	71	67.6
20/40-20/50	14	13.3
20/60-20/80	9	8.6
20/100-20/200	6	5.7
20/400	2	1.9
F.C.	1	1.0
LP	2	1.9
TOTAL	105	100.0

The following associated ocular abnormalities were observed in each group:

20/20-20/30: Five cystoid macular edema, two vitreitis, three transient corneal edema (one with peaked pupil), one irregular pupil, one glaucoma controlled with 4% pilocarpine drops, one filamentary keratitis, one early macular change

20/40-20/50: One cystoid macular edema with a surgically cured retinal detachment, one cystoid macular edema with a peaked pupil and edema of the upper one fifth of the cornea, one cystoid macular edema, one updrawn pupil, one chronic iritis, one hyphema, one vitreous hemorrhage, one retinal hemorrhage 6 weeks postoperatively

20/60-20/80: Two cystoid macular edema, one retinal detachment 2 years later, one bullous keratopathy with 2 degree glaucoma, one peaked pupil, two senile maculopathy, one 7.5 D astigmatism, one preoperative corneal scar

20/100-20/200: Three cystoid macular edema, two retinal detachments 2 years later, one corneal dendritic ulcer

20/400: One cystoid macular edema, one central retinal artery occlusion 2 years later

FC: One expulsive hemorrhage that preceded and caused the vitreous loss

LP: One retinal detachment, one expulsive hemorrhage that preceded and caused the vitreous loss

Final summary

Cystoid macular edema: 14 cases, or 13%; five cleared to 20/30, leaving 7% (two of these cleared to 20/40)

Retinal detachment: 5% (two occurred 1 year later, and one occurred 2 years later)

Transient corneal edema: 3%

Vitreitis: 2%

Chronic iritis: 1%

Excessive astigmatism: 1%

Bullous keratopathy plus glaucoma: 1%

When properly performed the aesthetic results speak for themselves (Fig. 11-9). If the pupil is round, it will remain so, and the peripheral iris openings will remain patent. If a sector iridectomy has been performed, there will be no tendency for the inferior pupillary edge to migrate upward.

Although one's surgical instinct reacts favorably to the technique of partial anterior vitrectomy, it is possible that a large series and a long-term follow-up will reveal serious complications such as vitreous hemorrhage, persistent iritis, persistent cystoid macular edema, and retinal detachment.

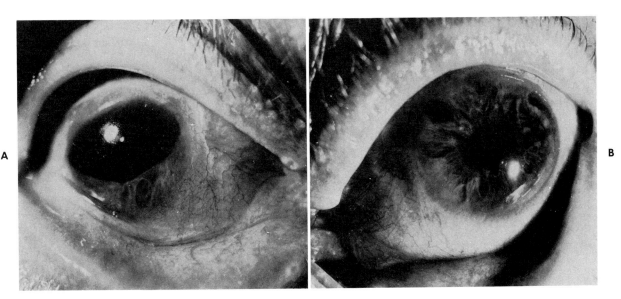

Fig. 11-9. This patient had cataract surgery in both eyes 6 years apart. In each instance, there was loss of formed vitreous. **A,** In first eye, vitreous was swept back into anterior chamber, and latter was filled with air. Sector iridectomy was not performed. Note marked distortion of pupil. Residual astigmatic error is 4.50 D. Cystoid macular edema was present for 2 years, followed by some residual degeneration of macula. Corrected visual acuity is 20/60. **B,** Second eye was managed by anterior vitrectomy. All formed vitreous was removed from anterior chamber. Small inferior sphincterotomy was performed. Note patency of peripheral iridotomies and lack of distortion of pupil. Residual astigmatic error is 0.75 D. Corrected visual acuity 2 years after surgery is 20/25. (From Jaffe, N. S.: The vitreous in clinical ophthalmology, St. Louis, 1969, The C. V. Mosby Co.)

Although others report more favorable results, I have adopted a more cautious attitude because I have observed retinal detachments in two patients and have knowledge of others and have observed vitreous hemorrhage in three patients. In spite of this I feel that this is the best way to manage operative loss of vitreous. The procedure must be correctly performed to avoid some of the complications seen earlier. It is most important to cut the vitreous at the level of the iris or slightly behind it to avoid excessive traction on the retina and its blood vessels.

Kaufman[48] has introduced a vitrector for the anterior segment surgeon, which he claims has advantages over the use of cellulose sponges. A disposable vitrector head comes in a separate Steri-pak that can be made instantly available. The principle of this instrument is simple. The vitreous is aspirated into the hole at the end of the instrument, and the fibrils are sheared by a rotary blade. The cutter is activated by pressing a knob on the handle, and the assistant applies suction, removing most of the solid vitreous. The main advantages of the instrument are that there is less chance of particulate contamination from shredding cellulose sponges, there is less danger of damaging the corneal endothelium by swollen sponges, and the procedure of vitrectomy is considerably shortened. However, it has not been emphasized that solid vitreous strands may be caught in the tip. This could cause marked traction on the retina. It is therefore important to use the instrument as a nibbler. The surgeon must carefully observe this precaution.

Some of these problems have been markedly lessened by a new version of this instrument called a Kaufman Vitrector II. The cutting mechanism has been improved so that there is less chance of catching vitreous strands in the tip of the instrument.

The very best devices for managing operative loss of vitreous are the more sophisticated vitrectomy instruments such as the Berkeley Ocutome, the Machemer VISC, the Douvas Roto-Extractor, and others. These are ideal, since they can be sterilized at the outset of the surgical day and autoclaved after each use. They all accomplish the desired effect rapidly with less chance of corneal damage or retinal traction than with sponges.

REFERENCES

1. Vail, D.: After-results of vitreous loss, Am. J. Ophthalmol. **59:**573-586, 1965.
2. Barraquer, J., Troutman, R. C., and Rutllán, J.: Surgery of the anterior segment of the eye, New York, 1964, McGraw-Hill Book Co., pp. 204, 281.
3. Richter, A. G.: A treatise on the extraction of the cataract. . . . Translated from the German with a plate and notes by the translator, London, 1791, J. Murray.
4. Smith, H.: The treatment of cataract, Calcutta, 1910, Thacker, Spink & Co., p. 100.
5. Vail, D. T.: Lantern demonstration of the unmodified "Smith" operation for cataract, Ophthalmoscope **9:**232-244, 1911.
6. Vail, D. C.: Loss of vitreous during cataract surgery, Highlights Ophthalmol. **11:**107-119, 1968.
7. Dunphy, E. B.: Loss of vitreous in cataract extraction, J.A.M.A. **89:**2254-2257, 1927.
8. Costomiris, G. A.: Du massage oculaire au point de vue historique et thérapeutique, et surtout du massage direct de la conjonctive de la cornée, Arch. Ophthalmol. **10:**37-79, 1890.
9. Donders, F. C.: Note in Zehender's Monatsbl., p. 302, 1872.
10. Pagenstecher, H.: Uber ide Massage des Auges und deren Andwendung bei verschiedenen Augenerkrankungen, Centralbl. prakt. Augenheilk. **2:**281-284, 1878.
11. Atkinson, W. S.: Local anesthesia on ophthalmology, Trans. Am. Ophthalmol. Soc. **32:**399-451, 1934.
12. Kirsch, R. E., and Steinman, W.: Digital pressure, an important safeguard in cataract surgery, Arch. Ophthalmol. **54:**697-703, 1955.
13. Hildreth, H. R.: Digital ocular compression preceding cataract surgery, Am. J. Ophthalmol. **51:**1237-1239, 1961.
14. Quinn, L. H., and Porter, J. C.: The removal of tritiated water from the vitreous of the dog, Trans. Am. Ophthalmol. Soc. **61:**181-195, 1963.
15. Robbins, R., Blumenthal, M., and Galin, M. A.: Reduction of vitreous weight by ocular massage, Am. J. Ophthalmol. **69:**603-607, 1970.
16. François, J., Gdal-On, M., Takeuchi, T., and Victoria-Troncoso, V.: Ocular hypotension and massage of the eyeball, Ann. Ophthalmol. **5:**645-662, 1973.
17. Curtin, B.: Tonometer compression as an efficient alternative to preoperative ocular massage. Am. J. Ophthalmol. **76:**472-474, 1973.
18. Jaffe, N. S., and Light, D. S.: Oral glycerin in cataract surgery, Arch. Ophthalmol. **73:**516-518, 1965.
19. Bucci, M. G., and Neuschüler, R.: Comportamento della profondità della camera anteriore dopo somministrazione di glicerolo per os, Boll. Oculist. **46:**116-127, 1967.
20. Bucci, M. G., and Neuschüler, R.: Indagini sul meccanismo d'azione ipotensiva oculare del glicerolo, Boll. Oculist. **42:**299-315, 1963.
21. Bucci, M. G.: Modificazioni ponderali del vitreo di coniglio dopo somministrazione orale di glicerolo, Boll. Oculist, **42:**569-577, 1963.
22. Robbins, R., and Galin, M. A.: Effect of osmotic agents on the vitreous body, Arch. Ophthalmol. **82:**694-699, 1969.
23. Bucci, M. G., and Virno, M.: Azione disidratante delle sostanze osmotiche sui tessuti oculari di coniglio, Boll. Oculist. **47:**407-416, 1968.
24. Iliff, C. E.: A surgically soft eye by posterior sclerotomy, Am. J. Ophthalmol. **61:**276-278, 1966.
25. Givner, I., Jaffe, N. S., and Teschner, B. M.: A lid retractor for cataract surgery, Am. J. Ophthalmol. **34:**108-110, 1951.
26. Best, C. H., and Taylor, N. B.: The physiological basis of medical practicee, ed. 3, Baltimore, 1943, The Williams & Wilkins Co., p. 43.
27. Ruiz, R. S., and Salmonsen, P. C.: Expulsive choroidal effusion: a complication of intraocular surgery, Arch. Ophthalmol. **94:**69-70, 1976.
28. Flieringa, H. J.: Procedure to prevent vitreous loss, Am. J. Ophthalmol. **36:**1618-1619, 1953.
29. van der Hoeve, J.: Ein Verfahren zur Vorbeugung von Glaskörpervorfall, Klin, Mbl. Augenheilk. **62:**791-794, 1919.
30. Brini, A., Bronner, A., Gerhard, J. P., and Nordmann, J.: Biologie et chirurgie du corps vitré, Paris, 1968, Masson & Cie., p. 411.
31. Girard, L. J.: Use of the scleral expander in intraocular surgery. In Emery, J. M., and Paton, D., editors: Current concepts in cataract surgery. Selected Proceedings of the Third Biennial Cataract Surgery Congess, St. Louis, 1974, The C. V. Mosby Co., pp. 231-237.
32. Andrews, J. A.: On the injection of a weak sterile solution of sodium chloride into collapsed eyes, Arch. Ophthalmol. **29:**50-53, 1900.
33. Starr, E. G.: On the injection of sterile salt solution into collapsed eyeballs. Report of two cases, Arch. Ophthalmol. **30:**418-419, 1901.
34. Knapp, H.: On the injection of a weak sterile salt solution into collapsed eyes, Arch. Ophthalmol. **28:**308-312, 1899.
35. Mayweg: Discussion of paper by Schreiber, L.: Ueber Glaskörperverlust und spontanen Glaskörperersatz, Ber. Dtsch. Ophthalmol. Ges. **40:**461, 1916.
36. Schreiber, L.: Ueber Glaskörperverlust und spontanen Glaskörperersatz, Ber. Dtsch. Ophthalmol. Ges. **40:**456-461, 1916.
37. Moutinho, H.: Discussion of paper by Séden, J., Farnarier, G., and Brégeat, P.: Les ectopies cristalliniennes; indications et techniques chirurgicales, Ann. Ther. Clin. Ophthalmol. **16:**210, 1965.
38. Miller, H. A., Perdriel, G., Graveline, J., and Manent, P.: Note préliminaire sur l'utilisation de gaz réfrigérants en

chirurgie oculaire, Bull. Soc. Ophtalmol. Fr. **64:**358-364, 1964.

39. Magdalena Castineria, J.: Profilaxis mediante el frio, de las pérdidas de vitreo en la operación de catarata, Arch. Soc. Oftalmol. Hisp.-Am. **25:**253-255, 1965.

40. Castroviejo, R.: Handling of eyes with vitreous prolapse, following cataract extraction, Am. J. Ophthalmol. **48:**397-399, 1959.

41. Maumenee, A. E.: Symposium: postoperative cataract complications. III. Epithelial invasion of the anterior chamber; retinal detachment; corneal edema; anterior chamber hemorrhages; changes in the macula, Ophthalmology (Rochester) **61:**51-68, 1957.

42. Maumenee, A. E.: Cited by Vail, D.: After-results of vitreous loss, Am. J. Ophthalmol. **59:**573-586, 1965, p. 583.

43. Castroviejo, R.: Cataract surgery: The handling of complications, Am. J. Ophthalmol. **58:**68-73, 1964.

44. Kasner, D.: The technique of radial anterior vitrectomy in vitreous loss. In Welsh, R. C., and Welsh, J.: The new report on cataract surgery, Miami, 1969, Miami Educational Press, pp. 1-4.

45. Gass, J. D. M.: Management of vitreous loss after cataract extraction, Arch. Ophthalmol. **83:**319-323, 1970.

46. Cerasoli, J.: The (Kasner) technique of radial anterior vitrectomy in vitreous loss (a 30 case follow-up). In Welsh, R. C., and Welsh, J.: The new report on cataract surgery, Miami, 1969, Miami Educational Press, pp. 5-9.

47. Kasner, D.: Personal communication.

48. Kaufman, H. E.: Vitrectomy from the anterior approach, Ophthalmic. Surg. **6:**58-65, 1975.

CHAPTER 12

Anterior chamber depth abnormalities

This opening chapter on anterior chamber depth abnormalities is general. The next three chapters consider the most important clinical situations associated with abnormalities of anterior chamber depth: hypotension, choroidal detachment, and aphakic pupillary block.

Of all the postoperative cataract complications, loss or shallowing of the anterior chamber is undoubtedly responsible for more poor visual results than any other. The problems connected with the restorative processes associated with the repair of surgical decompression are numerous and complex. The different pathogenesis of some of these problems appears obvious but helps to explain the many variations in healing patterns that arise. In considering alterations in anterior chamber depth after cataract surgery, some repetition of what is discussed in the sections on aphakic pupillary block, choroidal detachment, epithelial invasion of the anterior chamber, and hypotension is unavoidable. However, frequent references to these subjects will be made.

These alterations are conveniently classified as follows:

1. Delayed restoration of the anterior chamber
2. Late alterations in anterior chamber depth
   a. Late loss of the anterior chamber
   b. Late shallowing of the anterior chamber

The importance of abnormal anterior chamber depth is underscored by the fact that ophthalmologists have considered the depth of the anterior chamber the most important indicator of the state of repair of surgical decompression.

PATHOPHYSIOLOGY

The eye is a relatively inelastic sphere containing two chambers filled with noncompressible aqueous and vitreous. The chambers are conveniently separated by the iris and intercommunicate through the pupil. The smaller of the two, the anterior chamber, whose morphology is defined by the contour of its anatomic boundaries, normally contains aqueous humor. The larger of the two is the posterior chamber, which contains aqueous, and the vitreous cavity, filled with formed gel and an aqueous-like fluid. The posterior chamber may undergo wide variations in shape. The vitreous cavity remains relatively fixed in volume, although considerable alterations in the distribution of its constituents may occur.

Once surgical decompression occurs, the mechanism of repair is initiated and is oriented toward ensuring normal anatomic relationships within the anterior chamber until healing is complete. To consider that a leaking wound is sufficient to explain all flattening or shallowing of the anterior chamber is convenient but not accurate. Under normal circumstances the pressures within the two compartments of the globe are equal, since aqueous flows freely within the globe. The pressure within the entire globe varies with the rate of aqueous production and resistance to its outflow. If the outflow apparatus is obstructed, an increase in pressure results, which is transmitted evenly throughout the entire globe. The pressure in the vitreous chamber may be higher than that in the anterior chamber if there is failure of communication between the true posterior chamber and the anterior chamber (pupillary block). The pressure in the anterior chamber can never be higher than that in the vitreous compartment, since resistance to aqueous flow is downstream to both. Thus during the ear-

274

ly reparative phase, while the processes of aqueous secretion and filtration are being restored, the rate of restoration of aqueous volume exerts some influence on the filling of the anterior chamber. However, once wound healing is complete, neither the rate of aqueous secretion nor the rate of outflow can alter the depth of the anterior chamber unless some other anatomic abnormality exists.

The role of a wound leak is often difficult to assess. Many ophthalmologists think the presence of a wound leak ensures a flattening of the anterior chamber. They would be shocked if they tested the operative wound for leaks 24 hours after surgery. Most wounds leak considerably at this stage, yet the anterior chamber is of full aphakic depth. In some eyes with a wound leak a conjunctival bleb is present, and in others, where a filtering procedure is performed, there is usually no flattening or shallowing of the anterior chamber. Therefore a wound leak cannot be the only cause of this flattening. However, if the

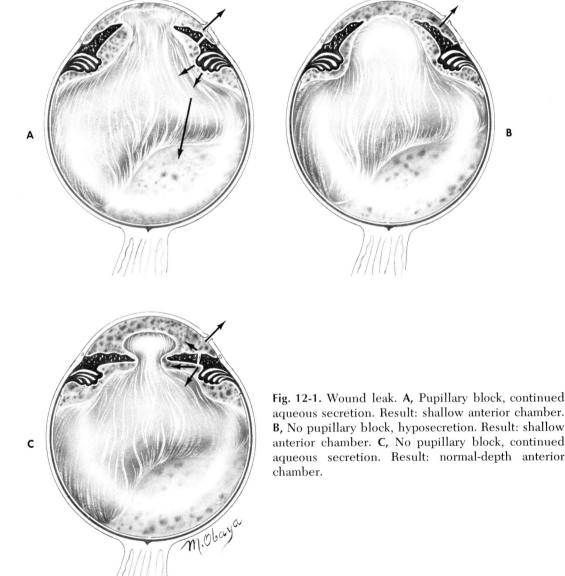

Fig. 12-1. Wound leak. **A,** Pupillary block, continued aqueous secretion. Result: shallow anterior chamber. **B,** No pupillary block, hyposecretion. Result: shallow anterior chamber. **C,** No pupillary block, continued aqueous secretion. Result: normal-depth anterior chamber.

wound leak is associated with an interference in aqueous flow between the posterior and anterior chambers or causes such interference, the pressure in the anterior chamber will fall below that exerted against the posterior surface of the iris, and this will result in a forward displacement of the iris (Fig. 12-1, *A*). If a wound leak is present and aqueous secretion has ceased, the anterior chamber is likely to be flat or shallow without the added factor of pupillary block (Fig. 12-1, *B*). In those eyes with a wound leak, with free communication of aqueous between the anterior and posterior chambers, and with normal-depth anterior chambers, aqueous production apparently is unimpaired (Fig. 12-1, *C*).

It is therefore apparent that the depth of the anterior chamber in a patient with a wound leak depends on whether there is continued aqueous secretion and pupillary block. A convenient summary follows:

	Wound leak	Aqueous secretion	Pupillary block	Depth of anterior chamber
A	Yes	Yes	Yes	Shallow
B	Yes	No	No	Shallow
C	Yes	Yes	No	Normal

Thus one can see that the wound leak may play a variable role in the pathogenesis of anterior chamber depth alterations. It may cause the iris diaphragm to move forward and initiate a pupillary block, which produces the flat or shallow anterior chamber. If there is no wound leak, a pupillary block may cause a wound leak by the elevation of intraocular pressure. However, the latter is much more rare than the former. A summary of clinical situations based on factors such as wound leak, intraocular pressure, anterior chamber depth, and ciliary body detachment is presented on p. 286.

Christensen[1] has outlined some factors that in his opinion are responsible for shallowing or flattening of the anterior chamber. For the iris diaphragm to be displaced forward, work must be performed. A source of energy must be available to perform the work. The potential sources of such energy are the following:

1. Pressure from misdirected, trapped aqueous behind the iris diaphragm
2. Pressure of an expanding vitreous because of hemorrhage

3. Displacement pressure of an expanding choroid
4. Displacement pressure of an invaginated wall of the globe.

These forces act on the iris through the medium of gelled vitreous, and unless this is present, no pressure can be exerted (except in the case of intravitreal hemorrhage, which is an infrequent factor). Furthermore, the gelled vitreous must have an intact anterior face, since if it is liquefied or if its face is broken, no pressure disparity will occur because the vitreous will course through the pupil and will apply pressure equally on both sides of the iris. A striking example of this is the immediate deepening of the anterior chamber after lens extraction because of rupture of the vitreous face. The iris may also be moved forward by aqueous dammed behind it (iris bombé), as seen in some cases of pupillary block.

In my opinion, a leaking wound is the most important primary factor responsible for the shallowing or flattening of the anterior chamber. The vitreous moves forward against the iris and factors aqueous flow in a posterior direction. The factors cited by Christensen may then come into play.

PATHOGENESIS

In general, a wound leak plays a principal role in the genesis of delayed restoration and late loss of the anterior chamber, whereas late shallowing may or may not be associated with a wound leak.

There are numerous causes of a wound leak, which is the principal cause of delayed reformation of the anterior chamber. These causes are the following:

1. *Inadequate incision*, including irregularities of the incision, are more commonly found in a scissors-enlarged section than in one made with a knife.
2. *Inadequate suturing*, including a perforating suture, which favors wound leakage; a deep suture, which may be converted to a perforating suture by necrosis of the deep portion of the wound; a superficial suture, which may cause posterior gaping; and an excessively tight suture, which favors necrosis. In general, these technical errors apply to larger sutures such as 6-0 and 7-0 silk and catgut. Monofilament nylon, 10-0, may

be inserted deeply and probably through full thickness of the wound margins. Deep necrosis does not occur.

3. *Accidental sclerectomy and excessive cauterization.*
4. *Incarceration of material*—iris, lens fragments, vitreous, lint, rubber, glass, suture pieces, and cilia—between the lips of the wound.
5. *Poor coaptation of the wound margins* because of variations in the depth of the suture, poor spacing of the sutures, and jagged wound edges.
6. *Accidental trauma,* which causes wound separation.
7. *Poor ocular structure,* including the thin scleral coats of highly myopic and juvenile eyes.
8. *Elevation of intraocular pressure,* which can occur with or without the use of alpha-chymotrypsin during cataract surgery.

The relationship between wound leak and wound incarceration is such that the leak may initiate wound incarceration or be caused by it.

Late loss of the anterior chamber occurs in an eye whose anterior chamber is initially formed during the first few postoperative days. The causes of this include those enumerated earlier as well as the following:

1. Sloughing out of a suture, too rapid absorption of a catgut suture, or necrosis around a suture
2. Later trauma, including suture removal
3. Inhibition of aqueous secretion associated with wound leakage and choroidal detachment

The most common cause of late flattening of the anterior chamber is external pressure exerted against the wound.

Late shallowing of the anterior chamber may be identical with late loss of the anterior chamber, the difference being one of degree. However, it is more commonly associated with pupillary block, which may be initiated by one of the several mechanisms discussed on p. 302. As a result of blockage of aqueous flow from the posterior to the anterior chamber, aqueous becomes misdirected into the vitreous or behind it, so that the mounting pressure exerted against the posterior surface of the iris causes shallowing of the anterior chamber. Pupillary block is discussed in Chapter 15.

INCIDENCE

Because of the wide variations in techniques of cataract extraction practiced by ophthalmologists the world over, statistics on the incidence of delayed restoration and late loss of the anterior chamber are meaningless. Unquestionably this complication was seen with far greater frequency before the advent of modern suturing techniques.

After cataract extraction the anterior chamber probably reaches full aphakic depth in a few hours in an overwhelming percentage of cases. It is rare to find a flat anterior chamber on the first postoperative dressing at 24 hours. The incidence of late flattening of the anterior chamber will vary with the frequency of postoperative examinations. Since most of these late flattenings are attributable to wound leaks that are self-limiting and that close in about 48 hours, they will be missed if the patient is seen weekly during the second to the fourth weeks after surgery. As Welsh,[2] emphasized there is ample evidence that wound leak has occurred between office visits, since "calling cards" are left by these leaks in the form of iris incarcerations in the wound. It is only when the chamber flattening becomes prolonged that they are recognized. However, it is possible for a postoperative rupture of the anterior hyaloid membrane to cause peripheral anterior synechias because of fibroplasia of the vitreous strands. This may be unrelated to a wound leak.

The method of wound closure probably has a great influence on the incidence of late flattening of the anterior chamber. It is my impression that corneoscleral sutures exteriorized through a limbus-based conjunctival flap cause a higher incidence than do sutures buried under a flap, limbus- or fornix-based. When catgut sutures are used, it makes a great difference whether the sutures are covered or exposed. When exposed, catgut sutures fragment early and tend to give rise to more wound leaks. The number of sutures used to close the wound is probably unimportant once one gets beyond five sutures if 6-0 or 7-0 material is used. More sutures are necessary with 8-0 to 10-0 material.

The method of making the incision likewise

influences the incidence of flattening of the anterior chamber. I have the impression that a beveled incision causes fewer wound leaks than a perpendicular incision. A half-lap or mitered incision is probably best of all.

SIGNS AND SYMPTOMS

In most instances of delayed re-formation of the anterior chamber and late loss of the anterior chamber, the iris comes in contact with the cornea. There may be a slight crescent-shaped separation, which varies in thickness from day to day. The intact anterior face of the vitreous may touch the back of the cornea. In cases of shallowing of the anterior chamber, the depth of the chamber may show variations on each examination. There also may be an irregularity to the depth, since fluid trapped in the posterior chamber in one area may cause a localized bulge in the iris in this location. This is particularly associated with pupillary block.

The patient may be aware of the onset of late loss of the chamber. There may be a sudden pain and sensation of moisture. However, it is just as likely for the event to be unattended by any revealing symptoms.

The conjunctiva overlying the area of wound leak may show a bogginess. However, in some cases the conjunctival flap may appear as a wide bleb. This bleb may also be seen with a fornix-based flap, especially when it is so well anchored that aqueous does not escape easily from under it.

The wound between two sutures may show a deep furrow to indicate that healing is impaired. The margins of the wound in this location may appear swollen. There may be some necrosis at a suture site.

The eye is usually markedly hypotonic except for cases associated with pupillary block. A choroidal detachment is usually found in those cases where the anterior chamber does not spontaneously re-form within 48 hours. In most instances the wound leak precedes the detachment. If the patient is examined frequently during the first 3 weeks after surgery, the flat chamber may be observed before the onset of the choroidal detachment. It may then be possible to prevent the detachment by re-forming the chamber medically as Welsh[2] suggested. The mechanism of

choroidal detachment in these cases is discussed on p. 296.

SEQUELAE

Loss of the anterior chamber is inconsistent with normal ocular function, and its continued presence will surely initiate one of several major consequences. The length of time a chamber may remain flat before it becomes pathologically organized is variable, although 5 to 7 days is a generally accepted average. The depth of the anterior chamber is somewhat dynamic at first, but if the etiology remains unattended, the stage is set for the activation of one or more pathologic mechanisms that may finally seal the fate of the globe.

Glaucoma

Glaucoma is the most common sequel of delayed restoration or late loss of the anterior chamber, and there may be one or more mechanisms responsible for it.

Peripheral anterior synechias may exist. As a result of persistence of iris contact with the angle structures and the cornea, permanent adhesions that effectively block angle drainage may result. There is some correlation between the duration of the flat chamber and the incidence of glaucoma. Kronfeld[3] combined two series[4,5] of cases of flat chamber and reported an incidence of glaucoma of 12.1% occurring after chamber absence for 5 to 8 days. The incidence rose sharply to 44% when the chamber remained flat for 9 to 12 days. A follow-up study[6] of 32 cases in which the chamber had been absent for 9 or more days revealed an incidence of glaucoma of 53%. The glaucoma is mild in many of these cases in the sense that the intraocular pressure is not very high and the eyes responded to miotics, especially to the cholinesterase inhibitors. Response to treatment is determined by the extent of the anterior synechias. In cases unresponsive to medical therapy, surgery (cyclodialysis, for example) is indicated.

Pupillary block may result from the firm apposition of the intact anterior face of the vitreous to the back of the iris. As the pooling of retrovitreal aqueous mounts, the iris is pushed forward with greater force, thus favoring anterior synechias and permanent angle obstruction.

Epithelial invasion of the anterior chamber is

favored by malunion of the wound (p. 514). Lining of the trabecular meshwork by epithelium increases the chance of glaucoma.

Hypotension

Since wound leakage sets the stage for ciliochoroidal detachment (p. 297) and cessation of aqueous production, hypotension results. Although this pathologic mechanism is usually reversed spontaneously or with the help of surgery, an occasional persistent and intractable hypotension may result.[7]

Inflammation and infection

Eyes whose anterior chambers show delayed re-formation or late loss usually exhibit increased congestion and a greater disposition to infection. There is a certain degree of normal postoperative inflammation, but when the iris adheres to the cornea and angle structures, inflammation is usually increased.

When the wound shows dehiscences, an open portal of entry for microorganisms is created. This may occur at any stage during the postoperative period. When wound incarcerations or prolapse occurs, the chance for such infection increases. An iris prolapse, particularly when uncovered by conjunctiva, makes the eye vulnerable to infection and probably increases the risk of sympathetic ophthalmitis. Ruiz[8] has emphasized this in pointing to vitreous prolapse through small breaks in the wound late in the postoperative course (p. 441). He terms this the "vitreous wick syndrome." This syndrome consists of microscopic wound breakdown with subsequent vitreous prolapse, which creates a tiny vitreous wick from the inner eye to the external surface. In some cases, severe intraocular inflammation that resembles endophthalmitis develops. The infection appears to gain entrance into the eye by way of the vitreous wisk.

Keratopathy

Persistent corneal edema from vitreocorneal adherence is usually an early complication of cataract surgery (p. 340), occurring in the first few postoperative days when the corneal endothelium is still suffering from the operative trauma and the bulge of the anterior hyaloid membrane is greatest. The most important etiologic factor in this complication is pupillary block secondary to a wound leak. This may favor a forward displacement of the vitreous until contact is made with the cornea. Patients with cornea guttata are particularly susceptible to this occurrence. These eyes must be observed very closely, and action must be initiated if the vitreous remains in contact with the cornea. The management of this complication is discussed on p. 343.

Epithelial downgrowth or fibrous ingrowth

These serious complications are discussed in Chapters 26 and 27. When the wound margins are poorly united and iris is adjacent to the wound and hypotension exists, a favorable climate for epithelial invasion of the anterior chamber is created. An epithelial cyst or downgrowth of epithelium along the posterior surface of the cornea, the angle structures, the iris, and the anterior face of the vitreous may occur. Such a situation also predisposes the globe to ingrowth of fibrous tissue elements from the margins of the incision or subepithelial connective tissue.

CLINICAL EXAMINATION

1. Search for a wound leak is usually performed with the aid of the slit lamp, using 2% fluorescein solution, which provides a greater concentration than fluorescein paper strips. The entire incision is scrutinized, using the cobalt filter. One must be patient when the chamber is flat, since there is little or no aqueous to leak out. At the site of a leak a trickle of aqueous will produce an area of green stain that contrasts with the orange color of the fluorescein around it. It may be helpful to place a drop of anesthetic solution in the eye and then gently stroke the cornea with the tip of a muscle hook while observing with the slit lamp. This part of the examination should be performed with great care. Posner[9] has suggested testing for a leak by holding a filter paper strip approximately 5 mm wide (the type used for Schirmer's test) in contact with the area suspected of containing the leaking would or suture track. If a leak is present, the filter paper becomes soaked with aqueous. In questionable cases a search for a wound leak is best performed in the operating room. Greater manipulation is possible, and corrective measures can be undertaken more effectively.

2. Fundus examination is performed to establish whether a clinically significant choroidal detachment exists.

3. Slip lamp examination is helpful in detecting anterior and posterior synechias, thickening of the anterior face of the vitreous, and herniation of vitreous into the anterior chamber.

4. Tonometry helps differentiate a flat chamber associated with wound leak from one caused by pupillary block.

PROPHYLAXIS

The incision should be correctly made by avoiding jagged margins. There are several methods of making the incision, and surgeons should carefully examine their own techniques if they encounter a high incidence of delayed re-formation and late loss of the anterior chamber.

Sutures should be correctly spaced, inserted to the proper depth, and not tied too tightly. Preplaced sutures are superior to postplaced ones if the microscope is not used. In my experience, corneoscleral sutures tied over the conjunctival flap produce more flat chambers than sutures buried under the flap. Catgut sutures are particularly liable to early fragmentation when exposed.

Excessive thermal cauterization should be avoided, especially close to the incision. The most satisfactory method for obtaining hemostasis is the Wet-Field Coagulator (p. 45). Additional hemostasis may be obtained by pressing an epinephrine-soaked cellulose sponge over the limbus for 1 minute before making the incision.

Meticulous attention must be directed to proper toilet of the wound. The iris should be entirely free of the wound. It may be helpful to complete the suturing after the lens is delivered by placing air in the anterior chamber to ensure that the iris is well away from the wound margins. If formed vitreous is lost, an anterior vitrectomy is the only procedure that ensures that the wound will be free of vitreous. Modern surgical drapes minimize contamination of the operative field with lint and cotton fibers. To eliminate particulate debris from solutions injected into the eye during surgery, disposable Millipore filter units are useful (p. 446).

The operated eye should be protected with a plastic or aluminum shield for the first 2 weeks and for a longer period during sleep.

Acetazolamide may be helpful in combatting elevations in intraocular pressure during the first few postoperative days, with or without the use of alpha-chymotrypsin. There is some question about the effectiveness of acetazolamide in this situation.

The eye should be examined frequently so that flattening or shallowing of the anterior chamber is promptly detected to enable early medical treatment. Excessive intraocular inflammation should be treated to avoid posterior synechias and thickening of the anterior face of the vitreous.

A sufficient number of iris openings should be made to ensure against pupillary block. In this regard a sector iridectomy is better than one peripheral iridectomy or iridotomy, but two transverse iridotomies are extremely effective.

Excessive physical activity on the part of the patient should be avoided. Tranquilizers and sedatives may be helpful for the highly nervous patient.

TREATMENT

If the anterior chamber is flat 24 hours after surgery, a firm pressure dressing is applied to the operated eye, and the opposite eye is patched. The patient is kept sedated and tranquilized. A strong, short-acting mydriatic is placed in the eye before the dressing is applied. Although long waits are rarely necessary, one may wait as long as 5 to 7 days before taking more drastic steps, provided that the cornea is clear and the eye is quiet. If the eye is known to have cornea guttata or endothelial dystrophy or if the cornea becomes increasingly edematous, earlier intervention is mandatory. At this earlier postoperative stage, it is best to institute reparative measures under general anesthesia after administering mannitol by the intravenous route. I prefer to place a bubble of air in the anterior chamber through a limbal stab wound inferotemporally. A useful instrument for this purpose is a Rizzuti-Spirizzi 27-gauge keratome cannula attached to a syringe containing sterilized air. Air is sterilized by collecting it in a syringe from the operating room atmosphere through a Millipore filter. A sharp disposable 1/2-inch 27-gauge needle is also effective in a soft globe with a flat anterior chamber. The wound is tested by the air bubble in the anterior chamber. If there is a dehiscence, it will be detected, and it can be repaired. If the leak is not immediately apparent, stroking the center of the cornea with a muscle hook will usually push air through the leak. In another technique a weak solution of fluorescein is injected into the anterior chamber. The dye points out the leak as it leaves the anterior chamber.

Air is left in the anterior chamber, both eyes are patched, and glycerin is given by mouth twice daily for at least 2 days. The air is replaced by aqueous over the next few days. By rising to the top of the anterior chamber, the air bubble probably blocks further leakage by interposing itself between the wound and the forming aqueous.

The situation is somewhat more grave if the anterior chamber has formed in the first few postoperative days and empties between the ninth and twentieth days. If frequent examinations are being performed, the chamber flattening will be detected at an early stage, and early detection may be of real benefit to the patient. If the chamber is flat or shallow, I assume that a wound leak has occurred and treat it as such. The pupil is dilated, a full dose of glycerin is administered orally, and both eyes are patched for 45 minutes. If the anterior chamber forms fully, I apply a pressure dressing to the eye and see the patient again the next day. The patient is advised to patch the unoperated eye after reaching home. As Welsh[2] pointed out, this is effective in most cases, since constant binocular patching eliminates, or greatly suppresses, the binocular blink reflex. Even if the anterior chamber does not form well after this regimen, a trial of a pressure dressing on the operated eye and a patch on the opposite eye is made for 1 day. It is likely that a lower incidence of choroidal detachment will be encountered if the flat chamber is detected and treated promptly. Generally the choroidal detachment is not observed until 2 days after the chamber flattens, although this is not constant, as witness its occasional immediate appearance during flattening of the chamber as a result of suture removal. If the patient is examined infrequently, the ophthalmologist is more likely to observe the flat chamber and the choroidal detachment at the same time.

If the patient suffers a late flattening of the anterior chamber and a choroidal detachment has already occurred, I treat the eye as if a wound leak is present, as outlined earlier. However, in my experience, there is less chance that this conservative regimen will result in a rapid cure at this stage. The treatment of choroidal detachment is fully discussed on p. 300.

The eye may suffer a late shallowing of the anterior chamber, which may have been initiated by a wound leak, intraocular inflammation, or some other cause, but the mechanism of pupillary block has supervened. It is important to bear in mind that, although this situation is usually associated with a normal or elevated intraocular pressure, hypotension may be present. In addition, a choroidal detachment does not rule out the possibility of pupillary block. The treatment of aphakic pupillary block is discussed on p. 312.

Postoperative cataract complications involving alterations in anterior chamber depth are potentially serious, and it will not be long before the young ophthalmologist has encountered a sufficient number of cases to be provided with adequate clinical experience to act with efficiency in bringing the problem to a successful conclusion.

The next three chapters deal with well-defined entities associated with alterations of anterior chamber depth.

REFERENCES

1. Christensen, L.: Postoperative flat chamber. In Symposium on cataracts, New Orleans, 1964, St. Louis, 1965, The C. V. Mosby Co., pp. 212-218.
2. Welsh, R. C.: Late flat anterior chambers following cataract surgery. In Welsh, R. C., and Welsh, J.: The new report on cataract surgery, Miami, 1969, Miami Educational Press, pp. 142-152.
3. Kronfeld, P.: Delayed restoration of the anterior chamber. In Fasanella, R. M.: Management of complications in eye surgery, Philadelphia, 1957, W. B. Saunders Co., pp. 194-209.
4. Pearlman, M. D.: Personal communication to Kronfeld, P. (ref. 3).
5. Bellows, J., Lieberman, H., and Abrahamson, I.: Flattened anterior chamber, Arch. Ophthalmol. **54:**170-178, 1955.
6. Kronfeld, P. C.: Delayed restoration of the anterior chamber, Am. J. Ophthalmol. **38:**453-464, 1954.
7. Chandler, P. A., and Maumenee, A. E.: A major cause of hypotony, Ophthalmology (Rochester) **65:**563-575, 1961.
8. Ruiz, R. S., and Teeters, V. W.: The vitreous wick syndrome, a late complication following cataract surgery, Am. J. Ophthalmol. **70:**483-490, 1970.
9. Posner, A.: Postcataract glaucoma associated with shallow anterior chamber, Int. Ophthalmol. Clin. **4:**1029-1043, 1964.

CHAPTER 13

Hypotension

The mechanism and significance of postoperative ocular hypotension have come into sharper focus in recent years. Although it causes less concern than hypertension because it is less severe and generally carries a more favorable prognosis, its recognition may prevent an unhappy ending to an otherwise successful cataract extraction.

Accurate definition of ocular hypotension by assigning a lower limit to the normal range of intraocular pressure is difficult. The height of this pressure in any population follows an asymmetrical curve of distribution around a mean of 14 to 16 mm Hg.[1] Leydhecker[2] measured the tension of 10,000 apparently normal eyes and found that in 95.5% the pressure lay between 10.5 and 20.5 mm Hg; it was below 10 mm Hg in about 2% of the population. He suggested that a pressure below 6.5 mm Hg be considered abnormal. However, such a guideline meets with the same objections as does a guideline for an upper limit to the normal range of intraocular pressure. Therefore, one can only define ocular hypotension as a level of intraocular pressure inconsistent with the normal functioning of the eye.

PATHOGENESIS

There are numerous causes of ocular hypotension, but in general, prolonged changes in the intraocular pressure may be produced by one of three factors[3]:

1. Changes in the resistance to the outflow of aqueous
2. Changes in the rate of formation of aqueous
3. Changes in the episcleral veins

Although the last is of little clinical importance, the first two factors are highly significant.

Changes in the resistance to the outflow of aqueous

Changes in aqueous-outflow resistance are caused by the incisional decompression of the globe attendant to intraocular surgery. Under normal circumstances, it is of short duration. However, if restoration of the anterior chamber is prolonged because of the numerous factors outlined on p. 276, a series of events leading ultimately to a more serious and enduring hypotension may ensue. In the presence of a wound leak, if aqueous secretion equals aqueous drainage, the anterior chamber may be of normal depth, choroidal detachment may be absent, and hypotension may be minimal (Fig. 12-1, C). However, wound breakdown is generally accompanied by hypotension, a net aqueous loss, shallowing or absence of the anterior chamber, choroidal detachment and its associated suppression of aqueous secretion (Fig. 12-1, B).

Changes in the rate of formation of aqueous

As a result of the incisional hypotension, the resulting decompression of the posterior segment of the globe may result in a hemorrhagic or serous ciliochoroidal detachment. Usually this is of short duration, terminating when the wound heals sufficiently. However, if the ciliary body remains detached, a pathologic organization of the pericyclitic hemorrhage or transudate may result in permanent hypotension.

The role of surgical trauma in causing hypotension is poorly understood. It is apparently vasomotor in origin and is probably associated with an increased capillary permeability. However the hypotension is usually not profound or of long duration, so its clinical significance is small.

ROLE OF CILIOCHOROIDAL DETACHMENT IN OCULAR HYPOTENSION

Chandler and Maumenee[4] have presented evidence suggesting that postoperative hypotension, at least in some cases, is attributable to hyposecretion of aqueous caused by a detachment of the choroid and ciliary body. Observations made from the role played by a cyclodialysis operation in lowering intraocular pressure are meaningful in explaining the hypotension in some eyes after a cataract extraction.

Eye surgeons formerly accepted that the lowering of intraocular pressure after a successful cyclodialysis procedure is the result of opening a supraciliary portal of aqueous filtration with subsequent absorption by the choroidal vessels. This theory meets with formidable objections. Currently the generally accepted mechanism is that the ciliary body detachment is the cause of the suppression of aqueous formation. There is a steadily growing weight of evidence in support of this concept.

Treacher Collins[5] observed a separation of the ciliary body up to the scleral spur in every case of persistent hypotension after severe contusion of the globe. He was able to produce hypotension in rabbits by repeated paracentesis and found separation of the ciliary body in these eyes.

Hudson[6] earlier concluded that serous detachment of the choroid and ciliary body is the natural accompaniment of considerable reduction of intraocular pressure and that its recurrence is the rule in every case of sustained reduction of pressure. He added that the degree of detachment varies with the degree of reduction of intraocular pressure.

Evidence favoring theory of hyposecretion hypotension

1. In some eyes whose intraocular pressure is well controlled by cyclodialysis, the detection of any gonioscopic evidence of a cleft may be impossible. When a cleft is present, its circumferential width often bears little relationship to the effectiveness of the surgery in lowering intraocular pressure. This fact suggests that the pressure-lowering effect of cyclodialysis is unrelated to the extent to which the ciliary body is detached from the scleral spur.

2. When the pressure becomes hypotensive after a cyclodialysis or some other intraocular operation, a total detachment of the ciliary body is not necessarily present. This may be proved by the following in vivo experiments: If a cleft is present, a weak solution of fluorescein injected into the anterior chamber will be detected by making a supraciliary incision well away from the cleft. This is the result of a complete circumferential ciliary body detachment. When a cleft is not present, the fluorescein will not find its way into the supraciliary space, but fluid will be found in this space when it is tapped (Fig. 13-1).

3. Chandler and Maumenee[4] provided further evidence of hyposecretion in four patients who had hypotension as a result of glaucoma surgery performed years previously. They were given 5 ml of a 10% solution of fluorescein intravenously. In one patient the fluorescein was visible

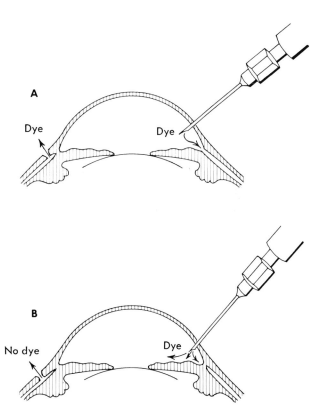

Fig. 13-1. **A,** In presence of cyclodialysis cleft, fluorescein injected into anterior chamber will be recovered by making supraciliary incision well away from cleft. **B,** When cleft is not present, fluorescein will not find its way into supraciliary space, although in hypotensive eyes fluid may be found in this space.

in the anterior chamber of the soft eye for approximately 48 hours but cleared from the opposite (normotensive) eye in about 10 hours. In the other three patients a similar, but less marked, stagnation of aqueous in the soft eye was observed.

4. Further in vivo observations lend support to the theory of hypotension being induced by ciliary body detachment, which inhibits aqueous secretion. In an eye with a wound fistula and a normal-depth anterior chamber, a scleral incision made over the ciliary body will not lead to trapped fluid, since there is no detachment of the ciliary body. Since aqueous production exceeds the outflow through the fistula, there is no net deficit of aqueous, and the anterior chamber is formed. In an eye with a small fistula and a flat anterior chamber, it is likely that aqueous production has ceased. An associated detachment of the ciliary body is present, and it can be proved by performing a supraciliary sclerotomy.

5. Additional circumstantial support of the theory of hyposecretion is derived from some eyes with flat anterior chamber and hypotension after cataract extraction in which there is no evidence of a wound leak. The angle appears blocked by iris, particularly in eyes with a round pupil. One would expect an elevated intraocular pressure in such an eye. However, a sclerotomy made over the ciliary body may reveal fluid.

6. Hogan[7] examined a number of eyes removed because of malignant glaucoma and found no detachment of the ciliary body in any of them. Chandler and Maumenee,[4] on the basis of findings in one eye removed because of malignant glaucoma, concluded that the anterior part of the ciliary body adjacent to the scleral spur must be separated for hyposecretion hypotension to occur. In this eye, there was a shallow choroidal separation attributable to hemorrhage, but the separation did not extend as far forward as the scleral spur.

7. Dellaporta and Obear[8] provided experimental support of the hyposecretion hypotension theory. They produced a flat detachment over the entire choroid and ciliary body up to the scleral spur by injecting citrated blood into the suprachoroidal space in rabbits. The hypotension created appeared significant when compared with control eyes.

As the result of these clinical and laboratory

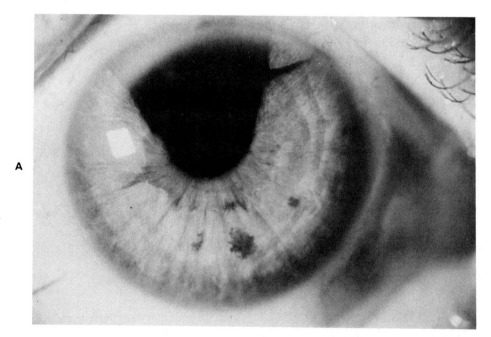

Fig. 13-2. Eye of 71-year-old patient who underwent uneventful intracapsular cataract extraction with sector iridectomy in 1969. During annual examinations, visual acuity was corrected to 20/20 and intraocular pressures were normal. In 1977, visual acuity decreased to 20/70, and applanation pressure was 2 mm. **A,** Appearance of eye in 1977. Note loose strand of pigment over iris at 1 o'clock.

observations, the hyposecretion hypotension hypothesis expressed earlier appears valid. Therefore, when cataract surgery is complicated by persistent hypotension in the absence of a wound leak, it is likely that an inadvertent cyclodialysis was created that resulted in a detachment of the ciliary body (Fig. 13-2). It is not difficult to imagine this occurring while the iris is grasped close to its root during the performance of an iridectomy or iridotomy.

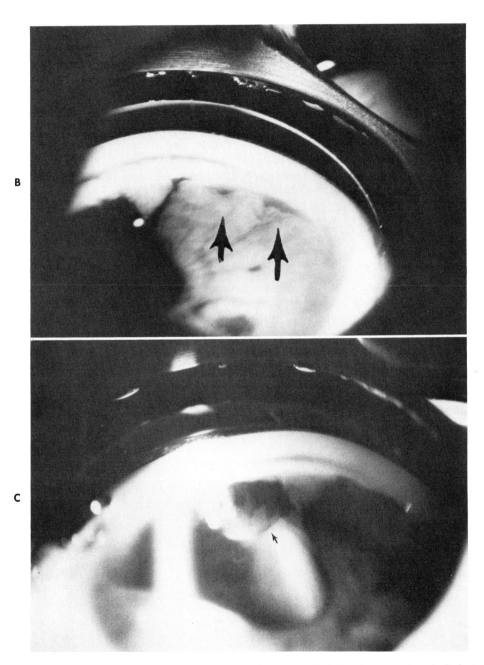

Fig. 13-2, cont'd. B, Gonioscopic view reveals two well-defined areas of cyclodialysis *(arrows)*. **C,** Detachment of ciliary body *(arrow)*. This extended behind iris in region of cyclodialysis clefts.

CLINICAL FINDINGS

According to the theory of hyposecretion hypotension just expressed a variety of clinical situations might be encountered. These are summarized as follows:

Wound leak	Intraocular pressure	Depth of anterior chamber	Ciliary body detachment
Yes	Hypotension	Normal	No
Yes	Hypotension	Shallow	Yes
No	Hypotension	Shallow	Yes
No	Normal or high	Shallow	No

In the first situation the depth of the anterior chamber is normal, although a wound leak is present. There is no net aqueous loss because of continued aqueous secretion. Thus the ciliary body is not detached. In the second the depth of the anterior chamber is shallow and is associated with a wound leak. There is a net aqueous loss due to hyposecretion. A ciliary body detachment is likely to be found. The third situation may represent a later stage of the second after disappearance of the wound leak. If the depth of the anterior chamber remains shallow, hyposecretion persists and the ciliary body remains detached. In these three situations the intraocular pressure is very low. In the fourth situation, if there is no wound leak and there is a shallow anterior chamber, a normal or high intraocular pressure points to a diagnosis of pupillary block (Chapter 15). There is continued aqueous secretion, and therefore the ciliary body is not detached.

This summary table might be compared with that on p. 276 where aqueous secretion and pupillary block are substituted for intraocular pressure and ciliary body detachment. It emphasizes the variety of situations encountered after cataract surgery that involve variations in anterior chamber depth.

The patient with ocular hypotension may have no unusual symptoms, and the eye may retain its function indefinitely. However, in most cases, signs of irritation and ciliary congestion associated with an irritative iridocyclitis may become evident. The eye may become intermittently painful. If the eye becomes phthisic, the pain, especially if associated with iridocyclitis, may become intense.

The cause of the blurred vision is still controversial. It has been attributed to macular edema, which has been reported in numerous cases of hypotension.[9] Gass[10] has challenged this view. He has observed that in some instances, patients with intraocular hypotension will develop loss of central vision secondary to marked irregular folding of the choroid and pigment epithelium. Initially, vision is affected primarily by virtue of the distortion of the overlying pigment epithelium and retinal receptors that follow the inner contour of the choroidal folds. Later, organic changes in the neuroepithelial layers may occur.

At first these folds are rather broad and not sharply delineated. They tend to radiate outward in a branching fashion from the optic disc temporally, whereas nasal to the disc they tend to be arranged concentrically or irregularly. The choroidal folds produce alternate yellow and dark streaks. Biomicroscopy reveals that the elevated portions or crests of the choroidal and pigment epithelial folds appear yellow, in contrast to the darker appearance of the troughs, or depressions, of these layers (Figs. 13-3, A, and 13-4, A). Papilledema may be produced by swelling of the choroid surrounding the optic nerve head together with circumpapillary retinal folding. However, papilledema may be present without these changes (Fig. 13-5). The papilledema may be due to protrusion of the optic nerve into the soft, easily deformable globe. Irregular retinal folds that do not parallel exactly the choroidal folds are observed. The retinal vessels are often tortuous and engorged. In the macula the retina is thrown into a series of radiating or stellate folds around the fovea that are not identical with folding of the underlying choroid. Gass[10] attributes this unusual parafoveal retinal wrinkling to central displacement of the normally very thick retina surrounding the very thin fovea by the partial collapse of the ocular wall posteriorly and swelling or folding of the underlying choroid. Cystoid retinal edema is not usually present (Figs. 13-3 and 13-4). Prolonged hypotension leads to prominent loss of pigment from the pigment epithelium along the crest of the choroidal fold and hyperpigmentation along the trough of the fold.

Fluorescein angiography is useful in detecting these folds, which in relatively mild degrees may be overlooked. Hyperfluorescent lines corre-

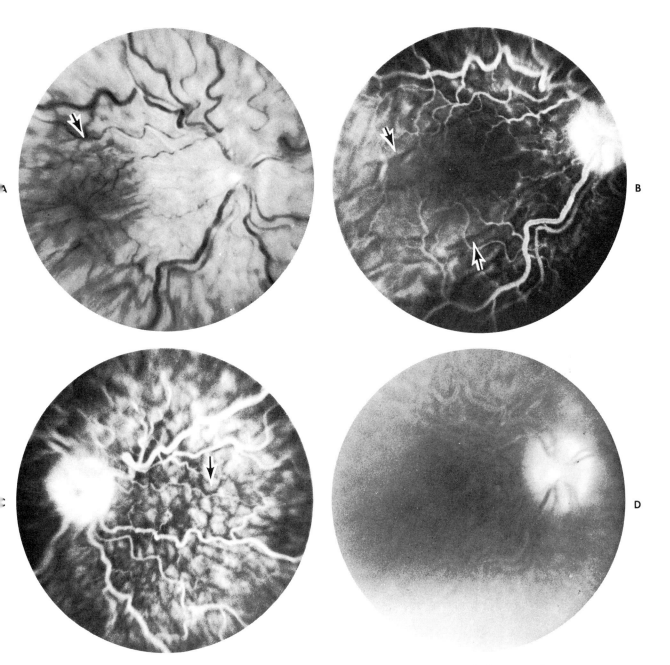

Fig. 13-3. A, Chorioretinal wrinkling caused by hypotension in patient who began to develop loss of central vision 4 months after cataract extraction and secondary operation to remove vitreous from wound during early postoperative period. Hypotension was result of unintentional cyclodialysis. Patient's visual acuity at time of photograph was 20/200. Note marked tortuosity of retinal vessels, which is particularly prominent within 2 disc diameters from optic disc. Retina is thrown into irregular folds that do not exactly parallel irregular folds of choroid, which are best seen just superior to macular region *(arrow)*. Crest of choroidal folds is yellow. Note stellate retinal folds radiating from foveal area. Note elevation of optic disc margins. **B,** Dark lines *(arrows)* are troughs separating broad choroidal folds radiating temporally from optic disc. **C,** Irregular pattern of dark lines *(arrow)* is indicative of multiple irregular folds nasal to optic disc. **D,** Late angiogram shows no evidence of dye leakage from retinal vessels and minimal evidence of papilledema. (From Gass, J. D. M.: Stereoscopic atlas of macular diseases. A funduscopic and angiographic presentation, St. Louis, 1970, The C. V. Mosby Co.)

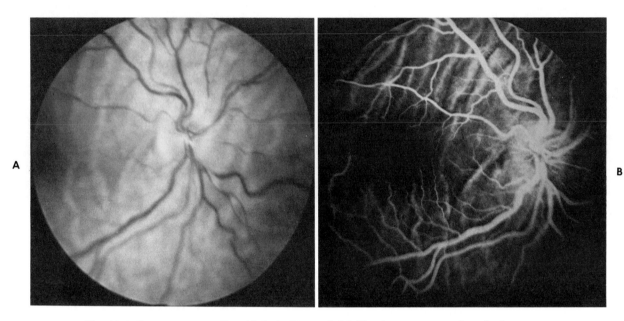

Fig. 13-4. Same eye as in Fig. 13-2. **A,** Choroidal folds characteristic of ocular hypotension. **B,** Folds are high-lighted during fluorescein angiography. Hyperfluorescent lines correspond to crests of folds. Hypofluorescent (dark) lines correspond to troughs of folds. There is no evidence of leakage of dye into macula.

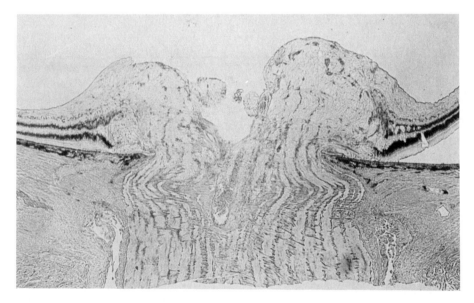

Fig. 13-5. Papilledema caused by hypotension. (×48, AFIP No. 283414.) (From Hogan, M. J., and Zimmerman, L. E.: Ophthalmic pathology. An atlas and textbook, ed. 2, Philadelphia, 1962, W. B. Saunders Co.)

sponding to the yellow lines observed in the fundus are plainly visible. They are the result of the relative thinning of the pigment epithelium on the crest, the greater thickness of the pool of choroidal dye beneath the crest, and the shorter course of the incident blue and reflected yellow-green light through the pigment epithelium on the crest.[10] The troughs of the folds appear relatively hypofluorescent (Figs. 13-3 and 13-4).

The alternating yellow and dark lines seen in the fundus are typical of hypotension retinopathy, but they are by no means pathognomonic. They are seen in other conditions such as high degrees of hypermetropia (Figs. 19-24 and 19-25) and intraocular neoplasms. Newell described similar folds in 16 patients, eight with orbital tumors and eight with a variety of ocular diseases: Graves' disease, ocular hypotension, hypermetropia, papilledema, disciform degeneration, and uveitis.

PATHOLOGY AND CONSEQUENCES OF HYPOTENSION

Unless the external filtration of the operative wound can be terminated and the normal secretory ability of the ciliary body restored, a sequence of events that may end the functional capacity of the eye will ultimately supervene.

It is the hypotension itself that, if permitted to persist, will cause severe alterations in the integrity of the globe. The most notable effects are observed in the vascular coats of the eye, the choroid, and the retina.

As stated on p. 293, the ease with which transudation occurs from the choroidal vessels is partly due to the nature of the veins of the anterior uvea. Anatomically, they are blood sinuses with a single-layer endothelial wall with no muscular coat and practically no connective tissue fibrillae. The release of external pressure from hypotension leads to their engorgement, and transudation through their thin walls then occurs easily. Associated with the effusion of fluid between the lamellae of the perichoroidal space, there is a marked congestion and dilatation of the uveal vessels. The fluid contained in the supraciliary and suprachoroidal space may be serous or hemorrhagic.

The yellow lines observed clinically are caused by prominent chorioretinal folds that may radiate in a stellate fashion from the macula but

that also involve the entire posterior portion of the globe. Partial collapse of the ocular wall posteriorly occurs, and the choroid and retina are thrown into these irregular folds. If the folds persist, changes in the pigment epithelium occur that are responsible for the hyperfluorescent lines seen with fluorescein angiography. Histopathologic examination of tissues from an eye with choroidal melanoma and choroidal folds has suggested to Norton[11] that the dark lines may be due to the inclination of the pigment epithelium in the valleys of folds, which effectively causes an increased thickness of pigment epithelium that blocks the transmission of choroidal fluorescence. Kroll and Norton[12] observed histologically that congestion of choroidal vessels and edema of the choroid are found in association with choroidal folds. They postulated that a localized increased thickness of the choroid may make the overlying Bruch's membrane redundant, forcing it and the overlying pigment epithelium into folds. They suggested that these folds might best be termed Bruch's membrane folds, occurring as they do with congestion and edema of the choroid in a manner analogous to Descemet's membrane folds, which occur with edema of the corneal stroma. Treacher Collins[13] noted histopathology in ocular hypotension quite similar to this as early as 1917.

Although the fundamental cause of choroidal folds is still conjectural, it appears safe to accept that they are produced by redundant choroid. Schepens[14] observed that spontaneously occurring choroidal folds are much more frequent around the posterior pole, particularly temporal to the disc. One reason for this is that the choroid is anchored around the disc at each point that a short ciliary vessel perforates the sclera. Because of this, redundant or swollen choroid has no freedom to adjust itself except by forming folds. Finally, Newell[15] attributed these folds to adhesions of Bruch's membrane to the underlying choriocapillaris combined with congestion of the choriocapillaris. When this adhesion is not present and when the choroid is congested, the pigment epithelium slips easily over the choriocapillaris, and folds are not produced.

Other less common findings are seen if the situation deteriorates. There may be thickening of the corneoscleral coat. The cornea may show superficial double contour lines attributable to folds in Bowman's membrane and wrinkling of Descemet's membrane, resulting in the clinical picture of striate keratopathy. Finally, the entire cornea may collapse into folds.

If this decompressive congestion becomes extensive and unrelenting, a serious pericyclitic organization may result, leading to circulatory stagnation with a permanent pool of nonabsorbable exudate, hemorrhage, and debris. Fibroblastic membranes, macrophages, epithelioid cells, giant cells, and cholesterol crystals may be found between the anterior uvea and the sclera.

As a final note of disintegration, general atrophy may set in, wherein the globe becomes soft and shrunken but retains its general internal architecture. However, a disorganization usually occurs, giving rise to the pathologic picture of phthisis bulbi.

TREATMENT

If an external fistula is present, it might be closed by applying a pressure dressing over the operated eye. It may be advisable in a resistant case to occlude the opposite eye also for a few days. If the anterior chamber is partially formed, gentle pressure on the globe will reveal the leak if the wound is first swabbed with a solution of 2% fluorescein and then examined through the cobalt filter of the slit lamp. The wound in this area should then be resutured and the anterior chamber partially filled with air. The search for a wound leak is usually more successful when performed in the operating room.

The treatment of hyposecretion is usually more complex. Unless dangerous signs such as extensive chorioretinal folds at the macula and decreased vision appear, it is best to simply observe the eye and not treat it. If one is compelled to intervene, the following approach may be adopted.

A search for a cyclodialysis cleft is made by use of a gonioscopic lens. This is best done with the pupil constricted. A painstaking examination is necessary, since the opening may be no more than a pinhead in width. If none is found the anterior chamber is filled with balanced salt solution to increase the intraocular pressure and deepen the chamber. This facilitates gonioscopy with a Koeppe lens and the surgical microscope.

The cleft is more easily located in this manner. If it is still not located, a weak solution of fluorescein (2% fluorescein diluted three or four times with normal saline solution) is injected into the anterior chamber. A scratch incision is made through the sclera over the ciliary body perpendicular to the limbus in the inferior temporal quadrant. If the fluid that escapes is tinged with fluorescein, a cleft must be present (Fig. 13-1). If it is not, all the fluid should be milked out by exerting pressure on the globe well away from the incision while the lips of the incision are spread with fine forceps. Air or balanced salt solution may then be placed in the anterior chamber through a limbal wound. This may terminate the hypotension if the ciliary body becomes reattached. If a cleft is present but cannot be located, the anterior chamber is again filled with balanced salt solution and another search made.

Once the cleft is located, it may be closed in the following manner, as Maumenee[9] suggested. After the fluid over the ciliary body in the inferior temporal quadrant is drained, the cyclodialysis cleft is sealed off with diathermy punctures applied over the sclera around the entire extent of the cleft. Maumenee recommends using cyclodiathermy pins 1.5 to 2 mm in length with the Walker diathermy machine set at approximately 30 units to obtain sufficient coagulation of the tissues. A semicircular area of perforations should be made directly through the sclera, beginning about 1 mm from the limbus and extending back at the greatest arc of the semicircle about 5 mm. The diameter of the semicircle at the limbal area should be at least 1 to 2 mm greater than the cyclodialysis cleft. The purpose of this treatment is to produce adhesions between the ciliary body and sclera beyond the area of the cyclodialysis cleft. If a second cleft is present, the fluorescein solution will continue to pass out of the sclerotomy opening. Further diathermy to include this cleft is placed.

After sufficient diathermy punctures have been made, air is injected into the vitreous either through the pars plana, if the patient's lens is present, or through the anterior chamber, if the patient is aphakic, so that the bubble of air will press the ciliary body against the sclera to ensure adequate chorioretinal adhesions during the postoperative period.

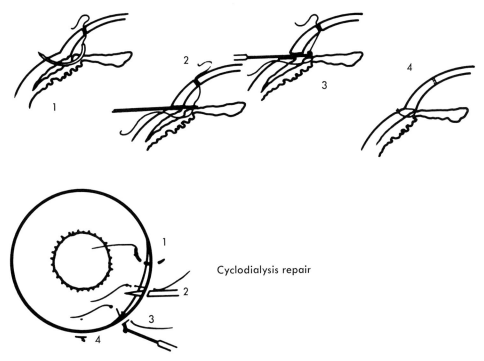

Fig. 13-6. McCannel method of cyclodialysis repair. Four monofilament nylon 10-0 sutures are placed across cleft, starting with intracorneal entry. Needle is directed down through clear cornea and in toward angle so that it engages iris root before it passes out through corneoscleral junction under small conjunctival flap, *1*. It emerges approximately 1 mm posterior to corneoscleral junction. After placing sutures, vertical cornea-to-iris suture is retrieved with small, blunt hook through narrow corneoscleral stab incision beside exiting suture, *2* and *3*. Sutures thus retrieved are brought out and exteriorized as loop. After loop is made, suture is cut off flush on surface of cornea, and continued pulling brings single suture strand out at limbal incision, *4*. Result is 10-0 nylon suture around iris root and cyclodialysis cleft and out corneoscleral exit. Suture is tied firmly and cut short under conjunctival flap. (From McCannel, M. A.: Ophthalmic Surg. **7**(2):98-103, 1976.)

Another technique of repair of cyclodialysis-induced hypotension was reported by Portney and Purcell.[16] Although the technique was used in a phakic eye with a cyclodialysis, it may be used as well in an aphakic eye with hyposecretion hypotension. It involves the placement of a scleral buckle over the region of the cyclodialysis cleft.

The technique that I favor is one suggested by McCannel.[17] The steps of the procedure are illustrated in Fig. 13-6. To this may be added cyclocryothermy over the area of the cleft. Some prefer this as the primary procedure.

One may justifiably conclude that the factors responsible for postoperative hypotension are now sufficiently understood so that a more rational approach to the problem has evolved.

REFERENCES

1. Duke-Elder, S.: System of ophthalmology. Vol. XI. Diseases of the lens and vitreous; glaucoma and hypotony, St. Louis, 1969, The C. V. Mosby Co., p. 726.
2. Leydhecker, W.: Symposium on glaucoma. VI. Clinical studies of the onset of simple glaucoma, Doc. Ophthalmol. **13**:357-388, 1959.
3. Duke-Elder, S.: System of ophthalmology. Vol. IV. The physiology of the eye and of vision, St. Louis, 1968, The C. V. Mosby Co., p. 243.
4. Chandler, P. A., and Maumenee, A. E.: A major cause of hypotony, Am. J. Ophthalmol. **52**:609-618, 1961.

5. Collins, E. T.: An experimental investigation as to some of the effects of hypotony in rabbits' eyes, Trans. Ophthalmol. Soc. U.K. **38:**217-227, 1918.

6. Hudson, A. C.: Serous detachment of the choroid and ciliary body as an accompaniment of perforating lesions of the eyeball, R. Lond. Ophthalmol. Hosp. Rep. **19:**301-310, 1913.

7. Hogan, M. J.: Personal communication to Chandler, P. A., and Maumenee, A. E.: A major cause of hypotony, Am. J. Ophthalmol. **52:**609-618, 1961.

8. Dellaporta, A., and Obear, M. F.: Hyposecretion of hypotony; experimental hypotony through detachment of the uvea, Am. J. Ophthalmol. **58:**785-789, 1964.

9. Maumenee, A. E.: Glaucoma. Hypotony, Highlights Ophthalmol. **9:**28-53, 1966.

10. Gass, J. D. M.: The cause of visual loss in hypotony. In Welsh, R. C., and Welsh, J.: The new report on cataract surgery, Miami, 1969, Miami Educational Press, pp. 162-164.

11. Norton, E. W. D.: A characteristic fluorescein angiographic pattern in choroidal folds, Proc. R. Soc. Med. **62:**119-128, 1969.

12. Kroll, A. J., and Norton, E. W. D.: Regression of choroidal folds, Ophthalmology (Rochester) **74:**515-526, 1970.

13. Collins, E. T.: Intraocular extension. I. The sequellae of hypotony, Trans. Ophthalmol. Soc. U.K. **37:**281-302, 1917.

14. Schepens, C. L.: Discussion of Kroll and Norton (ref. 12).

15. Newell, F. W.: Choroidal folds, Am. J. Ophthalmol. **75:**930-942, 1973.

16. Portney, G. L., and Purcell, T. W.: Surgical repair of cyclodialysis induced hypotony, Ophthalmic Surg. **5:**30-32, 1974.

17. McCannel, M. A.: A retrievable suture idea for anterior uveal problems, Ophthalmic Surg. **7**(2):98-103, 1976.

CHAPTER 14

Choroidal detachment

Von Graefe[1] in 1858 was the first to make the clinical diagnosis of choroidal detachment with the ophthalmoscope, although several anatomic reports existed prior to this time. Iwanoff[2] in 1865 reported the first postoperative choroidal detachment in an eye enucleated 3 weeks after an iridectomy for glaucoma. Reuling[3] in 1870 made the first clinical diagnosis after intraocular surgery.

Duke-Elder[4] correctly indicates that the name "choroidal detachment" is a terminologic inexactitude, since the condition affects not only the choroid but the ciliary body as well. He therefore suggests the name "ciliochoroidal detachment." We will, however, continue to use the more usual nomenclature.

PATHOPHYSIOLOGY

A study of the anatomy of sclerochoroidal relationships reveals that the perichoroidal space is a very narrow cleft that lies between the inner surface of the sclera and the outer surface of the uvea. It extends from the ciliary spur anteriorly to the optic nerve posteriorly, although the space probably ceases altogether some distance in front of the nerve, especially on the temporal side in the region of the fovea.[5] The choroid and ciliary body are bound to the sclera by suprachoroidal and supraciliary lamellae that ramify throughout the perichoroidal space in an almost random distribution, which provides a system of intercommunicating spaces.

The topography of a ciliochoroidal detachment is determined by the nature of the attachment of the uvea to the sclera. Moses[6] studied some of the anatomic and physical features of the choroid and ciliary body that predispose to their separation from the sclera in eye bank eyes less than 72 hours post mortem. The attachments were much more secure posteriorly than anteriorly (Fig. 14-1) and, except at the ciliary body, were slightly greater at the ora, and again almost absent from the ora to just posterior to the equator. They were most dense posterior to this. The more secure posterior relationship is attributed to the vortex veins, short posterior ciliary arteries, and nerves passing between sclera and choroid, which augment the suprachoroidal lamellae in holding the posterior choroid to the sclera. The attachment of sclera to choroid is also secure at the optic nerve. Anteriorly, the attachment is negligible, since here the long, thin suprachoroidal lamellae run in a very oblique manner. Thus the transudate from the choroidal vessels becomes distributed mainly throughout the supraciliary space and posteriorly between the choroid and sclera to the entrance of the vortex veins.

Spaeth and DeLong[7] have shown by microscopic sections correlated with the ophthalmoscopic findings that so-called choroidal detachment in most instances is a massive choroidal edema. The choroid becomes tremendously thickened, with the lamellae so widely separated by hydrops that a profound elevation occurs. Pau[8] concurs in this and observes that when the suprachoroidal lamellae become separated by the transudate, a "spongiosis choroideae" exists.

The ease with which transudation occurs in these regions is partly caused by the nature of the veins of the anterior uvea. They are anatomically blood sinuses with a single-layer endothelial wall with no muscular coat and practically no connective tissue fibrillae. A sudden release of external pressure leads to their engorgement, and transudation through their thin walls is easy. Associated with the effusion of fluid between the lamellae of the perichoroidal space is a marked congestion and dilatation of the uveal vessels.

The fluid in a serous detachment is a transudate, since it is albuminous, containing fibrin and some red blood cells and coagulating readily, and its content of electrolytes and proteins, including both albumin and globulin, corresponds to that of serum.[9]

There are three main forces influencing the transudation of fluid from the choroidal vessels:

1. *Intraocular pressure* acts against transudation. During surgical decompression of the globe, this pressure falls to that of the atmosphere.

2. *Intravascular pressure* favors transudation. Since transudation occurs chiefly at the capillary level, the pressure in the choroidal capillaries is to be considered. Blood pressure at the arterial end is about 32 mm Hg, whereas at the venous end it is 12 mm Hg.[10]

3. *Intravascular oncotic pressure or colloid osmotic pressure* is an osmotic force exerted by

the protein colloids of the plasma and tends to draw fluids from the tissues into the vascular tree. The oncotic force is especially active at the venous end where the plasma is more concentrated in colloids because water and electrolytes are forced out at the arterial end. The fluid transudate (because it has the same constituents as plasma) tends to reenter the vascular bed at the venous end without the air of lymphatics. The normal oncotic pressure measures 25 to 30 mm Hg.

Capper and Leopold,[11] using rabbit eyes, studied the effects of hypotension, trauma, and a combination of both on the production of a serous choroidal detachment. They simulated hypotension in one group by cutting out a rectangular piece of cornea near the limbus, trauma in a second group by making groove incisions in the sclera and a 180-degree groove around the limbus, and both conditions in a third group. They found that either hypotension or trauma alone is incapable of producing a serous detachment, but a combination of the two will readily produce it, a conclusion reached 12 years earlier by Spaeth

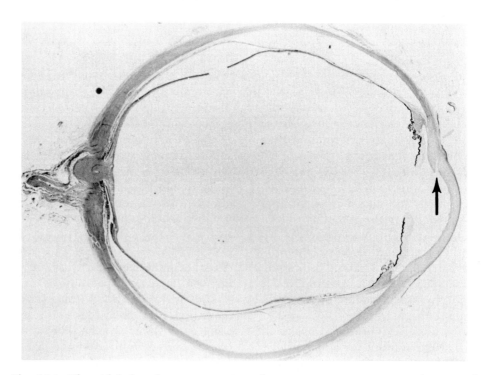

Fig. 14-1. Choroidal detachment occurring after cataract extraction. Attachments of choroid are much more secure posteriorly than anteriorly. Note postmortem dehiscence at site of cataract incision (*arrow*).

and DeLong[7] on a purely clinical basis. Hypotension from decompression or fistulization will raise the intravascular oncotic pressure, since more water and electrolytes are forced out at the arterial end, whereas the plasma colloids are retained. Trauma causes capillary damage with leakage of colloids. This lowers the intravascular oncotic pressure.

To emphasize the role of the three pressures in the mechanism of a serous choroidal detachment, one may consider the effects of hypotension, trauma, and a combination of the two in its production. The figures presented here, suggested by Capper and Leopold,[11] are merely for illustration. There are so many variables in human eyes that they do not represent an accurate guide to what occurs in these eyes.

Hypotension alone

Capillary blood pressure (BP)	
at arterial end	= 32 mm Hg out
Intraocular pressure	= 10 mm Hg in
Favors transudation	= 22 mm Hg out
Capillary BP at venous end	= 12 mm Hg out
Intraocular pressure	= 10 mm Hg in
Intravascular oncotic pressure	= 35 mm Hg in
Favors fluid return to blood	= 33 mm Hg in
Result	= 11 mm Hg in

Trauma alone

Capillary BP at arterial end	= 32 mm Hg out
Intraocular pressure	= 25 mm Hg in
Favors transudation	= 7 mm Hg out
Capillary BP venous end	= 12 mm Hg out
Intraocular pressure	= 25 mm Hg in
Intravascular oncotic pressure	= 10 mm Hg in
Favors fluid return to blood	= 23 mm Hg in
Result	= 16 mm Hg in

Combination of hypotension and trauma

Capillary BP at arterial end	= 32 mm Hg out
Intraocular pressure	= 10 mm Hg in
Favors transudation	= 22 mm Hg out
Capillary BP at venous end	= 12 mm Hg out
Intraocular pressure	= 10 mm Hg in
Intravascular oncotic pressure	= 10 mm Hg in
Favors fluid return to blood	= 8 mm Hg in
Result	= 14 mm Hg out

Moses[6] found that the elasticity of the choroid is such that in the enucleated human eye about 2 mm Hg pressure is necessary to distend the uvea against the sclera. The fact that the choroid retracts implies that even in the dead eye it is under tension. Further, the elasticity of the ciliary body and choroid suggest that when the intraocular pressure falls to atmospheric, as during a cataract extraction, the pressure in the suprachoroidal potential space falls to as much as 2 mm Hg below atmospheric pressure. Thus it is not surprising that transudate appears in the space in many such cases. Hudson[12] also pointed to the fact that the nearly spherical sclera tends to maintain its domed shape when the intraocular pressure drops to atmospheric. Miller[13] and Hagen[9] emphasized the loss of elasticity of the sclera, giving age as a reason that choroidal detachment is often seen with hypotension in older adults but not often in the young. Thus it has been suggested[6] that the thinness and elasticity of the rabbit's sclera may account for the lack of choroidal detachment on fistulization of the anterior chamber alone, found by Capper and Leopold.

FUNDUS ALTERATIONS ASSOCIATED WITH LONG-STANDING CHOROIDAL DETACHMENT

Lobular choroidal detachments are separated by deep valleys, probably caused by anchorages

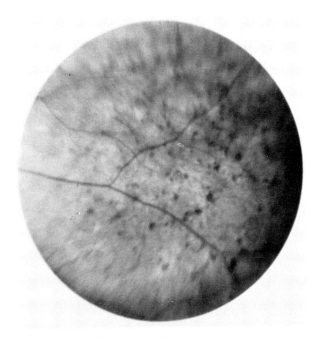

Fig. 14-2. Atrophy of retinal pigment epithelium with clumping of pigment confined to area of prior choroidal detachment.

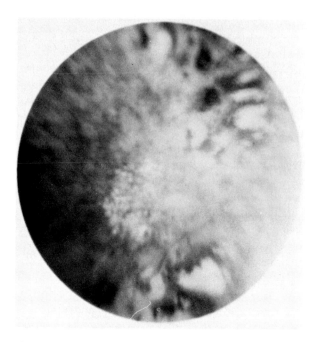

Fig. 14-3. Widespread atrophy of retinal pigment epithelium with some clumping of pigment confined to area of prior choroidal detachment.

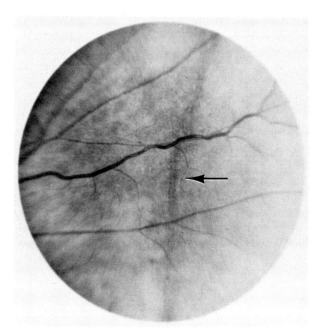

Fig. 14-4. Characteristic pigment streak *(arrow)* observed some time after subsidence of choroidal detachment.

of vortex veins. If a choroidal detachment persists for a long time, two types of pigmentary disturbances may be observed on fundus examination. One consists of widespread atrophy of the retinal pigment epithelium, with clumping of pigment confined to the area of the choroidal detachment (Figs. 14-2 and 14-3). A second consists of streaks of pigment that may appear even after the lesion has subsided for some time (Fig. 14-4). They are said to be pathognomonic of this condition.[14] Their cause is not definitely known, but Fuchs[15] thought they were due to depressions in the choroid formed by the pigment epithelium after the dome of the detachment subsided. Verhoeff[16] thought that the effect was due to a ridgelike hyperplasia of the pigment epithelium that had accumulated in the creases formed in the choroid during detachment.

MECHANISM OF HYPOTENSION IN CHOROIDAL DETACHMENT

Chandler and Maumenee[17] suggested that the cause of the hypotension often seen in patients with choroidal detachment, in whom there is no external filtration, is a serous detachment of the

ciliary body. The evidence supporting this theory is outlined on p. 283. This detachment apparently prevents aqueous secretion. The reason for this is not entirely clear. However, it is possible that the severe edema of the ciliary processes may prevent arterial blood from getting to the portion of the processes that manufacture aqueous. The resulting venous engorgement continues to permit loss of fluid from the vessels from the venous side. The ciliary body regains its function after the fluid is removed surgically or disappears spontaneously because of normalization of ocular hemodynamics.

The depth of the anterior chamber in hypotensive eyes after cataract extraction may show unexpected variations. In some eyes with an obvious wound leak, the anterior chamber may remain deep and no choroidal detachment is found. In others without apparent wound leak, the anterior chamber may be very shallow. Chandler and Maumenee[17] have explained this seeming discrepancy by the rate of aqueous formation. In the former situation, a separation of the choroid is not seen. Aqueous is being formed at a normal rate, as evidenced by its continual escape from the anterior chamber. If the fistula is small, the rate of aqueous inflow will balance the rate of outflow. In the latter situation, there is retardation of aqueous formation because of detachment of the ciliary body and choroid. There may be no recognizable wound leak. This may be diagnosed by ophthalmoscopy or by obtaining fluid through a suprachoroidal tap (if the detachment cannot be seen).

The cause of a flat or shallow anterior chamber in an eye without a wound leak but with a choroidal detachment is not always clear. Theoretically, for the anterior chamber to become shallow in these situations, the iris has to move forward, and it must be pushed from behind by some force exerted against it (p. 276). When a large bullous choroidal detachment is present, it is not difficult to imagine that the mass compresses the vitreous, which in turn pushes the iris forward. However, what about those eyes in which a thin suprachoroidal cleft is present? The answer may be found in an observation made by Grant.[20] In a normal enucleated human eye the cornea was excised, an iridectomy was done, and the lens was removed. A needle was passed obliquely through the sclera, just over the ciliary body. Fluid was injected, resulting in a moundlike ciliochoroidal elevation, which was observed with a dissecting microscope. After a while the fluid diffused into a thin layer over a wide area so that the large elevation could not be seen. More fluid was injected, and another elevation occurred and again disappeared after awhile. However, Grant observed through the iris coloboma that the ciliary processes had rotated and lay in the plane of the cornea. This rotation of the ciliary body may be a cause of shallowing of the anterior chamber.

To this may be added the observations of Moses,[6] discussed on p. 295, that the ciliary structures are under tension, and when the intraocular pressure is reduced, they tend to cause the ciliary body to curl inward.

CLASSIFICATION OF CILIOCHOROIDAL DETACHMENTS

1. Spontaneous serous
2. Postoperative
3. Exudative
4. Traumatic
5. Hemorrhagic
6. Purulent
7. Caused by traction in phthisic eyes

Postoperative ciliochoroidal detachments may occur typically at three different intervals after cataract surgery. The condition may be seen immediately after surgery, 7 to 21 days after surgery, or it may be delayed, occurring months or years after surgery.

Immediate choroidal detachments have been considered very common after cataract surgery. The incidence is uncertain, but O'Brien[21] found them in 86 of 92 cataract extractions, which were uneventful and where the fundus was visible. This is an incidence of 93%. Other have likewise reported a very high incidence. In some instances the detachment may become more apparent several days later.[22] These are most commonly found in the inferior quadrants. They appear as a dark, slightly elevated line with its convexity directed posteriorly. They are usually flat and not always easy to see. Several peripheral areas may be found at one time. Generally these detachments disappear, although some persist or get worse so that they resemble the next type of detachment.

I have not observed a high incidence of immediate choroidal detachment. Kirsch and Singer[23] have also challenged O'Brien's findings. They observed striking fundus changes immediately after delivery of the lens, using binocular indirect ophthalmoscopy and fluorescein angiography. These consisted of full-thickness infoldings in the sclera, choroid, and retina. They were not choroidal detachments. They closely resembled the appearance of buckles in scleral-buckling procedures. There was no evidence of suprachoroidal fluid extravasation, the infoldings did not increase in size, and they disappeared as a result of various anterior segment maneuvers. They attributed the phenomenon to ocular hypotension. These folds have also been observed with open-sky partial anterior vitrectomy but not with closed-system vitrectomy (Machemer). This was not considered a possible cause of operative loss of vitreous, since the anterior vitreous face was observed to be very concave in most cases (Fig. 14-5).

Postoperative choroidal detachments may occur 7 to 21 days after surgery. They may be a persistence of the immediate type or occur later

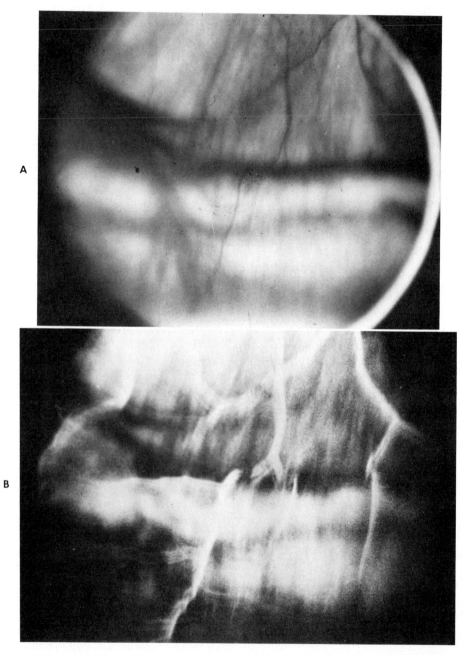

Fig. 14-5. A, Infolding of eye immediately after cataract extraction. Infolding of posterior ocular coats closely resembles appearance of buckles produced in scleral buckling procedures for retinal detachment. **B,** Fluorescein angiogram of same eye immediately after cataract extraction. (From Kirsch, R. E., and Singer, J. A.: Arch. Ophthalmol. **90:** 460-463, 1973. Copyright 1973, American Medical Association.)

because of a wound leak, delayed wound healing, or a rupture of an inadequately healed wound. Before the popularization of fine sutures and more effective closure of the wound, the incidence of this type of choroidal detachment was probably about 5% to 8%. It appears to be much less now.

They may or may not be associated with a shallow anterior chamber. However, as a rule, the first sign is some shallowing of the anterior chamber, which directs one to the associated hypotension. The lobular choroidal detachment may not be observed for several days, although I have seen it immediately after disruption of the wound during suture removal. Not infrequently a wound leak may be demonstrated, using fluorescein (Seidel's test).[24] The detachment is usually found anterior to the equator, although it may extend more posteriorly. As mentioned earlier, several lobes may exist, usually separated by the vortex veins. I have never seen it reach the macula or the disc, nor have I ever observed the retina overlying it detached. Its ophthalmoscopic appearance is that of a dark elevated mass, which usually offers no diagnostic problem in postoperative cases (Fig. 14-6). However, it has been mistaken for a retinal detachment, although it has a smooth surface that is not wavy or mobile, and for a tumor from which it may be differentiated by transillumination. There may be exaggerated lighting of the sclera over a choroidal detachment.[9] Nevertheless, many eyes with a choroidal detachment have been enucleated with the mistaken diagnosis of melanoma. The appearance of a dark mass in an eye with hypotension and a shallow anterior chamber 1 to 3 weeks after cataract surgery is nearly always attributable to a choroidal detachment.

Symptoms are not prominent, since the patient's eye has not yet been refracted, and the tested visual acuity is usually not depressed unless the lobes of the detachments nasally and temporally obscure the visual line ("kissing choroidals").

The course is usually benign, with the detachment subsiding in 2 to 3 weeks, although I have seen it persist for as long as 7 months.

The main complication concerns the possibility of anterior iris adhesions with permanent angle damage and secondary glaucoma if it persists

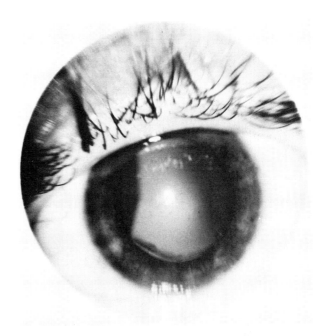

Fig. 14-6. Ophthalmoscopic appearance of choroidal detachment showing dark, elevated mounds.

too long. I usually do not wait more than 8 days to treat the problem surgically if the angle is closed. If a wound leak is demonstrated and medical means (binocular patch) have failed to heal the wound, it should be resutured. The fundus picture that may result after the subsidence of a prolonged choroidal detachment has been described on p. 295.

Delayed choroidal detachment occurs some months or years after cataract extraction. The mechanism is unclear, although some cases seem to be associated with trauma, with a reopening of the wound being likely. There may be a sudden onset of decreased vision, ocular irritability, tearing, and a shallow or absent anterior chamber.

Expulsive choroidal effusion may occur as a complication of intraocular surgery.[25] This rare condition involves a massive serous choroidal effusion, which resembles in some respects an expulsive hemorrhage. Some of the predisposing factors of these two entities may be shared: atherosclerosis, hypertension, and sudden surgical decompression. During surgery a sudden loss of vitreous occurs, and this is followed by the appearance of a large choroidal detachment. As with expulsive hemorrhage, the treatment consists of rapid closure of the wound, drainage of

suprachoroidal effusion through a posterior sclerotomy site, and injection of a physiologic solution into the anterior chamber to tamponade the
leaking vessels and restore normal intraocular
anatomic relationships. It is interesting that in
one of the two cases reported by Ruiz and Salmonsen[25] and in my most recent case, very little
fluid was found after performing the posterior
sclerotomy. It is also interesting that in both of
these cases a retinal detachment occurred several
weeks after the surgery. Also, in both cases the
detachments involved the ora. Unfortunately,
my patient's eye rapidly progressed to massive
vitreous retraction before surgical reattachment
could be performed. Although the events during
surgery parallel those of expulsive hemorrhage,
the prognosis for visual recovery following expulsive choroidal effusion is much more favorable.

TREATMENT OF POSTOPERATIVE CHOROIDAL DETACHMENT

Most postoperative choroidal detachments
subside within 3 weeks and therefore require no
treatment unless the anterior chamber remains
shallow.

Prophylactic treatment

Prophylaxis is important, since a poorly made
cataract incision, an inadequately sutured incision, and the inclusion of material between the
lips of the wound (iris, lens remnants, vitreous,
and particulate debris) predispose to fistulization
and choroidal detachment. The avoidance of a
precipitous fall in intraocular pressure during
surgical decompression is probably of value. The
methods of achieving a soft eye are discussed on
p. 256. It may also be of some benefit to fill the
anterior chamber at the conclusion of surgery
with balanced salt solution, with or without a
small air bubble.

Medical treatment

Cycloplegic agents are theoretically indicated,
since by relaxing the ciliary muscle, tension on
the uvea is minimized. Acetazolamide is often
used but with little rationale, since hyposecretion and stagnation of aqueous already exist. If
there is a wound leak, one may argue that healing
will be hastened if aqueous does not filter

through the wound defect. I have not found acetazolamide useful.

Not infrequently a wound leak will precipitate
a forward movement of the iris and vitreous as
the anterior chamber empties. A ciliochoroidal
detachment may occur. At the same time,
aqueous may be misdirected posteriorly so that
the element of pupillary block enters the picture
in the presence of a choroidal detachment. The
systemic administration of a hyperosmotic agent
plus the topical administration of a cycloplegic
will often deepen the chamber and permit
aqueous to be directed into the anterior chamber.
However, if hyposecretion is present, this will be
ineffective.

Surgical treatment

The presence of a choroidal detachment in itself is of no serious consequence. The dangers of
permanent angle damage from anterior iris adhesions and secondary glaucoma are another matter. Probably one should not procrastinate for
more than 8 days before attempting a surgical
correction. The best surgical procedure consists
of the following:

1. Performing a suprachoroidal tap
2. Placing air in the anterior chamber
3. Repairing the leak, if it is found

A small meridional incision is made through
the sclera in the region of the choroidal detachment. This can be made anywhere between the
pars plana and the equator. An escape of yellow-
tinged fluid occurs. With the tip of a muscle hook
or the end of an iris spatula the sclera is stroked
toward the incision to milk out additional fluid. If
this is continued, other bullous areas will finally
empty through the same opening. I usually wait 1
to 2 minutes before resuming the gentle pressure
on the sclera. It is surprising how much more
fluid can be stroked out this way.

Formerly, I prepared a limbal stab wound before incising the sclera for the suprachoroidal tap.
I no longer find this necessary. After the subchoroidal fluid is evacuated, fixation of the globe is
sometimes very difficult because of the extreme
hypotension. A fine suture can be placed 1 mm
posterior to the limbus, and the globe is pulled
up while the anterior chamber is entered with a
25-gauge Rizzuti-Spirizzi cannula needle attached to a syringe filled with sterile air (p. 446). The

anterior chamber is completely filled with an air bubble. A sharp disposable 25- or 27-gauge needle may do as well. Air may indicate the site of a wound leak. The pupil may be constricted with acetylcholine placed directly in the anterior chamber before the needle is withdrawn, or pilocarpine solution and eserine ointment may be applied topically. I prefer the pupil miotic when air is left in the anterior chamber. In most instances, this treatment will handle the situation. The ciliary body resumes aqueous secretion, and the anterior chamber deepens. However, on more than one occasion I have had to repeat the procedure. When the air is placed in the anterior chamber, the wound should be inspected for a leak. If found, it should be repaired. An alternate method of searching for a wound leak is to inject a weak fluorescein solution into the anterior chamber as described earlier for the introduction of air. The dye will be detected escaping through the opening in the wound.

REFERENCES

1. von Graefe, A.: Vereinzelte Beobachtungen und Bemerkungen, Graefe Arch. Ophthalmol. 4(Abt. 2):211-276, 1858.
2. Iwanoff, A.: Zur Abösung der Choroidea, Graefe Arch. Ophthalmol. 11:191-199, 1865.
3. Reuling, G.: Ablösung der Choroidea in Folge von Cataract-Operation mit Glaskörperverlust, Arch. Augenheilk. 1(Abt. 2):186-191, 1870.
4. Duke-Elder, S.: System of ophthalmology. Vol. IX. Diseases of the uveal tract, St. Louis, 1966, The C. V. Mosby Co., pp. 940, 949.
5. Salzmann, M.: The anatomy and histology of the human eyeball in the normal state, its development and senescence. Translated by E. V. L. Brown, Chicago, 1912, University of Chicago Press, p. 48.
6. Moses, R. A.: Detachment of the ciliary body—anatomical and physical considerations, Invest. Ophthalmol. 4:935-941, 1965.
7. Spaeth, E. B., and DeLong, P.: Detachment of the choroid. A clinical and histopathologic analysis, Arch. Ophthalmol. 32:217-238, 1944.
8. Pau, H.: Über die Amotio Chorioideae (Spongiosis Chorioideae), Klin. Mbl. Augenheilk. 130:347-371, 1957.
9. Hagen, S.: Die seröse postoperative Chorioidealablösung

und ihre Pathogenese, Klin. Mbl. Augenheilk. 66:161-211, 1921.
10. Best, C. H., and Taylor, N. B.: The physiological basis of medical practice, ed. 3, Baltimore, 1943, The Williams & Wilkins Co., p. 43.
11. Capper, S. A., and Leopold, I. H.: Mechanism of serous choroidal detachment; a review and experimental study, Arch. Ophthalmol. 55:101-113, 1956.
12. Hudson, A. C.: Serous detachment of the choroid and ciliary body as an accompaniment of perforating lesions of the eyeball, R. Lond. Ophthalmol. Hosp. Rep. 19:301-310, 1914.
13. Meller, J.: Ueber postoperative und spontane Chorioidealabhebung, Graefe Arch. Ophthalmol. 80:170-205, 1912.
14. Plocher, R.: Ueber Pigmentstreifenbildung nach postoperativer Aderhautablösung, Klin. Mbl. Augenheilk. 59:610-623, 1917.
15. Fuchs, E.: Ueber Pigmentstreifen im Angenhintergrunde, Klin. Mbl. Augenheilk. 60:797-801, 1918.
16. Verhoeff, F. H.: The nature and origin of the pigmented streaks caused by separation of the choroid, J.A.M.A. 97:1873-1877, 1931.
17. Chandler, P. A., and Maumenee, A. E.: A major cause of hypotony, Am. J. Ophthalmol. 52:609-618, 1961.
18. Dellaporta, A., and Obear, M. F.: Hyposecretion hypotony; experimental hypotony through detachment of the uvea, Am. J. Ophthalmol. 58:785-789, 1964.
19. Barkan, O.: Cyclodialysis: Its mode of action. Histologic observations in a case of glaucoma in which both eyes were successfully treated with cyclodialysis, Arch. Ophthalmol. 43:793-803, 1950.
20. Grant, M.: Personal communication to Chandler, P. A., and Maumenee, A. E.: A major cause of hypotony, Am. J. Ophthalmol. 52:609-618, 1961.
21. O'Brien, C. S.: Further observations on detachment of the choroid after cataract extraction, Arch. Ophthalmol. 16:655-656, 1936.
22. Bernard, P.: Le décollement de la choroïde, Bull. Soc. Ophthalmol. Fr. (suppl.,) 1963.
23. Kirsch, R. E., and Singer, J. A.: Ocular fundus immediately after cataract extraction, Arch. Ophthalmol. 90:460-464, 1973.
24. Seidel, E.: Weitere experimentelle Untersuchungen über die Quelle und den Verlauf der intraokularen Saftströmung. VI. Die Filtrationsfähigkeit, eine wesentliche Eigenschaft der Scleralnarben nach erfolgreicher Elliotscher Trepanation, Graefe Arch. Ophthalmol. 104:158-166, 1921.
25. Ruiz, R. S., and Salmonsen, P. C.: Expulsive choroidal effusion: a complication of intraocular surgery, Arch. Ophthalmol. 94:69-70, 1976.

CHAPTER 15

Aphakic pupillary block

HISTORICAL BACKGROUND

Reference to pupillary block appeared in the literature as early as 1865 when Bowman[1] described obstruction of the pupil by lens remnants. Dupuy-Dutemps[2] in 1904 and Hudson[3] in 1911 referred to pupillary block by vitreous, but it was not until Chandler and Johnson described their concept of this postoperative complication in 1947 that the problem was clarified.[4] Although there still remains some controversy over portions of the mechanism, their explanation has been subsequently confirmed by others.[5-10]

By definition, pupillary block refers to a failure of communication of aqueous between the anterior and posterior chambers caused by obstruction of the pupil and surgical openings in the iris.

PATHOGENESIS

Causes of pupillary block after cataract extraction are the following:

1. Leaky wound
2. Postoperative iridocyclitis
3. Posterior vitreous detachment associated with pooling of retrovitreal aqueous
4. Dense, impermeable anterior hyaloid membrane
5. Pupillary block by air
6. Inadequate iris openings
7. Swollen lens material behind the iris
8. Choroidal detachment and hemorrhage
9. Scleral collapse
10. Free vitreous block
11. Anterior chamber hemorrhage

Leaky wound. A leaky wound is probably the most frequent cause of early pupillary block. A wound leak permits the anterior hyaloid membrane to adhere to the iris and to any surgical openings made in the iris. It may be caused by inadequate wound closure associated with faulty technique, by external pressure on the globe as a result of squeezing of the eyelids, or by sneezing or coughing. Chandler[11] considered delayed reformation of the anterior chamber a definite predisposing factor to pupillary block. In fact, a flat anterior chamber caused by wound leak, associated with hypotension and a choroidal detachment, is often followed by pupillary block. Teng and co-workers[12] suggested that aqueous may exert a destructive effect on the collagen of the wound, whereas Posner[13] stated that aqueous inhibits fibroblastic proliferation. A wound leak may in turn be caused by pupillary block, especially if the intraocular pressure is elevated. A marked elevation of intraocular pressure may be associated with the use of alpha-chymotrypsin, as suggested by Kirsch,[14] and this may separate the lips of an inadequately closed wound. In my experience a shallow anterior chamber associated with pupillary block is very rarely associated with a filtering bleb, and when such a bleb occurs after cataract surgery, a shallow or flat anterior chamber is seldom found.

Postoperative iridocyclitis. Postoperative iridocyclitis is a frequent cause of a relatively late pupillary block. The normal inflammatory reaction that accompanies a routine intracapsular lens extraction may under certain conditions cause the anterior hyaloid membrane to adhere to the iris and block any iris openings. The more intense the iridocyclitis, the greater the likelihood of iris-vitreous synechias. The pattern of these synechias is of importance in surgical management, as described on p. 312. The vitreous may adhere to the iris only at the pupillary bor-

302

der (sphincteric pupillary block) or it may line the entire posterior surface of the iris.

Posterior vitreous detachment associated with pooling of retrovitreal aqueous. Although most patients who come to cataract surgery already have a complete posterior vitreous detachment with collapse, the removal of the lens increases the sagittal diameter of the vitreous cavity and favors anterior displacement of the residual formed vitreous. Because of a mechanism described on p. 308, a pooling of retrovitreal aqueous that favors such an anterior displacement may occur.

Dense, impermeable anterior hyaloid membrane. There are times when the anterior hyaloid membrane appears unusually thickened. This condition may be attributable to an occlusion membrane associated with postoperative inflammation, it may follow a hyphema, or it may occur after a rupture of the anterior hyaloid membrane followed by an unusually dense recondensation of its surface. In such cases, aqueous may direct itself into the vitreous itself, where it pools. A free exchange of water and electrolytes between the vitreous and the anterior chamber aqueous is prevented. This mechanism was emphasized by Schlossman, Posner, and Theodore.[15]

Pupillary block by air. Although the dangers of placing an excessive amount of air in the anterior chamber have been known for some time, the possibility of air-block glaucoma has increased as a result of the growing popularity of the preoperative use of hyperosmotic agents. This dehydration, combined with the dehydration of the vitreous afforded by digital massage, permits a considerable volume of air to be placed in the anterior chamber after lens extraction or allows an inordinate amount to inadvertently enter the chamber as the lens is delivered. When the preoperative volume of the vitreous is resumed, the air may be severely compressed. A portion may get behind the iris and exert an acute rise in intraocular pressure. This danger has been stressed by Jaffe and Light.[16]

Inadequate iris openings. The danger of a nonperforating iridectomy is obvious. Occasionally the two layers of the iris are not closely applied, so that the superficial layer is grasped and cut, leaving an intact posterior layer. Swan[9,17] emphasized the importance of a properly performed peripheral iridectomy or iridotomy. He found the incidence of shallow or flat anterior chamber after cataract extraction to be 5% when the iris opening did not extend to within 1 mm of

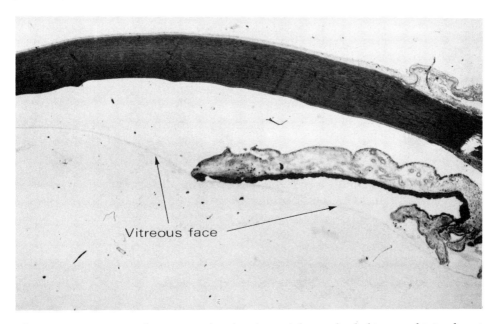

Vitreous face

Fig. 15-1. Persistence of posterior chamber in periphery of aphakic eye obtained post mortem. Ciliary body and processes prevent vitreous from contacting extreme periphery of iris. (From Swan, K. C.: Arch. Ophthalmol. **69:**191-202, 1963.)

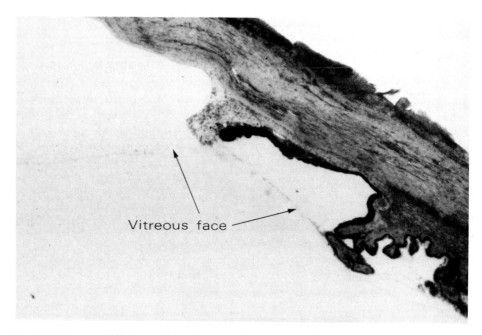

Vitreous face

Fig. 15-2. Vitreous block resulting from inadequate peripheral iris opening. Vitreous is adherent to edges of pupil and coloboma, but posterior chamber is present. Ciliary body and processes might have prevented vitreous from blocking peripheral iris opening. (From Swan, K. C.: Arch. Ophthalmol. **69:**191-202, 1963.)

the base but less than 2% when the opening was basal. Vitreous herniation into truly basal iris openings seldom was found. He demonstrated that in aphakic eyes the face of the vitreous usually was blocked from contact with the extreme periphery of the iris by the ciliary processes and the ciliary body (Figs. 15-1 to 15-3). Therefore, if a cataract incision is made anterior to Schwalbe's line, iris and vitreous will more likely become adherent to the incision, and a basal coloboma is more difficult to obtain.

Swollen lens material behind the iris. The presence of swollen lens fibers and capsular material behind the iris after an intended or unintentional extracapsular cataract extraction may cause the iris to bulge irregularly. This favors anterior synechias and obstruction of the surgical iridectomies. What may be even more important is the greater amount of postoperative intraocular inflammation induced by residual lens debris. This favors adherence of the iris to the anterior hyaloid membrane, thus favoring pupillary block.

Choroidal detachment and hemorrhage. As discussed on p. 293, the ease with which transu-

dation occurs in this area is partly attributable to the nature of the veins of the anterior uvea. Anatomically, they are blood sinuses with a single-layer endothelial wall with no muscular coat and practically no connective tissue fibrillae. A sudden release of external pressure leads to their engorgement, and transudation through their thin walls is facilitated. Associated with the effusion of fluid between the lamellae of the perichoroidal space is a marked congestion and dilatation of the uveal vessels. When a large bullous choroidal detachment is present, it is not difficult to visualize that the mass compresses the vitreous, which in turn pushes the iris forward. The fluid, instead of being a transudate, may consist of blood and thus is a subchoroidal hemorrhage. A postoperative choroidal detachment observed 7 to 21 days after surgery may be a persistence of an earlier one or may be caused by a rupture of the inadequately healed wound.

Scleral collapse. The factor of scleral collapse is probably of importance only at surgery or during the immediate postoperative period. It is more significant in a young person, whose sclera is less rigid and therefore tends to collapse when

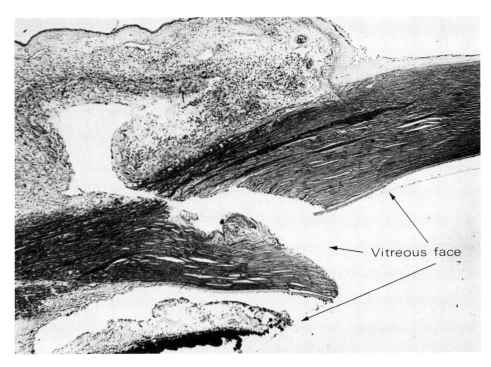

Vitreous face

Fig. 15-3. Postmortem specimen obtained 11 days after cataract extraction, complicated by shallow chamber, hypotension, and choroidal detachment. Incision entered anterior chamber too far forward, and iridectomy was not basal. Vitreous is adherent to edge of coloboma and pupil, with resultant obstruction of aqueous flow. Wound separation by trauma of enucleation. (From Swan, K. C.: Arch. Ophthalmol. **69:**191-202, 1963.)

the globe is decompressed. This is discussed on p. 263. It may cause operative loss of vitreous or cause a compression of the main vitreous mass against the iris, which favors pupillary block.

Free vitreous block. Free vitreous in the anterior chamber may fill the pupillary space, obstruct the surgical iridectomies, and incite a fibroplastic interference with aqueous drainage. A similar situation arises with a subluxated lens when vitreous fills the space between the lens and the iris, thus interfering with aqueous passage into the anterior chamber.

Anterior chamber hemorrhage. If there is repeated bleeding into the anterior chamber, some of the blood may become organized and form a membrane over the anterior hyaloid membrane, which makes free passage of water and electrolytes more difficult. It may also block the iris openings.

PATHOPHYSIOLOGY

Since Chandler and Johnson's[4] explanation of the mechanism involved in aphakic pupillary block, considerable attention has been directed to this postoperative complication, which is responsible for so many lost eyes. A clearer picture of the pathophysiology has arisen, although some controversial points remain. The uncertainty is probably attributable to the fact that the clinical picture may appear in a variety of ways.

It appears certain that in concert with the pathogenic factors just listed the intact anterior hyaloid membrane moves forward and blocks the pupil and any surgically made iris openings. At this juncture a number of variations in the appearance of the iris, anterior chamber, and posterior chamber may be observed. Although the anterior chamber in aphakic pupillary block is classically thought of as being shallow, it will be seen this is not necessarily so. Moreover, the posterior chamber may undergo wide variations in size.

1. If, because of intraocular inflammation the entire pupillary margin become adherent to the anterior hyaloid membrane and the peripheral surgical openings become obstructed by exudate,

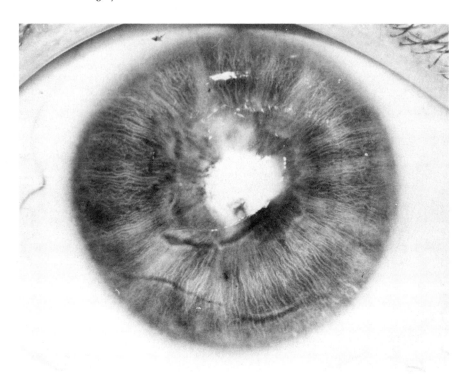

Fig. 15-4. Iris bombé after extracapsular cataract extraction complicated by phacoana-phylactic uveitis.

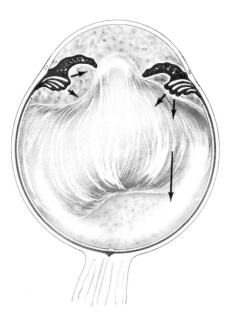

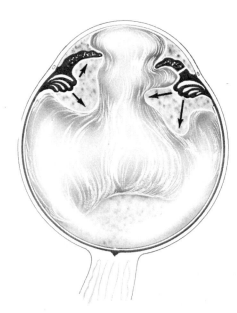

Fig. 15-5. Iris bombé. Anterior chamber is of normal depth in center but shallow peripherally, where iris is most convex *(left)*. Posterior chamber is also of uneven depth; deep on left but shallow on right.

Fig. 15-6. Marked bulge of vitreous into anterior chamber caused by compression of its central core by enlargement of posterior chamber.

the picture of iris bombé will be observed. This is caused by a marked distention of the posterior chamber (Fig. 15-4). The anterior chamber may be deep in the center but shallow peripherally where the iris is most convex (Fig. 15-5). In some eyes there may be a marked bulge of vitreous into the anterior chamber attributable to compression of its central core by the enlargement of the posterior chamber (Fig. 15-6).

2. If, because of intraocular inflammation the entire posterior face of the iris become lined by the anterior hyaloid membrane, a uniform shallowing of the anterior chamber usually results, and there may be a total absence of the posterior chamber (Fig. 15-7). If a pocket of aqueous accumulates in one portion of the posterior chamber, there may be a localized iris convexity in this area. Usually the aqueous is misdirected posteriorly by a route to be discussed on p. 308. A marked pooling of retrovitreal aqueous occurs, which favors an anterior displacement of the solid vitreous and the iris.

3. If vitreous blocks the pupil and the iris

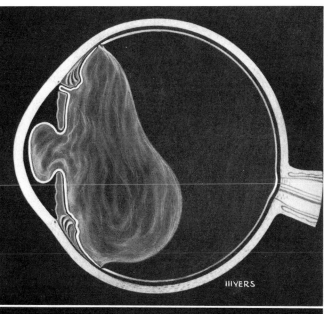

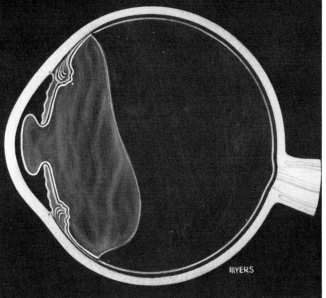

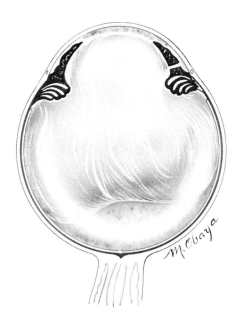

Fig. 15-7. Aphakic pupillary block associated with uniform marked shallowing of anterior chamber. Entire posterior surface of iris adheres to anterior hyaloid membrane. This may prevent bulge of vitreous into anterior chamber. There is complete absence of posterior chamber.

Fig. 15-8. A, Aphakic pupillary block associated with anterior chamber of normal depth. Vitreous with intact anterior hyaloid membrane bulges in mushroom fashion into anterior chamber. B, Aphakic pupillary block associated with shallowing of anterior chamber. Vitreous with intact anterior hyaloid membrane bulges in mushroom fashion into anterior chamber. (From Jaffe, N. S.: The vitreous in clinical ophthalmology, St. Louis, 1969, The C. V. Mosby Co.)

openings without synechia formation, the force created by the pooled retrovitreal aqueous may herniate the vitreous in bullous fashion through the pupil, thus providing a relatively deep anterior chamber. The chamber will be less deep if the vitreous herniation is less (Fig. 15-8).

The differences in the depth of the anterior chamber depending on whether vitreous is herniated into the anterior chamber or remains entirely behind the iris are emphasized by the mechanisms involved in air-block glaucoma. If all the air is located in the posterior chamber, the anterior chamber will be shallow. If a portion of the bubble is in the anterior chamber and a portion in the posterior chamber, the anterior chamber will be deeper. The anterior chamber will be very deep if all the air is in the anterior chamber (Fig. 15-9). Thus it is clear that the depth of the anterior chamber cannot be used as a reliable indicator of the presence of pupillary block. Furthermore, it is a pity that we do not yet possess accurate means of determining the presence or absence of the posterior chamber, since this could aid us greatly in deciding on the proper surgical approach in pupillary block. Surgical approaches are discussed on p. 312.

The manner in which aqueous humor pools in the retrovitreal space is still open to question.

Shaffer[6] explained the process as follows. Once the communication of aqueous between the anterior and posterior chambers is blocked (partially or completely), aqueous accumulates in the posterior chamber, which becomes so distended that the vitreous becomes detached from its base (ciliary detachment of the vitreous), and this detachment permits passage of aqueous to the posterior portion of the globe. This posterior pooling of aqueous pushes the residual formed vitreous forward against the iris. However, it is known that the vitreous may also become adherent to the entire ciliary body, thus obliterating the posterior chamber just anterior to the vitreous base, where the ciliary detachment presumably occurs. The aqueous can still pass behind the vitreous into the retrovitreal space despite this attachment. Besides, a ciliary detachment of the vitreous is virtually unknown without a traumatic avulsion of the vitreous base. Therefore it is assumed that aqueous gains the retrovitreal space by passing through the vitreous itself.

My own impression of the preceding process is as follows: Most patients who come to cataract surgery have a posterior vitreous detachment with collapse. Thus the formed (collapsed) vitreous is separated from the retina by a pool of fluid. This fluid likely arises from the vitreous

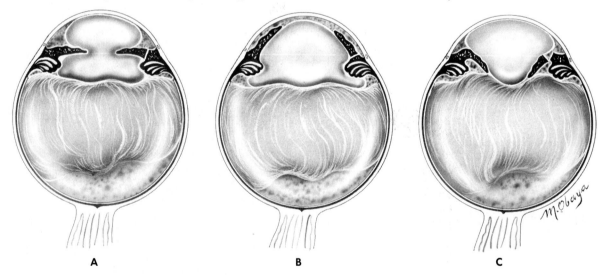

A **B** **C**

Fig. 15-9. Air-block glaucoma. **A,** Portion of air bubble is in anterior chamber and portion in posterior chamber, resulting in relatively normal-depth anterior chamber. **B,** Entire air bubble is located in posterior chamber, resulting in shallow anterior chamber. **C,** Entire air bubble is located in anterior chamber, resulting in very deep anterior chamber.

itself, since the phenomenon of posterior vitreous detachment with collapse occurs after a rupture of the thinned or partially liquefied posterior limiting border of the vitreous. Fluid from lacunae within the vitreous rapidly empties into the retrovitreal space as the vitreous framework collapses, folds, and sinks. This fluid does not create a force that pushes the residual formed vitreous forward, since it is equal in volume to what was contained within the vitreous prior to the posterior vitreous detachment. Thus this degenerative phenomenon is not associated with an elevation of intraocular pressure or a shallowing of the anterior chamber. It is the pooling of additional aqueous in the retrovitreal space in the presence of a relative or complete pupillary block that causes the clinical picture that is now well known. The aqueous flow is misdirected posteriorly because it cannot gain access to the anterior chamber. I believe it reaches the retrovitreal space by perfusing the vitreous (Fig. 15-10). I have had sufficient opportunity to examine patients with aphakic pupillary block, using a three-mirror lens, to satisfy myself that the vitreous mass does not detach from its base. Once sufficient pooling of aqueous occurs, a force sufficient to move the main vitreous mass forward (Fig. 15-11) is set up.

The vital role played by the pooling of vitreous in the retrovitreal space in aphakic pupillary block is emphasized by considering the same mechanism in malignant glaucoma and acute narrow-angle glaucoma in phakic eyes.

In malignant glaucoma the anterior chamber remains very shallow or absent, and the intraocular pressure is high after a peripheral iridectomy, a basal iridectomy, a cyclodialysis, or a filtering procedure. The lens-iris diaphragm moves anteriorly. The vitreous likewise moves forward and may lie anterior to the lens equator and even the ciliary processes. Removal of the lens is usually insufficient to remedy the situation, since the vitreous then occupies the space formerly held by the lens, and the pupil remains blocked. Aqueous continues to pool behind the vitreous. Shaffer[6] injected fluorescein into the anterior

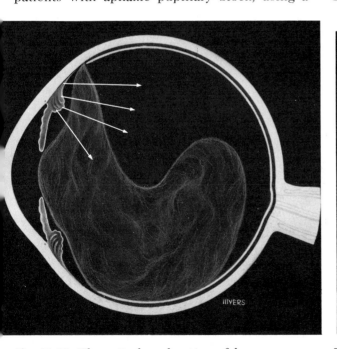

Fig. 15-10. Theoretical explanation of how aqueous gains retrovitreal space. Posteriorly directed force has been set up (by pupillary block), which causes aqueous to perfuse formed vitreous. (From Jaffe, N. S.: The vitreous in clinical ophthalmology, St. Louis, 1969, The C. V. Mosby Co.)

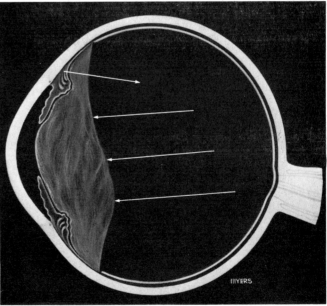

Fig. 15-11. Aqueous is directed posteriorly into retrovitreal space *(upper arrow)*. Pooling of retrovitreal aqueous creates force that pushes residual formed vitreous forward. (From Jaffe, N. S.: The vitreous in clinical ophthalmology, St. Louis, 1969, The C. V. Mosby Co.)

chamber in such a situation, but the anterior chamber did not form and the intraocular pressure remained elevated. He then tapped the retrovitreal space and recovered fluorescein. This proves the prompt transfer of fluid from the anterior segment to the retrovitreal space. Chandler[18] attempted treatment of malignant glaucoma by lens extraction and registered success only when the surgery was complicated by unintentional loss of vitreous. Thus apparently one must create a communication between the anterior chamber and the retrovitreal space where the misdirected aqueous has accumulated. He recommended a new surgical procedure[19,20] that involved a perilenticular incision of the vitreous, going through the anterior hyaloid membrane and the posterior limiting border of the vitreous. Thus a communication is again established between the anterior chamber and the retrovitreal space. This reemphasizes the role of retrovitreal pooling of aqueous. A recent impressive report[21] on an improvement in this technique and its results was presented. The operation was uniformly successful in all 14 phakic and 12 aphakic eyes in which it was tried. There were no serious complications. In phakic eyes, vitreous puncture and aspiration from a wound of entry 4 mm behind the limbus is performed, followed by air injection into the anterior chamber with marked deepening of the latter. In aphakic eyes with malignant glaucoma the procedure is the same, except that the wound of entry is made at the limbus, since there is no lens to be injured, and the needle is passed through an existing, or a newly made, coloboma of the iris (Fig. 15-17).

The fact that surgery of the vitreous body alone can relieve malignant glaucoma suggests that the vitreous play an important part in the pathophysiology of malignant glaucoma. The mechanism by which the described technique relieves the malignant glaucoma is still not precisely known. Its efficacy may be due to the piercing of the vitreous body through the anterior and posterior surfaces of the vitreous, which provides a channel for forward flow of posteriorly trapped aqueous. Since it is assumed that the normal vitreous and normal anterior hyaloid membrane do not provide a significant resistance to aqueous flow, one must postulate that in malignant glaucoma some portion of the vitreous body, the ante-

rior hyaloid membrane and/or the posterior border of the vitreous, shows abnormal resistance to aqueous flow. However, there is no evidence to support the concept of abnormal permeability of the anterior and posterior surfaces of the vitreous. The efficacy of the procedure may be due to several factors working in combination. The marked deepening of the anterior chamber with air may break a relative block to the anterior flow of aqueous in the region of the anterior ciliary body or may correct a relative posterior diversion of aqueous in this region by correcting the abnormal apposition of the anterior vitreous face to the anterior ciliary body. However, air injection alone will not cure the condition. It is necessary to simultaneously decompress the pocket of posteriorly trapped aqueous.

One would expect this procedure to be technically more difficult to perform in phakic eyes, since one must contend with the lens. The strikingly good results with the method suggest that even if a cataract is present in the eye at the time of the malignant glaucoma attack, it is safer to carry out a perilenticular incision of the vitreous combined with air injection into the anterior chamber than to remove the lens. Later, when the eye is quiet and the malignant glaucoma has been relieved, lens extraction can be undertaken in easier conditions should lens removal be required for vision.

Additional evidence for the mechanism of pooling of retrovitreal aqueous in pupillary block was offered by Christensen and Irvine.[22] They performed an instructive clinical experiment on two eyes of two patients with acute narrow-angle glaucoma. A 22-gauge needle was inserted into the posterior vitreous cavity, and approximately 0.5 ml of fluid was aspirated. Simultaneously, the pupils were dilated with phenylephrine (Neo-Synephrine) and atropine. The anterior chambers deepened considerably. For several days the intraocular pressures remained controlled, and anterior chambers remained deep. However, 8 to 10 days later, shallowing again occurred, and the pressures rose again to abnormal levels. Peripheral iridectomies were then performed, and the pressures were controlled. This demonstrates that when the posterior vitreous pool is tapped and the pressure against the vitreous diaphragm is relieved, the anterior chambers return to normal depth. Thus, the role played by the pooling of retrovitreal aqueous once communication with the anterior chamber is blocked is again emphasized. Therefore there is a similarity in the pathophysiology of the pupillary block mechanism in three clinical entities: aphakic pupillary block, malignant glaucoma, and acute narrow-angle glaucoma.

CLINICAL FINDINGS

In my experience the most frequent clinical course leading to aphakic pupillary block is as follows: The anterior chamber shallows or flattens either shortly after lens extraction because of delayed re-formation of the anterior chamber or 10 to 15 days later because of a wound leak. This shallowing is accompanied by ocular hypotension and choroidal detachment. The wound leak ceases, and the anterior chamber deepens slightly. The choroidal elevations subside. As aqueous secretion resumes, only to be misdirected to the retrovitreal space, the patient may complain of pain. Intraocular pressure may be normal or elevated. The iris is abnormally involved anteriorly and posteriorly. Anterior synechias may be mild or severe, according to the number of days the anterior chamber has been shallow or flat. The vitreous moves forward and rests firmly against the posterior surface of the iris. The pupil does not dilate readily. Posterior synechias may be found if there is an associated iridocyclitis.

There may be other findings according to the particular pathogenic factor. An occlusion membrane may be found after a severe iridocyclitis or a hyphema. The anterior chamber may be shallow or deep according to the position of the vitreous herniation through the pupil (p. 308). The chamber may not be of uniform depth, since one area may show a marked convexity of the iris because of accumulation of a pocket of aqueous behind it. If the iris is adherent to the vitreous at the pupillary margin only and if the iris openings are blocked, the picture of iris bombé may be seen.

The cornea may be edematous from elevation of intraocular pressure or because of vitreous adherence to its posterior surface. The cornea is more susceptible to edema associated with an elevated intraocular pressure after surgery, probably from trauma to the endothelium. When confronted with corneal edema after cataract extraction, the ophthalmologist must diagnose the cause. It may be necessary to clear the edema with a topically administered hyperosmotic agent to be certain it is not caused by a vitreocorneal adherence, since this requires early treatment (p. 343). If the elevation of pressure is from the use of alpha-chymotrypsin during the surgery, it is usually of short duration.

The presence of a normal or subnormal intraocular pressure does not rule out the possibility of pupillary block, since aqueous production may be absent or slowed. Also, the presence of a choroidal detachment should not deter one from diagnosing pupillary block. It is not unusual to find the transition from hypotension to normotension while the choroidal detachment is still present. The shallowness or absence of the anterior chamber may permit anterior synechia formation, so that when aqueous production is resumed, its flow is misdirected posteriorly. In the meantime the choroidal elevations may still be visible.

An interesting test for aphakic pupillary block was described by Ray and Binkhorst.[23] They injected 10 ml of a 5% aqueous solution of fluorescein into an antecubital vein. With the aid of the slit lamp the fluorescein can be observed passing into the anterior chamber within a short time (approximately 20 seconds) in a normal aphakic eye. With aphakic pupillary block the fluorescein accumulates in the posterior chamber or more posteriorly and may not appear in the anterior chamber, or else a small amount may trickle in after several minutes.

TREATMENT
Prophylaxis

The most satisfactory therapy for any complication is its prophylaxis. Adequate wound closure, reduction of postoperative inflammation, treatment of a leaking wound, no prolonged delay in restoring the anterior chamber when associated with choroidal detachment, avoidance of large amounts of air within the eye, and performance of adequate iris openings during cataract extraction are all likely to lessen the incidence of pupillary block. Despite these measures the surgeon will still encounter an occasional patient with aphakic pupillary block.

Medical treatment

Medical treatment consists of dilating the pupil as widely as possible. In an early case (Fig. 15-12), this will permit aqueous to enter the anterior chamber, thereby breaking the block. However, mydriasis may not be easy to achieve when the vitreous mass is closely apposed to the iris or when an adhesion exists. A potent mydriatic regimen[24] consists of 2-pyridine aldoxime methyl chloride (Protopam Chloride). This oxime causes regeneration of cholinesterase inhibited by phosphate ester. The effect is more dramatic when echothiophate (Phospholine Iodide) is first placed in the eye. A rebound type of response is obtained. The method consists of placing two drops of 0.25% echothiophate in the eye. Protopam, 0.1 to 0.2 ml of a 5% solution, is then injected subconjunctivally. Atropine sulfate solution, 1%, is then dropped in the eye to block acetylcholine; 10% phenylephrine is used to stimulate the iris dilator muscle. I have found it equally effective to soak pledgets of absorbent cotton with Protopam and place them in the upper and lower conjunctival fornices. The Protopam must be freshly prepared.

In resistant cases a systemically administered hyperosmotic agent may be used as an adjunct to mydriasis. This was reported by Jaffe and Light.[25] Two patients with aphakic pupillary block were cured by such agents when mydriasis alone was ineffective. The dehydration of the vitreous, which results from these agents, may cause a posterior displacement of the anterior hyaloid membrane from its closely apposed position against the back of the iris.

Mechanical treatment

Mechanical rupture of iris adhesions to vitreous at the pupillary margin is occasionally possible with a technique suggested by Swan[17] (Fig. 15-13). Gentle point pressure applied to the iris through the anesthetized cornea is performed at the slit lamp or with the operating microscope. The lubricated tip of a glass rod is placed on the cornea midway between the pupillary margin and the limbus. Pupillary adhesions may be seen to separate and the anterior chamber to re-form within 2 to 3 minutes in some cases.

Surgical treatment

Surgical therapy is applied when medical treatment fails. It should not be unduly delayed, lest permanent angle damage occur. From what has been mentioned in discussing the pathogenesis of aphakic pupillary block, it should be apparent that there is no single approach to therapy in all cases.

Iridectomy. Iridectomy is probably the most frequently performed surgical procedure for

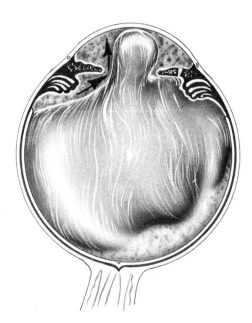

Fig. 15-12. Relief of aphakic pupillary block by mydriasis. Permits trapped aqueous in posterior chamber to enter anterior chamber.

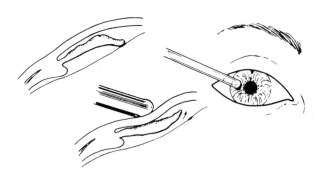

Fig. 15-13. Mechanical rupture of iris adhesions to vitreous at pupillary margin. With topical anesthesia cornea and underlying iris are gently indented with lubricated tip of glass rod. (From Swan, K. C.: Arch. Ophthalmol. **69:**191-202, 1963.)

aphakic pupillary block. It works best when fluid is trapped in the posterior chamber (Fig. 15-14). The peripheral iridectomy is placed at a site other than the previous cataract incision to avoid anterior synechias. It is usually placed anywhere below the horizontal meridian of the iris. The anterior chamber is then filled partially with air and partially with balanced salt solution. In some cases the anterior chamber will become flat again because the block is not broken. Theoretically one should be able to predict a failure in the following manner: After the iridectomy is performed, the anterior chamber should spontaneously re-form without the use of air or balanced salt solution. If it does not, it indicates that all the trapped aqueous is in the vitreous or behind it.

Incision of anterior hyaloid membrane. In cases where the anterior hyaloid membrane appears unduly thickened or is covered by a membrane after iridocyclitis or hyphema, a simple incision of the anterior vitreous face will release a gush of pooled aqueous and terminate the block (Fig. 15-15).

Through-and-through incision of the vitreous. More frequently the fluid is trapped behind the vitreous. The vitreous from the anterior hyaloid membrane to the retrovitreal space through an inferior limbal approach is penetrated with a 22-gauge 1.5-inch needle attached to a 2 ml syringe. When the latter space is reached, aspiration of fluid into the syringe is possible. The needle is then moved up and down as it is withdrawn to create a wide communication between the anterior chamber and the retrovitreal space. Aqueous will then gush into the anterior chamber (Fig. 15-16). Air and balanced salt solution are then placed in the anterior chamber.

Cyclodialysis or cyclocryothermy. When permanent angle damage has occurred, none of the procedures just described will be of benefit. Cyclodialysis appears to offer the best chance for cure. It may conveniently be combined with a peripheral iridectomy through the same incision made inferiorly. An alternative to cyclodialysis, whose benefit is frequently of short duration, is cyclocryothermy. It has the advantage that it is an external procedure and can be repeated several times.

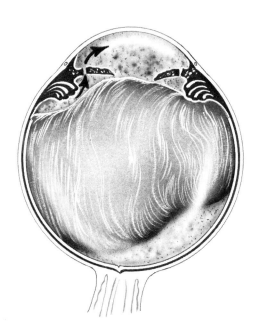

Fig. 15-14. Relief of aphakic pupillary block by peripheral iridectomy inferiorly *(left)*. This is effective if aqueous is trapped in posterior chamber.

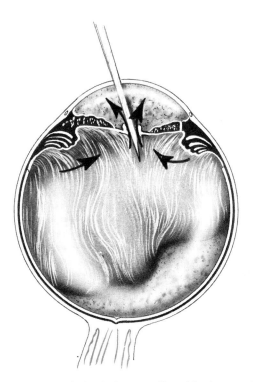

Fig. 15-15. Relief of aphakic pupillary block caused by dense, impermeable anterior hyaloid membrane by incising anterior face of vitreous. Aqueous pooled within vitreous gushes into anterior chamber.

Suprachoroidal tap. If a choroidal detachment is associated with aphakic pupillary block, the sclerochoroidal space should be tapped, an iridectomy performed, and a partial air bubble placed in the anterior chamber.

Although these techniques offer varied approaches to the surgical management of aphakic pupillary block, it is not always easy to decide which technique to apply. As mentioned earlier (p. 310), Chandler[26] recommended an approach to the treatment of malignant glaucoma that might be applied here. As an alternative to lens extraction plus through-and-through vitreous incision, he recommended a perilenticular incision of the vitreous, going through the anterior hyaloid membrane and the posterior limiting border of the vitreous, combined with a peripheral iridectomy. With this in mind, Meisekothen and Allen[27] performed a peripheral iridectomy combined with a vitreous incision, since the anterior chamber will not spontaneously reform in some eyes with aphakic pupillary block after the peripheral iridectomy. They recommended the following technique: A limbal stab wound is made temporally. A peripheral iridectomy is performed

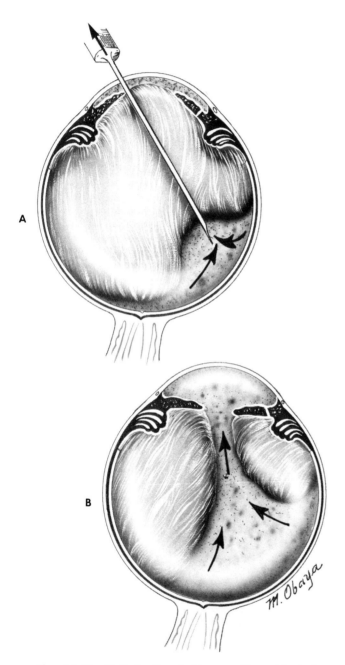

Fig. 15-16. Relief of aphakic pupillary block by through-and-through incision of vitreous. **A,** Aspiration of pooled aqueous from retrovitreal space. **B,** Communication created between anterior chamber and retrovitreal space.

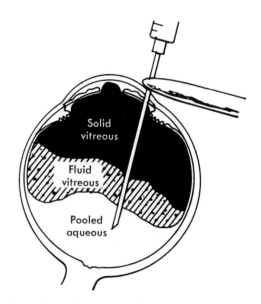

Fig. 15-17. Procedure to be followed if anterior chamber does not re-form after peripheral iridectomy. Small hemostat is clamped on 18-gauge needle with blunt point, 17 mm back from tip. A 2 ml syringe is attached, and needle is inserted through iridectomy and directed toward posterior pole of globe. Liquid vitreous is aspirated. (From Meisekothen, W. E., and Allen, J. C.: Am. J. Ophthalmol. **65:**877-881, 1968.)

at 5 or 7 o'clock under a small limbal-based flap. If the anterior chamber fails to re-form, a small hemostat is clamped on an 18-gauge needle with a blunt point, 17 mm back from the tip. A 2 ml syringe is attached, and the needle is inserted through the iridectomy with care to direct it toward the posterior pole of the globe (Fig. 15-17). One milliliter of liquid vitreous or aqueous is withdrawn. The incision is then closed. Ringer's lactate solution, 0.25 ml, followed by a 6 mm bubble of air is then injected into the anterior chamber with a 27-gauge cannula through the temporal stab wound. The eye is purposely left soft, as Chandler[26,28] suggested. He believed that if excess fluid is injected, some of it might go back through the same wound in the anterior hyaloid membrane and run behind the vitreous, causing a flat anterior chamber and elevation of intraocular pressure. I concur in this belief because I have seen it happen more than once. Meisekothen and Allen state that whether the 18-gauge needle forms a new channel for aqueous flow anteriorly or the solid vitreous falls back long enough for the aqueous to set a new pattern of flow anterior to the solid vitreous is a matter of speculation. My own experiences indicate that a peripheral iridectomy is followed in most cases by a spontaneous re-formation of the anterior chamber after the incision is closed; when re-formation occurs, the pupillary block mechanism is broken. If the anterior chamber does not re-form, a through-and-through vitreous incision through the iridectomy usually results in re-formation of the anterior chamber. I prefer to slash the anterior vitreous through the peripheral iridectomy as the tip of the needle is withdrawn to the level of the iridectomy.

Pars plana vitrectomy. In some cases these methods may fail to cure the aphakic pupillary block. A more drastic procedure that may correct the abnormality is a partial vitrectomy through the pars plana using one of the automated vitrectomy devices. This procedure, while highly effective, carries a higher risk of complications than those just described.

REFERENCES

1. Bowman, W.: On extraction of cataract by a traction-instrument with iridectomy, with remarks on capsular obstructions, and their treatment, R. Lond. Ophthalmol. Hosp. Rep. **4**:332-368, 1865.
2. Dupuy-Dutemps: Du glaucome consécutif à l'extraction du cristallin, Ann. Oculist **132**:93-100, 1904.
3. Hudson, A. C.: Injury to the vitreous body as a factor in the production of secondary glaucoma, R. Lond. Ophthalmol. Hosp. Rep. **18**:203-228, 1911.
4. Chandler, P. A., and Johnson, C. C.: A neglected cause of secondary glaucoma in eyes in which the lens is absent or subluxated, Arch. Ophthalmol. **37**:740-771, 1947.
5. Reese, A. B.: Herniation of the anterior hyaloid membrane following uncomplicated intracapsular cataract extraction, Trans. Am. Ophthalmol. Soc. **46**:73-95, 1948.
6. Shaffer, R. N.: The role of vitreous detachment in aphakic and malignant glaucoma, Ophthalmology (Rochester) **58**:217-231, 1954.
7. Sugar, H. S.: Pupillary block in phakic and aphakic eyes, J. Int. Coll. Surg. **33**:312-318, 1960.
8. Sugar, H. S.: Pupillary block and pupillary block glaucoma following cataract extraction, Am. J. Ophthalmol. **61**:435-443, 1966.
9. Swan, K. C.: Relationship of basal iridectomy to shallow chamber following cataract extraction, Arch. Ophthalmol. **69**:191-202, 1963.
10. Etienne, R.: Le blocage pupillaire et ses conséquences: le glaucome secondaire de l'aphake, Ann. Oculist. **200**:729-744, 1967.
11. Chandler, P. A.: Symposium: cataract extraction. Complications after cataract extraction: clinical aspects, Ophthalmology (Rochester) **58**:382-396, 1954.
12. Teng, C. C., Chi, H. H., and Katzin, H. M.: Aqueous degenerative effect and the protective role of endothelium in eye pathology, Am. J. Ophthalmol. **50**:365-379, 1960.
13. Posner, A.: Postcataract glaucoma associated with shallow anterior chamber, Int. Ophthalmol. Clin. **4**:1029-1043, 1964.
14. Kirsch, R. E.: Glaucoma following cataract extraction associated with the use of alpha-chymotrypsin, Arch. Ophthalmol. **72**:612-620, 1964.
15. Schlossman, A.: Complications in the immediate postoperative period, Int. Ophthalmol. Clin. **4**:815-837, 1964.
16. Jaffe, N. S., and Light, D. S.: The danger of air pupillary block glaucoma in cataract surgery with osmotic hypotonia, Arch. Ophthalmol. **76**:633-634, 1966.
17. Swan, K. C.: Relationship of basal iridectomy to shallow chamber following cataract extraction, Trans. Am. Ophthalmol. Soc. **60**:213-235, 1962.
18. Chandler, P. A.: Malignant glaucoma, Am. J. Ophthalmol. **34**:993-1000, 1951.
19. Chandler, P. A., and Grant, W. M.: Lectures on glaucoma, Philadelphia, 1965, Lea & Febiger, p. 202.
20. Balakrishnan, E., and Abraham, J. E.: Chandler's operation for malignant glaucoma, Arch. Ophthalmol. **82**:723-725, 1969.
21. Simmons, R. J.: Malignant glaucoma, Br. J. Ophthalmol. **56**:263-272, 1972.
22. Christensen, L., and Irvine, A. R., Jr.: Pathogenesis of primary shallow chamber angle closure glaucoma, Arch. Ophthalmol. **75**:490-495, 1966.
23. Ray, R. R., and Binkhorst, R. D.: The diagnosis of pupillary block by intravenous injection of fluorescein, Am. J. Ophthalmol. **61**:481-483, 1966.

24. Byron, H. M., and Posner, I.: Clinical evaluation of Protopam, Am. J. Ophthalmol. **57:**409-418, 1964.

25. Jaffe, N. S., and Light, D. S.: Treatment of postoperative cataract complications by osmotic agents, Arch. Ophthalmol. **75:**370-374, 1966.

26. Chandler, P. A.: A new operation for malignant glaucoma, Trans. Am. Ophthalmol. Soc. **62:**408-419, 1964.

27. Meisekothen, W. E., and Allen, J. C.: Treatment of pupillary block caused by aqueous pooling in vitreous, Am. J. Ophthalmol. **65:**877-881, 1968.

28. Chandler, P. A.: The vitreous in anterior segment surgery, Audio-Digest Tape, Vol. 5, No. 10, 1967.

CHAPTER 16

Glaucoma in aphakia

Glaucoma is a frequent companion, or ultimate sequel, of many of the postoperative cataract complications described elsewhere. It is mainly of a secondary etiology, in which a variety of factors, acting alone or in concert with other complications, obstruct aqueous flow or block aqueous drainage from the chamber angle. It is responsible for the largest number of eyes enucleated after cataract surgery. It usually is the final obstacle in the surgeon's attempt to thwart the thrust of an overwhelming postoperative complication.

Since glaucoma is associated with many postoperative syndromes, its pathogenesis in relation to the inciting complication will be discussed. To avoid repetition, when a specific entity has been fully described elsewhere, the glaucomatogenic capacity of the postoperative complication is only briefly mentioned.

PRIMARY OPEN-ANGLE GLAUCOMA

Primary open-angle glaucoma is not caused by cataract surgery. When present, it may be at any stage in its development when the cataract extraction is done. The surgeon may be aware of its presence before surgery or may first recognize it after surgery. Cataract surgery may exert a beneficial or a damaging effect on its development, but usually it does not influence its course. Glaucoma in the aphakic eye can be called primary only when by gonioscopy it is evident that the chamber angle is entirely or almost entirely open and there are no other abnormalities in the angle. It should not be called aphakic glaucoma, since this implies that the glaucoma is caused by the lens extraction.

The impression exists that primary open-angle glaucoma is favorably influenced by cataract surgery, since less or no treatment is required postoperatively in many cases. This view, however, has not yet been supported by adequate data, but several factors are responsible for its origin.

During the first week after cataract surgery, there may be a transient rise in intraocular pressure. This may be associated with the use of alpha-chymotrypsin, although it may occur in eyes where the enzyme has not been used. Kirsch[1] found an abnormal elevation of intraocular pressure during the first week in 39 of 165 eyes (23.6%) without alpha-chymotrypsin, compared with 129 of 178 eyes (72.5%) with the enzyme. Kaufman[2] found an intraocular pressure of 22 mm Hg or more in 11 of 25 eyes without alpha-chymotrypsin during the first week. Most of the pressure elevations occurred on the first postoperative day. This is in line with a recent report[3] that recorded ocular hypertension in 20 consecutive uncomplicated cataract extractions without alpha-chymotrypsin. Intraocular pressures rose acutely to a maximum level 2.4 times the preoperative level (range 26 to 50 mm Hg) at a mean time of 6.8 hours after surgery. Pain and corneal edema were observed at the time of the rise in the intraocular pressure but did not continue despite persistent high intraocular pressures. It was emphasized that this phenomenon is made manifest by watertight incision closure and that less secure incision closure may permit this rise in pressure to be a factor in common postoperative complications. This watertight closure associated with a phase of rapid aqueous formation occurring during the very early postoperative period may account for this early rise in intraocu-

317

Table 16-1. Average Schiøtz scale readings (5.5 g weight)

	Outset	Ending	Minutes of massage
Extracapsular cataract extraction	5.70	12.33	6.24
Phacoemulsification	5.27	12.35	6.80
Intracapsular cataract extraction	5.73	12.53	6.75

lar pressure. In this series, final pressures were recorded from 23½ to 30 hours after surgery. The maximum mean value of intraocular pressure was 39.3 mm. The mean of measurements at the end of the observation period was 23.1 mm.

My co-workers and I[4] studied 145 cases of cataract extraction to determine the postoperative pressure as a function of the type of surgery performed, the presence of an intraocular implant lens, and the type of suture material used. There were 77 extracapsular cataract extractions, 30 phacoemulsifications, and 38 intracapsular cataract extractions. A Shearing posterior chamber lens was used in some of the extracapsular and phacoemulsification cases. A Binkhorst 4-loop implant was used in some of the intracapsular cases. Intermittent digital massage was given and frequent Schiøtz pressure readings were taken before starting the surgery. The pressure-lowering effect of this massage is shown in Table 16-1.

Alpha-chymotrypsin was used in all intracapsular cases. Acetazolamide, 500 mg, was given intramuscularly in all cases 1 hour after surgery. Applanation pressures were measured between 1 and 7 hours postoperatively, the morning after surgery, and at each examination thereafter.

After the first day, no difference existed as a result of the type of surgical approach or the presence of a pseudophakos. This study showed that, in spite of the use of alpha-chymotrypsin in all intracapsular cases, there was no difference in intraocular pressure from the extracapsular cases (including phacoemulsification) where no enzyme was used. It also showed the ineffectiveness of acetazolamide in preventing early elevation of intraocular pressure. For example, 41% of extracapsular cases had a pressure greater than

25 mm Hg between 1 and 7 hours after surgery. There was no significant difference in postoperative pressure in eyes with an intraocular lens and eyes without an intraocular lens, with one exception. Cases of intracapsular cataract extraction with a lens implant had significantly lower pressures during the first 7 hours than those without an implant, but this effect did not persist. By the day after surgery, all patients with low tension (less than 10 mm Hg) in all groups had normalized intraocular pressure. Likewise those with higher pressures (greater than 25 mm Hg) had normalized pressure by the third day. In all groups, there was no statistical difference in the pressures 1 to 7 hours and 1 day postoperatively with 10-0 nylon and 9-0 silk.

The cause of this pressure elevation (without enzyme) is not entirely clear, but it may be due to swelling of the trabecular meshwork fibers or to breakdown of the blood-aqueous barrier. However, as stated earlier, the combination of a rapid phase of aqueous formation with a watertight wound closure may account for this pressure rise. It has been felt that most eyes are hypotonic immediately after surgery, but this may be a reflection of outdated methods of wound closure. I have been able to demonstrate wound leakage during the first few postoperative days when using larger and fewer sutures. Newer sutures and techniques of closure have virtually eliminated this. Those eyes showing an initial pressure rise (with or without alpha-chymotrypsin) during the first day or two also tend to reveal low intraocular pressures later. This is probably due to cessation or reduction of aqueous secretion, which may last for several weeks. Miller and Morin[5] found that hypotension with pressures less than 8 mm Hg lasted about 4 weeks in 24 eyes of 23 patients after cataract extraction. In one third, it was still present 8 weeks after. Hilding[6] found that after the twelfth postoperative day the intraocular pressure after cataract extraction was reduced in nearly all of 134 eyes. He stated that the pressure may remain very low for up to 3 weeks. In practice I have found that the pressure in some eyes may remain low for many months.

This prolonged period of subnormal intraocular pressure may give one the impression that the cataract extraction has had a very favorable influence on the course of the patient's primary open-angle glaucoma. Coupled with this is the known tendency for some of these eyes to respond better to the stronger, long-acting miotics than do phakic eyes. Some eyes have an open angle with a superimposed narrow-angle component. The removal of the lens and the creation of iris openings benefit these eyes.

Occasionally an eye whose primary open-angle glaucoma is well controlled before cataract surgery falls out of control some months after surgery. This loss of control may be due to the natural progression of the disease. However, complications after the surgery, such as prolonged iridocyclitis, flat anterior chamber with subsequent anterior synechias, pupillary block and so on, may further embarrass an outflow mechanism whose facility is already marginal. Also, when subjected to cataract extraction, some eyes with functioning filtering blebs are subsequently afflicted with an elevated intraocular pressure. In many of these the bleb becomes fibrotic and ultimately closes. In my experience, this process is more likely to occur if the cataract incision is made superiorly through the cornea and less likely if the incision is made below. Bleb closure is probably the result of postoperative inflammation, but it may also result from a wound leak that may cause angle closure or adherence of vitreous to the wound. If the intact anterior hyaloid membrane adheres to the posterior edges of a corneal incision, it may give rise to a fibrous ingrowth, resulting in closure of the bleb (p. 543).

The impression that filtering blebs may fail after cataract extraction has been emphasized by Maumenee.[7] He found that only about 50% of blebs continued to function, no matter where the incision was made. As for the cause of failure, he feels that during the phase of hypotension, when there is no fluid flowing through the bleb, fibrin from the secondary aqueous precipitates onto the bleb. Fibroblastic invasion of this layer of fibrin makes it impermeable. The fibrin extends on to the back of Tenon's capsule and creates an impermeable barrier between the sclera and Tenon's capsule.

Chandler[8] stresses that cataract extraction has no known permanent influence on the development of primary open-angle glaucoma. He feels that this type of glaucoma may be at any stage of development when the cataract is extracted. It may already be evident at the time of operation or may become evident postoperatively. The surgery merely lowers the intraocular pressure for a few weeks or months after surgery. This view is not universally shared. For example, Sédan and Ourgaud[9] reported the results of cataract extractions in two series of cases (235 and 75 cases) brought under glaucoma control by medical or surgical treatment. Their study stressed the constantly favorable role of cataract extraction on the evolution of the glaucoma. Bigger and Becker[10] studied the effects of uncomplicated intracapsular cataract extraction on the control of intraocular pressure in a series of 100 consecutive patients with primary open-angle glaucoma. The diagnosis of glaucoma was based on the presence of characteristic visual field loss or spontaneous intraocular pressure greater than 30 mm Hg. All patients had been on glaucoma therapy for at least 1 year prior to cataract extraction. Twenty eyes were controlled adequately without medication postoperatively. Forty-eight eyes required less therapy than before surgery, and only two eyes required increased medication 1 year later. Only two eyes required subsequent glaucoma surgery during the first 1½ years after cataract extraction. They concluded that in most cases, it is reasonable to perform cataract extraction alone as the primary procedure in the patient with primary open-angle glaucoma and cataracts, regardless of the status of the patient's intraocular pressure control. Linn[11] reached a similar conclusion in a series of 85 cataract operations in patients with glaucoma that was adequately controlled by mild to maximum therapy. The glaucoma in a significant number of patients was more easily controlled after cataract surgery, and few patients presented any problem in medical management.

In spite of this optimistic note regarding the beneficial effect of a cataract extraction on the control of primary open-angle glaucoma, there are patients whose eyes show marginal or poor medical control before cataract surgery and are not improved after cataract surgery. In these patients there are various surgical options available to the surgeon. These are discussed on p. 231. At this time a simultaneous glaucoma and cataract extraction has become the most popular approach to this problem.

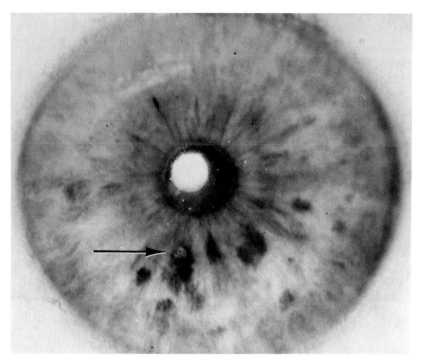

Fig. 16-1. Pseudoexfoliation. Light gray amorphous material at pupillary border and coiled piece adherent to cornea *(arrow)*.

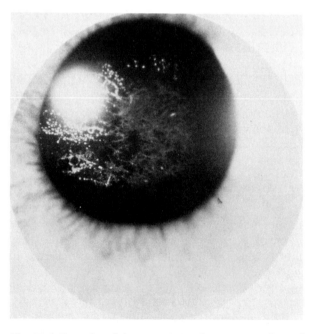

Fig. 16-2. Pseudoexfoliation material seen on surface of anterior hyaloid membrane after intracapsular lens extraction.

GLAUCOMA ASSOCIATED WITH PSEUDOEXFOLIATION IN APHAKIA

The influence of aphakia in glaucoma associated with pseudoexfoliation is similar to its influence in primary open-angle glaucoma. The glaucoma may not be permanently improved after cataract extraction, although the intraocular pressure may remain low after the surgery. My intention is not to discuss this entity fully, but the influence of cataract surgery on the development of this glaucoma is pertinent.

When the signs of pseudoexfoliation are observed before cataract surgery, they usually persist after surgery. The light gray amorphous material (Fig. 16-1) is still present at the pupillary border and in the chamber angle. It is also present on the posterior surface of the iris and may be observed directly on the ciliary processes and zonular remnants through an iridectomy and on the anterior hyaloid membrane (Fig. 16-2).

We still do not know whether psuedoexfoliation with glaucoma ever develops after cataract extraction. Chandler[8] states that he has not recog-

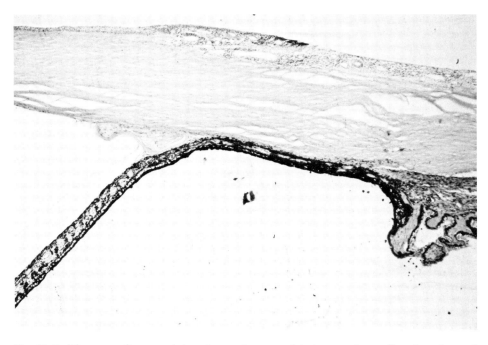

Fig. 16-3. Glaucoma from peripheral anterior synechia in eye that suffered prolonged absence of anterior chamber after cataract extraction.

nized a case in which glaucoma attributable to pseudoexfoliation has developed after the eye has been rendered aphakic.

GLAUCOMA FROM PERIPHERAL ANTERIOR SYNECHIAS

Of all the secondary glaucomas to be described here and later, peripheral anterior synechia formation is the most frequent and important pathogenic mechanism resulting in glaucoma (Fig. 16-3). This formation may be caused by a number of complications, including operative loss of vitreous, iris prolapse, and incarceration of iris or capsule in the wound. However, most frequently there is a history of delayed re-formation of the anterior chamber or late loss of the chamber. This condition is usually associated with wound leakage. Hypotension favors a ciliochoroidal detachment with its accompanying cessation of aqueous production. If the anterior chamber remains flat for a prolonged period, permanent peripheral anterior synechias result. If they have not formed during the period of hypotension, they may form as a result of pupillary block that is not promptly relieved.

When peripheral anterior synechias are present in an aphakic eye, the extent of their involvement is not always an indication of the severity of the glaucoma. When gonioscopy is performed after the anterior chamber re-forms, most of the angle may appear closed by the synechias. Frequently, some eyes with the most ominous-appearing angles are simple to manage for glaucoma control. They may respond readily to the stronger miotics combined with epinephrine. Chandler[8] suggested that some peripheral anterior synechias that extend to Schwalbe's line, or even anterior to it, may actually bridge the trabecular meshwork and not be attached to the filtration area of the meshwork, so that aqueous may have access to at least a portion of the angle behind the synechias.

It is also difficult to determine by gonioscopic appearance whether eyes with postoperative peripheral anterior synechias have permanently closed angles. At times, a peripheral iridectomy or a through-and-through incision of the vitreous will open the angle, particularly if the peripheral anterior synechias are the result of pupillary block. At other times, especially when they result from postoperative iridocyclitis, the angle is permanently sealed. In these instances, cyclocryothermy or cyclodialysis offers the best hope for combating the glaucoma. As a rule the glaucoma in these patients is discovered before the optic nerve head becomes cupped or atrophic.

GLAUCOMA FROM PUPILLARY BLOCK IN APHAKIA

As a result of the various pathogenic mechanisms described on p. 302, an obstruction to communication of aqueous between the anterior and posterior chambers results. In some eyes with aphakic pupillary block glaucoma, the anterior chamber depth may be normal, but in most it is shallow. Peripheral adhesions of the iris to the cornea and trabecular meshwork result if the condition is neglected.

GLAUCOMA ASSOCIATED WITH EPITHELIALIZATION OF THE ANTERIOR CHAMBER

The mechanism of glaucoma in this postoperative complication is varied (p. 524). It may result from epithelium lining the angle structures. In some eyes the chamber angle is already closed by anterior synechias, the epithelium covering this "false" angle created by these adhesions. A particulate type of obstruction of the trabecular meshwork may occur by desquamating epithelium.[12] Since the epithelial invasion involves the anterior surface of the vitreous in many cases, pupillary block glaucoma may result, as suggested by Chandler.[8]

GLAUCOMA ASSOCIATED WITH FIBROUS INGROWTH

Glaucoma associated with fibrous ingrowth (Chapter 27) is characterized by an ingrowth of connective tissue elements from the margins of the cataract wound, aided and abetted by poor wound healing and incarceration of tissues, such as vitreous, iris, or lens remnants, into the surgical incision. The fibroplasia may also result from metaplastic corneal endothelial cells that convert to fibroblasts. Glaucoma is a frequent finding, since the fibrous tissue elements usually invade and cover the angle structures. The incidence of glaucoma is high, especially in eyes with fibrous ingrowth that come to enucleation.

GLAUCOMA ASSOCIATED WITH PHACOANAPHYLAXIS

The complication of glaucoma with phacoanaphylaxis may arise when lens cortex is left in the anterior chamber as a result of an intentional or unintentional extracapsular lens extraction (p. 494). The intraocular response to the retained lens material appears to be related to autosensitization to exposed lens proteins. The evidence favoring the allergic nature of the phacoanaphylactic reaction is discussed on p. 492. The inflammatory membranes that result may cause pupillary block glaucoma, and the trabecular meshwork may become clogged by floating lens debris, lens-laden macrophages, or inflammatory exudate. The treatment depends on its early recognition and its differentiation from sympathetic uveitis. Irrigation of the lens remnants from the anterior chamber often yields dramatic improvement.

HEMOLYTIC GLAUCOMA IN APHAKIA

The recently recognized entity of hemolytic glaucoma in aphakia (p. 417) may occur as a result of a postoperative intraocular hemorrhage. It is most often associated with a vitreous hemorrhage. A macrophage response is elicited by blood-breakdown products that pass into the anterior chamber. A fine anterior chamber cellular response, with the cells often being yellow tinged, is observed. This has been referred to as hemophthalmitis.[13] The macrophages may accept a Prussian blue stain because of hemosiderin engulfed within them. These cells may clog the trabecular meshwork, causing glaucoma. This condition has been termed hemolytic glaucoma by Fenton and Zimmerman.[14] Thus the mechanism is analogous to that seen in phacolytic glaucoma where macrophages laden with lens protein similarly clog the drainage apparatus.

Medical treatment consists of glaucoma control. Steroids are of little value. In most cases the process is self-limiting. As the cellular response subsides, the elevated intraocular pressure diminishes. The process often commences 2 to 3 weeks after cataract surgery and may last for weeks or months. Although I have not had an opportunity to resort to this, if the glaucoma becomes intractable, one might irrigate the anterior chamber, as in phacolytic glaucoma.

GLAUCOMA FROM PROLONGED POSTOPERATIVE INFLAMMATION IN APHAKIA

The mechanism causing elevation of intraocular pressure is no different from that occurring in the phakic eye after prolonged inflammation. The glaucoma may be due to obstruction of the trabecular meshwork by inflammatory debris, peripheral anterior synechias, or pupillary block. The treatment is mainly prophylactic, since intensive therapy usually controls postoperative iridocyclitis. Any residual glaucoma after the inflammation has subsided can usually be controlled medically unless an element of pupillary block exists. Occasionally cyclodialysis or cyclocryothermy becomes necessary.

GLAUCOMA ASSOCIATED WITH FREE VITREOUS IN THE ANTERIOR CHAMBER

Glaucoma with free vitreous in the anterior chamber is usually innocuous and results when vitreous fills the anterior chamber and blocks the trabecular meshwork.[15] This condition is usually seen during the first few weeks after cataract surgery when most postoperative ruptures of the anterior hyaloid membrane occur. It may, however, occur months or even years after surgery. On gonioscopy the angle appears open but is filled with vitreous fibrils. The response to miotics is unpredictable. Mydriatics are usually more effective. Generally the conglomerate mass of vitreous recedes from the angle and anterior chamber toward the pupillary space. When recondensation occurs the angle structures become less obstructed, and intraocular pressure gradually falls. Acetazolamide is helpful during the period of elevated intraocular pressure. Surgery is rarely necessary. However, if the rupture of the anterior face of the vitreous is associated with wound separation, iris incarceration or prolapse, hyphema, epithelialization of the anterior chamber, or fibrous ingrowth, the problem becomes much more complex.

GLAUCOMA ASSOCIATED WITH PROGRESSIVE IRIS ATROPHY IN APHAKIA

A progressive iris atrophy occurs in some patients after cataract surgery. Pigment is dispersed and fills the chamber angle, especially inferiorly. Defects in the pigment epithelium are observed on slit lamp examination by transillumination. This entity does not resemble essential iris atrophy as far as the appearance of the iris is concerned. It is seen in diabetics and in other patients who show a predilection for pigment dispersion. It also occurs more frequently after other postoperative complications such as iridocyclitis, hyphema, and pupillary block. It is an occasional postoperative complication after cataract extraction with insertion of a plastic intraocular lens. The response to miotics, especially the longer acting miotics, is usually satisfactory.

GLAUCOMA ASSOCIATED WITH HYPHEMA

A small hyphema usually is absorbed spontaneously and creates no problem. It is only with a massive hyphema, especially with repeated bleeding, that elevation of intraocular pressure results. The blood may pass into the vitreous or cause bloodstaining of the cornea if the process is not brought under rapid control. The elevation of intraocular pressure may be treated with acetazolamide. A hyperosmotic agent (glycerin, mannitol) may be useful in a marked elevation of pressure associated with prolonged pain. Certain blood dyscrasias may require antihemorrhagic therapy. Surgical treatment is described on p. 413.

ZONULYTIC GLAUCOMA

The introduction of alpha-chymotrypsin, a proteolytic enzyme having a specificity of action at certain peptide bonds, as an adjunct to intracapsular lens extraction has been enthusiastically hailed by ophthalmic surgeons during the past two decades. Its discovery is attributed to Barraquer,[16] who injected the enzyme into the eye of a patient in an unsuccessful attempt to dissolve a vitreous hemorrhage. Observing that the patient's lens had become dislocated, he readily recognized its potential value in cataract surgery. The use of alpha-chymotrypsin has become so widespread that it is surprising how few well-documented reports have appeared in the literature regarding complications arising from its application. Kirsch[1] was the first to recognize elevated intraocular pressure (glaucoma) as a side effect of the use of alpha-chymotrypsin in cataract extractions in humans.

Characteristics of enzyme glaucoma

Enzyme glaucoma typically appears 2 to 5 days after cataract extraction. The patient may complain of pain. Corneal edema is usually present, the anterior chamber is of normal aphakic depth, and the angle is wide open. The intraocular pressure is usually mildly elevated, although it may be as high as the 60s and 70s. Kirsch[17] demonstrated that pilocarpine lowered the intraocular pressure and increased aqueous outflow except during the peak of the pressure rise, when it has little effect. This suggests that the outflow mechanisms are so impaired at this stage that they are unresponsive to miotics. The response to pilocarpine improves as the peak of tension rise passes. Bloomfield[18] found that the incidence of enzyme glaucoma after cataract extraction was not reduced by the postoperative use of acetazolamide, pilocarpine, subconjunctival steroids, or corneal placement of the incision. Galin[19] also found a significant increase in the incidence of postoperative hypertension when alpha-chymotrypsin was used. The use of acetylcholine at the conclusion of the surgery does not reduce the incidence of pressure elevation. Tonography reveals no evidence of hypersecretion.[17] Serial tonography and perilimbal suction-cup analysis reveal no alteration in intraocular dynamics up to 6 months after surgery in patients exhibiting postoperative pressure elevations.[19]

Kirsch[20] demonstrated a dose relationship of alpha-chymotrypsin in the production of glaucoma after cataract extraction. Eighty nonglaucomatous eyes were subjected to intracapsular cataract extraction with enzymatic zonulysis by doses of alpha-chymotrypsin (1:5000 dilution) varying from 0.25 to 1.5 ml. A dose as small as 0.25 ml produced glaucoma in 55%. The peak pressure rose with increased dose of enzyme. With the use of 1.5 ml, 70% developed an abnormal pressure.

Alpha-chymotrypsin also produces glaucoma experimentally in monkeys.[21-26] Kalvin and co-workers[21] found that they could produce glaucoma in owl monkeys (Aotus trivirgatus) if the enzyme was injected into the posterior chamber but not if the enzyme was injected only into the anterior chamber. This difference suggested that an interaction between the enzyme and something in the posterior chamber was necessary for the production of glaucoma.

Etiology of enzyme glaucoma

Enzyme glaucoma is unrelated to pupillary block glaucoma or to glaucoma secondary to uveitis, air block, lens remnants, or hyphema. However, when these are present the glaucoma may be exaggerated by the use of alpha-chymotrypsin. Thus when pupillary block glaucoma occurs, it will respond to mydriatics, and then the enzyme glaucoma will supervene on the third day or later. It is also unrelated to preexisting open-angle glaucoma or to aphakic glaucoma caused by peripheral anterior synechias.

It is interesting that Kirsch[1] considered the possibility of particulate obstruction of the trabecular meshwork by aggregates of undissolved enzyme or other debris. He filtered the enzyme preparation through a Millipore filter, but this did not prevent or minimize the enzyme glaucoma. He also performed skin tests, which revealed no hypersensitivity to alpha-chymotrypsin, confirming an earlier report by Sallman,[27] who demonstrated the low allergenicity of the enzyme in animals.

Referring to the work of Kalvin and co-work-

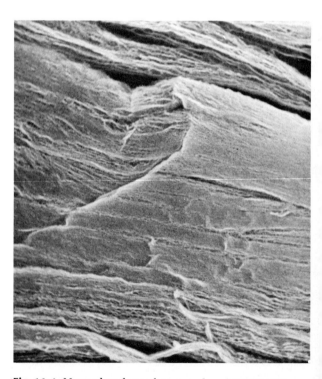

Fig. 16-4. Normal owl monkey zonules. (×1000.) (From Anderson, D. R.: Am. J. Ophthalmol. **71:**619-625, 1971.)

ers,[21] Anderson[28] believed that an obvious and plausible explanation of enzyme glaucoma is that fragments of the digested zonule may clog the trabecular meshwork. To examine this theory, he studied the trabecular meshwork of owl monkeys with enzyme glaucoma by the then new technique of scanning electron microscopy[29] (Fig. 16-4). This technique allows the examination of relatively large pieces of unsectioned material. This is possible because, unlike with the conventional transmission electron microscopy, the illuminating electrons do not pass through a thin section of the specimen. Instead, backscattered (reflected) and secondary electrons are viewed from the same side of the specimen that is showered by the illuminating electrons. The resulting image is a view of the surface of the specimen, and it has a three-dimensional quality because of the presence of shadows and highlights. The scanning electron microscope does not achieve quite the same resolution or magnification as the transmission electron microscope. However, it yields much greater magnification than can be achieved by a dissecting microscope.

Using the new technique, Anderson examined the trabecular meshwork of the monkeys and compared it with that of the human. There were some apparent minor species variations, but the overall pattern was the same. The trabecular meshwork consisted of a uveal portion with large openings, a corneoscleral portion with smaller openings, and a juxtacanalicular portion without apparent openings.

Anderson[28] produced enzyme glaucoma in one eye of each of four owl monkeys. The eyes were enucleated and examined by scanning electron microscopy. They dramatically demonstrated that white particulate matter obstructed some of the openings in the trabecular meshwork that overlies Schlemm's canal. White particulate mat-

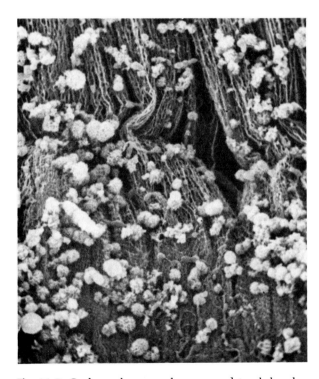

Fig. 16-5. Owl monkey zonules exposed to alpha-chymotrypsin. Zonules are somewhat disaggregated, and fluffy particles are seen as product of reaction between zonules and alpha-chymotrypsin. (×1000.) (From Anderson, D. R.: Am. J. Ophthalmol. **71:**619-625, 1971.)

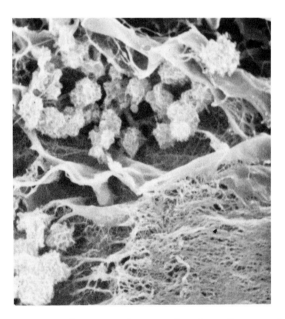

Fig. 16-6. Higher magnification of owl monkey zonule exposed to alpha-chymotrypsin. In lower right corner is relatively intact normal zonule, but rest of field shows lysed zonule with fluffy spherical particles remaining as product of reaction between zonule and alpha-chymotrypsin. (×4375.) (From Anderson, D. R.: Am. J. Ophthalmol. **71:**470-476, 1971.)

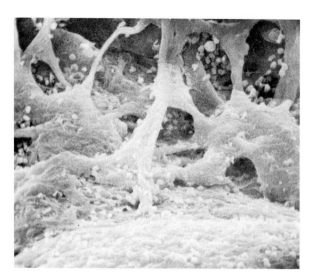

Fig. 16-7. Recess of filtration angle of owl monkey with zonulytic glaucoma after zonulysis by injection of alpha-chymotrypsin into posterior chamber. Anterior iris surface is visible in lower one fourth of field, and above is surface view of uveal meshwork. Spherical particles of type shown in Figs. 16-5 and 16-6 are seen in meshwork, presumably obstructing outflow through smaller openings in underlying corneoscleral meshwork. (×200.) (From Anderson, D. R.: Am. J. Ophthalmol. **71:**470-476, 1971.)

ter was also found within the cavernous spaces of the uveal meshwork that fills the angle recess (Figs. 16-5 to 16-7). The particles were not all the same. Most were of irregular shape and resembled zonular fragments typically formed by the action of alpha-chymotrypsin on the zonule. Transmission electron microscopy confirmed that the particles were clumps of filaments of the kind that make up zonular fibers. Such clumps of filaments were not seen in the trabecular meshwork of control eyes that had received a saline injection into the posterior chamber instead of the enzyme. The particles bore no resemblance to alpha-chymotrypsin itself when examined by scanning electron microscopy. No normal ocular structure, including the lens, that has been examined so far by this technique looks like these particles. Close scrutiny shows that there are also some erythrocytes and leukocytes present.

From the specimens examined, it appeared obvious at once that the particles of zonular fragments could reasonably be expected to impede

aqueous outflow and account for the elevated intraocular pressure. Furthermore, it is probably safe to conclude that these findings in monkey's eyes apply equally to humans where cataract extraction facilitated by enzymatic zonulysis is performed. On a clinical level the enzyme glaucoma in humans appears to be self-limited, presumably because the zonular fragments are finally pushed through the trabecular meshwork. In monkeys the glaucoma is more severe and longer lasting, possibly because the passageways in the corneoscleral meshwork are smaller, as Anderson[28] suggested.

One cannot but admire the excellent research of Kirsch, who first recognized enzyme glaucoma, and of Anderson, who discovered its cause.

Complications of enzymatic zonulysis

Shortly after the introduction of alpha-chymotrypsin in 1958,[16,30] numerous references to possible complications arising from its use appeared in the literature. Maumenee[31] demonstrated the deleterious effect of the enzyme on the retina of rabbits. The supporting structure of the retina (Müller's fibers) appeared to be more sensitive to the enzyme than the neural cells, medullated nerve fibers, and blood vessels. However, the concentration and duration of exposure to the enzyme far exceeded the concentration and duration of exposure used in cataract surgery. Other reports[32-34] that pointed to a similar destructive effect of the enzyme on the retina followed. Some doubt is cast on the importance of such an effect under clinical conditions, since there has been no increase in the incidence of detachment of the retina after cataract extraction aided by enzymatic zonulysis during the past 15 or more years.

A number of other complications attributed to the enzyme have been observed. They include defects of wound healing, iridocyclitis, depigmentation of the iris, pigmentary glaucoma, prolapse of vitreous into the anterior chamber, striate keratitis, corneal opacification, and others.

After Kirsch discovered the pressure-elevating effect of alpha-chymotrypsin, it became apparent that at least some of the complications were caused by the stress inflicted on the healing wound by the high intraocular pressure.[17] The infrequency of wound complications during the first postoperative week is surprising, since the intraocular pressure is at its peak then. Kirsch[17] pointed to the early edema of the tissues between the sutures contributing to the watertight integrity of the incision as a possible explanation. This integrity could diminish as the edema lessens, allowing operation of the phenomena that delay healing. If glaucoma does cause, or contribute to, poor wound healing, the mechanism of its action is still unknown. Nevertheless, it is suggested that the elevated intraocular pressure, and not the proteolytic action, of the enzyme causes defects in wound healing.

It is likely that some of the other complications are attributable to defects in the commercial preparation of the enzyme. Particulate contamination is discussed on p. 433. The occurrence of several consecutive cases of immediate corneal clouding on instilling the enzyme solution in the eye must be blamed on faulty preparations or errors in diluting the enzyme. The increased incidence of striate keratopathy, if it does exist, is probably attributable to mechanical factors associated with the introduction of the enzyme into the eye or to the forward displacement of the lens-iris diaphragm associated with enzymatic zonulysis, which makes intraocular manipulations more difficult. The possibly increased incidence of postoperative rupture of the anterior hyaloid membrane is discussed on p. 407.

Prophylaxis

Since a 1 : 10,000 dilution of the enzyme affords as much zonulytic effect as a 1 : 5000 dilution, this concentration is preferable. The enzyme should be left in the eye for no more than 2 minutes, and no more than 2 ml should be instilled. Much less is effective.

Lee and Lam[35] say that thorough washing of the enzyme from the eye is not of benefit. They performed quantitative analyses of the proteolytic activity in animal eyes occurring after lens extraction with alpha-chymotrypsin. The analyses indicated that the enzyme is lost or inactivated by the antichymotrypsin activity of the eye itself within a few minutes after injection. Therefore repeated washing during surgery and the use of agents that inhibit alpha-chymotrypsin are of little help in reducing postoperative complications. There is probably more to be lost from repeated irrigation. However, the work of Anderson[28] suggests that thorough washing of the anterior chamber may rid the eye of some of the zonular particles.

Since increased stress is placed on the wound as a result of zonulytic glaucoma, Kirsch[17] recommended using an increased number of sutures when the enzyme is employed.

REFERENCES

1. Kirsch, R. E.: Glaucoma following cataract extraction associated with the use of alpha-chymotrypsin, Arch. Ophthalmol. **72:**612-620, 1964.
2. Kaufman, I. H.: Letter to the editor: intraocular pressure after lens extraction, Am. J. Ophthalmol. **59:**722-723, 1965.
3. Rich, W. J., Radtke, N. D., and Cohan, B. E.: Early ocular hypertension after cataract extraction, Br. J. Ophthalmol. **58:**725-731, 1974.
4. Arkfeld, D., and Jaffe, N. S.: Postoperative intraocular pressure. Presented at Bascom Palmer Eye Institute Annual Residents' Day, Miami, June 1979.
5. Miller, J. R., and Morin, J. D.: Intraocular pressure after cataract extraction, Am. J. Ophthalmol. **66:**523-528, 1968.
6. Hilding, A. C.: Reduced ocular tension after cataract surgery, Arch. Ophthalmol. **53:**686-693, 1955.
7. Maumenee, A. E.: Opinion, Highlights Ophthalmol. **12:**124-137, 1969.
8. Chandler, P. A., and Grant, W. M.: Glaucoma in aphakia. In Lectures on glaucoma, Philadelphia, 1965, Lea & Febiger, pp. 234-243.
9. Sédan, J., and Ourgaud, A. G.: L'extraction de la cataracte chez le glaucomateux normalisé, Ann. Oculist **201:**385-399, 1968.
10. Bigger, J. F., and Becker, B.: The effect of uncomplicated cataract extraction of glaucoma control, Ophthalmology (Rochester) **75:**260-272, 1971.
11. Linn, J. G., Jr.: Surgery for cataract complicated by glaucoma, Ophthalmology (Rochester) **75:**273-280, 1971.
12. Terry, T. L., Chisholm, J. F., Jr., and Schonberg, A. L.: Studies on surface-epithelium invasion of the anterior segment of the eye, Am. J. Ophthalmol. **22:**1083-1110, 1939.
13. Duke-Elder, S.: System of ophthalmology. Vol. IX. Diseases of the uveal tract, St. Louis, 1966, The C. V. Mosby Co., p. 23.
14. Fenton, R. H., and Zimmerman, L. E.: Hemolytic glaucoma, an unusual cause of acute open-angle secondary glaucoma, Arch. Ophthalmol. **70:**236-239, 1963.
15. Grant, W. M.: Open-angle glaucoma associated with vitreous filling the anterior chamber, Trans. Am. Ophthalmol. Soc. **61:**196-218, 1963.
16. Barraquer, J.: Totale Linsenextraktion nach Auflösung der Zonula durch α-Chymotrypsin-enzymatische Zonulyse, Klin. Mbl. Augenheilk. **133:**609-615, 1958.
17. Kirsch, R. E.: Further studies on glaucoma following cataract extraction associated with the use of alpha-chymotrypsin, Ophthalmology (Rochester) **69:**1011-1023, 1965.

18. Bloomfield, S.: Failure to prevent enzyme glaucoma. A negative report, Am. J. Ophthalmol. **65:**405-406, 1968.

19. Galin, M. A., Barasch, K. R., and Harris, L. S.: Enzymatic zonulolysis and intraocular pressure, Am. J. Ophthalmol. **61:**690-696, 1966.

20. Kirsch, R. E.: Dose relationship of alpha-chymotrypsin in production of glaucoma after cataract extraction, Arch. Ophthalmol. **75:**774-775, 1966.

21. Kalvin, N. H., Hamasaki, D. I., and Gass, J. D. M.: Experimental glaucoma in monkeys. I. Relationship between intraocular pressure and cupping of the optic disc and cavernous atrophy of the optic nerve, Arch. Ophthalmol. **76:**82-93, 1966.

22. Kalvin, N. H., Hamasaki, E. I., and Gass, J. D. M.: Experimental glaucoma in monkeys. II. Studies of intraocular vascularity during glaucoma, Arch. Ophthalmol. **76:**94-103, 1966.

23. Hamasaki, D. I., and Fujino, T.: Effect of intraocular pressure on ocular vessels filling with India ink, Arch. Ophthalmol. **78:**369-379, 1967.

24. Zimmerman, L. E., de Venecia, G., and Hamasaki, D. I.: Pathology of the optic nerve in experimental acute glaucoma, Invest. Ophthalmol. **6:**109-125, 1967.

25. Lampert, P. W., Vogel, M. H., and Zimmerman, L. E.: Pathology of the optic nerve in experimental acute glaucoma. Electron microscopic studies, Invest. Ophthalmol. **7:**199-213, 1968.

26. Lessell, S., and Kuwabara, T.: Experimental α-chymotrypsin glaucoma, Arch. Ophthalmol. **81:**853-864, 1969.

27. von Sallmann, L.: Experimental studies of some ocular effects of alpha-chymotrypsin, Ophthalmology (Rochester) **64:**25-32, 1960.

28. Anderson, D. R.: Experimental alpha chymotrypsin glaucoma studied by scanning electron microscopy, Am. J. Ophthalmol. **71:**470-476, 1971.

29. Anderson, D. R.: Scanning electron microscopy of primate trabecular meshwork, Am. J. Ophthalmol. **71:**90-101, 1971.

30. Barraquer, J.: Enzymatic zonulolysis: contribution to the surgery of the crystalline lens (preliminary note), Acta Ophthalmol. **36:**803-806, 1958.

31. Maumenee, A. E.: Effect of alpha-chymotrypsin on the retina, Ophthalmology (Rochester) **64:**33-36, 1960.

32. Müller, H. K.: Résumé de la discussion de la table ronde sur la zonulolyse enzymatique, Ann. Inst. Barraquer **2**(1): 103, 1961.

33. Lugossy, G.: Complications rétiniennes de la zonulolyse enzymatique, Bull. Soc. Franc. Ophthalmol. **77:**238-251, 1964.

34. Sekiguchi, K.: Histological studies on the ocular toxicity of α-chymotrypsin, Jpn. J. Ophthalmol. **4:**104-116, 1960.

35. Lee, P. F., and Lam, K. W.: Alpha-chymotrypsin and cataract surgery. An experimental study, Am. J. Ophthalmol. **66:**528-532, 1968.

CHAPTER 17

Corneal edema

Corneal edema is one of the most serious complications of cataract surgery. When one considers that until approximately 15 to 20 years ago, this was one of the most hopeless sequelae of a cataract extraction, there is some sense of relief that a medical and surgical approach to this problem has finally evolved, made possible by the enormous increase in our knowledge of the pathophysiology of corneal edema over the past decade. Therefore an updating of modern concepts is presented in this chapter. I hope it will serve as a sound basis for the diagnosis and treatment of this unfortunate complication of cataract extraction.

PATHOPHYSIOLOGY

The major site of the refractive power of the eye is the cornea. Its smooth surface and structural regularity permit free passage of light with minimal scattering. As long as the cornea remains transparent, it allows the formation of an optically clear image on the retina.

The most important part of the refractive function of the cornea occurs at its anterior surface between the air and the tear film. The refractive power here is +49 D, whereas at its posterior surface it is −6 D. Thus irregularities at the anterior surface such as epithelial edema will have a far greater effect on visual acuity than posterior surface irregularities. They readily reduce visual acuity because of a marked irregular astigmatism. In the normal epithelium the intercellular space is very narrow (100 to 200 Å). When epithelial edema exists, however, these spaces become greatly dilated. The cells nevertheless cling to each other by their attachment bodies, the desmosomes. Therefore the dilated intercellular spaces become pools of fluid, perhaps a few microns in diameter. Light is diffracted from the surface of these droplets, rendering the epithelium hazy. This is the anatomic basis of epithelial haze or edema. Stromal edema has relatively little effect on visual acuity unless it is complicated by opacification.

The corneal stroma consists of fine collagen fibrils (190 to 340 Å in diameter) that are disposed parallel to each other, closely packed, with a minimum of interweaving or cross-linking.[1,2] These fibrils are embedded in a matrix of proteins and polysaccharides. When the stroma swells, the added fluid is absorbed by this ground substance while the fibrils retain their diameter.[3,4] Because of this anatomic arrangement, the corneal stroma shows a remarkable ability to swell, unlike most other connective tissues where more interweaving of coarser collagen fibrils seems to prevent marked swelling.[5]

Swelling forces are mostly electrostatic, rather than colloid osmotic,[6] since conditions that alter the ionization of the macromolecules (polysaccharides) cause swelling in the stroma. The polysaccharides in the cornea (keratin sulfate and chondroitin sulfate) occur in only small amounts, —about 3% of the dry weight based on hexosamine determinations[7]—yet they seem to play the principal role in stromal swelling. If the acid radicals of the polysaccharides are blocked in situ (ionically cross-linked) with cetyl-pyridium chloride, the swelling of the stroma is markedly depressed.[8] It is suggested that swelling is due to the negatively charged acid radicals (the carboxyl groups and, possibly, the sulfate groups) along the polysaccharide chain repelling one another.

329

Corneal stromal swelling results in a pressure exerted against Descemet's membrane and the endothelium, which measures 50 to 60 mm Hg in the normal state.[9] Like the vitreous the stroma is likened to a solid framework filled with fluid.[10] The more the ground substance is compressed, the higher the swelling pressure. The more the stroma swells (from expansion of the ground substance), the lower the swelling pressure.[5]

Since the swelling pressure of the cornea is dependent on hydration, it has been correlated with corneal thickness.[11] Thus if the corneal thickness is known, as measured with a pachymeter, the stromal swelling pressure can be calculated. The pressure of the interstitial fluid of the stroma (in contrast to the stromal solids) that draws fluid in is normally negative,[12] and the magnitude of the fluid pressure is equal to the difference between the swelling pressure and the intraocular pressure. Since the stromal fluid pressure is negative, the stroma tends to imbibe fluid from the surrounding tears, limbal vessels, and aqueous. The limiting cellular layers (epithelium and endothelium) have a very high resistance of the flow of fluid and thus serve as an effective barrier against the flow of fluid into the stroma. However, this in itself is not sufficient to maintain corneal dehydration, since some fluid eventually gains access to the stroma through these limiting layers and across the limbus. Thus a dehydrating mechanism or a pump is also necessary and appears to be supplied by the endothelium.[13-17] The epithelium to date has not demonstrated any pumping or fluid transport ability. The exact mechanism of the dehydration process is still not clear, although some form of metabolic activity is involved. I predict that investigators will eventually show that the process involves an ion exchange as in other parts of the body.

The endothelium tends to pump fluid posteriorly, while the intraocular pressure works in the opposite direction. In the normal state the endothelial pump pressure exceeds the intraocular pressure, thereby creating a negative fluid pressure in the stroma.[18] Clinically, it has been known for some time that endothelial damage has a far greater effect on corneal edema than does epithelial damage. Epithelial damage permits access of fluid to the stroma (from the tears),

but this is resisted by the intraocular pressure[19] and pumped out by the endothelium. Endothelial damage, on the other hand, permits free access to the stroma, which condition is favored by the intraocular pressure, and the defective pump mechanism is little able to cope with the edema.

The mechanism involving epithelial edema as a result of endothelial dystrophy or glaucoma has recently been investigated.[20] It was found that an increase in stromal fluid pressure from negative to positive is probably the direct cause of epithelial edema. Thus in patients with endothelial dystrophy or glaucoma, the epithelium does not become edematous if the stromal fluid pressure remains negative, since fluid is not pushed into the epithelium.[21]

The pathophysiology of bullous keratopathy is better understood after consideration of these factors. The first change occurs in the mechanism when, from whatever cause (surgical trauma, vitreocorneal adherence, glaucoma), fluid gains access to the stroma. When the stromal fluid pressure becomes positive as just described, the epithelium becomes edematous, the edema beginning in the basal cell layers, then spreading through the epithelium, and occasionally resulting in subepithelial bullae. For the epithelium to be pushed off the stroma or for it to appear as if it is, the following obstacles must be overcome: (1) the epithelial attachment to Bowman's membrane by the desmosomes must be severed and (2) the negative pressure of the stromal tissue, which draws the epithelium to the underlying tissue, must become positive.

In the early stages the stroma is edematous. After months to years, opacification occurs in an irregular, stellate fashion, just anterior to Descemet's membrane. Folds in Descemet's membrane that persist for a long period become fixed scars. The effect of this opacification decreases visual acuity, but it is not the main factor, since epithelial edema is usually present long before opacification of the stroma occurs.

The changes in the endothelium as a result of dystrophy, or other causes, is now histologically well understood. The cells normally appear low and rectangular in cross section. When damage occurs, they become flattened, enlarged, and attenuated. Their concentration decreases, and eventually they disappear. At some critical time, the pumping activity of the endothelium becomes so ineffective that stromal edema, and finally epithelial edema, ensue. The clinical picture may be characterized by exacerbations and remissions until eventually a persistent corneal edema results. The epithelium loses its surface regularity. It becomes irregular in number of layers, edematous, vacuolated, and loosely adherent to the underlying tissue.[22]

Until now little consideration has been given to Descemet's membrane. Fuchs in 1917 first suggested that the endothelium produces Descemet's membrane.[23] The endothelial cells contain intracytoplasmic vacuoles of electron-dense material that are released into the region of Descemet's membrane.[24-27] They can lay down a basement membrane similar to Descemet's membrane in tissue culture[27-29] and in ectopic intraocular locations. The chemical composition and structural organization of Descemet's membrane are similar to that of other mammalian basement membranes.[30,31]

Descemet's membrane, like a typical basement membrane, is a compact connective tissue consisting of small-diameter collagen fibrils and filaments bonded to a matrix of glycoproteins.[32-34] The collagen shows some differences from typical connective tissue collagen, a modification beneficial for both filtration and structural support. However, the endothelial cell, as just stated, is the main barrier regulating the flow of water and molecules in and out of the cornea. Descemet's membrane is 15 times more permeable than the endothelium, permitting passage of relatively large molecules and particles.[35]

Waring and co-workers[36] have pointed to three characteristic properties of Descemet's membrane that account for many of the pathologic changes seen clinically and histologically.

1. *Elasticity.* The distensibility of Descemet's membrane permits stretching, or distortion, followed by return to its original shape. When the stroma imbibes fluid and the cornea thickens, the increased volume is distributed posteriorly, producing bowing and folding of Descemet's membrane, while the anterior cornea retains a fixed curvature. If the stroma is thin, stretching of Descemet's membrane may result in a descemetocele. Part of the resistance of Descemet's membrane to perforation is due to its compact

collagen structure and distensibility, but the pressure developed within the descemetocele is also an important factor. Since the tension on the wall of a sphere is proportional to the pressure exerted times the radius of the sphere, the short radius of the descemetocele reduces the pressure on its wall to about $\frac{1}{25}$ that on the sclera, and the force of the intraocular pressure is partially dissipated (Laplace's law).[37] Nevertheless, the elasticity of Descemet's membrane is limited. Acute stretching (buphthalmos, keratoconus) may cause breakdown in Descemet's membrane. Recent, more sophisticated staining techniques and electron microscopy refute earlier claims that Descemet's membrane contains elastic fibers.[38,39] The reason for its elasticity is unknown, although other basement membranes such as lens capsule have a similar property.

2. *Barrier to penetration by cells and vessels.* Leukocytes and bacteria do not penetrate an intact Descemet's membrane, a property that confines them to the cornea in deep corneal ulcers until Descemet's membrane is ruptured or disrupted by action of proteolytic enzymes. Newly formed blood vessels do not penetrate this glassy membrane, and anterior synechiae adherent to it are unable to send vessels into the stroma.

3. *Resistance to autolysis.* Since Descemet's membrane is not digested by the autolytic processes of the body, it remains undisturbed indefinitely in ectopic locations or abnormal configurations (Fig. 28-4, *C*). Changes that occur in childhood are often observed during a routine examination years later.

There appear to be wide clinical variations in the onset of corneal edema in different patients in response to similar insults. Some patients show a severe corneal edema from a mild iritis, whereas others retain a normal cornea despite alarming elevations of intraocular pressure. These apparent discrepancies might be explained by an excellent study[40] that considered the normal variations in endothelial cell population. A striking similarity between the concentration of these cells in the two eyes of an individual but a marked difference in cellular concentration in the eyes of different individuals was found. In addition, endothelial cell population apparently decreases with age. Thus we might infer that these variations in cellular concentration indicate the levels of intraocular pressure that must be exceeded before corneal edema ensues. Thus some corneas under high pressure might show little or no edema, and others might show marked hydration at a low intraocular pressure. These wide variations in endothelial cell population might explain why a variety of insults such as iritis, vitreocorneal adherence, increased intraocular pressure, hyphema, and introduction of particulate matter into the anterior chamber will affect the normal cornea with a lower concentration of endothelial cells more severely.

The availability of the specular microscope for clinical examination of the corneal endothelium in vivo has created greater interest in studying endothelial cell population. With this technique, an extensive evaluation of the effects of age and surgical procedures on endothelial cell density is possible. As discussed on p. 177, corneas can remain clear with significant reduction in endothelial cell numbers. As yet, the minimum number of central endothelial cells per square millimeter required to maintain corneal dehydration cannot be determined. Eyes with fewer cells, however, may be more susceptible to corneal edema due to inflammation or trauma. The possible effect of further cell death with age is still unknown. Although many questions regarding the significance of endothelial cell density cannot be answered at this time, specular microscopy is becoming a valuable tool for monitoring the various maneuvers used in intraocular surgery. It has already resulted in changes in the technique of routine cataract extraction, phacoemulsification, and intraocular lens implantation.

Reduction in corneal endothelial cells is preceded by histologic cellular changes such as pleomorphism, vacuolization, and hyperchromatism. As the endothelial cells are destroyed, the neighboring cells enlarge and attempt to cover the surface defect caused by cell death. Pathologic specimens showing destruction of corneal endothelium usually show a thickening of Descemet's membrane. This thickening may be nodular, a characteristic finding in Fuchs' endothelial dystrophy, and gives the cornea the hammered silver appearance. Focal thickenings in the anterior endothelial cell wall have been called hemidesmosomes,[41,42] but more recent opinion[24,32,43] is that these are not sites of attach-

ment. Descemet's membrane is poorly adherent to both stroma and endothelium, allowing easy separation. Descemet's membrane increases in thickness throughout life, measuring 10 to 14 μm in the adult. The endothelium forms new basement membrane on the posterior surface of the banded embryonic Descemet's in a discontinuous pattern, resulting in a lamellar tree-ring appearance of the adult Descemet's membrane.[24,38,41,44-46] In addition the endothelium produces more basement membrane in some areas. These focal thickenings are called Hassall-Henle warts in the periphery, and cornea guttata centrally.

Regenerating endothelial cells produce new Descemet's membrane. Whereas stimuli to endothelial regeneration in childhood may provoke marked proliferation of endothelial cells and Descemet's membrane, in the adult an identical stimulus may produce barely enough response to maintain corneal integrity.[47-49] There are also wide species differences in regeneration; for example, rabbit endothelium has regenerative powers far in excess of those of humans.[50-52] Waring and co-workers[36] have emphasized that corneal endothelium responds to diverse types of pathology in a single fashion—by conversion to a fibroblast-like cell.[25,53] It produces a fibrous tissue that becomes incorporated into Descemet's membrane, resulting in a thickened, multilaminar, "regenerated Descemet's membrane." The term "fibroblast-like," which describes the cell resulting from this fibrous metaplasia, indicates that these cells possess features of both endothelial cells and fibroblasts. More severe insults result in fibroblast-like transformation. The fibroblastic characteristics include an increased amount of rough endoplasmic reticulum containing electron-dense substance, intracytoplasmic filaments that are probably collagen precursors, increased cortical densities adjacent to the cell surface, intracytoplasmic vacuoles, and lack of apical tight junctions.[54]

The corneal endothelium is really a mesothelium. It is mesodermally derived (as are fibroblasts) and can undergo fibroblastic metaplasia. This is in contrast to true endothelium, which is the lining of a vascular channel and usually does not convert to a fibroblast.[55] The fibroblast-like cell may redifferentiate into endothelial cells,[54] which resume the production of basement membrane similar to Descemet's, or regenerating endothelial cells may migrate in from undamaged areas and produce a layer of basement membrane. Thus the cells covering the posterior cornea may alternate between the fibroblast-like and endothelial types, each producing its own characteristic contribution to Descemet's membrane. The result is a multilaminar Descemet's membrane consisting of the original membrane anteriorly and the newly produced material posteriorly. This tree-ring lamination reflects the stresses experienced by the endothelium.

Glaucoma has an effect on the endothelium that may be influenced by subsequent intraocular surgery. The incidence of postoperative corneal edema is higher after an uneventful cataract extraction in a glaucomatous patient, and it is high when cataract surgery is performed subsequent to glaucoma surgery. Edema may occur, even though postoperative intraocular pressure may be normal or even low.

After surgery or endothelial damage, there is a tendency for the damaged and attenuated endothelial cells to form new endothelial cells, but rarely is a normal endothelium ever produced. The endothelium has a capacity to form a new Descemet's membrane. This is sometimes seen after the enlargement of the cataract incision where Descemet's membrane has peeled off and rolled some distance toward the center of the cornea. Endothelial proliferation is seen in a number of intraocular pathologic conditions (p. 551). It may proliferate along a vitreous strand to the cornea or operative wound, along a clump of zonular fibers attached to the wound, along fibrous tissue, and on the lens capsule. It may even line the entire anterior chamber and elaborate a glassy membrane. Irvine[22] has observed that the endothelial components of these strands are always flattened and attenuated and are never of normal configuration and that the pathologic states that accompany such proliferations are often associated with hemorrhage.

Corneal vascularization is sometimes observed after long-standing bullous keratopathy. A distinction is made between superficial and stromal vascularization of the stroma has been emphasized in many studies.[57-64] Normally the stroma is and Bowman's membrane. Connective tissue is

found around the vessels, and finally a thin membrane separates these two layers of cornea. In the latter the actively growing vessels advance in the interlamellar space from their point of entrance.[56] They are straight and brushlike. The vessels may assume a more random distribution if destruction of corneal tissue occurs.

The importance of limbal edema as a factor in vascularization of the stroma has been emphasized in many studies.[57-64] Normally the stroma is anatomically compact, but if the lamellae become separated, vascular invasion can occur. If limbal edema occurs, neovascularization is made possible. The factors that determine whether vessel ingrowth occurs are not clearly understood.

Maurice[4] theorized that corneal transparency is because of the orderly arrangement of collagen fibrils and because the diameter of each fibril is smaller than the wavelength of light. When the stroma swells, the arrangement of the fibrils is altered, and the amount of scattered light increases. If this increase is great enough, the contours of the retinal image become less distinct, and visual discrimination becomes more difficult. This represents the optic basis for decreased vision from stromal swelling and subsequent scarring.

PATHOGENESIS OF POSTOPERATIVE CORNEAL EDEMA

Any decompression operation may result in corneal edema. If clinically significant, it will be accompanied by folds in Descemet's membrane (striate keratopathy, Fig. 17-1). Generally this condition clears after a time. In my experience, if striate keratopathy or folds in Descemet's membrane occur in one eye after cataract surgery, they usually occur in the second eye after cataract surgery. I have frequently seen patients whose corneas showed no evidence of cornea guttata or other degeneration who, after cataract surgery on the first eye, suffered corneal edema involving all layers of the cornea. This persisted for several weeks to an alarming degree but finally cleared. At first I attributed this to some untoward event during the surgery such as inadvertent endothelial trauma or chemical injury. However, when the second eye had its cataract removed, a similar postoperative course ensued.

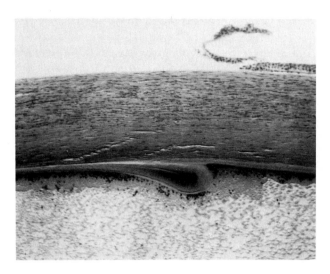

Fig. 17-1. Striate keratopathy. Fold in Descemet's membrane. (×75.) (AFIP No. 168089.) (From Hogan, M. J., and Zimmerman, L. E.: Ophthalmic pathology. An atlas and textbook, ed. 2, Philadelphia, 1962, W. B. Saunders Co.)

This pattern suggests that some inherent factor in the cornea exists in both eyes and causes the cornea to tolerate the trauma of cataract surgery poorly. It is likely that this factor involves the corneal endothelium. As mentioned earlier some patients have a low threshold for endothelial trauma because of a low endothelial cell concentration or some other subclinical factor. A study[65] of the effect of cataract surgery on the cornea revealed that 76% of uneventful cataract extractions caused a significant increase in corneal thickness. The unoperated eyes of these patients had a mean corneal thickness of 0.540 mm, the operated eyes 0.581 mm. If the intraocular pressure is normal after cataract extraction, epithelial edema is likely to appear at a corneal thickness of 0.70 mm (or 30% greater than normal). Although these findings are impressive, there have been contradictory findings by other observers. Although pachymetry used preoperatively may prove to be useful in predicting these corneas likely to suffer from corneal edema postoperatively, we still do not possess a reliable prognostic indicator.

That corneal edema after cataract extraction may be due to factors other than preexisting corneal disease and mechanical trauma during sur-

gery has been receiving greater attention. An excellent study by Edelhauser and co-workers[66] examined the effect of commonly used intraocular irrigating solutions on the corneal endothelium of rabbit and monkey corneas, using a specular microscope perfusion system and scanning and transmission electron microscopy. Corneas perfused with 0.9% NaCl swell at a rate of 60 to 90 μm/hour; endothelial cells separate from each other and show extensive degenerative changes (Fig. 17-2). Corneas perfused with a lactated Ringer's solution swell at a rate of 37 to 40 μm/hour; the endothelial cells show slower but progressive degeneration. Corneas perfused with commercial balanced salt solution (BSS; Alcon Laboratories, Fort Worth, Texas) swell at a rate of 24 to 31 μm/hour; degenerative changes become severe only after 2 hours (Fig. 17-3). Corneas perfused with a Ringer's solution containing bicarbonate, reduced glutathione, and adenosine do not increase thickness, and there is minimal deterioration of endothelial ultrastructure for periods up to 6 hours (Fig. 17-4). These data indicate that the endothelial cell damage observed during perfusion is related to the composition of the irrigating solutions. Balanced salt solution was better than either 0.9% NaCl or lactated Ringer's but was not as ideal as glutathione bicarbonate Ringer's solution, except when glutathione and adenosine were added to the BSS. Other studies have shown that calcium is essential for endothelial cell junctional protection. A bicarbonate buffer system is preferable because bicarbonate is the normal aqueous humor buffer, and glucose is necessary as a substrate for cellular aerobic metabolism. By accident, Dikstein and Maurice[67,68] found that the addition of reduced glutathione to a bicarbonate Ringer's solution improves the performance of the endothelial pump in corneas undergoing temperature reversal. The addition of adenosine (which was known from erythrocyte studies to drive the pentose shunt, which in turn increases the rate of ATP production) was also shown to improve the corneal endothelial pump mechanism. The mechanism by which adenosine and glutathione help to maintain normal corneal endothelial function is still under investigation.

It is not difficult to estimate the importance of these studies when one considers (as noted ear-

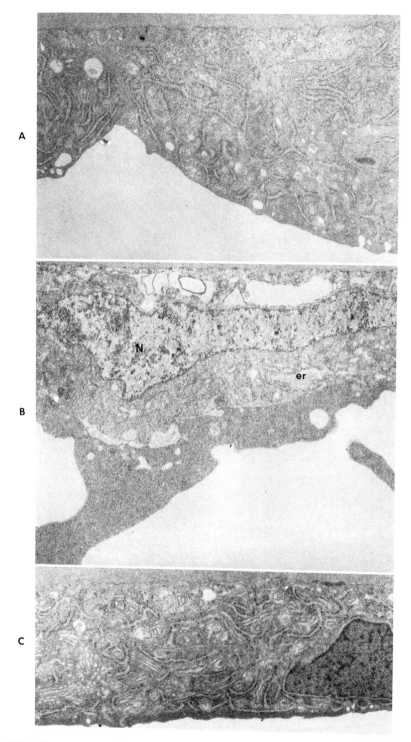

Fig. 17-2. Transmission electron photomicrographs of endothelium of rabbit corneas after perfusion with saline solution. **A,** For 50 minutes. (×14,500.) **B,** For 1.75 hours. Cytoplasmic bleb extends out from apical portion of cell and swelling of nucleus (*N*); cytoplasm and endoplasmic reticulum (*er*) are apparent. (×8700.) **C,** Glutathione-bicarbonate-Ringer solution (GBR) perfusion for 3 hours. (×13,500.) (From Edelhauser, H. F., Van Horn, D. L., Hyndiuk, R. A., and Schultz, R. O.: Arch. Ophthalmol. **93:**648-657, 1975. Copyright 1975, American Medical Association.)

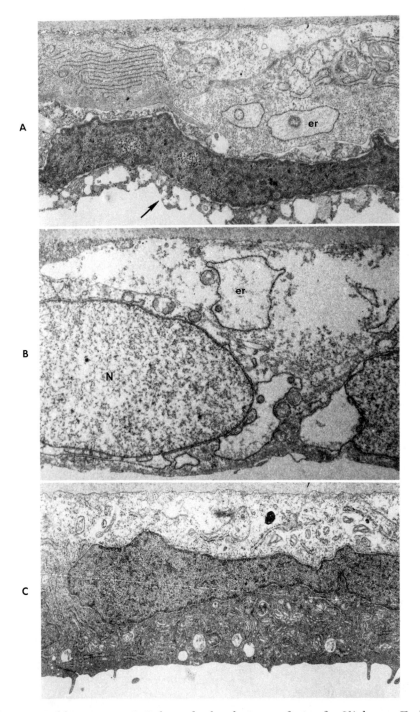

Fig. 17-3. Rabbit corneas. **A,** Balanced salt solution perfusion for 2½ hours. Endoplasmic reticulum *(er)* is dilated in one cell, and cell membrane is discontinuous. (×14,500.) **B,** Balanced salt solution perfused for 5 hours. Cytoplasm, nucleus *(N)*, and endoplasmic reticulum *(er)* are swollen, and posterior cell membrane is discontinuous. (×13,500.) **C,** Paired corneas perfused for 5 hours with balanced salt solution containing adenosine and reduced glutathione. (×15,500.) (From Edelhauser, H. F., Van Horn, D. L., Hyndiuk, R. A., and Schultz, R. O.: Arch. Ophthalmol. **93:**648-657, 1975. Copyright 1975, American Medical Association.)

lier) that a significant increase in corneal thickness may be present in 76% of the eyes of patients after successful intracapsular cataract surgery. This indicates that permanent endothelial damage has occurred, although stromal thickness increases less than 30%, and no epithelial edema or visual loss occurs.[65] Clinically manifest corneal edema and visual loss are significant problems after routine cataract extraction, especially in patients with preexisting endothelial disease or endothelial damage from previous intraocular surgery, inflammation, or trauma.[69] These studies may assume even greater significance in the future, since surgical procedures that employ the prolonged use of large volumes of intraocular irrigating solutions such as phacoemulsification and pars plana vitrectomy will undoubtedly be performed more frequently. In these procedures, corneal edema is a relatively frequent complication.[70,71]

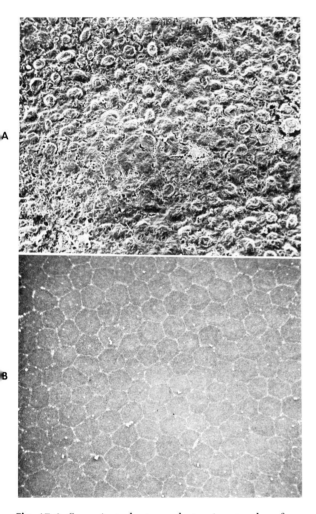

Fig. 17-4. Scanning electron photomicrographs of endothelial surface of monkey corneas following **A,** perfusion with saline for 1¼ hours. Cells have undergone necrotic changes and are pulling apart. (×500.) **B,** Perfusion of GBR for 3 hours. Normal mosaic-like pattern of endothelial cells is present, and their posterior surfaces are smooth. (×500.) (From Edelhauser, H. F., Van Horn, D. L., Hyndiuk, R. A., and Schultz, R. O.: Arch. Ophthalmol. **93:**648-657, 1975. Copyright 1975, American Medical Association.)

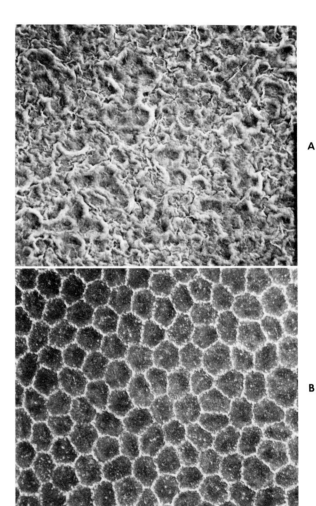

Fig. 17-5. A, Scanning electron micrograph of endothelium of rabbit cornea that had been perfused with epinephrine 1:1000 for 5 minutes. Posterior surface of cells is rough and irregular, and normal mosaic pattern of cell borders has been lost. (×600.) **B,** Scanning electron micrograph of endothelium of rabbit cornea perfused with epinephrine 1:5000 for 3 hours. Posterior surface of cells is flat, and normal masaic pattern of cell borders is maintained. (×600.) (From Hull, D. S., Chemotti, T., Edelhauser, H. F., Van Horn, D. L., and Hyndiuk, R. A.: Am. J. Ophthalmol. **79:**245-250, 1975.)

Hull and co-workers,[72] in another excellent study, showed that commercial epinephrine 1:1000 in its preservative, sodium bisulfite 0.1%, can cause chemically induced endothelial cell breakdown and functional disruption, leading to rapid corneal swelling. The importance of this is underscored by the fact that intracameral epinephrine has been advocated for treatment of iris bleeding and inadequate pupillary dilatation during intraocular surgery. Diluting commercial epinephrine fivefold (1:5000) or using freely soluble epinephrine bitartrate diluted 1:1000 prevented any detectable damage to the corneal endothelium of rabbits and monkeys during a continuous 3-hour perfusion (Fig. 17-5). The damaging effect of commercial epinephrine was found to be related to the preservative sodium bisulfite and not to the epinephrine. Sodium bisulfite is present as a preservative in most epinephrine preparations. At a 1:5000 concentration of commercial epinephrine, the sodium bisulfite was also diluted fivefold, and at this concentration, it was not damaging to the corneal endothelium of rabbits and monkeys.

These significant studies bear emphasis, since it is likely that the cornea of an older human patient with an already decreased endothelial cell population, cornea guttata, or Fuchs' dystrophy would show endothelial cell damage after a much shorter exposure time to the currently available intraocular irrigating solutions and the commercially available epinephrine preparations.

The causes of persistent corneal edema are as follows:

1. Preexisting corneal endothelial disease observed clinically (cornea guttata, Fuchs' dystrophy) or present on a subclinical level (low endothelial cell concentration, early degenerative changes); this may be the sole factor or be associated with any of the following causes
2. Trauma during surgery
3. Adherence of vitreous to the back of the cornea or incarceration in the operative wound
4. Adherence of some other ocular structure, such as iris or lens capsule to the back of the cornea or incarceration in the wound
5. Epithelial downgrowth
6. Endothelial proliferation
7. Fibrous ingrowth
8. Detachment of Descemet's membrane
9. Glaucoma
10. Uveitis
11. Chemical injury from alpha-chymotrypsin, acetylcholine, saline solution, balanced salt solution, epinephrine, pilocarpine, and so on
12. Foreign material introduced during surgery, including lint, rubber, glass, and other particulate matter that adheres to the back of the cornea

Preexisting corneal disease

At best, the surgeon can gain only a clinical impression of an endothelial dystrophy, which may range from a mild, hammered-silver appearance in the center of the cornea to an extensive involvement that includes stromal and epithelial edema and stromal opacification. There are two types of cornea guttata: the primary degenerative type and the postinflammatory type. These excrescences of Descemet's membrane appear as dew drops on the posterior surface of the central cornea and produce focal defects in the endothelial mosaic when viewed by specular reflection. Primary guttata are seldom seen in patients under 50 years of age, but they are present in about 10% of patients between 50 and 70.[73] Guttata alone pose no threat to vision, but when endothelial decompensation is severe, stromal and epithelial edema occurs (Fuchs' dystrophy). By light microscopy, guttata indent the underlying endothelial cells and display a mushroom-shaped configuration, so that a section through the broad flared portion that misses the narrower stalk gives the impression of a disconnected excrescence.[38,74] Descemet's membrane exhibits about three times its normal thickness (20 to 40 μm). In about 20% of cases of Fuchs' dystrophy, guttata are not visible by routine light microscopy.[75] However, phase contrast microscopy[38] or electron micrscopy[25,76] often reveals closely packed excrescences lying within the thickened lamellae with absence of posterior protrusion.

The endothelial cells undergo degeneration and alteration to fibroblast-like cells that become thinned or focally absent beneath the excrescences. There is an increase in rough endoplasmic reticulum and formation of intracellular vacuoles, which enlarge and rupture the cell wall, leading to cell death. These abnormal cells produce the thickened Descemet's membrane.[25,74,76,77] This material consists of three layers.[36] The first layer lies adjacent to the transformed endothelial cells, has a fibrillar appearance, and consists of fine lamellae of collagen and basement membrane substance. The second layer consists of both thin and thick collagen fibrils that may aggregate in bundles and of basement membrane material. The third layer lies adjacent to the original Descemet's membrane and is composed of a sheet of banded material similar to the normal anterior one third of Descemet's membrane, which is interspersed with fusiform bundles of long-spacing collagen. It is a focal thickening of this new banded layer that pushes posteriorly toward the anterior chamber and produces the guttate excrescences.[25] It has been postulated[25] that the fibroblast-like endothelial cells produce the larger collagen fibrils in the first fibrillar layer. These fibrils then become disintegrated into their smaller component fibrils in the second "border layer" but are later recompacted into sheets with the addition of fusiform bundles of long-spacing collagen in the third "posterior banded" layer. This has been interpreted[74] as an attempt by the degenerating endothelium to create a more compact Descemet's membrane and prevent corneal edema.

Secondary cornea guttata is of lesser importance to the cataract surgeon because the surrounding endothelial cells are usually capable of regeneration. when traumatized. A distinctive linear branching pattern is often present in interstitial keratitis.[29,56,60] Secondary guttata have been produced during experimental graft rejection[78] and have been observed in healed corneal wounds in human eyes.[79] They appear similar to primary guttata by electronc microscopy.[80,81] The pathogenesis of the branching linear configuration is still unknown. They do not follow the pattern of the overlying stromal vessels or nerves.[82-84]

Whenever cataract surgery is attempted on an eye with endothelial dystrophy, the surgeon must anticipate complications. There are several prophylactic measures as well as surgical techniques that may be used to lessen the possibility of persistent corneal edema. The surgeon must often make a difficult decision when faced with the problem of a disabling cataract and a moderately advanced endothelial dystrophy in the same eye. A distinction must be made between endothelial dystrophy without edema and one with edema. Generally in the former case a cataract extraction should be the primary procedure. In a dystrophy with persistent edema, cataract extraction combined with a penetrating keratoplasty is preferred. Some surgeons in this situation elect to perform a preliminary penetrating keratoplasty followed about 1 year later by a cataract extraction. My impression is that this latter approach is being abandoned because the risk of edema in a formerly clear graft after cataract surgery is higher, and the interval between procedures is long for some patients. The judgment of the surgeon is severely tested when a method of approach must be chosen to correct an endothelial dystrophy with little, or only intermittent, edema. Since there is no accurate means of evaluating the decompensation potential of the endothelium, the surgeon must make the decision and forewarn the patient of the consequences. Some clinicians depend on corneal thickness measurements to aid them in assessing the decompensation potential of the endothelium and therefore their choice of surgical procedure. For example, it has been suggested[85] that a measurement of 0.620 mm indicates abnormal corneal hydration bordering on decompensation. In such cases, cataract extraction alone as a primary procedure is likely to result in postoperative corneal edema. It is hoped that the specular microscope will eventually be useful in predicting which corneas will decompensate after cataract surgery. There is a tendency, however, for some surgeons to withhold cataract extraction from patients whose corneas show endothelial dystrophy without any signs of decompensation. In my experience, these eyes usually tolerate cataract extraction well if the safeguards here outlined are employed. The following surgical approach may be helpful in minimizing the risk of further corneal damage when cataract extraction is performed in the presence of endothelial dystrophy.

Measures to lessen the chances of operative loss of vitreous. These measures include surgery on a very soft eye. I make my incision only after the Schiøtz tonometer scale reading with a 5.5 g weight is 12 scale units or more (4.9 mm or less). This degree of hypotension is achieved by one or more of the following means (discussed on p. 257):

1. Giving the patient a hyperosmotic agent (glycerin orally or mannitol intravenously) 90 minutes before surgery[86]
2. Applying digital pressure to the globe for at least 5 minutes just before opening the eye
3. Performing a lateral canthotomy
4. Performing a posterior sclerotomy to release retrovitreal aqueous[87]

Surgical technique to minimize endothelial trauma. My personal preference is as follows: A scleral incision at the posterior limbal border is made. Since bleeding is more common here, episcleral vessels near the limbus are cauterized or constricted with epinephrine. The incision is enlarged to close to 180 degrees because a large incision requires less bending of the cornea. Three relatively large, transverse, nearly basal, iridotomies are performed to lessen the chance of pupillary block. I find that although cryoextraction permits the extraction through the smallest incision, one must keep in mind that an inadequate incision can do more harm than good. I use 0.5 ml (1:10,000) of alpha-chymotrypsin irrigated only through two of the iridotomies. To avoid possible endothelial trauma, the enzyme is not placed behind the iris inferiorly. Aside from this, irrigation of the anterior chamber is minimized. To avoid particulate matter contamination, the enzyme is instilled through a disposable Millipore filter unit. Extra sutures to minimize the risk of wound leak are used. I leave the anterior chamber half filled with air at the conclusion of surgery. A long-acting steroid preparation is injected subconjunctivally to minimize postoperative inflammation. I no longer use binocular patches in this situation because the patient is far more restless with them, and other problems often arise. Therefore a monocular dressing is used.

My preference for postoperative care

1. Acetazolamide, 750 mg daily, is prescribed in anticipation of an elevation of intraocular pressure caused by alpha-chymotrypsin. This regimen is continued for 6 days.
2. A sub-Tenon's injection (via the inferior cul-de-sac) of 40 mg of triamcinolone is performed at the conclusion of the surgery.
3. If the patient's physical condition permits, four tablets of a steroid are given daily for 1 week and tapered to zero during the second week.
4. Glycerin is administered by mouth every 12 hours for 4 days, commencing the first night after surgery. This is done to keep the vitreous well back from the cornea. In my experience, vitreocorneal adherence occurs soon after surgery; therefore glycerin has its greatest usefulness at this stage. This is discussed further later.
5. An antibiotic-steroid solution is instilled three times daily for several weeks.
6. A short-acting mydriatic (Cyclomydril) is instilled three times daily simultaneously with the antibiotic-steroid solution for 2 weeks. This minimizes the risk of pupillary block.
7. After the first 2 weeks, 2% pilocarpine solution is placed in the eye twice daily. My impression is that this decreases the incidence of postoperative rupture of the anterior hyaloid membrane with adherence of vitreous fibrils to the cornea. I continue this for 6 weeks or longer.
8. The eye is examined at frequent intervals. Particular attention is directed to the back of the cornea to be sure vitreous is not adherent to it. Vitreous, as well as blood, lint, and capsule remnants, adhere readily to this kind of cornea. If necessary, a topical hyperosmotic agent such as glycerin is used to lessen corneal edema to better visualize the anterior face of the vitreous.

If corneal deterioration is aggravated by the cataract extraction, penetrating keratoplasty or application of a soft contact lens may become necessary. These means are discussed later.

PERSISTENT CORNEAL EDEMA CAUSED BY VITREOCORNEAL ADHERENCE

Persistent corneal edema from vitreocorneal adherence may occur after an uneventful lens extraction (Fig. 17-6). Its incidence is higher if cornea guttata or endothelial dystrophy exists, since vitreous (intact anterior hyaloid membrane or loose vitreous fibrils) adheres easily to dam-

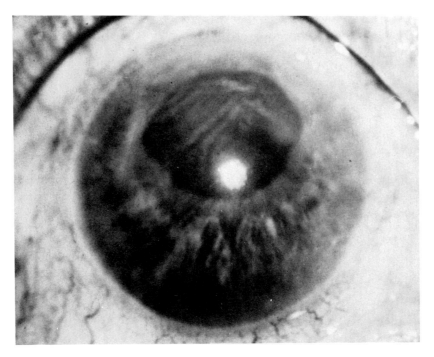

Fig. 17-6. Corneal edema after cataract extraction attributable to vitreocorneal adherence.

aged endothelium. The condition is particularly frustrating for both the patient and the surgeon, since it may follow a well-performed operation.

One cannot emphasize too strongly that the key to successful management of this complication is its early recognition. The treatment gets more complex, and the prognosis becomes worse, the longer this pathologic state exists.

In my experience, this condition is usually an early complication of cataract surgery, occurring in the first few postoperative days when the corneal endothelium is still suffering from surgical trauma and the bulge of the anterior hyaloid membrane is greatest.[88,89] However I have seen several late cases occurring 1 or more years after cataract surgery. In these a rupture of the anterior hyaloid membrane occurred at some time after surgery, and loose vitreous fibrils adhered to the back of the cornea. The cornea remained clear for a long time despite the adherence, but finally corneal edema ensued. As described earlier, sufficient endothelial cell damage results from the vitreous adhesion so that decompensation results.

Pathogenesis

The cause of this complication is varied. Chandler[90] emphasized the role of pupillary block. Either associated with this or independent of it is the occurrence of an early or late flat anterior chamber. In fact, Goar[91] reported the complication in 12 cases out of 300 intracapsular lens extractions. Eight had a late flat chamber, averaging 18 days after surgery. The condition of the corneal endothelium is also important. Damage to the corneal endothelium as a result of surgical trauma establishes a favorable environment for vitreocorneal adherence. However, the presence of corneal endothelial disease (endothelial dystrophy) prior to surgery likewise favors such an adherence. There are also a number of other factors difficult to assess. One must consider those factors such as pooling of retrovitreal aqueous that create a bulge of the anterior hyaloid membrane. I also have the impression that after chemical or mechanical zonulysis, the vitreous loses some of its support at the vitreous base. I do not believe that the vitreous ever detaches from its base, but the vitreous in this area possibly gains some freedom so that is compresses the central core of vitreous, creating a bulge. This is purely speculative. Paufique[92] suggested that these patients demonstrated a genetic fragility—a tempting thought, since it might explain bilateral cases. There appears to be a relatively high incidence of bilaterality with this complication.

Prognosis

When vitreocorneal adherence occurs postoperatively, I have found several prognostic factors useful. It is helpful to clear the cornea with topically administered glycerin to obtain a proper estimate of the vitreocorneal relationship at the slit lamp.

The following acronym helps one remember these prognostic factors: L-A-D-D-E.

1. **L**ocation of the contact. Generally, adherence of vitreous to the center of the cornea is far more serious than adherence to the periphery of the cornea (Figs. 11-1 and 11-2).

2. **A**rea of the contact. Generally, the greater the area of adherence, the poorer the prognosis. The area of contact usually appears larger than it actually is. The actual portions of the adherence are usually marked by lines of adherence oriented horizontally or obliquely. These lines appear as elevated ridges, as if the vitreous is tugging at the back of the cornea. The remainder of the area of contact is usually mere apposition and not true adherence. This may be demonstrated by having the patient look up and down. The vitreous may roll on and off the cornea with these movements.

3. **D**uration of the contact. The longer the persistence of the vitreocorneal adherence, the poorer the prognosis.

4. **D**ensity of the contact. Density is estimated by the ease with which mydriatics and systemically administered hyperosmotic agents effect a separation of the adherence.

5. **E**ndothelium. The status of the corneal endothelium is probably the most important prognostic factor. This includes preoperative corneal disease (endothelial dystrophy) as well as postoperative corneal alterations caused by surgical trauma. Clinical experience tells us that loose vitreous fibrils in contact with a normal cornea after postoperative rupture of the anterior hyaloid membrane do not cause persistent corneal edema, whereas if the endothelium is dis-

eased or damaged, this complication does result. However, many exceptions exist. Loose vitreous fibrils may cause this complication in one patient but not in another because of individual variations in endothelial cell concentration, as discussed previously. Materials such as blood, vit-

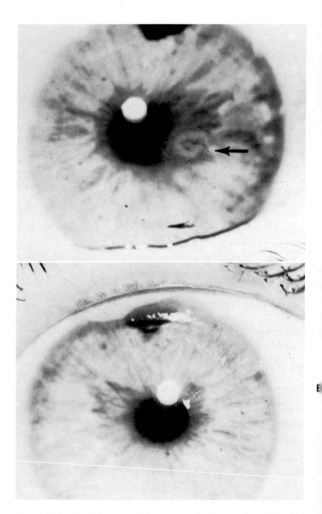

Fig. 17-7. A, Patient with corneal dystrophy (Fuchs' dystrophy), who underwent intracapsular lens extraction in her left eye and suffered vitreocorneal adherence just temporal to the pupil *(arrow).* This localized area of bullous keratopathy has persisted for 5 years without spreading across cornea. No postoperative oral glycerin was used. Visual acuity is 20/30. **B,** Right eye of patient in **A** with corneal dystrophy (Fuchs') after intracapsular lens extraction. Oral glycerin administered postoperatively for 4 days. No vitreocorneal adherence. Visual acuity is 20/30. (From Jaffe, N. S.: The vitreous in clinical ophthalmology, St. Louis, 1969, The C. V. Mosby Co.)

reous, lint, rubber, and suture material adhere with great ease to the dystrophic cornea. It is a pity that we have no reliable means of predicting which corneas with guttata will proceed to develop endothelial dystrophy of the Fuchs type.

Clinical course

The course of this problem is a relentless progression of corneal edema, bullous keratopathy, and late opacification. As described previously, when vitreous adheres to the cornea for a considerable period, the endothelial cells enlarge and eventually disappear, thus depriving the cornea of its pump mechanism. Stromal edema occurs and causes a positive stromal fluid pressure, which favors epithelial edema. Apparently, therefore, these cases must be discovered early, since late treatment is usually ineffective in reversing the corneal edema even if the vitreocorneal adherence is terminated. As an aid to early diagnosis, glycerin is applied topically to clear the cornea; in extreme cases the corneal epithelium may be denuded.

Prophylactic treatment

One might consider various prophylactic measures for patients in whom the first eye suffered this postoperative complication or where an early preoperative corneal dystrophy exists (Fig. 17-7). These are discussed on p. 339.

Medical treatment

When vitreocorneal adherence is detected early, medical therapy may be effective. I have occasionally been successful in terminating the adherence by administering a hyperosmotic agent (glycerin orally or mannitol intravenously).[93] These agents effect a posterior displacement of the anterior hyaloid membrane, presumably by a reduction of vitreous volume. Mydriatics are used in conjunction to minimize pupillary block.

Surgical treatment

Modified Leahey procedure. The best treatment in an early case is that recommended by Leahey[94] (Figs. 17-8 and 17-9). I prefer to use a 25-gauge Rizzuti-Spirizzi cannula needle attached to a syringe to perforate the sclera through the pars plana 5 mm from the limbus. While I aspirate on the syringe, the needle enters the vit-

reous in its posterior superior portion. When the needle penetrates the posterior limiting border of the vitreous, a gush of retrovitreal fluid enters the syringe. One to 2 ml is removed. The needle is removed, and the pars planotomy site need not be sutured. The need for a sharp needle is emphasized in Fig. 17-10. Air is then forced into the anterior chamber by the same cannula needle, which enters the anterior chamber through the limbus in the inferior temporal quadrant. If the bubble of air is fragmented by residual strands of adherent vitreous, one may need to break the adhesion with an iris spatula introduced through the enlarged limbal wound. I have found that this is rarely necessary. If pupillary block is present, a peripheral iridectomy or anterior vitrotomy may be performed through this incision. When the air has successfully separated the vitreous from the cornea, acetylcholine is introduced into the anterior chamber, and the large air bubble is left in place. The miosis is of benefit, since it lessens the chances of a readherence of vitreous to the cornea and of an air-block glaucoma due to air getting behind the iris and into the vitreous. The limbal wound is sutured with a single suture. Postoperatively, glycerin is administered orally every 12 hours for 4 days, and mydriatrics are prescribed.

This surgical approach is effective in early cases (Fig. 17-11) and in an occasional late case (Fig. 17-12). However, after 3 to 4 weeks the chances for a surgical success fall sharply.

Partial anterior vitrectomy via pars plana. A new, effective method of removing vitreous from the anterior chamber without opening the original cataract wound is via a pars plana approach. The instruments of either Machemer (VISC — vitreous infusion suction cutter) or Douvas (roto-extractor) promise to replace the Leahey procedure, since it can safely rid the back of the cornea of adherent vitreous through a relatively small pars plana incision. At this time I know of several successful applications of this method for this complication. It is not likely that this technique will suffer the fate of many promising modalities, since it has had several years of successful trials in the posterior vitreous for removal of opaque material such as organized hemorrhage and amyloid and for removal of traction bands in retinal detachment.

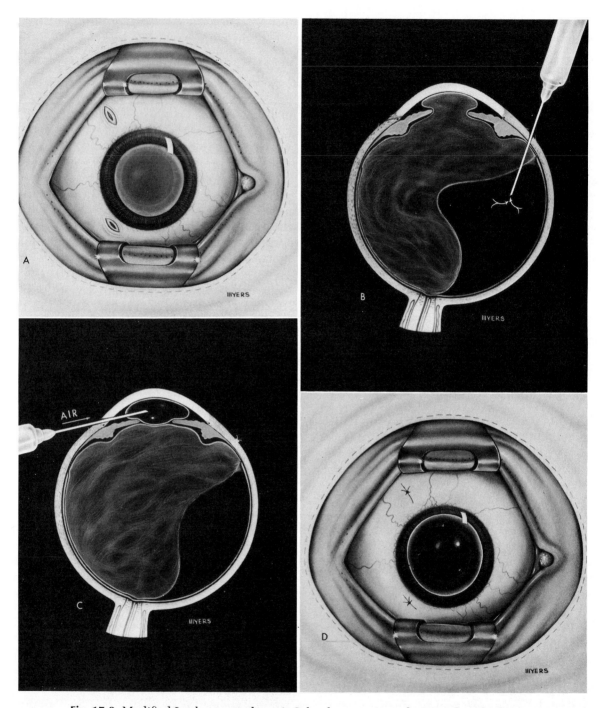

Fig. 17-8. Modified Leahey procedure. **A,** Scleral groove is made 2 mm from limbus in inferior temporal quadrant. **B,** Fluid is aspirated from retrovitreal space via pars planotomy through upper scleral incision with 18-gauge needle. **C,** Air is forcibly pushed into anterior chamber after lower scleral incision into anterior chamber is completed, as in cyclodialysis. **D,** Completion of procedure with air in anterior chamber and scleral incisions sutured. (From Jaffe, N. S.: The vitreous in clinical ophthalmology, St. Louis, 1969, The C. V. Mosby Co.)

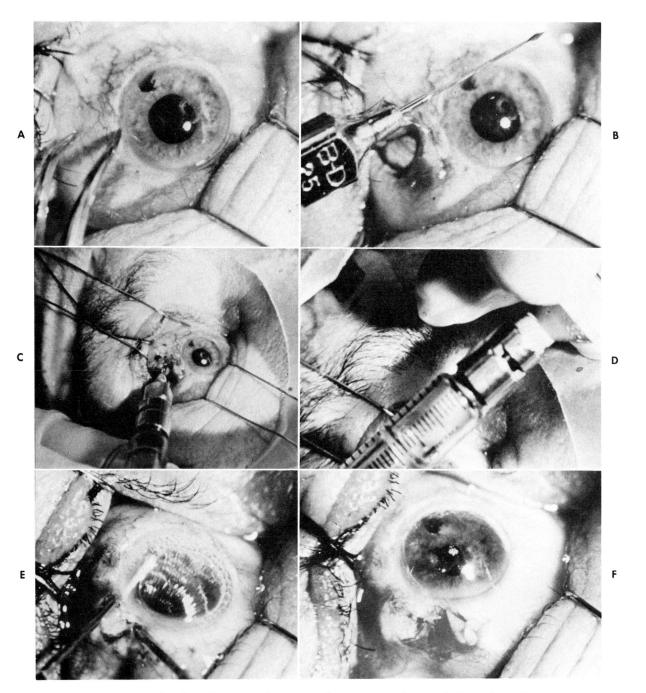

Fig. 17-9. Modified Leahey procedure for early treatment of corneal edema from vitreo-corneal adherence. **A,** Mark made 5 mm from limbus in superior temporal quadrant at site of posterior sclerotomy. **B,** Rizzuti-Spirizzi 25-gauge cannula needle. **C,** Aspiration of fluid vitreous from retrovitreal space. **D,** Air from operating room sterilized by collecting through Millipore filter. **E,** Air injected into anterior chamber through limbal wound. **F,** Miosis achieved after irrigation of acetylcholine solution into anterior chamber. Anterior chamber remains filled with air.

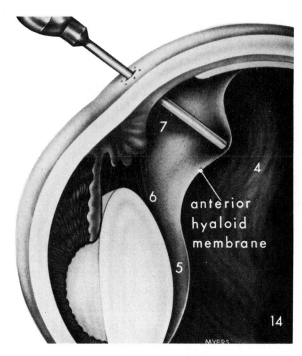

Fig. 17-10. Need for sharp-tipped rather than blunt-tipped needle is demonstrated in performing aspiration of fluid from retrovitreal space. *4,* Formed vitreous. *5,* Berger's space. *6,* Canal of Petit. *7,* Hyaloideo-orbicular space (Garnier). *14,* Retrovitreal space. (After Cibis, P. A.: Vitreoretinal pathology and surgery in retinal detachment, St. Louis, 1965, The C. V. Mosby Co.)

Cryotherapy. Drysdale and Shea[95] have recommended the use of a cryoapplicator applied to the cornea. This destroys the endothelium, permitting the vitreous to retract. Regeneration of the corneal endothelium occurs, resulting in a cure. If pupillary block is present, the cryoapplicator is combined with an iridectomy. They reported success in a single case. I have had no experience with this technique, but I would urge extreme caution, since it is possible to cause a permanent and total corneal decompensation. This technique has not gained much popularity in the 14 years following its introduction.

Partial anterior vitrectomy via open sky. I have occasionally seen patients who developed corneal edema 1 or more years after cataract extraction in whom a rupture of the anterior hyaloid membrane with adherence of loose vitreous strands to the back of the cornea had occurred soon after surgery. These eyes fare well for some

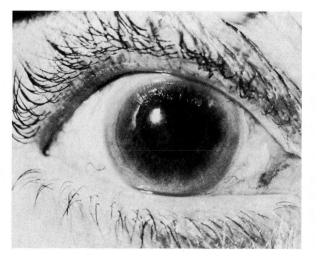

Fig. 17-11. Ideal patient for Leahey treatment. Right eye of patient 2 weeks after intracapsular lens extraction complicated by corneal edema and bullous keratopathy caused by vitreocorneal adherence. (From Jaffe, N. S.: The vitreous in clinical ophthalmology, St. Louis, 1969, The C. V. Mosby Co.; courtesy F. Blanton, Fort Lauderdale, Fla.)

time but then develop intermittent bouts of corneal edema. Close inspection reveals that the vitreous conglomerates in the anterior chamber have thickened, and their adhesions on the back of the cornea have become more apparent. It is typical for the occurrences of corneal edema to become more frequent and more prolonged for the reasons discussed earlier. In these late cases I have found the Leahey procedure useless. I have occasionally been successful in terminating the edema by performing an anterior vitrectomy. However, if the endothelial cell population is markedly attenuated, this procedure will be ineffective.

In performing this technique, a 180-degree section is made. The cornea is retracted with a retraction suture. The vitrectomy is performed by the open-sky technique. With cellulose sponges, bundles of formed vitreous are engaged and excised. As the vitreous is drawn out of the anterior chamber, strands peel off the back of the cornea. Vitreous is removed from the surface of the iris and from the pupillary area until the anterior surface of the remaining vitreous assumes a concave shape behind the level of the iris, and the iris drops back. A considerable amount of vitreous

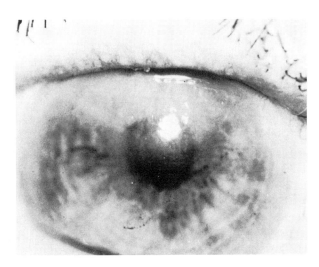

Fig. 17-12. Right eye of patient who underwent intracapsular lens extraction complicated by persistent corneal edema, bullous keratopathy, and almost total corneal opacification. Visual acuity was 10/400. Leahey procedure was performed 5 months after lens extraction. Lower half of cornea cleared, and visual acuity improved to 20/40. Photograph taken 1 year after Leahey procedure was performed. (From Jaffe, N. S.: The vitreous in clinical ophthalmology, St. Louis, 1969, The C. V. Mosby Co.)

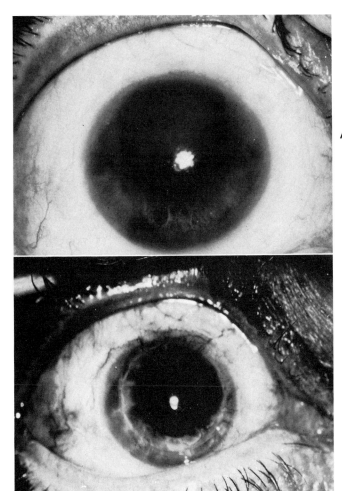

Fig. 17-13. A, Marked corneal edema after intracapsular lens extraction complicated by vitreocorneal adherence. Iris is adherent to cornea at 7 o'clock. **B,** Same eye. An 8 mm penetrating keratoplasty with removal of all vitreous from anterior chamber was performed. Corneal graft remains clear. (From Jaffe, N. S.: The vitreous in clinical ophthalmology, St. Louis, 1969, The C. V. Mosby Co.)

may be removed by this procedure. It is surprising how well the eye tolerates this manipulation. Postoperatively the anterior surface of the vitreous recondenses but usually does not readhere to the cornea.

In two patients the edema recurred 5 weeks and 4 months postoperatively respectively. In two others the corneas remained clear for more than 1 year after the surgery.

It is likely that this technique will be replaced by partial anterior vitrectomy through the pars plana approach.

Penetrating keratoplasty. In late cases with persistent corneal edema, a penetrating keratoplasty offers the best hope for visual rehabilitation. Twenty-five years ago, this would have been considered an unfavorable condition for keratoplasty. There is certainly no unanimity among ophthalmologists, and even among keratoplasty surgeons, that bullous keratopathy associated with vitreocorneal adherence is favorably managed by a corneal transplantation. My personal experience, corroborated by the experience of colleagues with whom I carry on a continuous

dialogue about this subject, indicates that 70% or more of these cases may be successfully grafted.

My impression is that the improvement in prognosis is attributable to (1) more satisfactory suture material, (2) better instrumentation, and (3) improved methods of preventing readherence of vitreous to the cornea. However, in estimating prognosis, one must bear in mind that these cases may be complicated by more than vitreous adherence. There may be extensive anterior iris adhe-

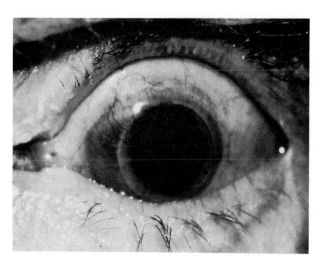

Fig. 17-14. A 7 mm penetrating keratoplasty was performed in eye with corneal edema, bullous keratopathy, extensive adhesions of iris to cornea, and extensive corneal vascularization after intracapsular lens extraction. Corneal graft remains clear. (From Jaffe, N. S.: The vitreous in clinical ophthalmology, St. Louis, 1969, The C. V. Mosby Co.)

sions (Fig. 17-13), corneal vascularization (Fig. 17-14), and glaucoma. If glaucoma is present, the outlook is gloomy. Anterior iris adhesions may be managed at surgery unless they are extensive. Corneal vascularization offers less hope for successful treatment.

Another impression I have gained is that these grafts show a tendency to late clouding. In these instances the recurrence of corneal edema is not usually associated with a readherence of vitreous to the back of the cornea. Although I am unaware of a reported series of cases, some eyes that were successfully grafted developed problems after 3 to 5 years. However, this is tempered by the fact that most of these patients are elderly, and a few years of good vision can be meaningful. Many late failures, in addition, may be successfully regrafted.

For some as yet unexplained reason, there appears to be a relatively high incidence of cystoid macular edema following aphakic keratoplasty. This was emphasized in a recent report[95] that stated that of 42 eyes, 14 had a combined cataract extraction and penetrating keratoplasty, and 28 had a penetrating keratoplasty some time after the cataract extraction. Twenty-seven of the

42 eyes (64%) had cystoid macular edema. It was stressed that eight eyes, which had had no vitreous manipulation during surgery or postoperative vitreous in the wound, had cystoid macular edema or a diffuse macular edema. I have also been aware of a relatively high incidence of cystoid macular edema in these patients. However, when the graft remains clear, the patient is usually pleased with his vision, since the preoperative visual acuity had improved to 20/800 in spite of hand motion and the postoperative acuity between 20/30 and 20/60, in spite of the presence of cystoid macular edema. I have experienced the opposite situation on at least two occasions. In two patients with aphakic bullous keratopathy and angiographically proven cystoid macular edema, there was no cystoid macular edema following penetrating keratoplasty and partial anterior vitrectomy. One of these is worthy of discussion. A 71-year-old man had phthisis bulbi in one eye following an expulsive hemorrhage several days after cataract extraction. The second eye had a cataract extraction that was complicated by persistent corneal edema, probably due to vitreocorneal adherence. When the patient was first seen by me 6 months after the second extraction, the visual acuity had improved to 20/800 in spite of relatively good clearing of the cornea with a topically administered hyperosmotic agent. Fluorescein angiography revealed 4+ cystoid macular edema. Since the eye was not painful, it was felt that a keratoplasty would not improve vision sufficiently to warrant the risk of surgery on this patient's only eye. Within 3 years the cornea opacified, and painful bullous keratopathy ensued. A bandage soft contact lens was fitted for continuous wear. There was no improvement in vision, and the cornea was invaded by vessels. After the vision decreased to hand motion at 6 feet, an 8 mm penetrating keratoplasty and partial anterior vitrectomy were performed. Postoperative visual acuity improved to 20/30 and has remained at this level for more than 5 years. There was no evidence of cystoid macular edema at any time during the postoperative course.

The technique I currently follow is to perform a 7 to 8 mm penetrating keratoplasty, using a Flieringa ring. The donor corneal button is excised with vitreous attached to its back surface. Vitreous may be removed from the anterior chamber with the aid of cellulose sponges (as previously described). However, an automated vitrectomy instrument is far more effective. Formed vitreous is removed from the angle, from the surface of the iris, and from the pupillary area (Fig. 17-15). When the iris falls back posteriorly, sufficient vitreous has been removed. I usually perform two or three peripheral iridotomies. The donor button is sutured in place, preferably with the aid of an operating microscope. The surgical results have been impressive (Figs. 17-16 to 17-20). I have achieved improved results with the following suture technique: Eight interrupted, uniformly separated, deeply inserted, edge-to-edge 10-0 nylon sutures are placed. Wide bites are taken, especially in the edematous host cornea. A continuous 10-0 nylon suture is then inserted, taking two bites between each interrupted suture. It is then tightened, one loop at a time, and tied at its origin. The interrupted sutures are removed in 4 to 6 weeks. The continuous suture is left in place permanently unless the cornea surrounding it becomes vascularized.

Many keratoplasty surgeons manage the vitreous differently. For example, Fine[97] removes vitreous through the pars plana. I prefer the method outlined earlier because I am more certain to evacuate the anterior chamber of vitreous. Condensation of the remaining vitreous usually occurs at the plane of the iris or behind it. It is rare for extensive readherence of vitreous to the back of the cornea, a serious complication, to occur after an anterior vitrectomy.

It is reemphasized that early recognition of this complication after cataract surgery and early reparative surgery will usually make extensive surgical therapy unnecessary.

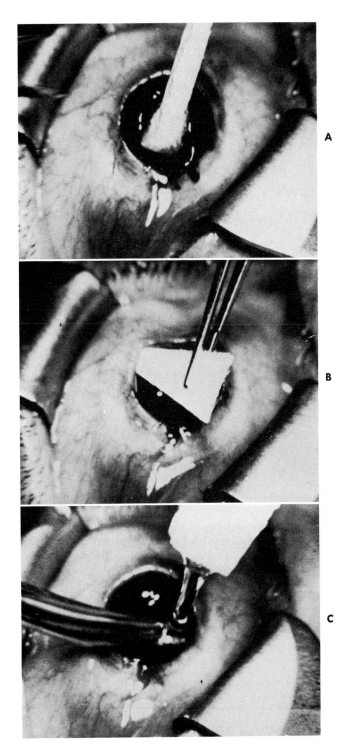

Fig. 17-15. A, Penetrating keratoplasty performed for persistent corneal edema caused by vitreocorneal adherence after lens extraction. Vitreous is excised from anterior chamber by cellulose sponges. **B,** Same eye. Vitreous is removed from angle of anterior chamber. **C,** Same eye. Formed vitreous picked up with cellulose sponge and excised with scissors. (From Jaffe, N. S.: The vitreous in clinical ophthalmology, St. Louis, 1969, The C. V. Mosby Co.; courtesy N. Sanders, North Miami Beach, Fla.)

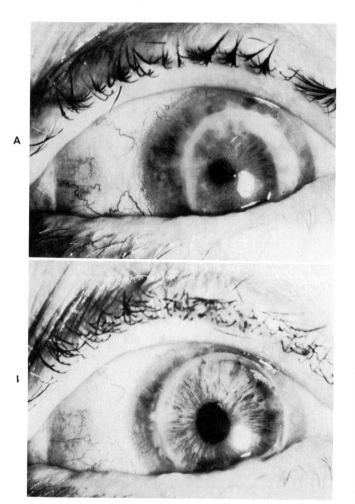

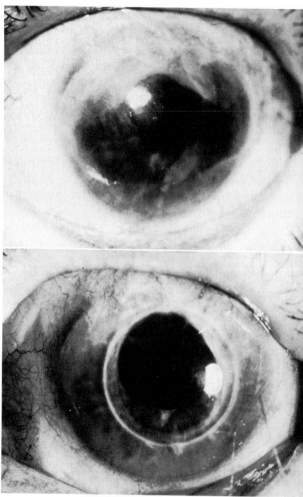

Fig. 17-16. A, Keratoplasty performed for persistent corneal edema caused by vitreocorneal adherence after lens extraction. In this case, vitreous was not excised from anterior chamber. Corneal graft became edematous. **B,** Keratoplasty performed again on same eye. Vitreous was completely removed from anterior chamber. Corneal graft remains clear. (From Jaffe, N. S.: The viteous in clinical ophthalmology, St. Louis, 1969, The C. V. Mosby Co.; courtesy N. Sanders, North Miami Beach, Fla.)

Fig. 17-17. A, Marked corneal edema and bullous keratopathy after intracapsular lens extraction complicated by vitreocorneal adherence. **B,** Same eye. A 7 mm penetrating keratoplasty with removal of all vitreous from anterior chamber was performed. Corneal graft remains clear. (From Jaffe, N. S.: The vitreous in clinical ophthalmology, St. Louis, 1969, The C. V. Mosby Co.; courtesy N. Sanders, North Miami Beach, Fla.)

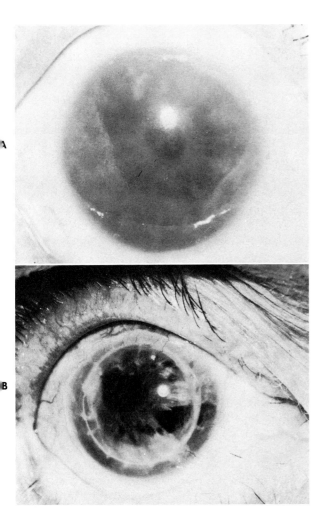

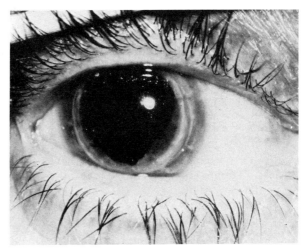

Fig. 17-19. An 8 mm penetrating keratoplasty was performed in 75-year-old woman who suffered persistent corneal edema associated with vitreocorneal adherence after intracapsular lens extraction. Portion of iris adherent to cornea inferiorly was excised. Photograph shows clear corneal graft 13 months after keratoplasty was performed. (From Jaffe, N. S.: The vitreous in clinical ophthalmology, St. Louis, 1969, The C. V. Mosby Co.)

Fig. 17-18. A, Persistent corneal edema 11 months after uneventful intracapsular lens extraction, right eye, in 71-year-old woman. Postoperative course was complicated by corneal edema associated with adherence of vitreous to central area of cornea. Iris was also adherent to cornea at 4 o'clock. B, Same eye after 8 mm penetrating keratoplasty. Portion of iris adherent to cornea at 4 o'clock was excised. Vitreous was removed from anterior chamber. Postoperative adherence of iris to keratoplasty incision at 10 o'clock. Photograph shows clear corneal graft 10 months after keratoplasty was performed. (From Jaffe, N. S.: The vitreous in clinical ophthalmology, St. Louis, 1969, The C. V. Mosby Co.)

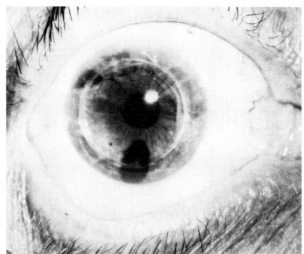

Fig. 17-20. A 7.5 mm penetrating keratoplasty was performed in 75-year-old man who suffered persistent corneal edema associated with vitreocorneal adherence after intracapsular lens extraction. Inferior iridectomy was performed 2 weeks after keratoplasty because of pupillary block. Photograph shows clear corneal graft 18 months after keratoplasty.

Treatment of painful bullous keratopathy

There are occasions when the surgeon must settle for something less than improvement in visual acuity. These are instances of painful bullous keratopathy. If the visual acuity in the opposite eye is satisfactory for the patient's needs, he may be satisfied with reduction of pain. Three methods of eliminating pain are useful.

Treatment with hydrophilic contact lenses. Although early enthusiasts of the bandage contact lens endorsed these lenses for improvement of visual acuity, I have found them disappointing in this regard in eyes with corneal edema. Unless the edema is confined to the epithelium, these lenses are usually ineffective in improving vision. Most of these eyes have corneal stromal involvement with some opacification. This is not lessened by hydrophilic lenses. However, they are frequently effective in reducing the pain of bullous keratopathy.

These lenses were first reported by Wichterle and Lim[98] in 1960. The lenses currently available in the United States are greatly improved over the original Czechoslovakian prototypes. Undoubtedly newer and better lenses will become available.

The bandage lens may be used in eyes that require topical medication. Hyperosmotic solutions may be used with the lens in situ. This may improve visual acuity to a small degree, although not to the extent originally advertised.

The material used in these lenses is 2-hydroxyethyl methacrylate (HEMA). A polymer results when pure HEMA is polymerized in the presence of bifunctional monomer such as ethylene glycol dimethacrylate (EGDM) to form a three-dimensional network of hydroxyethyl methacrylate chains crosslinked occasionally with diester molecules, approximately one every 200 monomer units as an average.

The following properties make them useful in ophthalmology:
1. Softness
2. Optic suitability
3. Water absorption ability, with a concomitant swelling to a soft mass of good mechanical strength
4. Complete transparency
5. Ability to retain shape and dimensions when equilibrated in a given fluid
6. Shape recovery after deformation

Although these lenses contain water, there is no satisfactory exchange of fluid and nutrients through them. These must come by tear flow and other means. They do not overcome astigmatism greater than 1.50 D. At this time, most normal eye medications can be used with the bandage lens, but fluorescein may permanently stain the lens. Not only is the anterior irregular astigmatism relieved, but the stromal swelling and haze, which can increase with an impermeable anterior surface barrier, are decreased when the soft lenses and hypertonic solutions are combined. Similarly the reduced corneal thickness with the hypertonic agents decreases the Descemet's folds and their interference with vision.[99]

For therapeutic purposes, soft hydrophilic contact lenses have been comfortably and successfully worn over pathologic and irregular corneal epithelium. Their beneficial effect in these cases has been attributed to the fact that they contain almost half their own weight in water. Therefore the hydrated lens used over the dry cornea acts as a precorneal source of fluid, besides protecting the cornea against exogenous trauma and eliminating the irregular astigmatism.[99]

The hydrophilic contact lens will provide the patient with bullous keratopathy rapid relief of pain. The mechanism by which soft lenses relieve pain in bullous keratopathy is not clear, but they are of unquestionable benefit in this regard. They may be worn day and night for long periods. Again, some of the initial enthusiasm for continuous wear must be tempered by the fact that a significant number of edematous corneas become dangerously vascularized. Also, there have been reports of corneal ulcers developing while the lenses were in place. The indications and results of these lenses will come into sharper focus in the very near future.

Cautery of Bowman's membrane. A second effective method of eliminating pain in aphakic bullous keratopathy is cautery of Bowman's membrane. An excellent, instructive report of this technique was recently provided.[100] The authors treated 100 eyes with painful bullous keratopathy. After scraping the corneal epithelium, they placed an average of 700 applications to Bowman's membrane with the Bovie electrosurgical unit. The unit was set for diathermy applications, and power controls were set to zero. A blunt tip diathermy probe was used. Light and electron microscopy demonstrated an extensive subepithelial connective tissue, probably formed by an extension of stromal connective tissue through breaks in Bowman's membrane. They suggested that the ground substance in this new tissue was responsible for an increased resistance to edema fluid and prevention of subepithelial bullae. Ninety-eight percent of their patients had marked to complete relief of pain.

Gundersen conjunctival flap. A thin Gundersen flap is another effective method of eliminating pain in this situation. Although effective for symptomatic relief, it usually leaves the patient with ptosis of the upper eyelid.

Peripheral corneal edema after cataract extraction

Brown and McLean[101,102] described an unusual form of peripheral corneal edema that spares the cornea between the 10 and 2 o'clock positions. The clinical characteristics of the entity are as follows:

1. The edema is both stromal and epithelial, extends to the limbus, and avoids the incision area and a central zone with a 5 to 7 mm diameter.
2. The edema may involve the central zone in the presence of cornea guttata. It is usually transient in these cases.
3. There is no associated corneal vascularization.
4. An orange punctate pigmentation of the posterior cornea behind the edematous area occurs in most cases.
5. Atrophy of the peripheral iris is seen by transillumination. This atrophy is probably not the result of liberation of iris pigment, since the trabecular mesh-work is not unduly pigmented in these cases.
6. There is nothing in the history of these patients to indicate that the edema is secondary to inflammation, synechia, or glaucoma.
7. The condition has not been seen earlier than 6 years after cataract extraction.
8. Women predominantly have this edema (11 of 13 patients).
9. It is usually bilateral if both eyes are aphakic.
10. It can occur after an extracapsular extraction,[50] although the authors at first stated

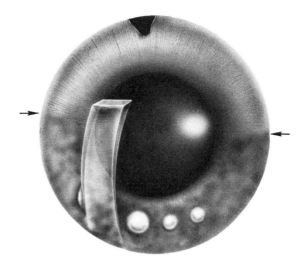

Fig. 17-21. Peripheral corneal edema observed many years after cataract extraction. Edema avoids incision area. *Arrows,* Transition between edematous and normal cornea.

that it always followed an intracapsular extraction.
11. Surgical trauma apparently is not the cause, since one patient with superior subluxation of both lenses showed the syndrome. However, this patient's anterior chambers were similar to those of an aphakic patient.
12. The cause is unknown, but the entity may be related to the prolonged presence of the aphakic type of angle.

I have observed the entity in four patients — three women and one man. The latter had had an extracapsular extraction of a congenital cataract 19 years earlier (Fig. 17-21).

REFERENCES

1. Schwarz, W.: Elecktronmikroskopische Untersuchungen über der Aufbau der Sklera und der Cornea des Menschen, Z. Zellforsch. **38:**26-49, 1953.
2. Jakus, M. A.: The fine structure of the human cornea. In Smelser, G. K., editor: The structure of the eye, New York, 1961, Academic Press, Inc., pp. 343-366.
3. François, J., Rabaey, M., and Vandermeerssche, G.: L'ultrastructure des tissus oculaires au microscope électronique. II. Étude de la cornée et de la sclérotique, Ophthalmologica **127:**74-85, 1954.
4. Maurice, D. M.: The structure and transparency of the cornea, J. Physiol. **136:**263-286, 1957.
5. Dohlman, C. H.: Corneal edema and vascularization. In King, J. H., Jr., and McTigue, J. H., editors: The Cornea

World Congress, London, 1965, Butterworth & Co. (Publishers), Ltd., pp. 80-95.

6. Kinsey, V. E., and Cogan, D. G.: The cornea. III. Hydration properties of excised corneal pieces, Arch. Ophthalmol. **28:**272-284, 1942.

7. Anseth, A.: Studies on corneal polysaccharides. III. Topographic and comparative biochemistry, Exp. Eye Res. **1:**106-115, 1961.

8. Hedbys, B. O.: The role of the polysaccharides in corneal swelling, Exp. Eye Res. **1:**81-91, 1961.

9. Hedbys, B. O., and Dohlman, C. H.: A new method for the determination of the swelling pressure of the corneal stroma in vitro, Exp. Eye Res. **2:**122-129, 1963.

10. Maurice, D. M.: The cornea and sclera. In Davson, H., editor: The eye, New York, 1962, Academic Press, Inc., p. 309.

11. Hedbys, B. O., and Mishima, S.: Flow of water in the corneal stroma, Exp. Eye Res. **1:**262-275, 1962.

12. Hedbys, B. O., Mishima, S., and Maurice, D. M.: The imbibition pressure of the corneal stroma, Exp. Eye Res. **2:**99-111, 1963.

13. Schwartz, B., Danes, B., and Leinfelder, P. J.: The role of metabolism in the hydration of the isolated lens and cornea, Am. J. Ophthalmol. **38**(part 2):182-194, 1954.

14. Davson, H.: The hydration of the cornea, Biochem. J. **59:**24-28, 1955.

15. Harris, J. E., and Nordquist, L. T.: The hydration of the cornea. I. Transport of water from the cornea, Am. J. Ophthalmol. **40**(part 2):100-111, 1955.

16. Langham, M. E., and Taylor, I. S.: Factors affecting the hydration of the cornea in the excised eye and the living animal, Br. J. Ophthalmol. **40:**321-340, 1956.

17. Donn, A., Maurice, D. M., and Mills, N. L.: Studies on the living cornea in vitro. I. Method and physiologic measurements, Arch. Ophthalmol. **62:**741-747, 1959.

18. Dohlman, C. H., and Boruchoff, S. A.: Corneal edema after cataract surgery, Int. Ophthalmol. Clin. **4:**979-998, 1964.

19. Anseth, A., and Dohlman, C. H.: Influence of the intraocular pressure on hydration of the corneal stroma, Acta Ophthalmol. **35:**85-90, 1957.

20. Ytteborg, J., and Dohlman, C. H.: Corneal edema and intraocular pressure. II. Clinical results, Arch. Ophthalmol. **74:**477-484, 1965.

21. Cogan, D. G.: Experimental production of so-called bullous keratitis, Arch. Ophthalmol. **23:**918-925, 1940.

22. Irvine, A. R., Jr.: Pathology of corneal endothelium. In King, J. H., Jr., and McTigue, J. W., editors: The Cornea World Congress, London, 1965, Butterworth & Co. (Publishers) Ltd., pp. 61-72.

23. Fuchs, E.: Erkrangung der hornhaut durch Schädigung von hinten, Arch. Ophthalmol. **92:**145-236, 1917.

24. Hogan, M. J., Alvarado, J. A., and Weddell, J. E.: Histology of the human eye, Philadelphia, 1971, W. B. Saunders Co.

25. Iwamoto, T., and DeVoe A. G.: Electron microscopic studies on Fuchs' combined dystrophy. I. Posterior portion of the cornea, Invest. Ophthalmol. **10:**9-28, 1971.

26. Kuwabara, T., Quevedo, A. R., and Cogan, D. G.: An experimental study of dichloroethane poisoning, Arch. Ophthalmol. **79:**321-330, 1968.

27. Perlman, M., and Baum, J. L.: Collagen reduction in mass cultures of rabbit corneal endothelial cells. Presented at meeting of Assoc. Res. Vision and Ophthalmol., Sarasota, Fla., May 3-7, 1973.

28. Kaye, G. I., Perlman, M., and Baum, J.: Fine structure and synthetic activity of rabbit corneal endothelium grown in vitro. Presented at meeting of Assoc. Res. Vision Ophthalmol., Sarasota, Fla., May 3-7, 1973.

29. Perlman, M., and Baum, J.: Synthesis of a collagenous basal membrane by rabbit corneal endothelial cells in vitro, Arch. Ophthalmol. **92:**238-239, 1974.

30. Kefalides, N. A.: Isolation of a collagen from basement membranes containing three identical α-chains, Biochem. Biophys. Res. Commun. **45:**226-234, 1971.

31. Kefalides, N. A.: The chemistry and structure of basement membranes, Arthritis Rheum. **12:**427-443, 1969.

32. Fine, B. S., and Yanoff, M.: Ocular histology. A text and atlas, New York, 1972, Harper & Row, Publishers, pp. 150-162.

33. Spiro, R. G.: Biochemistry of the renal glomerular basement membrane and its alterations in diabetes mellitus, N. Engl. J. Med. **288:**1337-1342, 1973.

34. Thiele, H., Flasch, R., and Joraschky, W.: Histolyse der Cornea. Descemet-membran, Albrecht v. Graefes Arch. Klin. Exp. Ophthalmol. **179:**157-174, 1970.

35. Boruchoff, S. A., and Kuwabara, T.: Electron microscopy of posterior polymorphous degeneration, Am. J. Ophthalmol. **72:**879-887, 1971.

36. Waring, G. O., Laibson, P. R., and Rodrigues, M.: Clinical and pathologic alterations of Descemet's membrane: with emphasis on endothelial metaplasia, Surv. Ophthalmol. **18:**325-368, 1973-74.

37. Davanger, M.: Descemetocele and the law of Laplace, Acta Ophthalmol. **49:**715-718, 1971.

38. Chi, H. H., Teng, C. C., and Katzin, H. M.: Histopathology of primary endothelial-epithelial dystrophy of the cornea, Am. J. Ophthalmol. **45:**518-535, 1958.

39. Cogan, D. G.: Applied anatomy and physiology of the cornea, Ophthalmology (Rochester) **55:**329-359, 1951.

40. Irvine, A. R., and Irvine, A. R., Jr.: Variations in normal corneal endothelium; a preliminary report of pathologic human corneal endothelium, Am. J. Ophthalmol. **36:**1279-1285, 1953.

41. Cogan, D. G., and Kuwabara, T.: Growth and regenerative potential of Descemet's membrane, Trans. Ophthalmol. Soc. U.K. **91:**875-894, 1971.

42. Jakus, M. A.: Further observations on the fine structure of the cornea, Invest. Ophthalmol. **1:**202-225, 1962.

43. Henderson, J. W., and Wolter, J. R.: Separation of Descemet's membrane in keratoplasty, Am. J. Ophthalmol. **65:**375-378, 1968.

44. Daicker, B.: Gewebliche Diskontinuitätszonen in der gesunden und pathologisch veränderten menschlichen Descemet's schen membrane, Ophthalmologica **161:**166-174, 1970.

45. Fehér, J., and Valu, L.: Über die struktur der Descemetschen membrane, Albrecht v. Graefes Arch. klin. exp. Ophthalmol. **179:**65-73, 1970.

46. Fränkl, G. C.: Argyrophile diskontinuitätsschichten der menschlichen Descemetschen membran. Albrecht v. Graefes Arch Klin. Exp. Ophthalmol. **178:**277-294, 1969.

47. Donaldson, D. D., and Smith, T. R.: Descemet's membrane tubes, Trans. Am. Ophthalmol. Soc. **64**:89-109, 1966.

48. Lauring, L.: Anterior chamber glass membranes, Am. J. Ophthalmol. **68**:308-312, 1969.

49. Wolter, J. R., and Fechner, P. U.: Glass membranes on the anterior iris surface, Am. J. Ophthalmol. **53**:235-243, 1962.

50. Flaxel, J. T., and Swan, K. C.: Limbal wound healing after cataract extraction. A histological study, Arch. Ophthalmol. **81**:653-659, 1969.

51. Klouček, F.: The corneal endothelium, Acta Univ. Carol. Medica, **13**:321-373, 1967.

52. Van Horn, D. L., Edelhauser, H. F., Aaberg, T. M., and Pederson, H. J.: In vivo effects of air and sulfur hexafluoride gas on rabbit corneal endothelium, Invest. Ophthalmol. **11**:1028-1036, 1972.

53. Capella, J. A.: Regeneration of endothelium in diseased and injured corneas, Am. J. Ophthalmol. **74**:810-817, 1972.

54. Matsuda, H., and Smelser, G. K.: Endothelial cells in alkali-burned corneas. Ultrastructural alterations, Arch. Ophthalmol. **89**:402-409, 1973.

55. Bloom and Fawcett, D. W.: A textbook of histology, ed. 9, Philadelphia, 1968, W. B. Saunders Co.

56. Ehlers, H.: Some experimental researches on corneal vessels, Acta Ophthalmol. **5**:99-112, 1927.

57. Cogan, D. G.: Vascularization of the cornea, its experimental induction by small lesions and a new theory of its pathogenesis, Arch. Ophthalmol. **41**:406-416, 1949.

58. Mann, I., Pirie, A., and Pullinger, B. D.: An experimental and clinical study of the reaction of the anterior segment of the eye to chemical injury, with special reference to chemical warfare agents, Br. J. Ophthalmol., Monogr. Suppl. 13, 1948.

59. Ashton, N., and Cook, C.: Mechanism of corneal vascularization, Br. J. Ophthalmol. **37**:193-209, 1953.

60. Langham, M.: Observations on the growth of blood vessels into the cornea. Application of a new experimental technique, Br. J. Ophthalmol. **37**:210-222, 1953.

61. Heydenreich, A.: Das Verhalten der Hornhautvaskularisation im Tierversuch, Klin. Mbl. Augenheilk. **127**:465-471, 1955.

62. Levene, R., Shapiro, A., and Baum, J.: Experimental corneal vascularization, Arch. Ophthalmol. **70**:242-249, 1963.

63. Cook, C., and Langham, M.: Corneal thickness in interstitial keratitis, Br. J. Ophthalmol. **37**:301-304, 1953.

64. Szeghy, G.: Die Rolle der Shädigung im Mechanismus der experimentellen Hornhaut-Vaskularisation, Graefe Arch. Ophthalmol. **162**:215-218, 1960.

65. Miller, D., and Dohlman, C. H.: Effect of cataract surgery on the cornea, Ophthalmology (Rochester) **74**:369-374, 1970.

66. Edelhauser, H. F., Van Horn, D. L., Hyndiuk, R. A., and Schultz, R. O.: Intraocular irrigating solutions. Their effect on the corneal endothelium, Arch. Ophthalmol. **93**:648-657, 1975.

67. Dikstein, S., and Maurice, D. M.: The metabolic bases to the fluid pump in the cornea, J. Physiol. **221**:29-41, 1972.

68. Dikstein, S.: Efficiency and survival of the corneal endothelial pump, Exp. Eye Res. **15**:639-644, 1973.

69. Dohlman, C. H., and Hyndiuk, R. A.: Subclinical and manifest corneal edema after cataract extraction. In Transactions of the New Orleans Academy of Ophthalmology. Symposium on the cornea, St. Louis, 1972, The C. V. Mosby Co., pp. 224-235.

70. Emery, J. M., and Paton, D.: Phacoemulsification. A survey of 2,875 cases, Ophthalmology (Rochester) **78**: OP 31-34, 1974.

71. Straatsma, B. R.: Summary, Symposium: Surgery of the vitreous body, Ophthalmology (Rochester) **78**:216-220, 1974.

72. Hull, D. S., et al.: Effect of epinephrine on the corneal endothelium, Am. J. Ophthalmol. **79**:245-250, 1975.

73. Kaufman, H. E., Capella, J. A., and Robbins, J. E.: The human corneal endothelium, Am. J. Ophthalmol. **61**: 835-841, 1966.

74. Kayes, J., and Holmberg, A.: The fine structure of the cornea in Fuchs' endothelial dystrophy, Invest. Ophthalmol. **3**:47-67, 1964.

75. Stocker, F. W.: The endothelium of the cornea and its clinical implications, ed. 2, Springfield, Ill., 1971, Charles C Thomas, Publisher.

76. Pouliquen, Y., et al.: Dystrophie congénitale de la cornée. Etude en microscopie optique et un microscopie électronique, Arch. Ophthalmol. **32**:391-414, 1972.

77. Jakus, M. A.: Ocular fine structure, Boston, 1964, Little, Brown, and Co.

78. Inomata, H., Smelser, G. K., and Polack, F. M.: Fine structure of regenerating endothelium and Descemet's membrane in normal and rejecting corneal grafts, Am. J. Ophthalmol. **70**:48-64, 1970.

79. Chi, H. H., Teng, C. C., and Katzin, H. M.: Histopathology of corneal endothelium. A study of 176 pathologic discs removed at keratoplasty, Am. J. Ophthalmol. **53**: 215-235, 1962.

80. Edmonds, C., and Iwamoto, T.: Electron microscopy of late interstitial keratitis, Ann. Ophthalmol. **4**:693-696, 1972.

81. Van Horn, D. L., and Schultz, R. O.: Electron microscopy of syphilitic interstitial keratitis (abstract), Invest. Ophthalmol. **10**:469, 1971.

82. Balavoine, C.: Les formations hyalines retrocornennes acquises, Ann. Oculist. **186**:111-140, 1953.

83. Vogt, A.: Lehrbuch und Atlas der Spaltlampenkikroskopie des Lebenden Auges. Vol. I, Berlin, 1930, Springer Verlag, pp. 260-261.

84. Wolter, J. R.: Secondary corneal guttata in interstitial keratopathy, Ophthalmologica **148**:289-295, 1964.

85. Farris, R. L.: Surgical precautions with the abnormal cornea, Datelines in Ophthalmology (Merck, Sharp, and Dohme) **2**(1):9, 1965.

86. Jaffe, N. S., and Light, D. S.: Oral glycerin in cataract surgery, Arch. Ophthalmol. **73**:516-518, 1965.

87. Iliff, C. E.: A surgically soft eye by posterior sclerotomy, Am. J. Ophthalmol. **61**:276-278, 1966.

88. Harrington, D. O.: Late changes in the vitreous following uncomplicated intracapsular cataract extraction, Am. J. Ophthalmol. **35**:1177-1184, 1952.

89. Goswami, A. P., Mathur, K. N., and Raizada, I. N.: Vitreous face after intracapsular lens extraction, Orient. Arch. Ophthalmol. **5**:42-46, 1967.

90. Chandler, P. A.: Complications after cataract extraction: clinical aspects, Ophthalmology (Rochester) **58**:382-396, 1954.

91. Goar, E. L.: Postoperative hyaloid adhesions to the cornea, Am. J. Ophthalmol. **45**:99-102, 1958.

92. Paufique, L., and Royer, J.: Complications post-opératoires survenant aprés une extraction du cristallin et dues au vitré antérieur, Ann. Oculist. **193**:545-560, 1960.

93. Jaffe, N. S., and Light, D. S.: Treatment of postoperative cataract complications by osmotic agents, Arch. Ophthalmol. **75**:370-374, 1966.

94. Leahey, B. D.: Bullous keratitis from vitreous contact, Arch. Ophthalmol. **46**:22-32, 1951.

95. Drysdale, I. O., and Shea, M.: Cryolysis of adhesion of anterior hyaloid membrane to corneal endothelium after uncomplicated cataract extraction, Arch. Ophthalmol. **76**:4-6, 1966.

96. West, C. E., Fitzgerald, C. R., and Sewell, J. H.: Cystoid macular edema following aphakic keratoplasty, Am. J. Ophthalmol. **75**:77-81, 1973.

97. Fine, M.: Keratoplasty in aphakia. In King, J. H., Jr., and McTigue, J. W., editors: The Cornea World Congress, London, 1965, Butterworth & Co. (Publishers), Ltd., pp. 538-552.

98. Wichterle, O., and Lin, D.: Hydrophilic gels for biological use, Nature **185**:117-118, 1960.

99. Gasset, A. R., and Kaufman, H. E.: Therapeutic uses of hydrophilic contact lenses, Am. J. Ophthalmol. **69**:252-259, 1970.

100. Farria, R. L., Iwamoto, T., and DeVoe, A. G.: Cautery of Bowman's membrane, Am. J. Ophthalmol. **77**:548-554, 1974.

101. Brown, S. I., and McLean, J. M.: Peripheral corneal edema after cataract extraction; a new clinical entity, Ophthalmology (Rochester) **73**:465-470, 1969.

102. Brown, S. I.: Peripheral corneal edema after cataract extraction, Am. J. Ophthalmol. **70**:326-328, 1970.

CHAPTER 18

Cystoid macular edema (Irvine-Gass syndrome)

We have known for some time that macular edema may occur sometime during the postoperative period of a cataract extraction. In 1952, Irvine[1] described a syndrome that now bears his name. By definition this included improvement of vision after cataract surgery, followed by diminution of vision associated with a postoperative rupture of the anterior hyaloid membrane, with or without adherence of vitreous to the surgical wound.

PATHOPHYSIOLOGY

Before an attempt is made to bring the clinical facts up to date, since Irvine's original description of this syndrome, the anatomic, pathologic, and physiologic properties of the macula will be considered.

The macula lutea is a shallow oval depression about the same size as the disc. Its center is located 3.5 mm lateral to the temporal edge of the disc and slightly below its middle. The side walls of the macula, its clivus, slope gradually toward its center, the fovea centralis. At the macula the ganglion cells are much more numerous than elsewhere in the retina, being arranged in several layers (five to seven). The outer plexiform layer is also thicker than elsewhere and is referred to here as the fiber layer of Henle. There is also a progressive disappearance of rods, which are replaced by cones. The pigment epithelial layer and the choriocapillaris are thicker at the macula, which is of significance, since the macula contains no retinal blood vessels.

The fovea centralis occupies the center of the macula and is the thinnest part of the retina, since it has no inner nuclear layer, inner plexiform layer or ganglion cells and practically no nerve fiber layer. At the fovea the layers of the retina are spread aside so that light may fall directly on the true percipient elements, the cones.[2] In the retina, each ganglion cell is connected to many visual cells (in up to 100 rods), whereas at the fovea, each cone is connected to only one ganglion cell. However, the latter has not been confirmed by electron microscopy.

At the center of the fovea the foveal cone cells, located in an area of about 50 μm in diameter, are separated from each other by relatively wide spaces of watery cytoplasm belonging to Müller's fibers. The basal lamina is extremely thin at the center of the fovea. The thinness of the basal lamina and the watery cytoplasm of Müller's fiber at the center of the fovea are most likely devices to help light to transpierce the retinal thickness.[3] The area is therefore largely made up of cone cells and Müller's fibers.

According to Wolff[2] the outer plexiform layer is made up of the arborization of the axones of the rods and cone granules with the dendrites of the bipolar cells. This layer also includes Müller's fibers and the processes of the horizontal cells. Elsewhere in the retina, this layer has a reticular structure, but as the macula is approached, it takes on a fibrous structure, hence the name Henle's fiber layer. The fibers at first run vertically, then obliquely near the macula, and finally parallel to the surface within the macular area. This layer is thickest at the macula but almost absent at the fovea.

The internal limiting membrane as seen by the

electron microscopist (going from in to out) has been resolved into the outermost vitreous fibrils, the basement membrane, and the outer cytoplasm of Müller's fibers. This layer is lost at the optic nerve head where it is continuous with the neuroglia forming the central connective tissue meniscus of Kuhnt. It undergoes a marked change as the macula is approached. The thickness of the basal lamina (basement membrane) at the macula is about 1.5 μm, as shown by Yamada's electron microscopic study.[3] At the periphery of the fovea it is 0.4 μm thick and at the foveal center, it is reduced to 10 to 20 mμm (Figs. 18-1 to 18-4).

The external limiting membrane at the macula is sometimes pushed inward, forming a concave depression that faces the choroid (fovea externa). However, electron microscopic studies[3] reveal that at the very center of the fovea, the external limiting membrane shows a slightly convex sur-

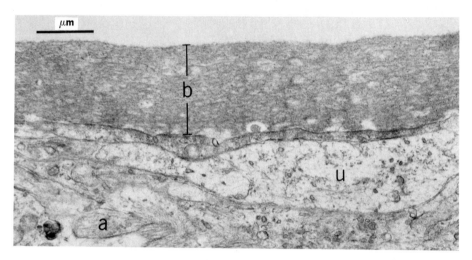

Fig. 18-1. Vitreal surface of retina at macular region. *b*, Basal lamina is about 1.5 μm thick; *a*, nerve fiber; *u*, process of Müller's fiber. (Reduced from ×17,400.) (From Yamada, E.: Arch. Ophthalmol. **82:**151-159, 1969.)

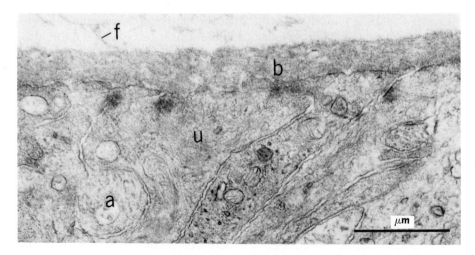

Fig. 18-2. Vitreal surface of peripheral fovea (*f*). *b*, Basal lamina is about 0.4 μm thick at this area; *a*, cross section of ganglion cell axon; *u*, foot process of Müller's fiber. (Reduced from ×29,000.) (From Yamada, E.: Arch. Ophthalmol. **82:**151-159, 1969.)

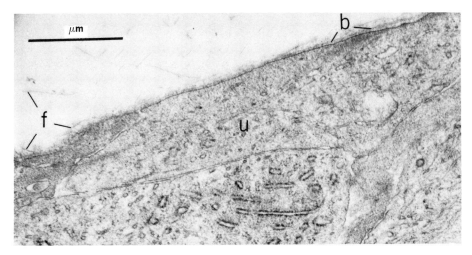

Fig. 18-3. Vitreal surface of fovea (*f*) at center. *b*, Basal lamina is extremely thin (10 to 20 mμm) in this area; floor of fundus is composed of processes from Müller's fibers, *u*. (Reduced from ×29,000.) (From Yamada, E.: Arch. Ophthalmol. 82:151-159, 1969.)

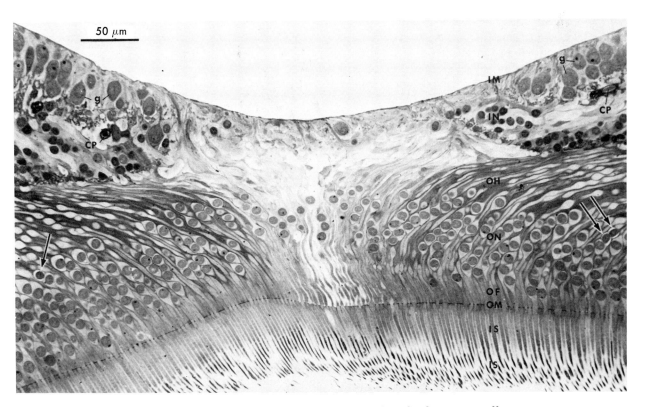

Fig. 18-4. Section through center of fovea. *Arrows*, Nuclei of rod receptor cells; remaining receptor cells are foveal cone cells; *g*, ganglion cell; *CP*, capillary; *IM*, internal limiting membrane; *IN*, inner nuclear layer; *OH*, outer fiber layer of Henle; *ON*, outer nuclear layer; *OF*, outer cone fiber; *OM*, external limiting membrane; *IS*, inner segment layer. (Reduced from ×400.) (From Yamada, E.: Arch. Ophthalmol. 82:151-159, 1969.)

face facing the choroid. Thus the fovea is deepest at the center (Fig. 18-4).

Müller's supporting fibers are long, complicated structures that traverse the entire thickness of retina, from internal limiting membrane to external limiting membrane. The nucleus of Müller's fiber is bipolar and is situated at the level of the inner nuclear layer. As stated earlier, the floor of the foveal center is abundant in Müller's fiber processes.

The main blood supply of the retina is provided by the central retinal artery. The branches of the artery on the temporal side of the disc arch over and under the macula (as do the nerve fibers) and send twigs toward the horizontal meridian. The macula is supplied by small branches of these twigs, but the fovea is entirely free of blood vessels. These small vessels run radially toward the macula and form a capillary loop that leaves an avascular center, 0.4 to 0.5 mm in diameter at the fovea.[2] The superior and inferior branches of the superior and inferior divisions of the central retinal artery supply the perifoveal capillaries almost equally.

The outer portion of the retina (rods, cones, and outer nuclear layer) is avascular and is nourished by the choriocapillaries. The outer plexiform layer is for the most part avascular but is fed partly from the choroidal and partly from the retinal vessels.

More knowledge is being accumulated about the microcirculation of the retina as a result of work by Michaelson and Campbell[4] and Henkind.[5] The peripapillary area is the thickest portion of the retina and also the most richly vascularized. The following layers of capillaries, derived from the smallest branches of the central retinal artery, have been described.[4]

1. Deepest layer, lying in the outer portion of the inner nuclear layer, forming a two-dimensional network
2. Two layers, both less well-defined and less dense than the deepest layer, with the second being in the deeper part of the nerve fiber layer
3. Superficial layer of radial peripapillary capillaries

The superficial layer of radial peripapillary capillaries is distinctive. Although these capillaries are superficial, they do not lie immediately adjacent to the internal limiting membrane. They pursue a long, straight, or slightly curved, path. Unlike in the deeper capillary networks, there are few anastomoses between adjacent radial peripapillary capillaries or the deeper capillaries. Henkind[5] observed that separate retinal arterioles are responsible for supplying various portions of this superficial bed, and these same arterioles also feed the deeper capillary nets (Figs. 18-5 to 18-7). This suggests that blood may be routed away from the superficial layer to the deeper layers when intraocular pressure is increased. The radial peripapillary capillaries drain into intraretinal venules or into venules lying in the optic nerve head. The distribution of

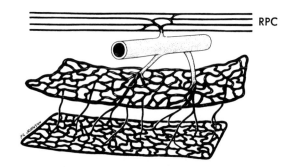

Fig. 18-5. Diagram of blood supply to retinal capillaries at posterior pole of eye. Retinal arteriole (*stippled vessel*) supplies both radial peripapillary capillaries, *RPC*, and deeper capillary networks. (From Henkind, P.: Ophthalmology (Rochester) **73:**890-897, 1969.)

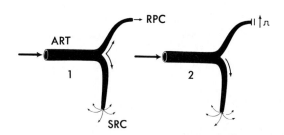

Fig. 18-6. Diagram of possible intraretinal vascular shunt mechanism. **1,** Under normal circumstances, arteriole, *ART*, distributes blood to radial peripapillary capillaries *RPC*, and to the other underlying capillary nets, *SRC*. **2,** Any situation that elevates resistance, *r*, in radial capillary bed may result in arteriolar blood being shunted to underlying capillaries. (From Henkind, P.: Ophthalmology (Rochester) **73:**890-897, 1969.)

these capillaries is seen in Fig. 18-7. It is likely that this network nourishes the superficially placed nerve fibers whose neurons apparently originate from ganglion cells of the posterior pole and enter the center of the nerve head.[6] They are the fibers probably involved in early glaucomatous field defects.

The vascular supply of the optic nerve head is derived from two separate systems. A circular anastomosis between two or more short posterior ciliary arteries that have penetrated the sclera on both sides of the optic nerve and the central retinal artery constitute the nerve head blood supply. The short posterior ciliary anastomosis is known as the circle of Zinn.[7]

Cystoid degeneration of the macula occurs in many conditions. These conditions have been outlined by Duke-Elder[8] as follows:

1. Senile degeneration
2. Cardiovascular disease such as arteriosclerosis, occlusion of the central retinal artery or vein, retinal periphlebitis, and hypertensive or diabetic retinopathy
3. Inflammatory conditions such as chorioretinitis or iridocyclitis
4. Degenerative conditions of the macula, retinal detachments, and retinal dystrophies

5. such as pigmentary dystrophy or Stargardt's disease
6. Trauma, usually in contusions or associated with the retention of a foreign body, and injury by radiation such as eclipse blindness
7. Glaucoma
8. Hereditary macular cystoid dystrophy

To this may be added the following: malignant melanoma, choroidal hemangioma, retinitis pigmentosa, epinephrine maculopathy, nicotinic acid maculopathy, retinal telangiectasis, after intraocular surgery such as cataract extraction, vitrectomy, penetrating keratoplasty, and glaucoma procedures.

These entities cause disturbances of particular elements of the posterior pole of the globe. For example, in branch vein occlusion and retinitis pigmentosa disturbance of retinal vasculature is seen. A predominant disturbance of the choroidal vasculature such as malignant melanoma, malignant hypertension, and senile macular degeneration with subretinal pigment epithelium neovascularization can cause a disruption of the retinal pigment epithelium. It is also possible for cystoid macular edema to be related predominantly to a disturbance of the retinal pigment epithelium or even to disturbances of all three of these elements.

Not infrequent is a secondary macular edema associated with ocular inflammations, usually affecting the anterior segment of the globe, especially if the ciliary body is involved. This is often associated with edema of the nerve head. That the macula is one of the main sites of predilection for edema is well known. This predilection is based on a number of anatomic facts considered earlier that include the following:

1. The fiber layer of Henle is thickest at the macula and because of its structure can absorb large quantities of fluid. This is a property shared by the retina around the disc, where the nerve fiber layer is thickest.[2,8] This layer is very liable to imbibe fluid and become swollen at the slightest provocation, both during life and as a result of postmortem or fixation changes.
2. The avascularity of the central area and the absence of capillaries limit absorption[9] of fluid.

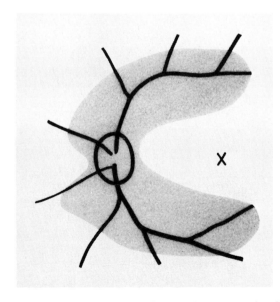

Fig. 18-7. Diagram of distributional pattern of radial peripapillary capillaries (*dark gray*). X, Fovea. (From Henkind, P.: Ophthalmology (Rochester) **73**:890-897, 1969.)

3. The thinness of the fovea, with its attenuated basal lamina necessary for light to gain easy access to the percipient elements, provides little protection against inflammatory exudates and their toxic products that pass through the vitreous.

The pathologic picture of cystoid macular edema includes the presence of cystoid spaces and lacunar cavities in the outer plexiform layer of Henle, which acts like a sponge, collecting the fluid. The fluid appears to arise from the perifoveal capillaries that show an incompetence. This differs from a true cyst, in which fluid accumulates progressively in a cavity with its own walls, producing a separation of the surrounding structures, which are damaged only by the pressure exerted on them. In cystoid macular edema the spaces may coalesce so that all retinal elements disappear except for the basal lamina. It is possible for this inner wall to disintegrate to form a lamellar hole. The inner wall may also detach or lie on the surface of the vitreous as an operculum. In some of these cases, vision may be surprisingly good because of the retention of some retinal elements. Favre[10] found 20/60 visual acuity or better in 50% of 44 eyes with such a lamellar hole.

CLINICAL FINDINGS

Nearly 30 years have elapsed since Irvine described this postoperative cataract syndrome. The mechanism involved in its production has only recently come into sharper focus, although there is still some controversy about it.

Irvine[1] postulated that the cause of the visual disturbance was either remote vitreous traction at the macula, initiated by adherence of vitreous to the operative wound, or vitreous opacities associated with iritis. Since techniques and instrumentation for biomicroscopic examination of the posterior vitreous were not well advanced at that time, he was not able to accurately define the pathologic picture. Years later the role of vitreous traction was strongly implicated by some[11,12] but denied by others.[13-15] However, painstaking observation of patients after cataract surgery and the development of techniques for observing the posterior vitreous and macula, including fluorescein photography, have clarified the problem greatly.

A more accurate picture of the Irvine-Gass syndrome has evolved as a result of observations made by Gass and Norton.[14,16] The typical patient undergoes an uneventful intracapsular cataract extraction. During the postoperative course, good visual acuity is attained. However, 1 to 3 months after surgery, visual acuity decreases to 20/50 to 20/100. The onset may be delayed. I have observed it more than 10 years after surgery. The eye may become irritable and photophobic and suffer recurrences and remissions of circumcorneal injection. Ophthalmoscopy (Fig. 18-8) reveals little except the loss of the foveal reflex and the presence of a yellowish reflex or spot that appears to lie deep in or behind the retina. The cystoid spaces are best seen by using red-free light, which renders their inner walls visible.

Biomicroscopic examination with a Hruby or fundus contact lens reveals a characteristic honeycomb lesion showing one or more larger cystoid spaces centrally, with any number of smaller oval spaces around them. The glistening section of the convex anterior walls of the cysts are seen overlying optically empty vesicles. They appear to be tightly packed together, with their interfaces presenting a spidery pattern (Figs. 18-9 and 18-10). Small perifoveal hemorrhages are not

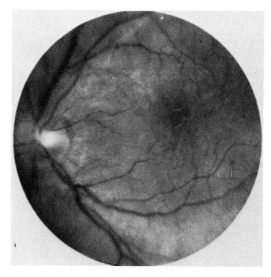

Fig. 18-8. Fundus in left eye of patient with cystoid macular edema after uneventful lens extraction. (From Jaffe, N. S.: The vitreous in clinical ophthalmology, St. Louis, 1969, The C. V. Mosby Co.)

uncommon. I have observed a level of blood on the floor of a relatively large central cystoid space. It persisted for many months. The retina may be markedly thickened, and the lesion may occupy an area as large as 1.5 to 2 disc diameters. An associated serous detachment of the macula has been described,[16] but in most cases the process appears to be entirely intraretinal. A wrinkling of the inner retinal surface (pucker) resulting from contraction of a semitranslucent preretinal membrane has been reported.[17] I have observed this several times in persisting cases of cystoid macular edema. Papilledema may occur in some cases, and it may be associated with peripapillary hemorrhages (Fig. 18-11).

As a diagnostic tool, fluorescein angiography has proved of great value. Within 1 to 2 minutes of an antecubital vein injection of 5 ml of 10% fluorescein or 10 ml of 5% fluorescein, leakage of the dye into the macula is observed. The macular pattern, which is well developed in most patients in 5 to 15 minutes, although it requires more than 30 minutes in others, consists of a stellate pattern with feathery margins (Fig. 18-12). The dark septa in the macular area, which compartmentalize the pattern, are probably attributable to Müller's supporting fibers of the retina. In many patients, there is considerable leakage of dye into the vit-

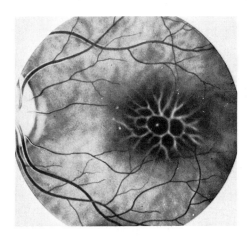

Fig. 18-9. Drawing of fundus in eye with cystoid macular edema after uneventful lens extraction. (From Gass, J. D. M., and Norton, E. W. D.: Arch. Ophthalmol. **76:**646-661, 1966.)

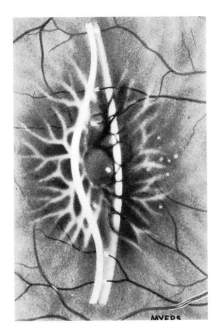

Fig. 18-10. Drawing of biomicroscopic appearance of cystoid macular edema after lens extraction. (From Gass, J. D. M., and Norton, E. W. D.: Arch. Ophthalmol. **76:**646-661, 1966.)

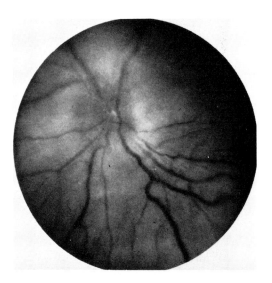

Fig. 18-11. Papilledema in eye with cystoid macular edema after lens extraction. (From Jaffe, N. S.: The vitreous in clinical ophthalmology, St. Louis, 1969, The C. V. Mosby Co.)

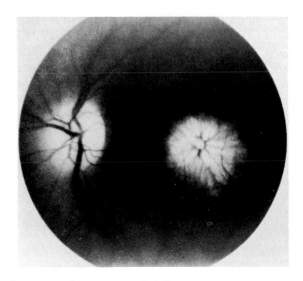

Fig. 18-12. Fluorescein ophthalmoscopic appearance of cystoid macular edema after lens extraction. One hour after injection, showing central dark figure surrounded by fluorescein pooled within intraretinal cystoid spaces. (From Gass, J. D. M., and Norton, E. W. D.: Arch. Ophthalmol. **76:** 646-661, 1966.)

reous and aqueous anteriorly, so that obscuration of fundus details occurs shortly after injection. However, the pattern becomes established and visible after a short time. In patients with papilledema, there may be leakage of dye into the optic nerve and peripapillary retina. Generally when edema of the macula and disc subside, fluorescein leakage ceases.

An elaborate photographic setup is not available to every ophthalmologist, nor is it required to make the diagnosis in this disorder. The typical fluorescein pattern may be observed with a Hruby lens or the ophthalmoscope, using a No. 47 or 47A filter (a Kodak Wratten filter). The macula will light up and become visible even in eyes where the fundus is difficult to see because of clouding of the media.

The pathogenesis of the visual disturbance appears to involve leakage of serous exudate from intraretinal capillaries in the perifoveal area and perhaps from the disc capillaries. The propensity of the macula for development of edema is based on its peculiar structure as outlined earlier. The exudate from the incompetent capillaries forms small puddles in the outer plexiform layer of Henle, which acts like a sponge. There are usually one or more large central cystoid spaces surrounded by numerous small ones.

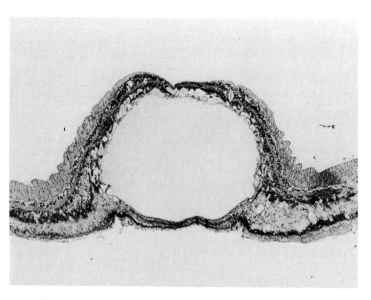

Fig. 18-13. Macular cyst after cataract extraction. (×40.) (AFIP No. 105-3425.) (From Maumenee, A. E.: Arch. Ophthalmol. **78:**151-165, 1967.)

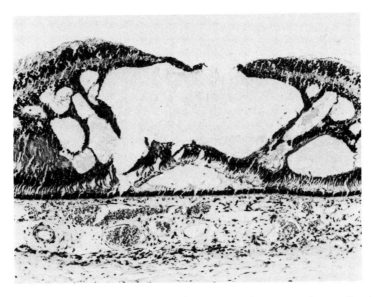

Fig. 18-14. Macular cyst after cataract extraction. Break in inner layer of retina is artifact. (×40.) (AFIP No. 119-145.) (From Maumenee, A. E.: Arch. Ophthalmol. **78:**151-165, 1967.)

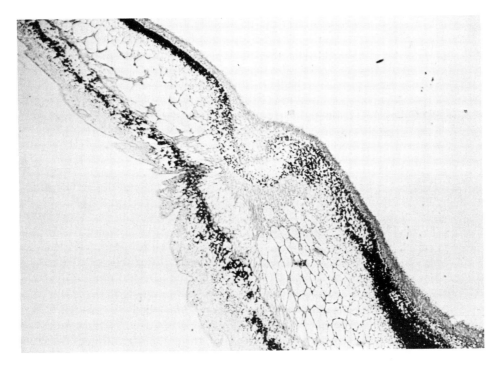

Fig. 18-15. Cystoid macular edema after cataract extraction in eye with long-standing postoperative iridocyclitis.

These spaces appear to intercommunicate (Figs. 18-13 to 18-15). If papilledema is present, it is probably due to a similar leakage of serous exudate into the optic nerve head.

When one examines the macula afflicted with cystoid macular edema, it is difficult to imagine that central vision is not completely lost. However, it is surprising how little visual function may be disturbed in the face of this ominous-appearing macula. Most patients recover, even after many months of morbidity, although permanent degenerative changes may result if the process continues unabated.

The clinical appearance of the macula is not pathognomonic of the Irvine-Gass syndrome, since it has been seen in pars planitis, venous thrombosis, chorioretinitis, telangiectasia of the retina, and acute nongranulomatous iritis. Kolker and Becker[18] observed it after after the use of topical epinephrine in aphakic patients with glaucoma. Their observation has now been confirmed. The fluorescein pattern in all of these situations likewise indicates cystoid macular edema. Fluorescein leakage into the macula generally does not occur in the vitreoretinal traction syndrome or with preretinal contraction membranes, an important differential point; however, there are exceptions.

The relationship between cystoid macular edema and the occasional association of wrinkling of the inner retinal layer because of contraction of a semitranslucent preretinal membrane is not entirely clear. Whether the wrinkling is caused by leaking retinal vessels (as Gass and Norton suggested),[17] whether it exists prior to cataract surgery, or whether either of these alternatives is possible is not yet established. I have observed such membranes in patients during the early postoperative period. Since they appeared well developed and since visual acuity at no time attained a satisfactory level, as in the Irvine-Gass syndrome, I have assumed that the maculopathy preceded the surgery.

In addition to the cystoid macular edema, there are important and significant accompanying signs. There is usually a prominent cellular infiltration in the vitreous along with vitreous opacities, most marked posteriorly and best viewed by retroillumination. I have also noted a disruption and loss of the usual smooth contour of the posterior limiting border of the vitreous in some patients. If the term is acceptable, this is the clinical picture of a "vitreitis." There is usually a circumcorneal injection, and cells are occasionally found in the aqueous. Intraocular pressure is usually normal.

It will be recalled that in the original definition of his syndrome, Irvine[1] stated that the anterior hyaloid membrane must be ruptured. However, the same pathologic process is found in eyes with an intact anterior hyaloid membrane or after an extracapsular lens extraction with an intact posterior capsule. Of 64 eyes with postoperative cystoid macular edema, Gass and Norton[17] observed an intact anterior hyaloid membrane in 34. In 30 eyes the anterior hyaloid membrane was ruptured, and in 25 of these, vitreous was attached to the posterior surface of the wound.

PATHOGENESIS

Some still consider the macular lesion to be the result of vitreous traction at the posterior pole. Most recent reports[13-16] have discounted this because it is extremely rare, even with the most careful technique of examination, to observe vitreous fibrils attached to the cystoid lesion at the macula.

One cannot but take notice of the high incidence of bilaterality in this disorder. It is perhaps too convenient to state that some patients are prone to capillary incompetence. In this regard, Gass and Norton[17] have made an interesting observation. Thirty-two of 48 patients with postoperative cystoid macular edema showed some evidence of existing or previous systemic hypertension. Five of these 32 also had mild diabetes. Of the 16 patients without evidence of hypertension, three had mild diabetes, one had congestive heart failure, and 12 had no history of cardiovascular disease. Thirteen of 14 patients with persistent macular edema for 1 or more years had evidence of cardiovascular disease. However, because of the age of the patients in this category, it is not known whether these observations are significant. Gass and Norton admit that a control series of patients without cystoid macular edema has not yet been studied for pertinent medical history. It is of interest to relate these observations to the occurrence of macular edema in aphakic patients receiving topical adrenergic medication for glaucoma, as first reported by Kolker and Becker.[18] Gass and Norton[17] observed six such patients. In four the edema disappeared shortly after the medication was discontinued, and in two it disappeared spontaneously, although the medication was continued.

It is apparent that the etiology of this maculopathy remains obscure, thus inviting speculation. I have the impression that vitreous traction at its base may be significant. Irritability at this site might be a causative factor in the same way that anterior segment inflammations involving the ciliary body are occasionally associated with cystoid macular edema. Biomicroscopic examination of the vitreous reveals the typical cellular infiltration, especially posteriorly. It is possible that these cells exert a toxic influence on the relatively unprotected macula. It will be recalled (p. 358) that the basal lamina at the fovea is very attenuated, almost nonexistent. The result may be incompetence of the capillaries at the macula. Equally speculative is a theory offered by Hawkins.[19] The vitreous body of 35 aphakic eyes with cystoid macular edema was studied prior to and following intravenous injection of fluorescein. Virtually all the eyes showed extensive syneresis and liquefaction of the vitreous gel and posterior detachment of the vitreous. This was not unexpected. Vitreomacular traction was not noted. Rupture of the anterior hyaloid membrane was present in 19 of the 35 eyes. The time required for fluorescein to appear in the anterior chamber averaged 2 minutes for the involved eyes as opposed to 10 minutes for the noninvolved eyes. Following its appearance within the aqueous, the fluorescein in most cases diffused into and became prominently concentrated within the collapsed vitreous gel. The findings suggested that aqueous humor proteins and electrolytes diffuse posteriorly throughout the collapsed vitreous gel. The liquefied vitreous (retrovitreal fluid) anterior to the retina assumes chemical and osmotic properties quite unlike those normally present. The result of such a change is an outpouring of fluid from the perimacular capillaries. Hawkins theorized that often after several weeks the perimacular capillaries adjust to the osmotic imbalance, and the edema clears. In those eyes in which the vitreous pathology is particularly severe, however, the edema is not likely to improve. One must wonder why myopic eyes with extensive syneresis and liquefaction of the vitreous gel do not show a higher incidence of cystoid macular edema if this theory is correct. Worst[20] has proposed a hypothesis, attributing a number of biotoxic effects to aqueous humor. A number of physiologic, anatomic, and pathophysiologic observations have given him reason to assume that aqueous humor contains biochemically active principles that manifest biotoxic effects when it leaves its natural reservoir. As a tentative name for these biotoxic principles, he proposed the name Aqueous Biotoxic Complex (ABC) factors. He attributes the lower incidence of cystoid macular edema after extracapsular lens extraction (compared with intracapsular extraction) to the presence of an intact posterior capsule that walls off the posterior portion of the eye from the effects of the ABC factors of the aqueous.

In recent years, considerable attention has been directed toward prostaglandins as the chemical mediator of intraocular inflammation and cystoid macular edema. This is the basis for the treatment of cystoid macular edema (described on p. 370). Many theories have been proposed for the role of prostaglandins in the pathogenesis of postoperative cystoid macular edema. Prostaglandins E_1 and E_2, isolated from the aqueous of the eye, are known to produce increased capillary permeability as well as signs of ocular inflammation such as increased protein concentration in the aqueous, miosis, vasodilation, and increased intraocular pressure. The action of these prostaglandins on the perimacular capillaries after lens extraction may explain the development of cystoid macular edema.

Prostaglandins are not stored in cells, and their presence in the aqueous is due to de novo synthesis. Since the eye does not contain the enzyme 15-prostaglandin dehydrogenase to deactivate prostaglandins, their removal is dependent on an active transport pump located in the ciliary epithelium. Bitot[21] has shown that this pump is inoperable for at least 3 weeks after ocular trauma. Indomethacin is one of the most potent antiprostaglandin synthetase inhibitors.

It should be apparent from reading this speculation how obscure the basic pathogenesis of cystoid macular edema is at this time.

The role of the posterior capsule, both intact and incised, has been related recently to the postoperative incidence of cystoid macular edema as well as to retinal detachment. Unfortunately some serious disparities still exist in several recent studies. A study by my co-workers and me[22] (p. 166) indicated that the presence of an intact posterior capsule lessens the incidence of cystoid macular edema in eyes with implants compared with eyes that have had intracapsular cataract extractions. Winslow and co-workers[23] showed a significantly lower incidence of this disorder in eyes after phacoemulsification when the posterior capsule was not incised. Kratz[24] and Chambless[25] reported similar findings. Moses[26] reported a much lower incidence of cystoid macular edema in eyes after phacoemulsification or planned extracapsular cataract extraction compared with intracapsular cataract extraction. However, he found that incising the posterior capsule did not increase the rate of cystoid macular edema. These results, along with others, suggest that the incidence of cystoid macular edema is lower after an extracapsular than an intracapsular cataract extraction if the posterior capsule is left intact. The effect of incising the posterior capsule is still undetermined.

INCIDENCE

Irvine[1] originally reported the incidence of this macular disorder to be around 2%. However, it is probably considerably higher, especially if searched for by performing almost daily visual acuity readings and frequent fundus and fluorescein evaluations. In some patients a transient cystoid macular edema occurs, causing little disturbance to the patient, who has not yet been given an aphakic correction. The process may subside in a few days. It is reasonable to assume that it occurs in at least 40% of normal cataract extractions and that if it is present in one eye, there is a high probability (around 70%) that it will occur in the second eye after lens extraction. If fluorescein angiography were performed daily, it would not surprise me to find at least some transient phase of cystoid macular edema after every cataract extraction.

Gass and Norton[17] followed 48 patients for at least 1 year after they developed macular edema. Forty-four of them were followed for 2 years or longer. Of these, 33 had bilateral cataract extractions. Macular edema occurred in both eyes of 16 patients and unilaterally in 17.

Although the role of vitreous traction at the macula is highly doubtful, the vitreous is implicated by the following considerations: There is a rise in the incidence of postoperative cystoid macular edema when vitreous has been lost at surgery, when there is a postoperative rupture of the anterior hyaloid membrane, and when there is adherence of vitreous to the operative wound, especially when it is associated with peaking of the pupil. In addition, cystoid macular edema is rarely encountered after glaucoma and retinal detachment surgery in which the lens is not removed and the vitreous cavity is minimally altered. However, it is becoming evident that this statement may no longer be valid. Cystoid macular edema is being observed and reported after retinal detachment and glaucoma surgery in phakic eyes. Ryan[27] described two cases of cystoid macular edema in phakic eyes after prophylactic procedures for treatment of retinal holes. It persisted in one patient. He also quoted Maumenee as having seen cystoid macular edema in phakic eyes after antiglaucoma filtering procedures. He suggested that it may cause a small residual central visual field to "snuff out" after surgery.

As previously pointed out (p. 348), there appears to be a high incidence of cystoid macular edema in aphakic eyes undergoing penetrating keratoplasty for corneal edema. While it is true that the vitreous is frequently manipulated during this type of surgery, 8 of 42 aphakic eyes with clear corneal grafts and cystoid macular edema had no vitreous manipulation during the surgery and no vitreous in the wound after the surgery.[28]

A low incidence of this disorder appears to occur in black patients, a fact difficult to explain.

PROGNOSIS

The prognosis for full restoration of visual acuity is generally good. In most instances the macular edema is transient, and vision recovers rapidly as the process subsides. However, in a significant number of patients the morbidity persists for a much longer period. When one examines the macula in a persistent case, the involvement may look so severe that it does not seem possible for full recovery to occur; yet, surprisingly, most of these patients do recover.

In the series reported by Gass and Norton,[17] resolution of macular edema occurred within the first 6 months in about half their cases. In 20%, 1 to 3 years passed before resolution, and in the remaining 30%, macular edema persisted. However, they suggest that this is probably not an accurate reflection, since the incidence of intractable macular edema is probably much lower. Patients with persistent edema are more likely to be referred for consultation and are followed more closely for longer periods.

Jacobson and Dellaporta[29] followed 28 eyes in 26 patients with cystoid macular edema after cataract extraction. The diagnosis was confirmed in all eyes by fluorescein angiography. There were 24 eyes that attained 20/30 or better visual acuity immediately after cataract extraction. Approximately 50% of these retained this vision for 6 months or more after surgery before it began to decrease. Twenty of the 28 eyes (71.4%) had a

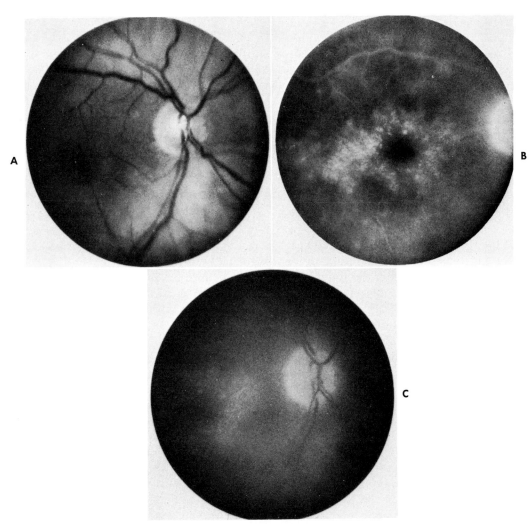

Fig. 18-16. A, Right eye of patient showing persistent macular edema and macular hole 3½ years after cataract extraction. Visual acuity is 20/70. **B,** Same eye. Fluorescein photograph showing intraretinal leakage of dye into macular region. **C,** Same eye. Fluorescein photograph, late stage, showing cystoid macular edema surrounding central nonfluorescent area in region of macular hole. (From Gass, J. D. M., and Norton, E. W. D.: Ophthalmology (Rochester) **73:**665-682, 1969.)

spontaneous resolution of the cystoid macular edema and achieved 20/30 or better vision. Seven of these required 6 months or longer to clear. Eight of the 28 eyes (28.6%) had 20/40 visual acuity or less. The patients were observed for 2 years or longer.

In most cases the macula regains a normal appearance after subsidence of the edema. However, instances of permanent macular degeneration will arise consecutive to prolonged persistent macular edema. Gass and Norton[17] have observed two patients who developed either lamellar or full thickness macular holes after persistent macular edema. In the absence of an operculum and in the absence of evidence of serous detachment, they assumed that a rupture in the inner retinal wall occurred secondary to the intractable edema. As mentioned earlier, the cystoid spaces at the macula may coalesce so that all retinal elements disappear except for the internal limiting membrane. When the latter disintegrates, a lamellar hole is formed. Such a hole may measure one fourth to one third of a disc diameter, which corresponds roughly to the size of the central avascular area. In the presence of a lamellar hole, visual acuity may be surprisingly good because of retention of some percipient elements. Occasionally it is difficult or impossible to determine biomicroscopically whether the inner layer of an apparent large foveal cystoid space is intact. Fluorescein angiography may be helpful in this situation. If the layer is intact the stellate figure with feathery margins, as described on p. 363, will become apparent. If a dehiscence exists, the dye will diffuse out into the vitreous cavity, and the sharply circumscribed area where there is a defect in the retina will appear relatively hypofluorescent, in contrast to the surrounding fluorescent cystoid spaces (Fig. 18-16).

In some cases, macular pucker results after subsidence of the cystoid macular edema. The pucker may be observed in some while fluorescein leakage into the macula may still be demonstrated. In these cases, fluorescein angiography usually eventually becomes negative, but the macular pucker persists. Retinal pigment epithelial changes may also be seen in cases after resolution of cystoid macular edema.

The presence of vitreous incarceration in the wound may have some bearing on the ultimate prognosis. Gass and Norton[17] noted that those patients with cystoid macular edema whose anterior hyaloid membranes remained intact recovered in an average of 6 months. Those with incarceration of vitreous in the posterior part of the wound required an average of 15 months for recovery. They reported an incidence of vitreous incarceration of 55% in those patients with persistent edema and 35% in those who recovered. My two most resistant cases were associated with operative loss of vitreous.

TREATMENT

As is usual with a disorder that shows a naturally high rate of recovery, a number of beneficial therapeutic remedies have been advocated. Systemic steroids and atropine applied topically may be of value, particularly in those cases with considerable cellular infiltration in the vitreous. In several patients I have used injection under Tenon's capsule of triamcinolone (Kenalog) and found that it improved vision. However, although its use is probably justified, to date I have not been overly impressed with steroids.

Tennant[34] has recently advocated the use of indomethacin (Indocin) in patients with cystoid macular edema. This nonsteroidal, anti-inflammatory compound is given orally in a dosage of 25 mg three times daily after meals. One should be alert to gastrointestinal disturbances, which occur in about 15% of patients taking this medication.

The basis for using indomethacin is its known action as an antiprostaglandin. Miyake[30] has used this agent topically in patients undergoing cataract surgery as a prophylaxis against the development of cystoid macular edema. He advocates a 1% solution of indomethacin in sesame oil. He found that the incidence and severity of cystoid macular edema were much milder in eyes treated in this manner than in the fellow untreated eye. Sholitan and co-workers[31] and Obstbaum,[32] however, reported no significant benefit from prophylactic indomethacin (oral administration) treatment for this disorder. Yannuzi and Klein[33] reported no difference between the use of indomethacin and a placebo in a controlled study of patients who had cystoid macular edema for 4 months or longer.

The manufacturer of indomethacin in the Unit-

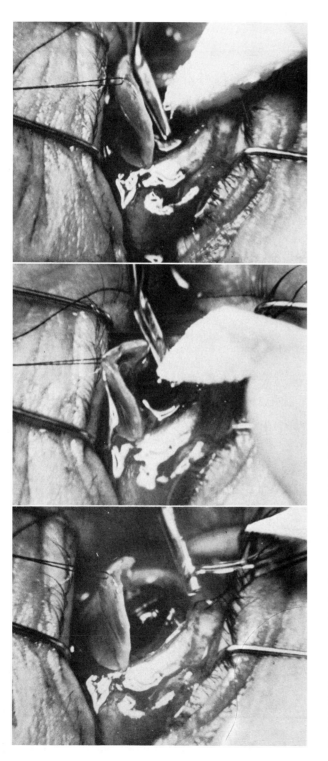

ed States (Merck, Sharp, and Dohme, West Point, Pennsylvania) has had little enthusiasm for encouraging further studies of the use of topical indomethacin. On the basis of two pilot studies carried out in the late 1960s and the mid 1970s, they concluded that the anti-inflammatory activity of topical indomethacin in humans was disappointing.[35]

In patients who show vitreous adherence to the surgical wound, especially with peaking of the pupil, separation of these adhesions may be of value. Iliff[36] has recommended incision of these adhesions by exteriorizing them with a bent 30-gauge cannula, which is inserted into the anterior chamber through a limbal stab wound so that one can cut them with scissors. Some report success with this procedure, whereas others observe no benefit. Too often, one is disappointed to find on biomicroscopic examination 1 or 2 days later that vitreous has readhered to the wound at the original site or to the region of the stab wound.

In some patients, solid vitreous may nearly fill the entire anterior chamber with widespread adherence to the wound. The procedure of Iliff cannot be used on these eyes. If the cystoid macular edema has persisted for a long time and visual acuity has dropped to 20/200 or less, an alternative procedure may be attempted. The wound is reopened to the extent of a cataract incision. The vitreous is removed from the anterior chamber with cellulose sponges (Fig. 18-17). The sponges are effective in engaging solid vitreous in the angle, over the anterior surface of the iris, and in the pupillary aperture. Large bundles of vitreous are picked up and cut with scissors. When sufficient vitreous has been removed, the iris will fall well posteriorly. The wound is then sutured in the usual manner. The eye tolerates this procedure surprisingly well. As a rule, a recondensation of the face of the remaining vitreous will occur at about the level of the iris.

Fig. 18-17. Vitrectomy performed in eye with cystoid macular edema associated with widespread adherence of vitreous to wound after lens extraction. Vitreous is picked up with cellulose sponge and cut with scissors. (From Jaffe, N. S.: The vitreous in clinical ophthalmology, St. Louis, 1969, The C. V. Mosby Co.)

This method of partial anterior vitrectomy is similar to that described for the management of vitreous loss during cataract surgery (p. 268) and in association with a penetrating keratoplasty for treatment of aphakic bullous keratopathy caused by vitreocorneal adherence (p. 343). This technique has not been replaced by the closed system type of partial anterior vitrectomy via the pars plana, using the VISC, the rotoextractor, or the Ocutome.

A pronounced trend to intervene surgically exists today when vitreous incarceration is associated with cystoid macular edema. The results achieved must be weighed against the decided tendency for spontaneous resolution of macular edema, even after prolonged periods. Whether early intervention will prove effective in preventing intractable cases is not yet known. I must reemphasize that vitreous surgery appears to be a drastic procedure for a disorder that shows a high rate of spontaneous recovery. It should probably be reserved for cases persisting for more than a year. I have had an opportunity to manage several cases of persistent cystoid macular edema treated in this manner. Some of these have shown a dramatic resolution of the pathologic process. However, others have shown no improvement. This method warrants further investigation.

In their series of 28 eyes in 26 patients with cystoid macular edema after cataract extraction, Jacobson and Dellaporta[29] concluded that no medical or surgical treatment has been demonstrated to improve the rate of natural, spontaneous resolution of cystoid macular edema after cataract extraction.

REFERENCES

1. Irvine, S. R.: A newly defined vitreous syndrome following cataract surgery interpreted according to recent concepts of the structure of the vitreous, Am. J. Ophthalmol. **36**:599-619, 1953.
2. Wolff, E.: Anatomy of the eye and orbit, ed. 6, revised by R. J. Last, Philadelphia, 1968, W. B. Saunders Co., pp. 122, 130, 139.
3. Yamada, E.: Some structural features of the fovea centralis in the human retina. Arch. Ophthalmol. **82**:151-159, 1959.
4. Michaelson, I., and Campbell, A. C. P.: The anatomy of the finer retinal vessels, and some observations on their significance in certain retinal diseases, Trans. Ophthalmol. Soc. U.K. **60**:71-112, 1940.
5. Henkind, P.: Microcirculation of the peripapillary retina, Ophthalmology (Rochester) **73**:890-897, 1969.
6. Wolff, E., and Penman, G. G.: The position occupied by the peripheral retinal fibres in the nerve fibre layer and at the nerve head. XVI Concilium Ophthalmologicum Acta London **1**:625-635, 1950.
7. Zinn, J. G.: Descriptio anatomica oculi humani iconibus illustrata, Göttingen, 1755, Abrami Vanderhoeck.
8. Duke-Elder, S.: System of ophthalmology. Vol. X. Diseases of the retina, St. Louis, 1967, The C. V. Mosby Co., pp. 125, 545.
9. Iwanoff, A.: Beiträge zur normalen und pathologischen Anatomie des Auges. 3. Das Oedem der Netzhaut, Graefe Arch. Ophthalmol. **15**(Abt. 2):88-105, 1968.
10. Favre, M.: Trou dans la macula et décollement de la rétine, Ophthalmologica **140**:94-98, 1960.
11. Tolentino, F. I., and Schepens, C. L.: Edema of posterior pole after cataract extraction: a biomicroscopic study, Arch. Ophthalmol. **74**:781-786, 1965.
12. Reese, A. B., Jones, I. S., and Cooper, W. C.: Macular changes secondary to vitreous traction, Trans. Am. Ophthalmol. Soc. **64**:123-134, 1966.
13. Jaffe, N. S.: Vitreous traction at the posterior pole of the fundus due to alterations in the vitreous posterior, Ophthalmology (Rochester) **71**:642-652, 1967.
14. Gass, J. D. M., and Norton, E. W. D.: Cystoid macular edema and papilledema following cataract extraction: a fluorescein funduscopic and angiographic study, Arch. Ophthalmol. **76**:646-661, 1966.
15. Maumenee, A. E.: Further advances in the study of the macula, Arch. Ophthalmol. **78**:151-165, 1967.
16. Gass, J. D. M., and Norton, E. W. D.: Fluorescein studies of patients with macular edema and papilledema following cataract extraction, Trans. Am. Ophthalmol. Soc. **64**:232-249, 1966.
17. Gass, J. D. M., and Norton, E. W. D.: Follow-up study of cystoid macular edema following cataract extraction, Ophthalmology (Rochester) **73**:665-682, 1969.
18. Kolker, A. E., and Becker, B.: Epinephrine maculopathy, Arch. Ophthalmol. **79**:552-562, 1968.
19. Hawkins, R. E.: Aphakic macular edema. In Emery, J. M., and Paton, D., editors: Current concepts in cataract surgery. Selected Proceedings of the Third Biennial Cataract Surgical Congress, St. Louis, 1974, The C. V. Mosby Co., pp. 339-342.
20. Worst, J. G. F.: Personal communication, 1977.
21. Bito, L. Z., and Salvador, E. V.: Intraocular fluid dynamics. 3. The site and mechanism of prostaglandin transfer across the blood intraocular fluid barriers, Exp. Eye Res. **14**:233-241, 1972.
22. Miami Study Group: Cystoid macular edema in aphakic and pseudophakic eyes, Am. J. Ophthalmol. **88**:45-48, 1979.
23. Winslow, R. L., Taylor, B. C., and Harris, W. S.: A one-year follow-up of cystoid macular edema following intraocular lens implantation, Ophthalmology **85**:190-196, 1978.
24. Kratz, R. P.: Results of phacoemulsification by Kelman and Girard techniques. In Transactions of the New Orleans Academy of Ophthalmology. Symposium on cataracts, St. Louis, 1979, The C. V. Mosby Co., pp. 196-200.

25. Chambless, W. S.: Phacoemulsification and the retina, Ophthalmology. (In press.)

26. Moses, L.: Cystoid macular edema and retinal detachment following cataract surgery, J. Am. Intraocul. Implant. Soc. **5**(4):326-329, 1979.

27. Ryan, S.: Cystoid maculopathy in phakic retinal detachment procedures, Am. J. Ophthalmol. **76**:519-522, 1973.

28. West, C. E., Fitzgerald, C. R., and Sewell, J. H.: Cystoid macular edema following aphakic keratoplasty, Am. J. Ophthalmol. **75**:77-81, 1973.

29. Jacobson, D. R., and Dellaporta, A.: Natural history of cystoid macular edema after cataract extraction, Am. J. Ophthalmol. **77**:445-447, 1974.

30. Miyake, K.: Prophylaxis of aphakic cystoid macular edema using topical indomethacin, J. Am. Intraocul. Implant. Soc. **4**(4):174-179, 1978.

31. Sholitan, D. B., Reinhart, W. J., and Frank, K. E.: Indomethacin as a means of preventing cystoid macular edema following intracapsular cataract extraction, J. Am. Intraocul. Implant Soc. **5**:137-140, 1979.

32. Obstbaum, S. A.: The whys and wherefores of cystoid macular edema. Presented at the U.S. Intraocular Lens Symposium, Los Angeles, Calif., March 15, 1978.

33. Yannuzi, L. A., et al.: Ineffectiveness of indomethacin in the treatment of chronic cystoid macular edema, Am. J. Ophthalmol. **84**:517-519, 1977.

34. Tennant, J. L.: Personal communication, 1978.

35. Katz, I. M.: Personal communication, 1978.

36. Iliff, C. E.: Treatment of the vitreous-tug syndrome, Am. J. Ophthalmol. **62**:856-859, 1966.

CHAPTER 19

Alterations at the posterior pole of the fundus

Failure to achieve improvement in vision after cataract surgery is disappointing to the patient and the surgeon. It may be due to any one of several alterations at the posterior pole of the fundus that predate or follow the surgery. Some of these changes are subtle and may be obscured by the lenticular opacity. For example, the visual acuity in an eye may be 20/60 when the cataract is first diagnosed. As a result of increasing opacity of the lens, it may drop to 20/400. At this point, fine fundus details are seen with difficulty. At a later date the visual acuity may only be good for counting fingers, and the surgeon may assume that the final decrease in vision is from the cataract, since macular and optic disc details may be difficult to see. The cataract is extracted, and despite uneventful surgery and an uncomplicated postoperative course, visual acuity does not improve to a satisfactory level. When the fundus can be carefully evaluated, the surgeon is disappointed to see that the disc is pale from ischemic optic neuropathy or that the macula shows marked puckering with a preretinal membrane.

The following alterations at the posterior pole of the fundus may be responsible for failure to achieve anticipated vision:

1. Cystoid macular edema (Irvine-Gass syndrome)
2. Acceleration or progression of senile macular degeneration
3. Inflammatory cystoid macular degeneration and optic neuritis
4. Ischemic optic neuropathy and temporal arteritis
5. Postoperative optic neuritis
6. Thrombosis of central retinal artery and vein
7. Macular changes from postoperative hypotension
8. Macular pucker and preretinal membrane
9. Vitreoretinal traction syndrome
10. Choroidal folds from high hyperopia

CYSTOID MACULAR EDEMA

Cystoid macular edema is by far the most frequent of the alterations at the posterior pole of the fundus. Although the pathologic process is self-limiting in most cases, persistent cases are by no means rare. This is discussed on p. 368.

SENILE MACULAR DEGENERATION

Whether cataract surgery can hasten the progress of senile macular degeneration is unknown. Although one may logically assume that the circulatory demands of borderline compensation made on the macula by cataract surgery may be sufficient to cause further degeneration, there is little evidence to support this thesis, in spite of an occasional report that makes this claim.[1] However, on numerous occasions I have observed eyes with mild senile macular degeneration over a period of years that showed rapid acceleration of the degeneration shortly after cataract extraction. Occasionally this consisted of a sudden hemorrhagic disciform degeneration. It may be difficult to implicate the surgery in some cases, since the changes at the macula may be the natural course of the disease in these eyes. I have the impression that some eyes with diabetic retinopathy show a hastening of the degenerative process after cataract surgery.

INFLAMMATORY CYSTOID MACULAR DEGENERATION AND OPTIC NEURITIS

Inflammatory complications involving the retina and optic nerve are uncommon but not rare after cataract surgery. They have been attributed, with little confirmatory evidence, to the diffusion of toxins toward the posterior pole of the eye with the fluid traffic in the vitreous.[2] Aseptic uveitis after cataract surgery may involve the vitreous as well as the anterior segment of the eye. In such cases, macular edema is frequently evident, sometimes with the appearance of cysts, a macular hole, and occasionally a retinal detachment. There may be an accompanying optic neuritis. A secondary retinal periphlebitis may occur, with sheathing and atrophy of the vessels and the appearance of neovascularization extending some distance from the posterior pole to the periphery of the fundus. After subsidence of the inflammation, extensive preretinal postinflammatory membranes may become visible. The macula may be involved in such a process.

ISCHEMIC OPTIC NEUROPATHY AND TEMPORAL ARTERITIS

Ischemic optic neuropathy occurs in older individuals and may be concealed by the presence of a cataract. It produces a sudden loss of vision, often appearing as an inferior altitudinal field defect. The field loss is usually permanent. Both eyes are often involved but not simultaneously. There may be a delay of several years between onset in the two eyes. Pain is rare. Ophthalmodynamometry reveals that ophthalmic artery pressures are usually equal in the two eyes. An ophthalmoscopic picture of the Foster Kennedy syndrome is frequently seen in the acute stage of involvement of the second eye.[3] Evidence of systemic vascular disease such as hypertension or arteriosclerosis is usually present.

The patient may be unaware of its occurrence, since he may be relying on the opposite eye for reading and other visual tasks. The disc is characteristically pale and swollen during the acute state. Splinter hemorrhages are frequent; exudates are rare. The exact vessel involved is still debated, but it is likely that the central artery of the optic nerve and the collateral circulation in the short posterior ciliary and pial vessels are involved. The focal ischemia causes swelling of the optic disc, which probably increases the ischemia in the adjacent nerve tissue. As further vascular stagnation occurs, papilledema increases.

The clinical picture does not differ much from that seen with temporal arteritis, which may be differentiated by an elevated erythrocyte sedimentation rate and a positive temporal artery biopsy. Classically, the latter disease may produce a constant, throbbing headache, painful palpable temporal arteries, fever, anorexia, malaise, amaurosis fugax, and weight loss. The erythrocyte sedimentation rate is almost always elevated, and biopsy of the temporal artery is usually positive. However, occult temporal arteritis is common and should be kept in mind. Blindness of one or both eyes occurs in 50% of all patients and is caused by ischemia of the optic nerve. The ophthalmoscopic picture usually does not differ from that seen with ischemic optic neuropathy, but on occasion temporal arteritis may appear as a central retinal artery occlusion or a retrobulbar neuritis.

POSTOPERATIVE OPTIC NEURITIS

The occurrence of optic neuritis as a late complication of cataract surgery received little attention in the literature until 1946, when Vila-Coro[4] reported 10 cases of optic atrophy in 5000 cataract extractions. Townes and co-workers[5] reported four cases in 1951. In 1958 Reese and Carroll[6] reported 17 such cases, and Carroll[7] recently added nine more. Since then, postoperative optic neuritis has been accepted as a rare, late complication unrelated to cystoid macular edema (Irvine-Gass syndrome), with or without papilledema and posterior pole changes from postoperative hypotension.

The problem generally does not arise shortly after surgery, and an initial period of good postoperative visual acuity usually occurs. Two to 4 months after surgery the patient notices a sudden onset of blurred vision in the operated eye. The visual acuity may be only slightly decreased, but in most cases it ranges from 20/70 to 20/200.

Visual field examination usually reveals depression of central vision from a central scotoma of 5 to 20 degrees. The scotoma is usually not pericentral. An altitudinal defect is probably the most characteristic feature. The patient generally can plot his own field defect on the Amsler chart.

The clinical findings consist of swelling of the optic disc with several adjacent, small, flame-shaped hemorrhages. The disc may appear pale even early in the course. One or more of the small arterioles near the disc margin may show a silver-wire appearance or perhaps just pallor. In some cases the disc may appear normal, but the presence of a central scotoma without any macular abnormality points to the possibility of a retrobulbar neuritis. Examination of the macula reveals no abnormality. Intraocular pressure is normal, uveitis is absent, and the vitreous appears unremarkable. Fluorescein angiography reveals leakage of dye from the disc, but the macula appears normal.

The clinical course is variable. Some patients, after an initial decrease in visual acuity, recover completely. However, in most there is a permanent reduction, which may range from 20/50 to complete blindness.

Probably this entity should be called "postoperative ischemic optic neuropathy," since it is no different from the ischemic process seen in phakic eyes, as just described. Since cataract surgery is performed on patients in the older age group, many of whom are hypertensive, it is not surprising that the condition is seen after surgery. It is unclear why there is usually a delay of weeks to months before the entity manifests itself. The surgery itself may place an additional burden on a patient with a marginal optic nerve blood supply, as suggested in the case of senile macular degeneration on p. 374. A recent report[8] suggested that this delayed form of optic neuropathy is due to a predisposing vascular insufficiency complicated by intracapsular lens extraction and possibly precipitated by a change in intraocular pressure during the postoperative period. However, one must consider the possibility that the surgery is coincidental and not at all related to the ischemic process. Carroll[7] considers the surgery more than coincidental. Of 17 patients who suffered an ischemic optic neuropathy after cataract surgery on the first eye, eight encountered the same problem after surgery on the second eye, an incidence of 47%. Relatively few in the combined series[6] of Reese and Carroll (26 patients) showed evidence of hypertensive cardiovascular disease. The complication was seen in eyes undergoing cataract extraction with either local or general anesthesia (with or without a retrobulbar injection). Carroll therefore speculated that there is at least a localized occlusive vascular process involving the blood supply to the optic nerve, that the operation tends to increase the occlusive disease over a period of weeks or months, and finally that an ischemic infarct suddenly occurs in the optic nerve. Unfortunately, there is no way of predicting whether the second eye will suffer the same fate as the first eye.

THROMBOSIS OF CENTRAL RETINAL ARTERY AND VEIN

Thrombosis of the central retinal vein may escape notice if the lenticular opacity is sufficiently dense. The patient is often unaware of the decrease in vision unless it is very great, and the surgeon may attribute it to the dense cataract. On the other hand, central retinal artery thrombosis rarely occurs without alerting the patient. However, I am aware of one patient whose vision was reduced to perceiving hand movements because of an almost fully mature cataract. Her surgeon recommended lens extraction, which the patient temporarily declined. She called 3 weeks later requesting that she be scheduled for surgery, since she could no longer see her hand moving before her eye. She was not reexamined before surgery. To the patient's and surgeon's chagrin, the eye had no light perception after surgery. The surgeon attributed this to possible optic nerve damage caused by the retrobulbar injection or to an occlusion resulting from digital pressure. I saw this patient in consultation. When she had called her surgeon's office, it was revealed, she could no longer see light, but she did not relate this to him because he had advised her that when she could not see her hand moving before her eye, her cataract was "absolutely ripe." Therefore she informed him only of this. Undoubtedly she had suffered an occlusion of the central retinal artery before the surgery.

Closure of the central artery may occur as a complication of the retrobulbar injection. When there are no clinical signs of a retrobulbar hemorrhage, the exact cause is obscure. It is usually attributed to one of the following: arterial spasm, mechanical tamponade, or increased intraocular pressure. Arterial spasm might be purely spontaneous or secondary to the anesthesia or to the trauma of the injection. If this were true, one would expect instances of central retinal artery closure after injection without retrobulbar hemorrhage. This has not been reported. Kraushar and co-workers[9] observed closure of the central retinal artery during retrobulbar hemorrhage in three patients who had been scheduled for photocoagulation treatment. Evidence from a retrospective study suggested that at least two of 28 patients (7%) who developed retrobulbar hemorrhage after injection of anesthesia for intraocular surgery may have suffered closure of the central retinal artery during the hemorrhage, with resultant visual loss. The central retinal artery is closed off during the retrobulbar hemorrhage as the eyeball reaches maximal proptosis, and the orbit, unable to accomodate more blood, transmits the increased pressure to the globe. They suggest that when the retinal circulation cannot be visualized, a lateral canthotomy should be performed immediately on diagnosis of retrobulbar hemorrhage to maintain retinal circulation and prevent retinal anoxia. Carroll[7] also reported this complication. It is surprising that it does not occur more frequently. It is known to the plastic surgeon involved in blepharoplasties where orbital bleeding is extensive. Direct injury to the nerve or its blood supply by the retrobulbar needle may also be a factor, but this is difficult to assess.

MACULAR CHANGES FROM POSTOPERATIVE HYPOTENSION

The macular changes associated with postoperative hypotension are described on p. 286.

A fuller discussion of macular pucker and preretinal membrane along with the vitreoretinal traction syndrome follows, since these entities cause subtle changes, which have only recently come into sharper focus.

MACULAR PUCKER AND PRERETINAL MEMBRANE

Although the condition of macular pucker and preretinal membrane is far less common than senile macular degeneration, it is one of the most frequent causes of failure to achieve anticipated vision after cataract surgery. It is not easily diagnosed before the surgery because the lesion at the posterior pole is often subtle and not readily visible in the presence of a moderately advanced cataract.

In my experience, this condition is much more often seen in phakic eyes, and when it is observed in the aphakic eye after cataract extraction, it probably predated the surgery.

Pathogenesis

The cause of preretinal membrane formation and its subsequent contraction is still unknown. Although it has been associated with specific ocular abnormalities such as diabetic retinopathy, hypertensive retinopathy, central vein thrombosis, posterior uveitis, vitreous hemorrhage (Fig. 19-1), retinal breaks, and rhegmatogenous retinal detachment (Fig. 19-2) and has been seen to occur after photocoagulation or cryopexy, it is frequently observed in eyes with no other evidence of intraocular disease or any other cause that would appear related to this process (Fig. 19-3).

I have suggested the following pathogenesis in apparently normal eyes.[10] The cells that normally inhabit the outer vitreous cortex along with the outermost fibrils may remain adherent to the internal limiting membrane after a posterior vitreous detachment. The origin of these cells is still unknown. Due to some unknown precipitating cause, cellular proliferation and contraction occur that result in wrinkling of the inner retinal surface because of the tangential traction created. The cells responsible for the preretinal membrane may also be derived from the retinal circulation or the ciliary body or may be wandering histiocytes.

Clinical findings

There may be an irregular wrinkling of the retina at the level of the internal limiting membrane. This wrinkling causes a pattern of light reflections from the inner layer of the globe that resembles the appearance of crinkled cellophane. Thus this entity is also called "cellophane macula." In this area a semitransparent membrane may be visible with a Hruby or fundus contact lens. One may then understand that this membrane is re-

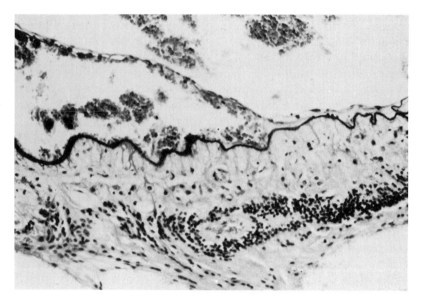

Fig. 19-1. Marked wrinkling of internal limiting membrane of retina with overlying membrane. Note vitreous hemorrhage and blood between membrane and retina on left. (From Jaffe, N. S.: The vitreous in clinical ophthalmology, St. Louis, 1969, The C. V. Mosby Co.; courtesy Dr. J. D. M. Gass, Miami, Fla.)

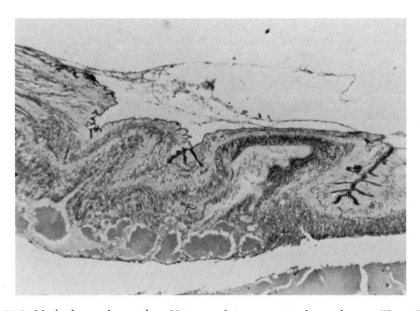

Fig. 19-2. Marked macular pucker. Note overlying preretinal membrane. (From Jaffe, N. S.: The vitreous in clinical opthalmology, St. Louis, 1969, The C. V. Mosby Co.; courtesy Dr. J. D. M. Gass, Miami, Fla.)

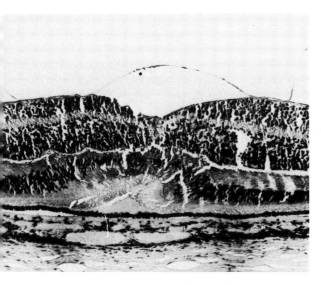

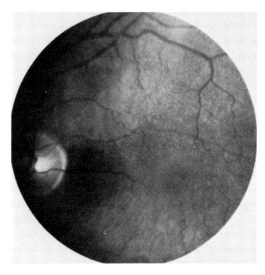

Fig. 19-3. Histologic section of macular area in eye enucleated for melanoma of ciliary body. Note membrané on surface of retina, with folds in underlying internal limiting membrane. (AFIP No. 122-2943.) (From Maumenee, A. E.: Arch. Ophthalmol. **78**:151-165, 1967.)

Fig. 19-4. Eye of 71-year-old man with wrinkling of inner layer of retina. Whitish gray membrane of irregular thickness is present. Haze is caused by lenticular nuclear sclerosis. Choroidal nevus is seen adjacent to disc. Visual acuity is 20/60 − 3. (From Jaffe, N. S.: Arch. Ophthalmol. **78**:585-591, 1967.)

sponsible for the disruption of the normally smooth contour of the internal limiting membrane. In about half the cases, a regular pattern of retinal folds that usually radiate out from the margin of the preretinal membrane is seen. One gains the impression that the contraction of the membrane causes these traction folds peripheral to it.

The location of the membrane is usually paramacular, often located above rather than below. Probably because of the peculiar anatomy of the macular region, the clinical appearance in this area shows several variations. The membrane may extend to one end of the macula and present the picture of an accentuated swirl of tissue at this edge, or else it may condense around the fovea without covering it and give the appearance of a macular hole. In some instances the membrane will cover the entire macula, which becomes lost to view within it. A paramacular membrane may be associated with retinal wrinkles that run through the macula.

Because of contraction of the membrane, the perimacular vessels show a marked tortuosity. The major arterioles on the temporal side of the

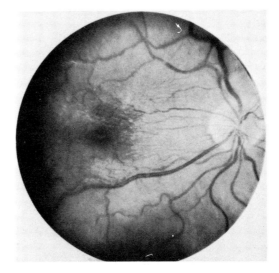

Fig. 19-5. Marked wrinkling of inner retinal layer in macular area in eye of 50-year-old man who underwent cataract extraction in eye 7 years earlier. Visual acuity is 20/25 − 3. (From Jaffe, N. S.: The vitreous in clinical ophthalmology, St. Louis, 1969, The C. V. Mosby Co.; courtesy Dr. E. W. D. Norton, Miami, Fla.)

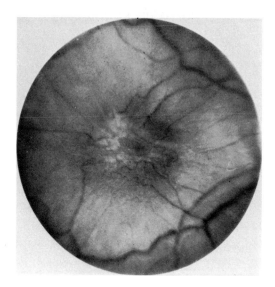

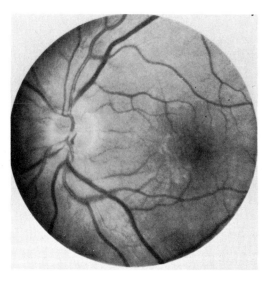

Fig. 19-6. Eye of 51-year-old man with history of sudden blurring of vision and metamorphopsia in 1959. Note marked wrinkling of macula with dense preretinal membrane just temporal to macula. Visual acuity is 20/80. (From Jaffe, N. S.: Arch. Ophthalmol. **78:**585-591, 1967.)

Fig. 19-7. Wrinkling of inner layer of retina at macula in eye of 57-year-old man. Note preretinal membrane just nasal to macula. (From Jaffe, N. S.: The vitreous in clinical ophthalmology, St. Louis, 1969, The C. V. Mosby Co.; courtesy Dr. J. D. M. Gass, Miami, Fla.)

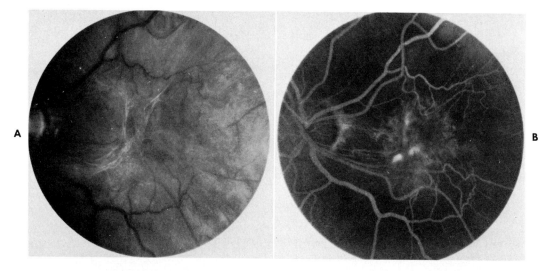

Fig. 19-8. A, Eye of 69-year-old man with wrinkling of inner layer of retina and extensive preretinal membrane. Visual acuity is 20/400. **B,** Same eye. Fluorescein fundus photograph reveals extensive leakage of dye into macular area. (From Jaffe, N. S.: The vitreous in clinical ophthalmology, St. Louis, 1969, The C. V. Mosby Co.; courtesy Dr. J. D. M. Gass, Miami, Fla.)

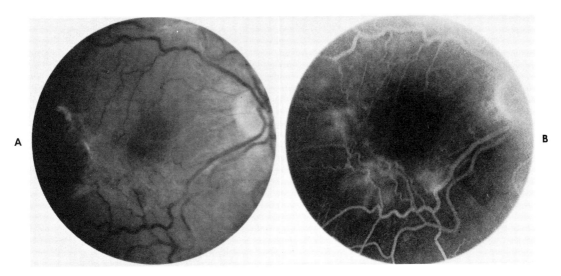

Fig. 19-9. A, Eye of 66-year-old woman with wrinkling of inner layer of retina and preretinal membrane formation. Visual acuity is 20/70. **B,** Same eye. Fluorescein fundus photograph reveals extensive leakage of dye into area of wrinkling. (From Jaffe, N. S.: The vitreous in clinical ophthalmology, St. Louis, 1969, The C. V. Mosby Co.; courtesy Dr. J. D. M. Gass, Miami, Fla.)

disc appear drawn to the fovea, so that the inferior and superior temporal arterioles become more closely approximated.

The membrane itself may show wide variations from a semitransparent and semitranslucent to a thick, grayish white, opaque tissue that causes major distortions of the retinal vessels (Figs. 19-4 to 19-7). Hemorrhages are occasionally seen and are usually of the splinter type. They are probably caused by the traction created on the walls of the vessels by the preretinal membrane.

It seems that the contraction, once begun, gains its final appearance in a relatively short time. It then does not appear to progress further for months or years. On rare occasions, such membranes may peel off or migrate to a new area. Maumenee[11] observed a preretinal membrane peel from the macular area and the patient's visual acuity return to normal. This was noted in a patient with pars planitis. Gass[12] has observed the spontaneous detachment and separation of such membranes in two patients.

The patient's visual acuity is usually relatively good (20/30 to 20/40) unless a dense preretinal membrane forms. Metamorphopsia may be present, and the patient may be aware of a definite scotoma.

The fluorescein angiographic findings, unlike those seen in cystoid macular edema, show little tendency for leakage of dye into the macula. Exceptions exist, especially in those patients with more marked retinal wrinkling and distortion. Gass[12] demonstrated that when alterations in the retinal capillary permeability to fluorescein occurred, the pattern of dye pooling was always irregular and appeared different from that seen in cystoid macular edema (Figs. 19-8 and 19-9). Fluorescein angiography also emphasized the tortuosity, dilatation, and central displacement of the paramacular vessels.

VITREORETINAL TRACTION SYNDROME

After lens extraction, alterations at the posterior pole of the fundus associated with vitreous adherent to the macula or disc are occasionally seen. In 1953 Irvine[13] ascribed the edema seen at the macula after cataract extraction to such a mechanism. This was restated more recently.[14] However, other observations[11,15,16] offer conclusive evidence that these are different entities (p. 366).

In my experience, vitreoretinal traction at the posterior pole of the fundus is seen far more frequently in phakic eyes because by the time patients come to cataract surgery, they are of an age when their eyes have usually undergone a posterior vitreous detachment. Whether alterations in the vitreous associated with the cataract surgery are responsible for the vitreoretinal traction at the macula is not known. However, it is theoretically possible for surgery-related alterations to occur, although I have the impression that when they are encountered after cataract surgery they usually predate the surgery.

Although the relationship of the vitreoretinal traction syndrome to cataract surgery remains unclear, the presence of the traction represents another cause of failure to achieve anticipated vision as a result of alterations at the posterior pole of the fundus.

It is not surprising that the relationship of the vitreous to the posterior pole has only recently become more clearly understood, at least on a clinical basis. The availability of more sophisticated means of examining the posterior vitreous and fundus with the slit lamp has enabled the clinician to recognize these relationships. Whereas I[16] reported 14 patients and Maumenee[11] reported seven patients with a macular pathologic condition resulting from the vitreoretinal traction syndrome, Goldmann[17] in 1958 stated that he had seen only one such case.

I repeat that if posterior pole alterations caused by vitreous traction are encountered after cataract surgery, they are probably not related to the surgery itself. Nonetheless, it is important to recognize and understand these changes so that they may be differentiated from other conditions that lend themselves to treatment and that a clearer picture of the ultimate prognosis may be obtained.

Pathogenesis

The cause of vitreoretinal adherence at the posterior pole is not known. It is probable that in the future a great deal more will be known about this condition, and we will consider these traction phenomena secondary vitreoretinal adherences. In some patients the condition may be caused by an unusually firm adherence of the vitreous to the macula. That the macula may be the site of such an adherence was noted by Grignolo,[18] who described a strong anatomic adhesion between the vitreous body and the retina in the

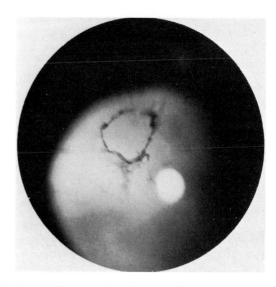

Fig. 19-10. Photograph of prepapillary opacity in eye with posterior vitreous detachment with collapse. (From Jaffe, N. S.: Arch. Ophthalmol. **78:**585-591, 1967.)

macular area. Schepens[19] stated that in the region of the disc and of the macula, it is difficult or impossible to separate the vitreous from the retina without breaking the surface layer or hyaloid membrane.

The exact anatomic nature of the vitreomacular relationship is still unknown. However, conclusions may be drawn from related histologic and clinical findings. The internal limiting membrane of the retina ends at the optic disc. It is not present over the nerve head. After a posterior vitreous detachment, a prepapillary ring is present in almost every case (Fig. 19-10). It is varied in shape, but in most instances a window exists where the posterior border of the vitreous appears absent. Presumably this window, or peephole, as Vogt[20] called it, corresponds to the area over the disc. Similarly, in some cases of posterior vitreous detachment, a round or oval premacular hole (Fig. 19-11) is also present. The edge of this hole is not thickened and irregular as is the prepapillary hole, probably because it is not surrounded by glial tissue. The internal limiting membrane is somewhat attenuated over the macula. This attenuation is substantiated by Yamada's[21] recent electron microscope observations that the basement membrane of the retina is

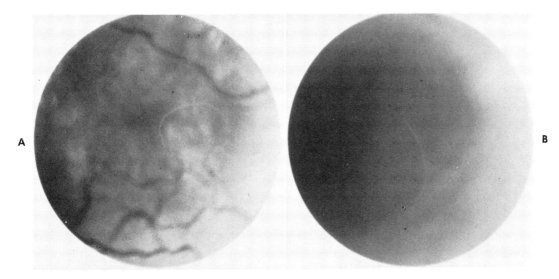

Fig. 19-11. A, Premacular hole in posterior border of detached vitreous in eye of 41-year-old man representing prior attachment of vitreous around macular area. **B,** Premacular hole in posterior border of detached vitreous in eye of 37-year-old woman with posterior uveitis. (**A** from Jaffe, N. S.: Ophthalmology [Rochester] **71:**642, 1967; **B** from Jaffe, N. S.: Arch. Ophthalmol. **78:**585-591, 1967.)

approximately 1.5 μm thick at the periphery of the macula, 0.4 μm thick at the edge of the fovea, and extremely thin (10 to 20 nm) at the foveal center. The outermost vitreous fibrils are attached to the basement membrane. A possible conclusion is that the vitreous is adherent to the macula around its periphery but may not have any attachment, or at best only a rudimentary one, to the center of the macula. The presence of a premacular hole in the posterior limiting border of the detached vitreous suggests this condition. Pathologic processes such as posterior uveitis, diabetes, and intraocular hemorrhage may cause a secondary vitreoretinal traction syndrome.

The vitreoretinal traction syndrome is a complication of posterior vitreous detachment rather than of cataract extraction. Posterior vitreous detachment may be a normal senescent process or may be associated with specific diseases such as posterior uveitis, diabetes mellitus.

Diagnosis

The diagnosis is made at the slit lamp with a Hruby or a fundus contact lens. The outline of the posterior vitreous detachment is traced. If the vitreous is detached from the disc, a prepapillary

opacity is usually found. This opacity occupies the posterior border of the detached vitreous. The residual vitreoretinal adherence is best viewed by making the angle between the light source and the observer as wide as possible. It is to be remembered that the normal vitreous strands are slightly greater than 100 Å in diameter, which is below the normal resolution of the light microscope. Thus some vitreoretinal strands will be missed. Dark adaptation is essential for the observer in identifying smaller fibrils.

Clinical findings

The vitreoretinal traction syndrome presents several signs and symptoms. The onset is abrupt; the patient complains of one or more of the following: painless blurring of vision, metamorphopsia, photopsia, entopsia, and micropsia.

Examination of the posterior vitreous and fundus reveals a posterior vitreous detachment with residual adherence of the vitreous to the posterior pole (Fig. 19-12). A mild cellular reaction may be present in the posterior vitreous. The macula appears under traction and may be somewhat thickened without a detachment of the sensory epithelium of the retina. Punctate and flame-

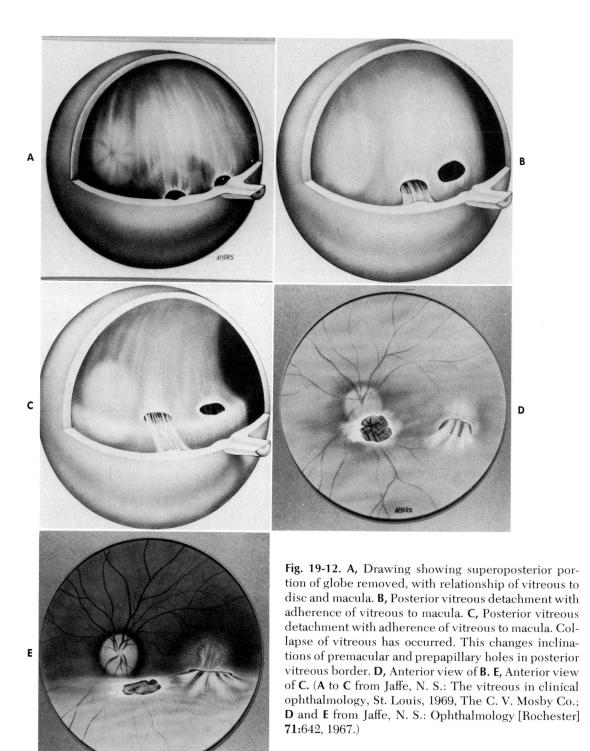

Fig. 19-12. A, Drawing showing superoposterior portion of globe removed, with relationship of vitreous to disc and macula. **B,** Posterior vitreous detachment with adherence of vitreous to macula. **C,** Posterior vitreous detachment with adherence of vitreous to macula. Collapse of vitreous has occurred. This changes inclinations of premacular and prepapillary holes in posterior vitreous border. **D,** Anterior view of **B. E,** Anterior view of **C.** (**A** to **C** from Jaffe, N. S.: The vitreous in clinical ophthalmology, St. Louis, 1969, The C. V. Mosby Co.; **D** and **E** from Jaffe, N. S.: Ophthalmology [Rochester] **71:**642, 1967.)

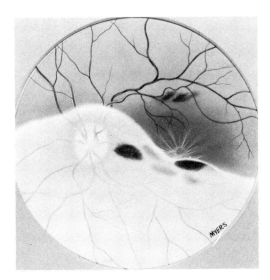

Fig. 19-13. Fundus drawing of eye of 65-year-old man with posterior vitreous detachment. There are two intraretinal hemorrhages superonasal to macula. There are five hemorrhages in posterior border of vitreous. Adherence of vitreous to macula is seen. Visual acuity is 20/70. Hemorrhages disappeared in 5 days, and visual acuity improved to 20/50. Three weeks later, vitreoretinal adherence separated, and visual acuity was 20/30. (From Jaffe, N. S.: Arch. Ophthalmol. **78:**585, 1967.)

shaped hemorrhages may occasionally be found in the retinal tissue (Fig. 19-13).

In my experience the adherence of vitreous to the posterior pole may appear in one of the following four ways:

1. As a distinct horizontal line of adherence, extending from the disc across the macula and out to the periphery (Fig. 19-14). The chronologic sequence of events in the pathogenesis of such a horizontal line of adherence was followed in a young adult who suffered a recurrence of a posterior uveitis (Fig. 19-15).

2. As a broad, irregular adherence to the posterior pole (Fig. 19-16). The sequence of events in such a lesion and its subsequent changes are shown in Fig. 19-17.

3. As a taut strand of vitreous, connecting the separated vitreous to the macula (Fig. 19-18).

4. As an adherence only to the disc, causing elevation with hemorrhages on or around the disc.

Fluorescein angiography usually reveals no leakage into the retinal tissue or into the subretinal space from the underlying choroid. This point is important in differentiating this condi-

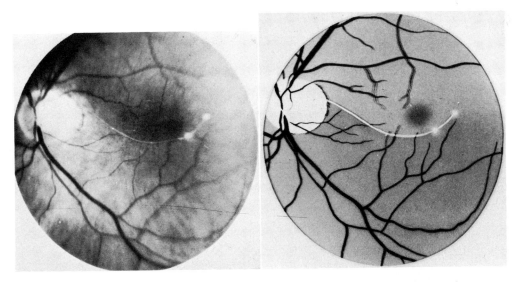

Fig. 19-14. Left eye of 67-year-old man with vitreoretinal traction syndrome, demonstrating horizontal line of adherence of vitreous to retina from disc across inferior portion of macular area. Sketch on right emphasizes line of adherence. (From Jaffe, N. S.: Arch. Ophthalmol. **78:**585-591, 1967.)

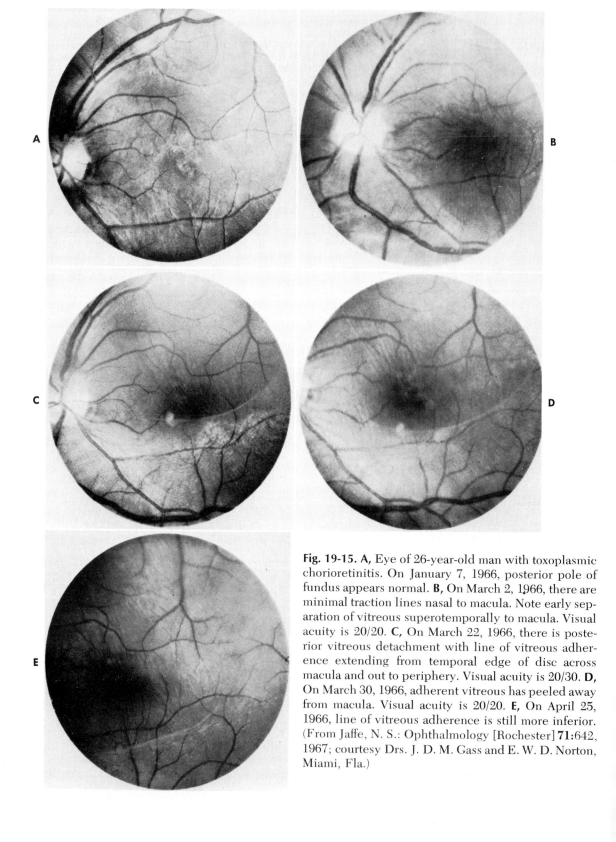

Fig. 19-15. A, Eye of 26-year-old man with toxoplasmic chorioretinitis. On January 7, 1966, posterior pole of fundus appears normal. **B,** On March 2, 1966, there are minimal traction lines nasal to macula. Note early separation of vitreous superotemporally to macula. Visual acuity is 20/20. **C,** On March 22, 1966, there is posterior vitreous detachment with line of vitreous adherence extending from temporal edge of disc across macula and out to periphery. Visual acuity is 20/30. **D,** On March 30, 1966, adherent vitreous has peeled away from macula. Visual acuity is 20/20. **E,** On April 25, 1966, line of vitreous adherence is still more inferior. (From Jaffe, N. S.: Ophthalmology [Rochester] **71:**642, 1967; courtesy Drs. J. D. M. Gass and E. W. D. Norton, Miami, Fla.)

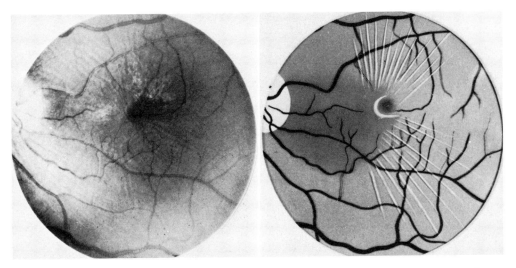

Fig. 19-16. Eye of 40-year-old man with posterior vitreous detachment. There is residual vitreoretinal adherence from disc to macula. Densest area of adherence is represented by swirl of vitreous on nasal and interior margins of fovea. Metamorphopsia is present. Visual acuity is 20/25. Sketch on right emphasizes broad area of vitreous adherence and swirl near fovea. (From Jaffe, N. S.: Ophthalmology [Rochester] **71**:642, 1967; courtesy Dr. J. D. M. Gass, Miami, Fla.)

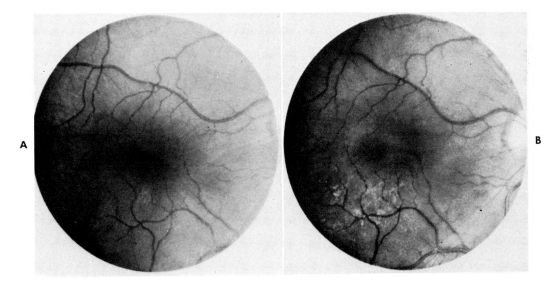

Fig. 19-17. A, October 11, 1965; right eye of 41-year-old man with posterior vitreous detachment and residual vitreoretinal adherence to paramacular area. Visual acuity is 20/70. Metamorphopsia is present. Densest area of adherence is superior and inferior nasal to macula. **B,** October 19, 1965; adherence had separated, and visual acuity had improved to 20/25 +3. Note irregular light reflexes inferior to macula as if smooth contour of inner layer of retina has been disturbed.

Continued.

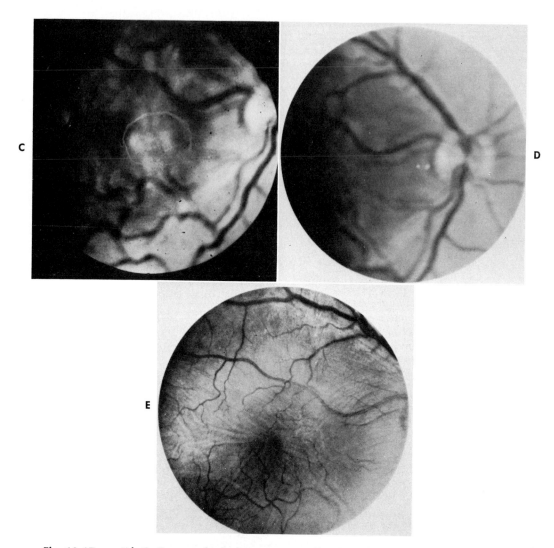

Fig. 19-17, cont'd. C, Premacular hole in posterior border of detached vitreous representing area of prior adherence to perimacular area. **D,** Note prepapillary opacity in front of disc and slightly temporal to it. **E,** One year later, fundus photograph reveals marked wrinkling of inner retina at level of internal limiting membrane. Visual acuity is 20/30, but patient complains of metamorphopsia. (**A** to **C** from Jaffe, N. S.: Ophthalmology [Rochester] **71:**642, 1967; **D** and **E** from Jaffe, N. S.: The vitreous in clinical ophthalmology, St. Louis, 1969, The C. V. Mosby Co.; **A** to **E** courtesy Dr. J. D. M. Gass, Miami, Fla.)

tion from the Irvine-Gass syndrome, serous detachment of the macula, and serous detachment of the pigment epithelium. As stated previously (p. 381), Gass[12] has observed that in those patients with a greater degree of retinal wrinkling and distortion, angiography occasionally demonstrated variable degrees of intraretinal leakage of dye (Figs. 19-8 and 19-9). He noted further that the pattern of dye pooling was always irregular and appeared quite different from the characteristic pattern seen in cystoid macular edema.

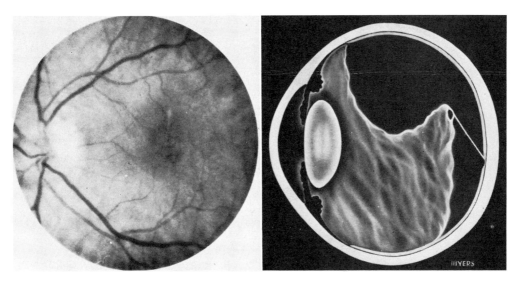

Fig. 19-18. Eye of 68-year-old man with taut strand of vitreous attached to macula at edge of macular hole. Strand originates from upper edge of premacular hole in posterior border of detached vitreous. Visual acuity is 20/100 +2. Sketch on right emphasizes residual vitreoretinal adherence. (From Jaffe, N. S.: Ophthalmology [Rochester] **71:** 642, 1967.)

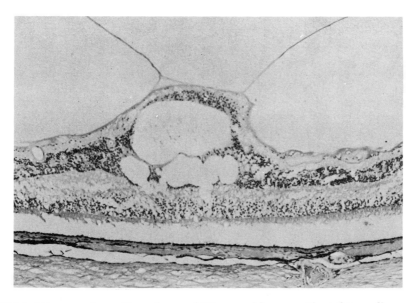

Fig. 19-19. Microscopic section of eye of 75-year-old man with striking adherence of vitreous to macula. Eye was phakic. Cystic macular edema was confined mainly to inner nuclear layer. (From Boniuk, M.: Surv. Ophthalmol. **13:**118, 1968.)

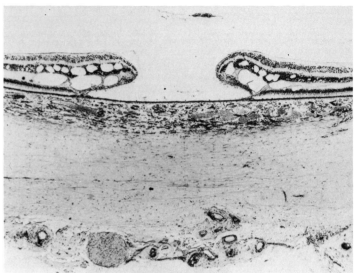

Fig. 19-20. Macular hole with operculum attached to overlying vitreous in eye of 41-year-old woman. Sympathetic ophthalmia after iridencleisis for glaucoma. No history of trauma other than operation. (From Maumenee, A. E.: Arch. Ophthalmol. **78:**151-165, 1967.)

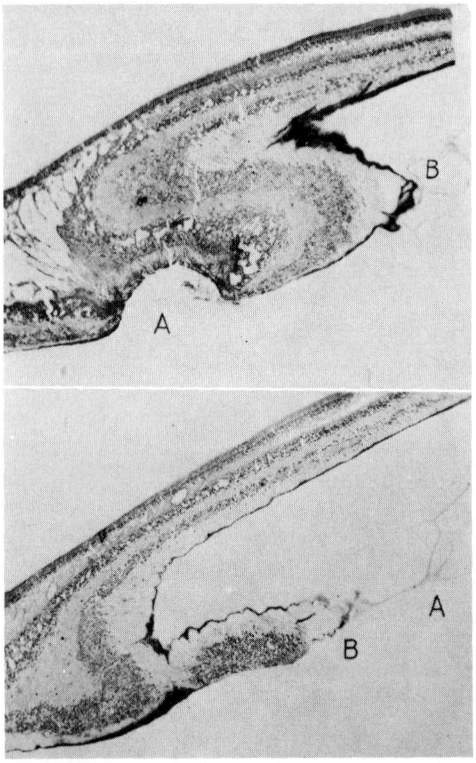

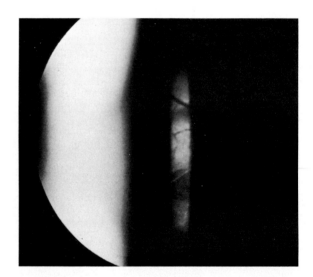

Fig. 19-21. Upper figure shows section through macular area prior to enucleation of eye for malignant melanoma of choroid. Macula is detached, edematous, and cystic. Fovea is shown as deep cut at *A*. There is traction at vitreomacular symphysis at *B*. Lower figure of same eye reveals tongue of tissue, *B*, being pulled away from detached macula by vitreous strands, *A*. There is edema of macula and cystic degeneration of inner nuclear layer. (From Reese, A. B., Jones I. S., and Cooper, W. C.: Trans. Am. Ophthalmol. Soc. **64:** 123, 1966.)

Fig. 19-22. Slit lamp photograph through Hruby lens demonstrating macular hole in left eye of 72-year-old man. Examination revealed posterior vitreous detachment with collapse complicated by residual adherence of vitreous to retina (seen 2 hole diameters above macular hole). Strand of this vitreous adherence is seen bridging macular hole 1:00 to 10:00 o'clock. (From Jaffe, N. S.: The vitreous in clinical ophthalmology, St. Louis, 1969. The C. V. Mosby Co.)

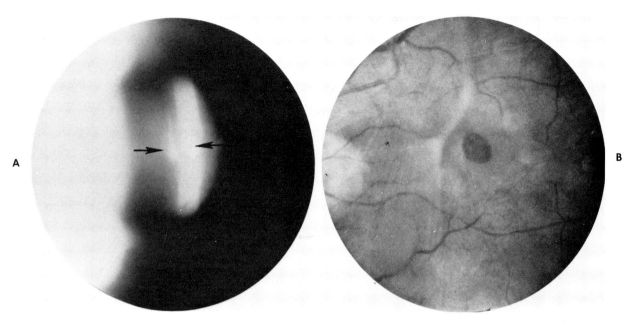

Fig. 19-23. A, Slit lamp photograph through Hruby lens demonstrating vitreous *(left arrow)* adherent to nasal edge of macular hole *(right arrow)* in left eye of 74-year-old man. **B,** In same eye, band of vitreous is seen 1 disc diameter nasal to macular hole with extension to nasal edge of hole.

Prognosis

In favorable cases the vitreous peels away from the retina, and the symptoms simultaneously disappear. However, in more intense cases, three important sequelae may result.

Cystic degeneration of the macula. When vitreous adheres to the retina for a considerable period, a cystic degeneration may ensue (Fig. 19-19). Boniuk[22] has differentiated a cystic macular edema confined mainly to the inner nuclear layer from the cystoid macular edema seen in the Irvine-Gass syndrome, which involves the outer plexiform layer of Henle. It is unknown if this is a valid differentiation.

Macular hole. Vitreomacular traction may cause a macular hole. I do not consider this a frequent cause, but when an operculum has been torn free from the macula and is adherent to a band of vitreous (Figs. 19-20 and 19-21), or when vitreous strands bridge or attach to the edge of a macular hole (Figs. 19-22 and 19-23), the evidence is compelling to consider this traction a probable cause of macular hole formation.

Macular pucker and preretinal membrane formation. After the vitreous separates from the pos-

terior pole, the symptoms usually disappear, and the fundus appearance may return to normal. However, one may be surprised at a later date to observe a wrinkling of the inner layer of the retina associated with a preretinal membrane of variable thickness. The clinical picture has been described on p. 377. The sequence of events in such a case is well exemplified in Fig. 19-17. The cause of the wrinkling and the preretinal membrane is still unknown. It may be related to the proliferation of vitreous cells in the vitreous fibrils that remain in contact with the retina after a posterior vitreous detachment, as discussed on p. 377.

CHOROIDAL FOLDS FROM HIGH HYPEROPIA

Patients with a high degree of hyperopia occasionally have choroidal folds, which may interfere with vision. The ophthalmoscopic appearance (Fig. 19-24) is similar to that seen with postoperative hypotension (p. 286). The choroidal folds produce alternate yellow and dark streaks, which often extend through the posterior pole of the eye. The direction of the folds may be horizontal, vertical, and oblique, and they tend to run

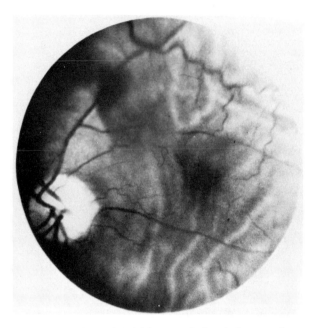

Fig. 19-24. Choroidal folds in aphakic left eye of 74-year-old woman with high degree of hyperopia (+22 D). Light streaks represent crests of folds. Valleys between folds appear dark.

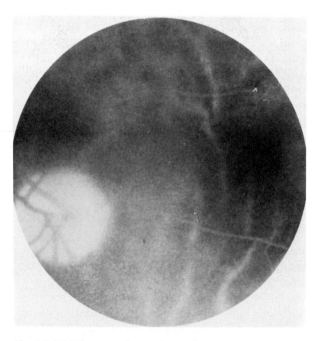

Fig. 19-25. Fluorescein angiography in same eye as in Fig. 19-24.

parallel to one another, although not exactly. Biomicroscopy reveals that the wrinkles involve the entire retina and choroid, not just the inner layer of the retina as in macular pucker. The crests of the choroidal and overlying pigment epithelial folds appear yellow, and the valleys between the folds appear dark.

Fluorescein angiography reveals streaks of hyperfluorescence that coincide with the yellow streaks seen with the ophthalmoscope (Fig. 19-25). This intensification of choroidal fluorescence is the result of the relative thinning of the pigment epithelium on the crest of the fold, the greater thickness of the pool of choroidal dye beneath the crest, and the shorter course of the incident blue and reflected yellow-green light through the pigment epithelium on the crest.[12] The dark troughs seen ophthalmoscopically appear relatively hypofluorescent. Angiography is helpful in differentiating these folds from finer folds in the retina that do not alter the background choroidal fluorescence.

Visual function is disturbed as a result of the distortion of the pigment epithelium and retinal receptors that overlie the crests of the choroidal folds. Later, organic changes in the neuroepithelium may occur. The effect on vision is greater if the folds run through the posterior pole of the eye.

The cause of choroidal folds in high hyperopia is not entirely clear. Obviously these cases are special, since folds are not constantly found in this condition. One might attribute the folds to excess choroid in relation to the sclera. This excess might be congenital or acquired.

REFERENCES

1. Oliver, M.: Posterior pole changes after cataract extraction in elderly subjects, Am. J. Ophthalmol. **62:**1145-1148, 1966.
2. Duke-Elder, S.: System of ophthalmology. Vol. IX. Disease of the uveal tract, St. Louis, 1966, The C. V. Mosby Co., p. 145.
3. Miller, G. R., and Smith, J. L.: Ischemic optic neuropathy, Am. J. Ophthalmol. **62:**103-115, 1966.
4. Vila-Coro, A.: Atrofia del nervio óptico después de la operación de cataracta, Arch. Soc. Oftalmol. Hisp.-Amer. **6:**901-904, 1946.
5. Townes, C. D., Moran, C. T., and Pfingst, H. A.: Complications of cataract surgery, Trans. Am. Ophthalmol. Soc. **49:**91-107, 1951.
6. Reese, A. B., and Carroll, F. D.: Optic neuritis following

cataract extraction. Ophthalmology (Rochester) **62:**765-770, 1958.

7. Carroll. F.: Optic nerve complications of cataract extraction, Ophthalmology (Rochester) **77:**OP 623-629, 1973.

8. Michaels, D. D., and Zugsmith, G. S.: Optic neuropathy following cataract extraction, Ann. Ophthalmol. **5:**303-306, 1973.

9. Kraushar, M. F., Seelenfreund, M. H., and Freilich, D. B.: Central retinal artery closure during orbital hemorrhage from retrobulbar injection, Ophthalmology (Rochester) **78:**OP 65-70, 1974.

10. Jaffe, N. S.: Macular retinopathy after separation of vitreo-retinal adherence, Arch. Ophthalmol. **78:**585-591, 1967.

11. Maumenee, A. E.: Further advances in the study of the macula, Arch. Ophthalmol. **78:**151-165, 1967.

12. Gass, J. D. M.: Stereoscopic atlas of macular diseases. A funduscopic and angiographic presentation, St. Louis, 1970, The C. V. Mosby Co., pp. 210-212, 100.

13. Irvine, S. R.: A newly defined vitreous syndrome following cataract surgery, interpreted according to recent concepts of the structure of the vitreous, Am. J. Ophthalmol. **36:**599-619, 1953.

14. Tolentino, F. I., and Schepens, C. L.: Edema of posterior pole after cataract extraction: a biomicroscopic study, Arch. Ophthalmol. **74:**781-786, 1965.

15. Gass, J. D. M., and Norton, E. W. D.: Cystoid macular edema and papilledema following cataract extraction: a fluorescein funduscopic and angiographic study, Arch. Ophthalmol. **76:**646-661, 1966.

16. Jaffe, N. S.: Vitreous traction at the posterior pole of the fundus due to alterations in the vitreous posterior, Ophthalmology (Rochester) **71:**642-652, 1967.

17. Goldmann, H.: Le corps vitré. In Busacca, A., Goldmann, H., and Schiff-Wertheimer, S. P.: Biomicroscopie du corps vitré et du fond de l'oeil, Paris, 1957, Masson & Cie, Editeurs, p. 97.

18. Grignolo, A.: Fibrous components of the vitreous body, Arch. Ophthalmol. **47:**760-774, 1952.

19. Schepens, C. L.: Clinical aspects of pathologic changes in the vitreous body, Am. J. Ophthalmol. **38**(part 2):8-21, 1954.

20. Vogt, A.: Handbook and atlas of the slit lamp microscopy of the living eye. Translation of vol. 3, ed. 2, Atlas of slit lamp microscopy, Zurich, 1941, Schweizer Druckund Verlagshaus, p. 992.

21. Yamada, E.: Some structural features of the fovea centralis in the human retina, Arch. Ophthalmol. **82:**151-159, 1969.

22. Boniuk, M.: Cystic macular edema secondary to vitreo-retinal traction, Surv. Ophthalmol. **13:**118-121, 1968.

CHAPTER 20

Vitreous changes

Before the popularization of the intracapsular method of lens extraction, postoperative alterations in the anterior vitreous excited little interest and created little anxiety. A well-performed, planned extracapsular extraction left an intact posterior lens capsule that occupied a position behind the level of the iris.

A brief reminder of pertinent anatomy will emphasize the great variation in the disturbance of morphologic relationships between the extracapsular and intracapsular lens extraction procedures.

The lens capsule has important relationships to the anterior vitreous and the zonular fibers. It will be recalled that the anterior hyaloid membrane is attached to the posterior capsule of the lens in the form of an 8 to 9 mm diameter circle known as the hyaloideocapsular ligament (Fig. 20-1). The zonular lamella forms the external layer of the lens capsule; it consists of an anterior insertion 1 mm from the equator and a posterior insertion 1.5 mm from the equator (Fig. 20-2).

EXTRACAPSULAR LENS EXTRACTION

In a planned extracapsular lens extraction the posterior capsule remains intact. It remains in contact with the anterior hyaloid membrane and retains some attachments to the zonular fibers. There may be some cortical remnants together with some proliferated lens epithelium (Elschnig's pearls). This is described on p. 481.

Frequently the thin posterior capsule becomes diaphanous. There may be a localized bulge of the vitreous covered by an intact anterior hyaloid membrane. In other cases the anterior hyaloid membrane ruptures, and loose vitreous fibrils course into the anterior chamber. However, in most instances the posterior capsule remains intact and prevents the vitreous from entering the anterior chamber. There is at least some theoretical advantage to confining the vitreous to a position similar to the position it occupies in the phakic eye and to preserving the zonular relationships to the ora serrata and to the capsule of the lens. These advantages are discussed on p. 368.

INTRACAPSULAR LENS EXTRACTION

After an intracapsular lens extraction, the anterior part of the vitreous is deprived of its support (lens and zonule). At the level of the patellar fossa, the anterior hyaloid membrane, previously concave, becomes convex. However, there are cases in which the membrane remains behind the level of the iris and retains a posterior chamber of sorts. Usually the anterior hyaloid membrane lies in contact with the posterior surface of the iris and the edge of the pupil and bulges somewhat into the anterior chamber.

Surface alterations of intact anterior hyaloid membrane

The anterior hyaloid membrane has the appearance of an opalescent sheet on whose surface are found pigment deposits and small white spots derived from organization of exudate. The latter are the residues of the slight inflammatory reactions accompanying an intracapsular lens extraction. Occasionally one finds bands of organized tissue with a fine fibrillary structure. They account for irregularities found on the surface of the anterior hyaloid membrane. The bands may cause a linear depression or cicatricial contraction in the membrane, the latter bulging forward

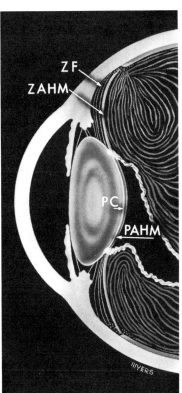

Fig. 20-1. Anterior hyaloid membrane, *AHM*, consists of two portions: a zonuler or extralenticular part, *ZAHM*, which covers secondary vitreous and extends from ora serrata to hyaloideocapsular ligament, and a patellar or refrolenticular part, *PAHM*, which covers the primary vitreous and is normally adherent to posterior lens capsule, *PC*, within Egger's line. Zonular fibers, *ZF*, are shown in posterior chamber just anterior to *ZAHM*. (From Jaffe, N. S.: The vitreous in clinical ophthalmology, St. Louis, 1969, The C. V. Mosby Co.)

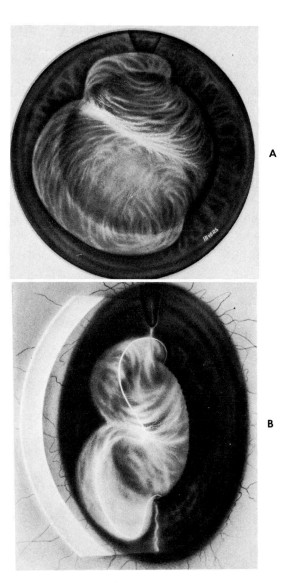

A

B

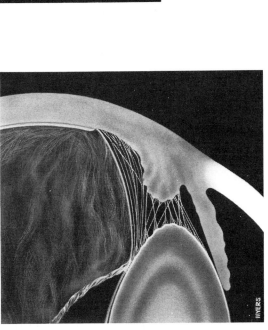

Fig. 20-2. Distribution of zonular fibers. Zonular lamella forms external layer of lens capsule consisting of anterior insertion 1 mm from equator and posterior insertion 1.5 mm from equator. (From Jaffe, N. S.: The vitreous in clinical ophthalmology, St. Louis, 1969, The C. V. Mosby Co.)

Fig. 20-3. A, Linear contraction of bulging intact anterior hyaloid membrane caused by organization of postoperative inflammatory exudate. **B,** By slit lamp. (From Jaffe, N. S., and Light, D. S.: Arch. Ophthalmol. **76:** 541, 1966.)

on both sides of the linear band (Fig. 20-3). If the inflammatory reaction is more severe, the iris may adhere to the anterior hyaloid membrane, either partially or wholly. As long as the surgical iridectomy is patent, the iris does not bulge forward. Similar morphologic changes may occur after partial organization of a hyphema. Generally the anterior hyaloid membrane bulges less after a significant inflammation or hyphema.

Occasionally the cicatrix will cover only a portion of the anterior hyaloid membrane; that portion remains flat while the remaining normal part of the membrane bulges considerably into the anterior chamber (Fig. 20-4). If the edge of the iris is adherent to the anterior hyaloid membrane as a result of inflammation, the synechias resemble the posterior synechias associated with iridocyclitis seen in phakic eyes.

Generally only the retrolenticular (patellar) portion of the anterior hyaloid membrane bulges forward. The extralenticular portion (zonular) is never visible through the normal pupil after round-pupil cataract surgery. It is visible through the one or more peripheral iridectomies and is

readily identified, since its surface reflects light more readily than the retrolenticular part as a result of its increased thickness. There is usually a distinct space between the iris and the membrane in this location. It practically never bulges through the peripheral surgical coloboma, although exceptions are seen (Fig. 20-5). If a sector iridectomy is performed, the transition between the retrolenticular and the extralenticular portions of the membrane is visible. The latter portion tends to remain flat as it courses posteriorly. It may even have a slight concavity superiorly. One should recall that the diameter of the circle outlined by Wieger's ligament on the posterior lens capsule is nearly 9 mm; therefore the transition zone is quite peripheral when viewed with the biomicroscope.

The factors responsible for the bulge and the grading system employed are discussed later. However, at this point it may be stated that the two eyes of the same person tend to show a similar bulge after bilateral cataract surgery.

Intracapsular lens extraction modifies the configuration of the anterior portion of Cloquet's

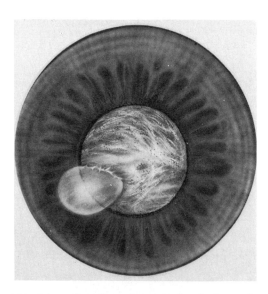

Fig. 20-4. Most of surface of anterior hyaloid membrane is covered by pigment and fibrous tissue, while one uninvolved area bulges considerably into anterior chamber. (From Jaffe, N. S., and Light, D. S.: Arch. Ophthalmol. **76:**541, 1966.)

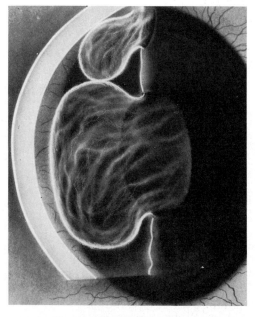

Fig. 20-5. Considerable elasticity of intact anterior hyaloid membrane is demonstrated. Bulge through peripheral iridectomy as well as through pupil is observed. (From Jaffe, N. S., and Light, D. S.: Arch. Ophthalmol. **76:**541, 1966.)

canal. It will be recalled that the anterior parts of the roof and floor of Cloquet's canal (superior and interior plicae) insert into the anterior hyaloid membrane at the hyaloideocapsular ligament. The superior plica remains in contact with the retrolenticular portion for some distance before it passes down and back. The inferior plica runs superiorly for a slight distance in contact with the membrane before it likewise swings down and back. After lens extraction the fixed parts of the plicae detach from the anterior hyaloid membrane except at its insertion, which is almost at the level of the insertion of the posterior zonular fibers. The superior plica, particularly, is well visualized and describes a somewhat more posterior course than in the phakic eye, where it runs almost vertically downward behind the lens. Thus the anterior funnel of Cloquet's canal appears more spacious in a sagittal direction. However, since the retrolenticular portion of the anterior hyaloid membrane bulges somewhat into the anterior chamber, the insertions of the superior and inferior plicas approach each other, and thus the funnel is narrowed.

Postoperative rupture of anterior hyaloid membrane

Holes in the anterior hyaloid membrane are frequent after an uneventful intracapsular lens extraction. They are associated with a variety of morphologic alterations in the anterior vitreous. There has been considerable confusion concerning the anatomic basis for the multitude of situations encountered. After reviewing a large postoperative series of cases, I have observed several characteristic patterns[1] that permit a classification of postoperative holes in the anterior hyaloid membrane. An attempt is made here to relate these changes to the facts of the anatomy of the anterior vitreous, considered previously.

Classification of holes in anterior hyaloid membrane

I. Hole in the anterior hyaloid membrane without vitreous coursing through
  A. Plugged by anterior limiting border of the vitreous
  B. Plugged by superior or inferior plica
II. Hole in the anterior hyaloid membrane with vitreous coursing through

A. Anterior contents of Cloquet's canal, covered by a "new" surface, coursing through hole
B. Anterior portion of Cloquet's canal, its plicae, and perhaps other membranes of secondary vitreous coursing through hole
C. Free vitreous that attaches to operative wound and cornea coursing through hole
D. Small amounts of free vitreous appearing like multiple loose strings in aqueous coursing through hole

Hole in anterior hyaloid membrane without vitreous coursing through. A hole in the membrane is visible, but at no time are vitreous fibrils found passing through the hole.

Plugged by anterior limiting border of vitreous. Recall that a layer of condensed vitreous

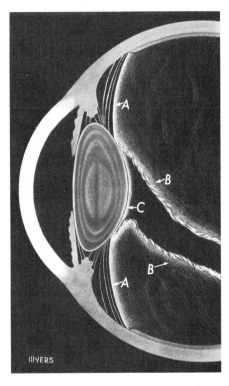

Fig. 20-6. Anterior limiting borders of anterior vitreous, consisting of layers of more closely packed vitreous fibers. Anterior limiting border of secondary vitreous, *A*, lines zonular portion of anterior hyaloid membrane and outer walls of Cloquet's canal, *B*. *C*, Anterior limiting border of primary vitreous. (After Busacca, A.: Biomicroscopie et histopathologie de l'oeil, vol. 3, Zurich, 1967, Schweizer Verlagshaus AG; from Jaffe, N. S.: The vitreous in clinical ophthalmology, St. Louis, 1969, The C. V. Mosby Co.)

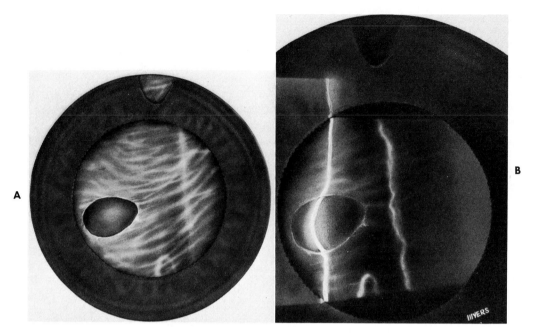

Fig. 20-7. Hole in anterior hyaloid membrane plugged by anterior limiting border of vitreous. Loose vitreous does not course through hole. Walls of Cloquet's canal are visible and appear normal. **B,** By slit lamp. (From Jaffe, N. S., and Light, D. S.: Arch. Ophthalmol. **76:**541, 1966.)

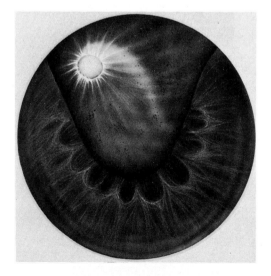

Fig. 20-8. Hole in anterior hyaloid membrane plugged by superior plica of Vogt. (From Jaffe, N. S., and Light, D. S.: Arch. Ophthalmol. **76:**541, 1966.)

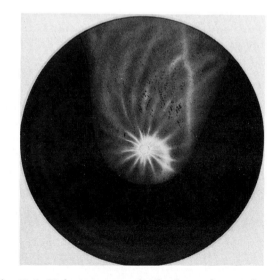

Fig. 20-9. Hole in anterior hyaloid membrane plugged by inferior plica of Vogt. (From Jaffe, N. S., and Light, D. S.: Arch. Ophthalmol. **76:**541, 1966.)

humor lines both portions of the anterior hyaloid membrane. Its thickness varies in different individuals. This layer represents the anterior limiting border of the primary vitreous at the anterior extremity of Cloquet's canal (Fig. 20-6). The membranes constituting the roof and floor of the canal remain undisturbed and do not project through or attach to the hole. The hole is easily visualized, since it is usually oval, and its margins tend to roll slightly outward (Fig. 20-7).

Plugged by vitreous membranes preventing loose vitreous fibrils from coursing through. The hole may be plugged by the superior plica (roof of Cloquet's canal, Fig. 20-8) or the inferior plica (floor of Cloquet's canal, Fig. 20-9). In neither case is free vitreous found in the anterior chamber at any time after the appearance of the hole. Around the hole and converging on it are found tension striae resembling the spokes of a wheel. That these membranes are indeed the walls of Cloquet's canal can be verified by tracing them posteriorly and observing their position and rela-

tionships on movements of the globe (ascension phenomenon).

Hole in anterior hyaloid membrane with vitreous coursing through

Anterior contents of Cloquet's canal, covered by a "new" surface, coursing through hole. At no time are loose vitreous fibrils found in the anterior chamber. The anterior contents of Cloquet's canal and its membranes herniate through the hole. One readily identifies the walls of the funnel, which approach each other when the hernia exteriorizes and separate more when it recedes. The "new" anterior hyaloid membrane is nothing more than the anterior limiting border of the vitreous, as Busacca[2] pointed out (Fig. 20-10). Purtscher[3] has contributed greatly to our knowledge of the anterior hyaloid membrane. He was able to study eyes histologically after an intracapsular lens extraction. He stated that the anterior hyaloid membrane (which he called *Grenzhaut*) is different from the condensation border or anterior limiting border of the vitreous (which he called *Grenzschicht*).

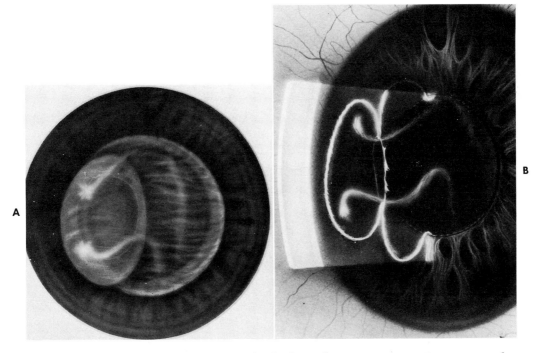

Fig. 20-10. A, Through hole in anterior hyaloid membrane course anterior contents of Cloquet's canal, lined by what appears to be new anterior hyaloid membrane. This may be anterior limiting border of vitreous. **B,** By slit lamp. (From Jaffe, N. S., and Light, D. S.: Arch. Ophthalmol. **76:**541, 1966.)

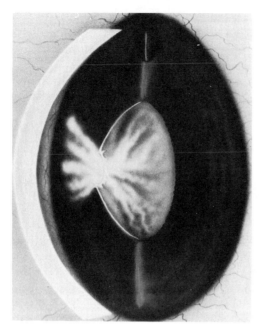

Fig. 20-11. Vitreous membranes course through hole in anterior hyaloid membrane, distorting normal relationships of anterior vitreous. (From Jaffe, N. S., and Light, D. S.: Arch. Ophthalmol. **76:**541, 1966.)

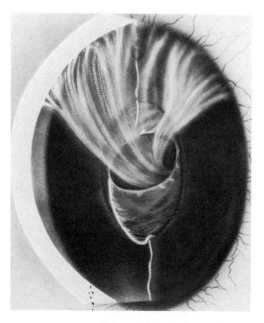

Fig. 20-12. Vitreous attached to operative wound. Eye exhibited Irvine-Gass syndrome. (From Jaffe, N. S., and Light, D. S.: Arch. Ophthalmol. **76:**541, 1966.)

Anterior portion of Cloquet's canal, its plicae, and other membranes of secondary vitreous coursing through hole. At some time after the appearance of the hole in the anterior hyaloid membrane, free vitreous is found in the anterior chamber. Later this conglomerate mass of vitreous recedes toward the hole. The surface of this mass becomes condensed, and tension striae are found on its surface. Since vitreous is a colloidal solution, its free surface will invariably suffer a condensation of this nature. The colloid particles become absorbed on its surface, where, being tightly packed and closely crowded together, the micelles become oriented in parallel lines and eventually are coagulated.[4] (The "skin" of boiled milk is an extreme example of such a surface condensation.) Eventually the hole may be lost to view. The normal relationships of the anterior vitreous become distorted and may be impossible to identify (Fig. 20-11).

Free vitreous that attaches to operative wound and cornea coursing through hole. These vitreous strands condense and become relatively opaque and tenacious (Fig. 20-12). They show little tendency to recede toward the hole in the anterior hyaloid membrane, as in the previous situation. They may cause peaking of a round pupil. Peaking is usually found in the first 3 to 4 months after lens extraction. After this time the vitreous does not readily attach itself to the area of incision. The anterior funnel of Cloquet's canal is obliterated. These "horsetail opacities" were emphasized by Irvine[5] in his elucidation of the syndrome that now bears his name. The contraction of these strands may exert an influence on the macula (cystoid macular edema) but not by direct traction at the macula (p. 366). A special situation exists when the corneal endothelium is dystrophic. Adherence to the cornea is thereby facilitated, and retraction of vitreous toward the hole does not occur.

Small amounts of free vitreous appearing like multiple loose strings in aqueous coursing through hole (Fig. 20-13). The relationships of the anterior vitreous remain relatively undisturbed. The anterior funnel of Cloquet's canal is easily identified, as are the superior and inferior plicae. The latter move freely on movements of the globe. These relatively small holes are usually located at or near the pupillary margin. They

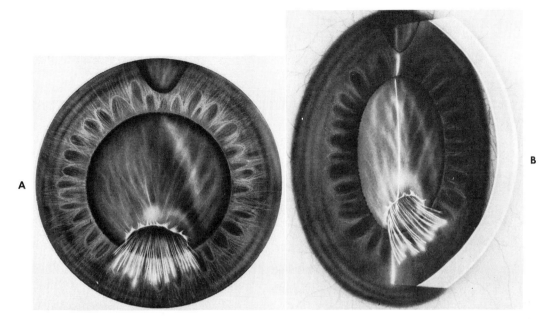

Fig. 20-13. A, Loose vitreous fibrils course through inferior hole in anterior hyaloid membrane with preservation of relationships of anterior vitreous. **B,** By slit lamp. (From Jaffe, N. S., and Light, D. S.: Arch. Ophthalmol. **76:**541, 1966.)

are frequent after an intracapsular lens extraction. Since they are small and not associated with striking morphologic changes in the anterior vitreous, they often remain undetected. The loose fibrils probably represent a portion of the superior or inferior plica or other membranes of the secondary vitreous, which may pass through a rent in the plica.

Holes in the anterior hyaloid membrane are outlined by a bluish white border that glistens and occasionally rolls slightly outward. They are usually round or oval, although their shape is not constant. They often appear at the edge of the pupil, suggesting that sphincteric action plays some role in their genesis. Fig. 20-14 shows three distinct holes at 3, 6, and 9 o'clock. However, holes are also found in the center of the exposed portion of the anterior hyaloid membrane, where sphincteric action probably exerts no influence (Fig. 20-15). It is my impression that holes are found with greater frequency if the pupil is kept widely dilated for 2 or more weeks after lens extraction. Holes are rarely found outside the retrolenticular portion of the anterior hyaloid membrane, possibly because the extralenticular por-

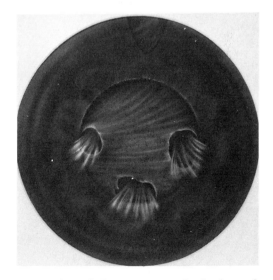

Fig. 20-14. Three holes in anterior hyaloid membrane in typical locations at iris border. (From Jaffe, N. S., and Light, D. S.: Arch. Ophthalmol. **76:**541, 1966.)

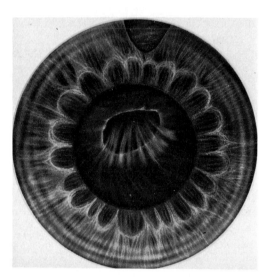

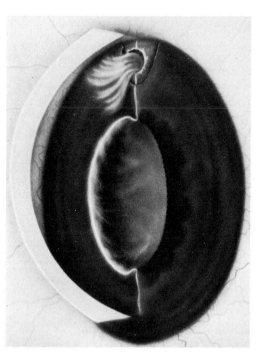

Fig. 20-15. Hole in central portion of anterior hyaloid membrane. (From Jaffe, N. S., and Light, D. S.: Arch. Ophthalmol. **76:**541, 1966.)

Fig. 20-16. Hole in anterior hyaloid membrane seen through peripheral iridectomy. (From Jaffe, N. S., and Light, D. S.: Arch. Ophthalmol. **76:**541, 1966.)

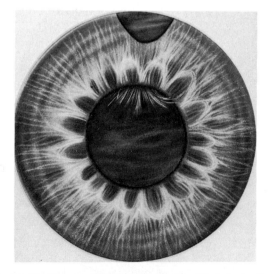

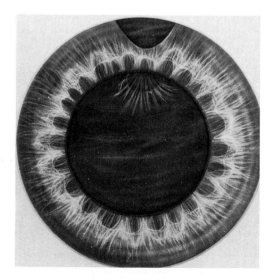

Fig. 20-17. Vitreous fibrils observed at 12 o'clock. Hole in anterior hyaloid membrane not visible. (From Jaffe, N. S., and Light, D. S.: Arch. Ophthalmol. **76:**541, 1966.)

Fig. 20-18. Same eye as in Fig. 20-17 after dilatation of pupil. (From Jaffe, N. S., and Light, D. S.: Arch. Ophthalmol. **76:**541, 1966.)

tion is thicker and not in contact with the iris. One interesting case (Fig. 20-16) showed a hole in the anterior hyaloid membrane, easily visible through the peripheral iridectomy. The edges of the iridectomy were ragged and appeared to be responsible for the hole. Nevertheless, almost all holes are confined to the patellar area. A total of 43 eyes with round pupils and no visible holes were dilated to search for holes behind the iris. None were found. In one case (Fig. 20-17), a small portion of a hole was seen at 12 o'clock, with fine strands of vitreous projecting through it. Dilatation of the pupil uncovered a hole that was originally 90% covered but still 10% exposed (Fig. 20-18).

Busacca and co-workers[2] have suggested that the residues of the hyaloid vessels adhering to the posterior face of the anterior hyaloid membrane might play a role in the production of holes. Since these remnants are usually found slightly nasal to the sagittal axis, most holes should occur here. This is not the case. Although residues of these embryonic vessels and the arcuate line of Vogt are often enough seen on the posterior lens capsule, I have been unable to demonstrate them on the anterior hyaloid membrane after lens extraction. Weber,[6] however, has observed them on the anterior hyaloid membrane after spontaneous senile anterior detachment of the vitreous.

In some patients the rupture of the anterior hyaloid membrane may be so extensive that the margins of the hole may be impossible to identify.

After a rupture of the anterior hyaloid membrane, changes in the prolapsed vitreous take place that sometimes make it difficult to state at a later time that a prior rupture of the membrane indeed existed. Careful examination of large numbers of these patients has revealed a group of characteristic patterns that provided me with the following clues that a postoperative rupture of the anterior hyaloid membrane existed:

1. Vitreous attached to the wound
2. Striae on the anterior face of the newly condensed surface
3. Loss of the anterior portion of Cloquet's canal
4. Loss of the free movements of anterior vitreous membranes

These clues are discussed in the following paragraphs.

Vitreous attached to the wound. In Fig. 20-19, the anterior hyaloid membrane has recondensed, but the vitreous is attached to the wound above. It is possible for an intact membrane to adhere to the superior portion of the wound even with a round pupil, but in the latter case the superior margin of the membrane can be traced posteriorly without interruption.

Striae on the anterior face of newly condensed surface. An almost constant finding is striae on the anterior face of the newly condensed surface. They probably result from traction (Fig. 20-20).

Loss of anterior portion of Cloquet's canal. One normal appearance of Cloquet's canal is shown in Fig. 20-21. Its contents usually empty after rupture of the anterior hyaloid membrane. The superior and inferior plicae are no longer identified or distinguished from other vitreous sheets and membranes (Fig. 20-22).

Loss of free movements of anterior vitreous membranes. The superior or inferior plica may become involved in the new surface condensation after rupture. This adhesion prevents the normal freedom of movement on ocular gaze up and down (Fig. 20-23).

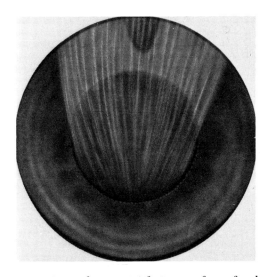

Fig. 20-19. Recondensation of vitreous face after large rupture of anterior hyaloid membrane. Vitreous remains attached to wound. (From Jaffe, N. S., and Light, D. S.: Arch. Ophthalmol. **76:**541, 1966.)

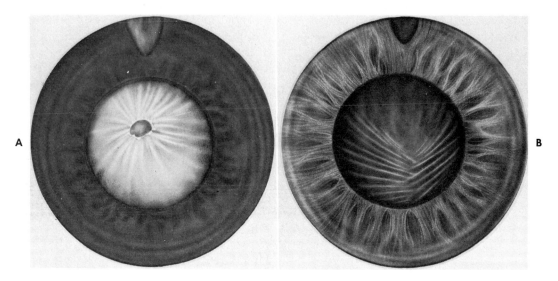

Fig. 20-20. A, Typical striae surrounding hole in anterior hyaloid membrane. **B,** Recondensation striae on anterior face of newly condensed anterior hyaloid membrane. (From Jaffe, N. S., and Light, D. S.: Arch. Ophthalmol. **76:**541, 1966.)

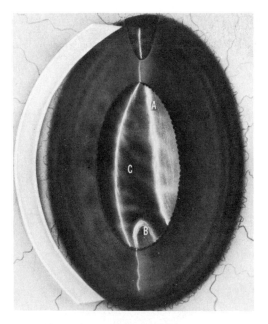

Fig. 20-21. Normal appearance of anterior vitreous after intracapsular lens extraction. *A,* Superior plica; *B,* inferior plica; *C,* Cloquet's canal. Intact anterior hyaloid membrane is clearly visible. (From Jaffe, N. S., and Light, D. S.: Arch. Ophthalmol. **76:**541, 1966.)

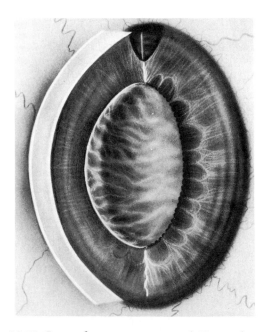

Fig. 20-22. Loss of anterior portion of Cloquet's canal after rupture of anterior hyaloid membrane with recondensation. (From Jaffe, N. S., and Light, D. S.: Arch. Ophthalmol. **76:**541, 1966.)

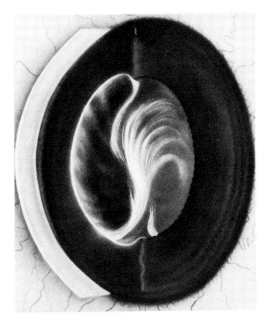

Fig. 20-23. Loss of free movements of walls of Cloquet's canal on ocular movements as result of their involvement in new surface condensation after rupture of anterior hyaloid membrane. (From Jaffe, N. S., and Light, D. S.: Arch. Ophthalmol. **76:**541, 1966.)

Incidence of postoperative rupture of anterior hyaloid membrane

From the preceding, one would expect a wide variation to exist in the reported incidence of postoperative rupture of the anterior hyaloid membrane, since it depends partly on how critical one is in diagnosing a rupture. However, the influence of alpha-chymotrypsin may be an additional factor. Thus Kirsch and Steinman[7] reported an incidence of 13.6%, Irvine[5] 23%, Goswami and co-workers[8] 23%, and Harrington[9] 21%. It would also be predicted that my series might show a higher incidence because of somewhat more rigid criteria. A rupture of the anterior hyaloid membrane includes any break in the continuity of the anterior hyaloid membrane, be it a small hole with little or no vitreous coursing through or a large rent obliterating all biomicroscopic remains of the membrane.

A careful study[1] was made from 1959 to 1965 of 1058 eyes undergoing an uneventful intracapsular lens extraction. Any untoward occurrence (such as capsule rupture and vitreous loss) or

Table 20-1. Status of anterior hyaloid membrane after uneventful intracapsular lens extraction

	Number	Percent
Anterior hyaloid membrane intact	560	67
Anterior hyaloid membrane ruptured	272	33
TOTAL	832	100

postoperative complication (such as marked hyphema, marked uveitis) eliminated the patient from the study.

To determine the postoperative status of the anterior hyaloid membrane, a series of 832 eyes was examined 6 months or more after an uneventful intracapsular lens extraction.

Table 20-1 shows that 33% of a large series of uneventful intracapsular lens extractions with an uneventful postoperative course demonstrated a rupture of the anterior hyaloid membrane 6 months or more after surgery.

To determine whether a rupture of the membrane was more than a chance occurrence, the incidence of rupture in both eyes of the same patient was examined. There were 328 patients studied in whom bilateral lens extraction had been performed. If the first eye had an intact anterior hyaloid membrane 6 months or longer after surgery (218 eyes), the second eye had an intact membrane after the same length of time in 182 patients (83%); the second eye showed a rupture in only 36 patients (17%). Note·that the overall incidence of rupture in 832 eyes was 33%, but if the first eye showed no rupture, there was a rupture in the second eye in only 17%. However, if the first eye in the series of 328 patients showed a ruptured anterior hyaloid membrane (110 eyes), the second eye had an intact membrane in only 28 patients (25%) and a ruptured membrane in 82 patients (75%). Note that the incidence of rupture increases from 33% in the overall series to 75% if the first eye demonstrated a rupture.

To emphasize further that the anterior hyaloid membranes in the two eyes of the same individual tend to behave in similar fashion, the following mathematical calculations are also presented: Of 328 patients who underwent bilateral lens extraction, 82 showed a bilateral rupture of the anterior hyaloid membrane. This is an incidence of 25%. If the incidence of rupture in one eye is 33% (overall series of 832 eyes, Table 20-1), the chance of rupture in the second eye is also 33% if local factors in the patient are ignored. This can be calculated to indicate that bilateral rupture should occur in 10.9% of bilateral cases (33% times 33%). However, our incidence of bilateral rupture was 25%. These figures demonstrate that whatever factors were responsible for the rupture in the first eye probably were present in the second eye as well.

For better understanding of the local factors involved in a patient, a system of grading an intact hyaloid membrane is of value (Table 20-2).

The two aphakic eyes of the same individual tend to show a remarkable symmetry of the position of the anterior hyaloid membranes. If one eye has a +2 anterior hyaloid membrane, the opposite eye tends to have the same. It is extremely rare, for example, for one eye to have a 0 position and its fellow eye +3. In the series of bilateral lens extractions referred to previously, there were only 14 patients who showed a difference of more than 1 grade unit (for example, −1 in one eye, and +1 in the second eye, or 0 in one eye and +2 in the second eye). In 8 of the 14, the difference was 2 grade units, in 6 it was 3 units. No patient showed a difference of 4 or more units.

To determine the possible relationship of sector iridectomy and peripheral iridotomy to postoperative rupture of the anterior hyaloid membrane (AHM), a further analysis of patients was undertaken. There were 122 eyes with a sector iridectomy and 710 eyes with one or more peripheral iridotomies. The results in Table 20-3 reveal little difference in the two.

A separate series of 44 eyes in which a prior antiglaucoma procedure (peripheral iridectomy or filtering operation) had been done was analyzed. The hyaloid membrane was intact in 18 eyes (41%); it was ruptured in 26 eyes (59%). Whether the high incidence of postoperative rupture in this series was a result of the glaucoma, the previous medical therapy, the effect of a second intraocular procedure, or a combination of factors is unclear.

To determine the time of occurrence of postoperative rupture of the anterior hyaloid mem-

Table 20-2. System of grading intact anterior hyaloid membranes

Position of membrane	Grade
At iris plane	0
Bulge to one-quarter depth of anterior chamber	+1
Bulge to one-half depth of anterior chamber	+2
Bulge to three-fourths depth of anterior chamber	+3
Touching cornea	+4
Slightly posterior to iris plane	−1
Moderately posterior to iris plane	−2

Table 20-3. Relationship of rupture of anterior hyaloid membrane to surgical method

	Peripheral iridotomy	Sector iridectomy
Intact AHM	484 (68%)	76 (62%)
Ruptured AHM	226 (32%)	46 (38%)
TOTAL	710 (100%)	122 (100%)

brane, an additional series of 182 uneventful intracapsular lens extractions was examined for the first 6 weeks after surgery. At the end of 6 weeks there were 45 ruptures (25%), whereas membranes were intact in 137 eyes (75%).

This series demonstrates that most of the ruptures occur in the first 6 weeks. Note that the overall incidence of rupture within 6 months was 33% of 832 eyes (Table 20-1). Thus it appears that approximately 76% of the ruptures occur within 6 weeks. The peak time of rupture was 14 to 28 days after surgery. Irvine[5] (1953) reported that 73% of 206 ruptures in membranes he studied occurred in the first 12 weeks. Of these, most occurred in the first 4 weeks.

A significant observation is the infrequent occurrence of vitreous traction bands attached to the surgical wound when the rupture of the anterior hyaloid membrane occurs more than 3 months after surgery. Numerous investigators have observed that the wound takes longer to heal than was previously thought, and vitreous adherence to the wound can occur up to 3 months or longer after surgery.

If the position of the anterior hyaloid membrane after an uneventful lens extraction is observed daily, one concludes that the anterior hyaloid membrane has a tendency to bulge out of the pupillary plane just after the operation, but later it recedes. Goswami and co-workers[8] reported that in 35 patients the intact vitreous face was in front of the pupillary plane, in 29 it was at the pupillary plane, and in two it was behind the pupillary plane on first examination. On subsequent examination the vitreous face came to the pupillary plane in 31 patients and behind it in 29. Of 31 cases in the pupillary plane, 19 were patients in whom the anterior hyaloid membrane had bulged on first examination, and only 12 were in the pupillary plane at the first examination. Of 29 patients in whom the anterior hyaloid membrane went behind the iris plane, 10 had prior bulge, and 17 had the membrane at the iris plane. Harrington[9] also noted the tendency for the vitreous to bulge after surgery and to gradually flatten subsequently.

The causes of bulging or rupture of the anterior hyaloid membrane remain speculative. The following are some of the factors to be considered:

1. Posterior vitreous detachment associated with enlargement of the vitreous cavity
2. Relative pupillary block
3. Hemorrhagic or serous ciliochoroidal detachment
4. Lessening of the tenacious attachment of the vitreous at its base as a result of zonulysis and loss of the lens (this may compress the central core of vitreous, promoting a bulge)
5. The influence of the iris (the pupillary margin may damage the anterior hyaloid membrane or movements of the iris over the membrane may cause it to rupture)
6. Inherent weakness of the anterior hyaloid membrane
7. Activity of the patient

The influence of alpha-chymotrypsin on the incidence of postoperative rupture of the anterior hyaloid membrane is still unsettled.

A group of 204 eyes were examined 6 months or longer after an uneventful intracapsular lens extraction and postoperative course. The surgery was performed in 1968 and 1969. In each instance, 2 ml of a 1:10,000 dilution of alpha-chy-

Table 20-4. Incidence of rupture of anterior hyaloid membrane by use of alpha-chymotrypsin

	Number	Percent
Anterior hyaloid membrane intact	94	46
Anterior hyaloid membrane ruptured	110	54
TOTAL	204	100

motrypsin was instilled into the posterior chamber for 2 minutes. The anterior chamber was then irrigated with saline or balanced salt solution. The status of the anterior hyaloid membrane was determined by the criteria discussed previously to decide the presence of a rupture. The results in Table 20-4 were obtained.

This seemingly increased incidence of rupture of the anterior hyaloid membrane (54%) after the use of alpha-chymotrypsin is difficult to explain. It may be caused by some as yet undetermined effect on the anterior hyaloid membrane itself. It may be associated with a higher incidence of wound leakage from defective wound healing when the enzyme is used. It may be caused by some trauma associated with the instillation of the enzyme. The increased incidence of postoperative rupture of the anterior hyaloid membrane from 33% in my earlier series to 54% in my later series may have nothing at all to do with the enzyme. In the later group, earlier ambulation and greater permissiveness in physical activity were allowed. Also, the use of cryoextraction was practiced in every case. I have not yet had the opportunity to compare a series of cases performed with and without the enzyme, with all other factors such as age of the patient, method of lens extraction, and postoperative management being identical.

REFERENCES

1. Jaffe, N. S., and Light, D. S.: Vitreous changes produced by cataract surgery: a study of 1,058 aphakic eyes, Arch. Ophthalmol. **76:**541-553, 1966.
2. Busacca, A., Goldmann, H., and Schiff-Wertheimer, S.: Biomicroscopie du corps vitré et du fond de l'oeil, Paris, 1957, Masson & Cie, Editeurs, p. 90.
3. Purtscher, E.: Histologische Frühuntersuchungen nach intracapsulärer Staroperation, Graefe Arch. Ophthalmol. **144:**669-697, 1942.
4. Duke-Elder, W. S.: Text-book of ophthalmology. Vol. I.

The development, form, and function of the visual apparatus, St. Louis, 1946, The C. V. Mosby Co., p. 117.

5. Irvine, S. R.: A newly defined vitreous syndrome following cataract surgery. Interpreted according to recent concepts of the structure of the vitreous, Am. J. Ophthalmol. **36:**599-619, 1953.

6. Weber, E.: Spaltlampenmikroskopische Untersuchungen über die vordere Glaskörperbegrenzung, und deren Beziehungen zur Linse, Klin. Mbl. Augenheilk. **108:**710-716, 1942.

7. Kirsch, R. E., and Steinman, W.: Spontaneous rupture of the anterior hyaloid membrane following intracapsular cataract surgery, Am. J. Ophthalmol. **37:**657-665, 1954.

8. Goswami, A. P., Mathur, K. N., and Raizada, I. N.: Vitreous face after intracapsular lens extraction, Orient. Arch. Ophthalmol. **5:**42-46, 1967.

9. Harrington, D. O.: Late changes in the vitreous following uncomplicated intracapsular cataract extraction, Am. J. Ophthalmol. **35:**1177-1184, 1952.

CHAPTER 21

Hemorrhage

The occurrence of an intraocular hemorrhage during or after cataract extraction is always a disturbing event. Even a hemorrhage from a minor cause may create anxiety for the patient, since it delays the ability to make out the characters on the vision chart during the early postoperative period. A vitreous hemorrhage that absorbs very slowly creates anxiety for both patient and surgeon. An expulsive hemorrhage is usually a disaster for all.

The following are the three most distinctive clinical entities associated with an intraocular hemorrhage:

1. Hyphema
2. Vitreous hemorrhage
3. Expulsive hemorrhage

HYPHEMA

Postoperative hemorrhage into the anterior chamber, a frequent occurrence before the popularization of corneoscleral suturing, has become less common and less serious after cataract surgery. Bleeding may arise from the operative wound, the iris, or the ciliary body. It usually occurs between the second and seventh days but may appear later. During this time, newly formed vessels bridge the incision in the process of healing. Any undue external pressure exerted on the eye may distort and rupture the wound to cause hyphema. It is likely that this factor is of far greater importance than the stress exerted on the wound from within, that is, the resumption of normal or slightly elevated intraocular pressure.

Causes

Defective wound healing. Defective wound healing may be the result of a poor incision or inadequate suturing. Therefore minor trauma disrupts such a wound more readily. Granulation tissue associated with increased vascularity is formed to excess in a poorly coapted wound. In such eyes hyphema is more likely.

Sutures. Catgut sutures incite a greater vascular response. In addition, they may absorb too rapidly, thus favoring wound disruption. Premature removal of silk sutures may do likewise.

Trauma. Trauma may cause an anterior chamber hemorrhage, even though wound closure is excellent.

Excessive scleral incision. Too great a scleral incision causes more bleeding at the time of surgery and in the early postoperative period as well. Corneal incisions tend to bleed less. An excessive scleral incision has been cited as a cause of late hyphema occurring months or years after cataract surgery[1,2] (Fig. 21-1). I have not been impressed with this as anything but a rare complication, since I have never recognized a case, in spite of favoring a posterior incision for many years.

Excessive cauterization of vessels that tend to bleed again during the early postoperative period. I am unaware of evidence favoring the concept that excessive cauterization causes further bleeding.

Damage to ciliary body. The ciliary body may be damaged while iridectomy is performed. Bleeding may occur from the annular artery. If this bleeding is copious at the time of surgery, there may be bleeding again during the early postoperative period.

Abnormal vascularization of the iris. Normally the iris does not bleed when cut. This is probably due to vasoconstriction mediated as an axon re-

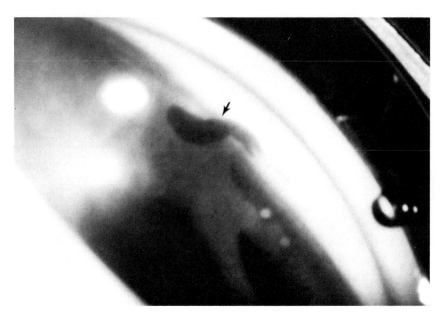

Fig. 21-1. Clot *(arrow)* attached to anomalous vessel within incision of eye, 4 years after cataract extraction. (From Watske, R. C.: Trans. Am. Ophthalmol. Soc. **72:**242-252, 1974.)

flex. However, the iris may be abnormal, as in rubeosis, heterochromic uveitis, iridocyclitis of unknown etiology, megalocornea, congenital glaucoma, Marfan's syndrome, and anterior chamber cleavage defects.

Blood dyscrasias. Among blood dyscrasias are hemophilia, thrombocytopenia, and polycythemia.

Anticoagulant therapy. Inadequate control of the prothrombin level may favor bleeding from the operative wound, the iris, or the ciliary body.

Pathology

The appearance of a hyphema of the anterior chamber is that of a bright red mass, usually with a fluid level. After repeated hemorrhage the hyphema may become stratified, the lower and older portion becoming reddish black, the upper part bright red.

Blood in the anterior chamber usually undergoes absorption by hemolysis in the same manner as blood in the retrovitreal space. It is rare for the blood to organize into a laminated connective tissue. However, the picture may be different if the anterior hyaloid membrane has ruptured and vitreous fibrils are present in the anterior chamber. Streaks of bright red blood may envelop clumps of vitreous membranules and retain this appearance for weeks or even months. Although the organization of blood in the anterior chamber is normally regarded as organization by mesothelial elements, Irvine[3] has observed that its occurrence in eyes that were experimentally injected with saccharated iron oxide and its intimate association with the endothelium of the cornea and the iris (the endothelium of the iris is continuous over its anterior surface in the rabbit) suggests a metaplastic origin from corneal, iris, or vascular endothelium. This makes the term "endotheliogenous connective tissue" more appropriate. Irvine has further observed that the similarities between this connective tissue and that producing an anterior capsular cataract, that forming a degenerative pannus in bullous keratopathy, and that making up the bulk of macular degenerations—that is, their peculiar, avascular, laminated appearance, the paucity and distribution of their cells, and their Schiff-positive reaction—suggest an origin by metaplasia from adjacent epithelial or endothelial tissues. Thus this fibrous tissue, which is secondary to hyphema, may apparently evolve from the presence of iron

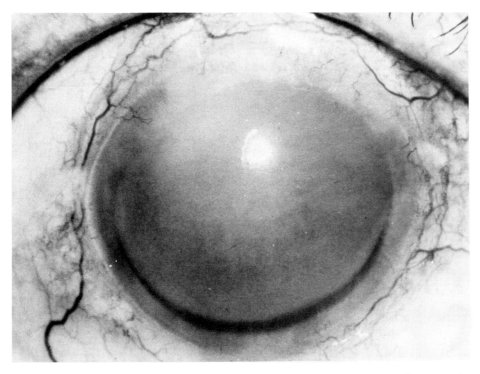

Fig. 21-2. Extensive bloodstaining of cornea after hyphema and elevated intraocular pressure after cataract extraction.

acting as a biologic catalyst in endothelial metaplasia.

The presence of blood in the anterior chamber may have a damaging effect on the cornea. Since a massive hyphema is often associated with glaucoma and iridocyclitis, one has difficulty determining whether endothelial damage is caused by the blood itself or by the associated problems. However, it is likely that all three factors may damage the endothelium, especially in those corneas with an attenuated endothelial cell population (p. 332). Bloodstaining of the cornea may occur, especially if there is repeated bleeding and the intraocular pressure remains elevated (Figs 21-2 to 21-4). These changes are generally associated with traumatic hyphema and are less frequently seen with hyphema after cataract surgery.

Blood in the anterior chamber may also give rise to a cellular response that may be mild to severe. This response is similar to that seen with a vitreous hemorrhage and is referred to as hemophthalmitis.[4] A macrophage response is elicited by the blood breakdown products, and these cells appear in the slit lamp beam as slightly yellow-tinged cells. The hemosiderin-laden macrophages often obstruct the trabecular meshwork, giving rise to a secondary glaucoma (hemolytic glaucoma).[5] In most instances the process is self-limiting; the intraocular pressure decreases as the macrophage response lessens (p. 417). Since vitreous hemorrhages absorb much more slowly and less completely than anterior chamber hemorrhages, hemophthalmitis is more severe and more prolonged with the former. Occasionally refractile bodies resembling cholesterol crystals associated with granulomatous masses located particularly in the iris and the filtration angle may be seen in the anterior chamber.[6,7] Tumor-like masses of granulation tissue may be seen particularly in the anterior chamber, the iris, and the ciliary body. They consist of monocytes, round cells, and fibroblasts, usually with an abundance of foreign-body giant cells, which are massed around the empty, slitlike spaces that are characteristic of the presence of cholesterol crys-

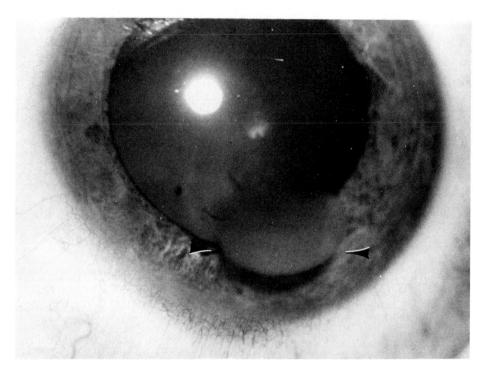

Fig. 21-3. Localized area *(arrows)* of bloodstaining of cornea after traumatic hyphema and elevated intraocular pressure.

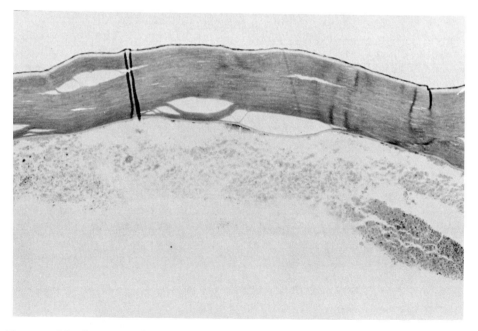

Fig. 21-4. Bloodstaining of cornea and striate keratopathy in eye that suffered repeated anterior chamber hemorrhage after cataract extraction.

tals. Klien[8] observed that necrotic areas are common in such tumors, around which round cell or polymorphonuclear infiltration is abundant.

Absorption of hyphema generally occurs through two routes. The first and most important is the canal of Schlemm. The second may be via the iris vessels, although the existence of this route is not at all certain. If the vessels of the iris are sclerosed or if the angle is damaged as in a uveitis, absorption may be delayed.

Prophylaxis

The best preventive measure for hyphema is the performance of adequate incision and closure of the wound. The proper methods of operative incisions are considered on p. 46. Multiple sutures are best to close the wound. They should be distributed evenly over the length of the incision. The newer, finer sutures may be buried beneath a conjunctival flap. This has the advantage of preventing the knots from rubbing against the palpebral conjunctiva and producing orbicularis spasm. Catgut sutures tend to fragment earlier if they are exposed. When they are well covered with either a limbus- or fornix-based flap, they persist longer. This flap provides greater comfort and better wound healing. Those surgeons old enough to recall the days when the wound was not sutured (conjunctival sutures were used) or when only two or three corneoscleral sutures were used will appreciate the role of a well-sutured incision in reducing the incidence of postoperative hyphema.

To avoid restlessness and agitation, the patient should be made as comfortable as possible, especially elderly patients. The principles of postoperative care have been described in Chapter 10.

Postoperative dressings should not be performed hastily, lest the patient squeeze and rupture a limbal vessel. A drop of anesthetic solution should be placed in the eye as the ocular secretions are cleansed. Since the patient sees the surgeon only infrequently during the hospital stay, this is the time to encourage the patient to be optimistic about his progress.

If thermal cauterization of vessels is performed at surgery, it should be limited to bleeding points only. Excessive cauterization may lead to bleeding from these vessels later. I have found it satisfactory to place a cellulose sponge soaked with epinephrine across the entire limbus and create pressure on the sponge for 1 or 2 minutes. This blanches the vessels adequately in most cases. Wet field coagulation of vessels (p. 45), far less traumatic than thermal cautery, is recommended.

With the aid of a hematology consultant, blood dyscrasias should be treated before surgery and during the postoperative period. The prothrombin level should be normal for those previously on anticoagulant therapy.

When the limbus appears excessively vascularized, it may be best to make the incision slightly corneally, bearing in mind that it may have to be made slightly larger. In these eyes a fornix-based flap is useful.

During the performance of the iridectomy or the iridotomy, injury to the ciliary body should be avoided. Injury can be prevented by not tearing the iris at its root as it is grasped with forceps and by not making the opening in the iris too basal.

Various plastic or aluminum shields are available to protect the eye against undue trauma. They should be used for at least 12 days during the day and for at least 3 weeks at night.

Treatment

The most important principle of management of a hyphema is conservatism. Most hyphemas absorb between 2 and 6 days after occurrence, although red blood cells may be seen with the slit lamp for a longer period. If the entire anterior chamber is filled with blood, it may be best to bandage both eyes for 1 or 2 days. The patient should be given sedatives and perhaps tranquilizers. Steroids may be of value because of the associated inflammation.

There is still no unanimity of opinion about the role of cycloplegics and miotics. One can argue that the ciliary body is put at rest by a cycloplegic and that a greater iris surface is available for absorption with miotic therapy. Since there is very little supporting evidence, I prefer to avoid both. Topical therapy is limited to an antibiotic-steroid solution.

If recurrent bleeding occurs, especially if it is associated with an elevated intraocular pressure, hyperosmotic therapy is probably of value. It may aid in opening the angle meshwork to permit escape of blood. It may favor aqueous flow, which aids in removal of the blood.

Acetazolamide may be of some benefit if there is an elevation of intraocular pressure. Its benefit may be nullified somewhat because it inhibits aqueous production, thereby providing less of a "washing out" effect from the anterior chamber.

Conservativism is the most prudent management of hyphema, but if surgical evacuation of blood from the anterior chamber is undertaken, one must bear in mind that the threat of a secondary hemorrhage is real. General anesthesia is usually necessary, since performing a retrobulbar injection of anesthetic solution only a few days after cataract surgery is hazardous. An adequate dose of mannitol by the intravenous route should be given before surgery. A small slanting paracentesis is performed inferiorly just within the limbus. Irrigation of the anterior chamber with balanced salt solution with or without fibrinolysin is performed. Under no circumstances should an attempt be made to irrigate out all or even most of the blood. Extraction of clotted blood with forceps is a dangerous procedure, since the risk of grasping iris or vitreous is great. An attempt to place air in the anterior chamber should be made, since air may be helpful in preventing a secondary hemorrhage. If necessary the lips of the paracentesis may be gently spread on a subsequent day to evacuate more blood if intraocular pressure rises again. This may be done with topical anesthesia at the bedside by depressing the posterior lip of the incision.

VITREOUS HEMORRHAGE

The occurrence of a hemorrhage into the vitreous that is large enough to seriously impair vision is uncommon after cataract surgery. However, lesser hemorrhages occur with a far greater frequency. The blood usually gravitates to the inferior part of the globe and has little or no effect on vision. It is not unusual to observe a bright red crescent of blood lining the anterior hyaloid membrane at the inferior portion of the pupil where the vitreous passes over the edge of the iris as it bulges into the anterior chamber. This is often thought to be a streak of blood from the anterior chamber resting on the anterior face of the vitreous. Actually this is intravitreal blood lining the anterior hyaloid membrane. It may persist

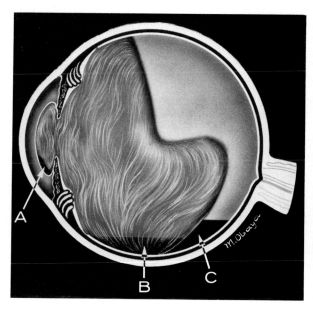

Fig. 21-5. Distribution of blood within vitreous after cataract extraction. *A,* Blood lining inner surface of anterior hyaloid membrane; *B,* blood lying on floor of formed vitreous; *C,* blood within retrovitreal space.

unchanged for several weeks or months. Within the first postoperative week, streaks of red blood may be visible with the slit lamp in the inferior part of the globe as the movement of the vitreous is observed when the eye moves up and down (ascension phenomenon). Blood from the vitreous may gain the anterior chamber through a rent in the anterior hyaloid membrane. Also, blood from the anterior chamber may reach the vitreous by the same route. I doubt that blood in the retrovitreal space may gain access to the anterior chamber as a result of ciliary detachment of the vitreous, as Cibis[9] suggested. The distribution of blood within the vitreous is depicted in Fig. 21-5.

Pathogenesis

Undoubtedly changes normally occur within the vitreous and its attachments to neighboring structures after lens extraction. The sagittal diameter of the vitreous cavity increases, and further separation of the vitreous from the retina occurs as the anterior vitreous bulges into the anterior chamber. There is also an additional strain placed on the tenaceous attachment of the vitre-

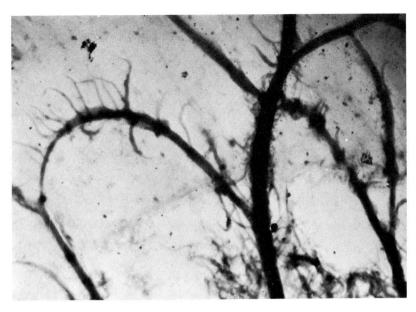

Fig. 21-6. Flat preparation of retina in area of lattice degeneration. Note vitreous fibrils attached to vessels in peripheral vascular arcade. (Hematoxylin and eosin.) (From Jaffe, N. S.: The vitreous in clinical ophthalmology, St. Louis, 1969, The C. V. Mosby Co.; courtesy Dr. D. Hunter, San Antonio, Tex.)

ous to its base at the pars plana and ora. Hyaloideoangioretinal adhesions (Fig. 21-6) may be severed during posterior vitreous detachment. Petechial hemorrhages may indicate the site of ruptured vessels. They disappear within a few days, but the blood within the vitreous may persist for a longer period. A retinal break may occur, but it is possible to encounter a vitreous hemorrhage without a retinal break.[10-12] Most intravitreal hemorrhages are caused by rupture of diseased blood vessels in connection with horseshoe breaks or large lacerations of the retina.[13] Usually the hemorrhage is small because the ruptured vessel is already partially obliterated. Blood may also leak from engorged vessels secondary to hypotonia. A posterior chamber hemorrhage arising from the ciliary body or an iridectomy may also pass into the vitreous.

A massive intravitreal hemorrhage may result from the rupture of a short posterior ciliary artery, a long posterior ciliary artery, or a choroidal artery. Usually this rupture causes an expulsive hemorrhage (p. 421). However, the hemorrhage may possibly remain confined to the vitreous.

Fate of blood within the vitreous

The fate of blood within the vitreous is varied. The blood may undergo absorption, resulting in little or no lasting damage, or it may cause highly destructive intraocular complications.

Absorption of blood from the vitreous is related to hemolysis and phagocytosis.[14] Depending on the size and location of the hemorrhage and the existence or nonexistence of associated ocular disease, the absorption may be a rapid or a gradual process. Generally blood clears from the retrovitreal space in a matter of days, whereas it may remain within the formed vitreous for much longer periods.

When the amount of blood in the vitreous is large and the fluid relatively little, phagocytosis of blood breakdown products plays a more important role than hemolysis. These products are hematoidin, hemosiderin, fats, and lipoids. A certain degree of laking is present where blood mixes with the vitreous. However, it is characteristic for blood to displace the vitreous structure, rather than to mingle with it.

With massive bleeding into the vitreous or

with repeated bleeding, absorption plays a lesser role than organization. Fibroblasts and glial tissue infiltrate the vitreous, invade the blood, and convert the hemorrhage into an amorphous mass wherein the identity of the erythrocytes is lost. Crystals of cholesterin may eventually separate out.

The fate of blood in the retrovitreal space (subhyaloid hemorrhage) is similar to that seen in a hyphema. The blood shows little tendency to coagulate and shifts its fluid level with movements of the patient's head. Subhyaloid hemorrhages absorb rapidly and usually completely. The cause of failure of this blood to coagulate is unknown; but Ballantyne and Michaelson[15] likened it to the occurrence of intravascular clotting when a vessel wall is damaged and to the absence of clotting when the endothelium is intact.

Complications

There are three main complications of intravitreal blood: fibroplasia, hemosiderosis, and hemophthalmitis. Fibroplastic and hemosideric responses are not separate entities, since hemosiderosis may result in fibroplastic reactions within the vitreous and retina.

Organization. It is remarkable how rapidly a hemorrhage within the vitreous organizes. Within 2 to 3 days, white membranous sheets replace the bright red blood, so that sometimes it is difficult to differentiate a vitreous hemorrhage from a severe exudative posterior uveitis. In performing the ascension phenomenon at the slit lamp, chunks of red blood intermingled with white sheets are thrust up from the floor of the globe, confirming the presence of a hemorrhage. In some eyes the blood absorbs rapidly and leaves little destruction behind, whereas in others extensive fibroplastic membranes develop that create traction on inner ocular structures and seriously impair vision. After a vitreous hemorrhage occurs, I have found the following test useful in estimating prognosis. The ascension phenomenon is observed at the slit lamp. If the membranes within the vitreous are motionless or if they spring up and down in a jerky staccato manner, fibroplasia is well developed. If the membranes rise and fall slowly, as they do in a normal eye, absorption will be rapid, and clearing may be anticipated.

The ultimate fate of a vitreous hemorrhage depends to some degree on the physical characteristics of the vitreous. If the vitreous is mostly fluid, the hemorrhage tends to absorb more rapidly and completely. If the membranous structure is more preserved, the blood tends to undergo organization and less absorption. In most instances of postoperative vitreous hemorrhages the blood clears from the vitreous within a short period. However, while the visual axis becomes unobstructed, it is surprising how opaque the vitreous remains in the inferior portion of the globe. Thick white sheets in the form of membranes cover the posteroinferior surface of the posterior limiting border of the vitreous. Because of the high density of the contents of the vitreous in this area, the "phenomenon of the rising of the lamellae," first described by Busacca,[16] may be seen. The anterior funnel of Cloquet's canal, instead of coursing in a posteroinferior direction, may run in a posterosuperior direction. This phenomenon is also observed in some cases of posterior uveitis where a large amount of organized exudate is present in the lower half of the globe.

Hemosiderosis oculi. Although the toxic effects of a retained intraocular iron foreign body are familiarly known to ophthalmologists as siderosis bulbi, a similar staining of ocular tissues may result after the release of blood pigments associated with an intravitreal hemorrhage. This is known as hemosiderosis oculi.

The role of iron in causing hyaloideochorioretinopathy is still not completely clear. Presumably hematogenous ferric ions bind themselves to siderophilic substances such as acid mucopolysaccharides, particularly abundant in the vitreous and perivascular tissue. Depolymerization of the mucopolysaccharides results in destruction of the vitreous framework and in sclerosis of the choroidal and retinal vessels. Blood in the subretinal space causes hemosiderosis of the pigment epithelial cells and destruction leading to retinopathy and subretinal fibroplasia. The end result of such an insult is loss of the pigment epithelium, disintegration of the lamina vitrea, and disappearance of the neural elements. The last are replaced by glial tissue.

The cause of retinal damage in hemosiderosis is controversial. Duke-Elder[17] attributed it to direct cytotoxicity by iron, whereas Cibis and co-workers[18] attributed it to vaso-obliteration caused by iron in the perivascular acid mucopolysaccharides. The current evidence favors cytotoxicity (with any vaso-obliteration being secondary to retinal degeneration), since Makiuchi and Dyamada[19] caused retinal necrosis with small amounts of intravitreal ferric citrate and Racker and Krimsky[20] inhibited the metabolism of neural tissue with iron ions. Wise[21] supplied other evidence that weighs against the vaso-obliteration theory. When iron ions enter the eye slowly from metallic iron, the electroretinogram can be diminished, and the iron staining of the epithelial cells can be marked at a time when the vessels and perivascular mucopolysaccharides show no staining. Also in siderosis the choroidal circulation remains unimpaired, whereas the retinal vessels are obliterated. This condition should produce a picture similar to occlusion of the central retinal artery with preservation of the outer retinal layer. However, it does not, since the entire thickness of the retina is damaged. Finally, when Cibis and coworkers[22] loaded the choriocapillaris with iron by intravenous injection of saccharated iron oxide, degeneration occurred in the retina and not in the choroid. Although current evidence favors a direct cytotoxic effect of iron, the final chapter may not yet be written.

Wise[21] outlined the pathogenesis of siderotic degeneration as follows: Free iron ions become loosely bound to acid mucopolysaccharides. These complexes, together with free iron ions, diffuse to various parts of the eye, where the iron is bonded to the cellular enzymes. The cell may then detoxify and store the iron, or degenerate and die, releasing iron pigments that are phagocytosed by macrophages. These iron pigments are presumed to be stable and nontoxic and are unable to release free iron ions again. The relatively resistant uvea stores the iron, while the retina, less able to detoxify it, is poisoned early.

In addition to the changes in the vitreous just described, there may be appreciable discoloration of the uveal tract. Orange or brown spots may be seen on the iris and perhaps over the ciliary processes through the iris openings.

Hemophthalmitis. Within 2 to 3 weeks after a vitreous hemorrhage, a cellular response may be observed in the anterior chamber. As stated earlier, this response has been termed "hemophthalmitis."[4] I have observed this entity on several occasions. When it is complicated by glaucoma, it has been referred to as "hemolytic glaucoma" by Fenton and Zimmerman.[5]

Hemophthalmitis is an established clinical entity that is most often but not exclusively observed after cataract surgery. After an uneventful cataract extraction the early convalescent course is unremarkable. Within 2 to 3 weeks an increased cellular response is observed in the anterior chamber. The cells may be yellow tinged. A whitish gray membrane may be observed adherent to the inner wall of the anterior hyaloid membrane. The clinical picture appears puzzling in view of the fact that the globe may appear remarkably uninflamed. Closer scrutiny reveals that there are few, if any, keratic precipitates, although the cells show a motility similar to that of the cells associated with an active iritis.

The intraocular pressure is usually normal. However, if the cellular response is great, a rise in pressure may occur, and the globe may become congested. Local or systemic steroids seem to have little effect on the course of the disease. Generally the process gradually subsides after weeks or months. Intraocular pressure falls as the cellular infiltration of the anterior chamber decreases. That this does not always happen is emphasized by a case report of Fenton and Zimmerman.[5] Hemophthalmitis probably represents the clinical counterpart of what they reported in a single pathologic case. They suggested the term "hemolytic glaucoma" to describe the intractable glaucoma that ensued in their case as a result of clogging of the trabecular meshwork by macrophages engorged with blood breakdown products (Fig. 21-7).

Erythrocytes in the vitreous stimulate a macrophage response with phagocytosis. The hemoglobin is broken down into hemosiderin and hematoidin. The latter is an iron-free pigment that is usually readily absorbed and excreted as bilirubin. The hemoglobin, not yet broken down into hemosiderin, is usually present in the vitreous, whose capacity to absorb and remove large collections of disintegrating red blood cells is relatively poor. This may be because of its avascularity and paucity of mesenchymal cells. The products of disintegrating erythrocytes are car-

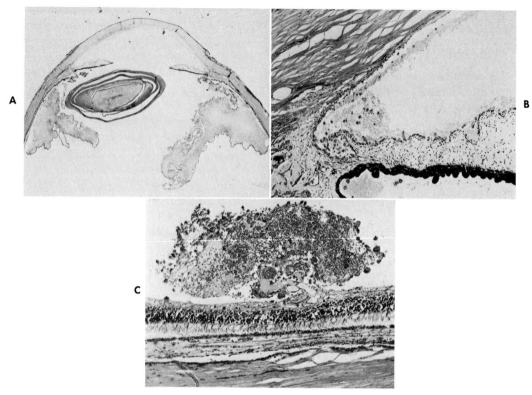

Fig. 21-7. A, Vitreous detached from retina posteriorly is diffusely impregnated with fine globules of light brown pigment, but almost no intact erythrocytes remain. Lens was subluxated during preparation of sections. **B,** Hemorrhagic debris and pigment-laden macrophages fill chamber angle and adhere to cornea, trabecular meshwork, and iris. **C,** Vascular channels originating from vessels in nerve fiber layer of retina protrude into vitreous body, where they are covered by fresh blood and pigmented macrophages. (Hematoxylin and eosin, reduced 8% from magnifications ×6, **A;** ×80, **B;** ×115, **C.**) (**A,** AFIP No. 62-5790; **B,** AFIP No. 62-5789; **C,** AFIP No. 62-6137.) (From Fenton, R. H., and Zimmerman, L. E.: Arch. Ophthalmol. **70:**236-239, 1963.)

ried by the intraocular fluids into the anterior chamber, where hemosiderin is found in the aqueous and in the outflow channels. The anterior chamber response to disintegrating red blood cells is analogous to that seen with morgagnian cataract, where macrophages laden with lens material fill the trabecular mesh-work and give rise to the picture familiarly known as phacolytic glaucoma[23] (p. 495) (Fig. 21-8). In hemolytic glaucoma, macrophages laden with iron-containing blood breakdown products engorge the angle drainage structures and give rise to an acute open-angle secondary glaucoma.

The appearance of the vitreous depends on the stage at which the entity is recognized. At first the vitreous appears filled with a material that resembles dilute tomato juice. Within a few days, white membranes appear and the red-appearing hemorrhage is difficult to find. This may raise a question of differential diagnosis. The observation of a relatively opaque vitreous after cataract extraction followed 1 week or more by the appearance of cells in the anterior chamber with relatively little external inflammation is typical of a fungus endophthalmitis.

The following diagnostic technique is relatively simple and easy to perform: A ½-inch 27-gauge disposable needle is attached to the male end of a disposable Millipore filter unit (Millipore Corporation, Bedford, Mass.) and a small syringe to

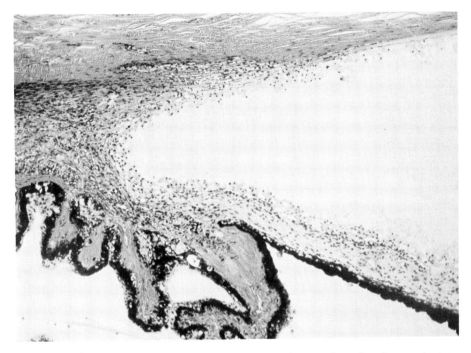

Fig. 21-8. Macrophages concentrated along surface of iris and in chamber angle in eye with phacolytic glaucoma. (From Hogan, M. J., and Zimmerman, L. E.: Ophthalmic pathology. An atlas and textbook, Philadelphia, 1962, W. B. Saunders Co.)

the female end. The filter unit contains millions of pores, each 0.22 μm in diameter (p. 446). An anterior chamber puncture is performed, and a small amount of fluid is aspirated into the syringe. The cells in the anterior chamber are larger than the micropores of the filter and therefore are collected on its surface. The Millipore filter is then removed from the unit and is ready for staining. Staining reveals macrophages. However, to reveal the presence of iron, the filter is stained with Prussian blue. Sometimes the nonreactive iron in the macrophages will not stain positively with this dye unless the process of microincineration[24] is performed. In this technique, protein-bound iron is converted to ferric oxide, which then becomes available for the Prussian blue reaction. The filter ensures that the cells will be laid out in a single layer and obviates the need for centrifugation, which may distort cellular morphology.

Treatment

Delayed absorption of blood from the vitreous may be a frustrating experience for the patient and surgeon, especially if the vitreous remains opaque. Until recently, there was little for the surgeon to do but wait and hope that vitreous transparency would be restored. Recent developments have offered a new approach to this vexing complication.

Intravitreal urokinase. An English report[25] has described the successful treatment of vitreous hemorrhage by the intravitreal injection of urokinase. This enzyme is a protein with a molecular weight of approximately 53,000 and is derived from human urine by a process of column fractionation. Urokinase is a plasminogen activator, and the conversion of gel-phase plasminogen to plasmin results in lysis of a fluid clot within a few minutes. Plasminogen is present in both the aqueous and vitreous humors. The improvement in vitreous transparency is due to the action of plasmin on the clot, thus allowing the normal mechanism of vitreous hemorrhage absorption to occur.

Eyes suitable for treatment are those with a visual acuity no better than for hand movements, in which no improvement in vitreous transparency has occurred over a period of 2 years and in which the anterior segment is healthy. Investigation of early treatment of vitreous hemorrhage is under way.

In a normotensive eye, it is impossible to inject urokinase solution without aspiration of an equal volume of vitreous. In three eyes with vitreous hemorrhage after aspiration of 0.5 ml of vitreous, 25,000 Ploug units of urokinase in 0.5 ml of sterile water were injected into the hemorrhage. Injection was through the pars plana, 6 mm from the limbus and inferior to the lower border of the lateral rectus muscle. In each case, lysis of the clot occurred, visual acuity improved from perception of light to 6/36, and fundus details became visible. No complications occurred, but in one eye the vitreous hemorrhage recurred 7 months later.[25] Another report[26] described the intravitreal injection of urokinase into five eyes with longstanding intravitreal hemorrhage. Whereas vision had previously been so poor as to render the eyes useless, after treatment with urokinase, there was a significant improvement in the visual acuity, and in one eye 6/6 vision was achieved. The most severe postoperative complication was a transitory anterior uveitis in two of the eyes.

Since surgical methods of treating persistent intravitreal clot have a high frequency of operative complications, this much less traumatic method of promoting clearance of intravitreal hemorrhage appears to have several advantages and might be attempted in the first place.

Closed system vitrectomy. The most promising, and currently most effective, method of evacuating unabsorbed intravitreal hemorrhage is the technique of vitrectomy through the pars plana.[27-29] A vitreous infusion suction cutter (VISC) was introduced by Machemer and is used for this purpose, as well as for other vitreoretinal problems. Initial reports indicate that vitreous opacities unconnected to the retina by proliferative changes are the easiest surgical cases and have the best prognosis for postoperative visual improvement. Cases of nondiabetic hemorrhages, amyloidosis, and opacities of unknown origin are said to be ideal for a beginner in vitrectomy.

The indication for removal of unabsorbed intravitreal hemorrhage is its lack of spontaneous absorption after 5 to 6 months. The technique consists of passing an automated virectomy device through a scleral incision made parallel to the limbus 4 to 4.5 mm from the limbus. The incision is 3.3 mm in length. In aphakic eyes the sclerotomy is located slightly more anteriorly (4 mm) than in phakic eyes (4.5 mm). The sclerotomy site is secured by a running 5-0 monofilament nylon suture, which has proven easier to place and to tighten than a mattress suture. Intraocular fiber-optic illumination[30] has been a major improvement over all previous illumination systems such as paraxial and slit lamp illumination. Old blood is often found behind a hemorrhagic detached vitreous. This blood consists of a sediment of blood cells, mainly erythrocytes. It is not coagulated and therefore accumulates easily in dependent parts of the eye and is easily stirred up. This may completely obscure visibility of the fundus structures, making work deep in the eye impossible. This has been solved with the VISC by employing a simple 22-gauge, 4 cm long hypodermic needle attached to a metallic tube 9 cm long. This tube acts as a handle for easy manipulation of the needle. The handle is connected to an infusion bottle of lactated Ringer solution via a plastic tube. No attempt is made to push the needle deep into the eye. Instead the stream of fluid is directed against the blood. The stream stirs the blood up, while suction is applied simultaneously with the VISC. This procedure has several advantages: Both instruments can be kept in the anterior part of the vitreous cavity, avoiding damage to any intraocular structure when visibility is extremely poor. The lavage is much more efficient because more cells are stirred up by the extra fluid available. When retrovitreal blood is not present, this two-instrument technique is not necessary. The opaque vitreous can be effectively removed solely by the VISC.

EXPULSIVE HEMORRHAGE

One of the most frightening and serious complications of cataract surgery is the sudden occurrence of an expulsive subchoroidal hemorrhage. Vail[31] referred to this as the "bête noire of the ophthalmic surgeon." Fortunately it is rare and will be witnessed only a few times by an ophthalmic surgeon.

Historical background

The first report of expulsive hemorrhage associated with cataract surgery is usually attributed to Wenzel,[32] who described it in 1786. However,

Münchow[33] reported such a description by Hellmann[34] in 1774. Verhoeff[35] reported the first instance of an eye that was saved, with retention of some vision, after an expulsive hemorrhage during the performance of a sclerectomy for glaucoma. His technique of scleral puncture for the evacuation of the blood has been repeated and reported by numerous authors since then.

Incidence

The fortunate rarity of this complication is attested to by the following reported statistics:

Author	Cataract extractions	Expulsive hemorrhage	Percent
Pau[36]	1,520	6	0.4
Gasteiger[37]	1,920	4	0.2
Owens and Hughes[38]	2,086	1	0.05
Pfingst[39]	2,500	2	0.08
Melanowski[40]	2,815	3	0.1
Goren[41]	2,907	8	0.3
Vail[42]	2,987	6	0.2
Jain[43]	3,000	3	0.1
Jaffe[44]	6,000	3	0.05
Newby[45]	12,000	17	0.1
DeVoe[46]	18,000	57	0.3
TOTAL	55,735	110	0.2

Pathophysiology

The source of the hemorrhage is one of the numerous arteries supplying the uveal tract. Most anatomic studies have implicated one of the short posterior ciliary arteries. The posterior ciliary arteries come off the ophthalmic artery as two trunks while it is still below the optic nerve. They divide into 10 to 20 branches, surround the nerve, and then enter the eyeball.[47] These terminal braches constitute the short posterior ciliary arteries, except for two, which pierce the sclera on the medial and lateral side of the nerve. These are the long posterior ciliary arteries. They enter the sclera somewhat farther anteriorly than the short ciliary arteries. After gaining the suprachoroidal space, they run forward to the ciliary muscle without giving off any branches. The short posterior ciliary arteries supply the choroid and break up into the capillary network or choriocapillaris. The larger branches extend to the ora serrata. Most of the larger short posterior ciliary arteries pierce the sclera lateral to the optic

nerve, while some smaller arteries enter the sclera all around but closer to the optic nerve.

Manschot[48] reported anatomic studies in six eyes removed because of an expulsive hemorrhage associated with cataract surgery. Five hemorrhages resulted from a ruptured necrotic posterior ciliary artery. In the sixth a choroidal artery was found that was largely dilated and obliterated by sclerosis and thrombosis. Müller[49] reported eight eyes with expulsive hemorrhage and found that the site of predilection was in the short posterior ciliary vessels, where they enter the suprachoroidal space from the sclera. Similar necrotic processes, however, may affect the rami of the long posterior ciliary artery. Choroidal vessels are affected to a lesser extent, and retinal vessels at the disc are seldom affected. It was Müller's impression that the venules are first and predominantly affected, but numerous arterioles also are destroyed by fibrinous necrosis and probably constitute the chief source of hemorrhage.

It is unknown whether the vessel rupture occurs at a site of previous necrosis or without previous pathologic condition. Manschot's study favors the former view, since he demonstrated that degeneration of the vessel wall was present before the onset of the hemorrhage. However, in cases where an explusive hemorrhage occurs during or after cataract surgery in infants and children (p. 422), vascular degeneration is an unlikely factor.

In considering the pathogenesis of necrosis of the vessel wall, one must understand the unique stresses exerted on blood vessels within the eye. The pressure acting on the blood vessel wall (from without) elsewhere in the body is atmospheric, whereas in the eye it is approximately 20 mm Hg (intraocular pressure). An analogous situation exists where the intracranial pressure is 10 to 12 mm Hg higher than the atmospheric pressure. The blood pressure falls about 20 mm Hg in going from the aorta to the small arteries, but the greatest fall in pressure occurs beyond these vessels, that is, during the passage of blood through the arterioles. The pressure drop in this part of the circulation is 50 to 60 mm Hg.[50] The pressure is much lower in the capillaries. As in any collapsible tube system, fluid can flow through the intraocular arterioles as long as the blood pressure within them is equal to or greater than the sum of the pressures exerted externally on the blood vessel. Thus the pressure of 20 mm Hg (intraocular pressure) must have some effect on the quantity and the speed of the blood that passes through the intraocular arterioles. This may explain why the vascular degeneration in cases of generalized vascular disease is often more severe within the eye than in other organs. Manschot[48] emphasized that this explains why the intraocular vascular degeneration is located by preference at the point where the vessels enter the eye, in other words, where the extravascular pressure changes from atmospheric to that of the intraocular pressure.

The nutrition of a blood vessel wall is supplied by (1) penetration of plasma constituents through the endothelium, (2) the vasa vasorum, and (3) penetration of extravascular tissue fluid.[48] Since arterioles do not possess vasa vasorum, the nutrition of the arteriolar wall is only accomplished by a penetration of fluid from inside and from outside the vessel wall. There is a diffuse penetration of the vessel wall with nourishing fluid, which is ultimately discharged into the perivascular tissue and not into the vascular lemun, as Lange[51] emphasized. His experiments have shown that every factor that impedes this intramural fluid circulation will cause a degeneration of the vessel wall.

At least on a theoretical basis, the factors that may cause degeneration of the walls of intraocular vessels are the following:

1. High blood pressure, causing arteriosclerosis
2. Generalized arteriosclerosis
3. Intraocular pressure

If intraocular pressure increases, it may cause interference with the intramural circulation by hampering the outflow of the circulating fluid. It will also diminish the passage of blood through the vessel wall. In glaucoma the intraocular pressure may exceed the arteriolar blood pressure. This favors collapse of the vessel wall. In the smallest arterioles, the pulse pressure will be reduced to nearly zero. The lumen therefore will not reopen during systole. Thus an ischemic necrosis of the vessel wall can occur. The practical significance of these considerations is emphasized in the intraocular vessel walls of glaucomatous eyes of patients with arterial hypertension or arteriosclerosis. This combination of factors may be important in vascular wall necrosis in some cases but certainly not in all cases.

When an expulsive hemorrhage occurs, the blood gathers preferentially anterior to the equator where the apposition of choroid to the sclera is weakest. This is particularly evident on the nasal and temporal sides, away from the anchorage of the vortex veins (Figs. 21-9 and 21-10).

The pathologic picture of an expulsive hemorrhage varies with the degree to which the intraocular contents are extruded. Usually, when untreated, vitreous humor, uveal tissue, and retina burst through the operative wound (Fig. 21-11). The globe should be examined histologically or its contents should be examined if an evisceration is performed, since an unsuspected melanoma may be present.[52]

Pathogenesis

This complication remains an enigma for the ophthalmic surgeon, since its exact cause is still unknown, and its consequences are so disastrous. At best, a varied approach to etiology must be taken, since reports that indict one particular factor are contradicted by other reports, and yet each report appears to be based on careful observations.

In Manschot's[48] cases, a necrosis of the arteriolar wall appeared to precede the rupture. Five of his six patients suffered from glaucoma. The role of glaucoma in causing vascular necrosis has been discussed earlier. Also, most cases of spontaneous expulsive hemorrhage (nonsurgical) have been associated with glaucoma.[53] The condition has also been described in glaucomatous eyes after a perforation of a corneal ulcer. However, in none of Jain's[43] three cases was glaucoma a factor, nor was it present in any of the six cases reported by François and co-workers.[54] Thus the role of glaucoma in this complication is not clear.

Most patients who have suffered this complication have been elderly and have been suitable candidates for arteriolar necrosis on the basis of arterial hypertension and arteriosclerosis. However, expulsive hemorrhage is also observed in young patients where these factors are inoperative. Cordes[55] reported four cases in 112 eyes enucleated because of complications arising from congenital cataract surgery. These patients

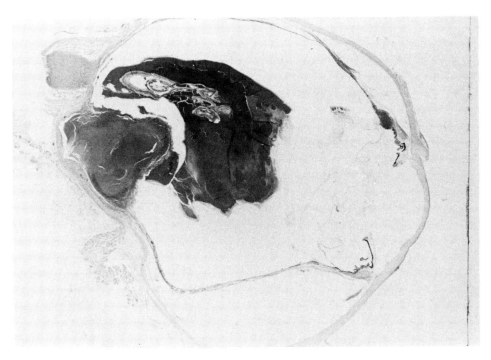

Fig. 21-9. Expulsive hemorrhage after cataract extraction. Hemorrhage appears to stem from one of the short posterior ciliary arteries.

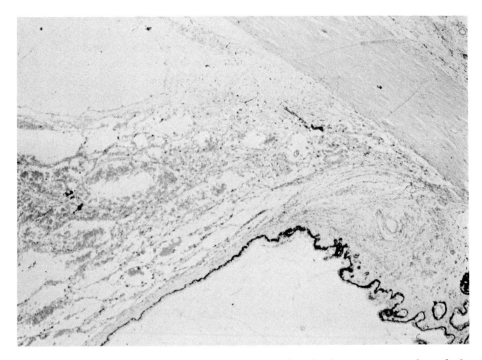

Fig. 21-10. Organized blood found between choroid and sclera in eye enucleated after expulsive hemorrhage.

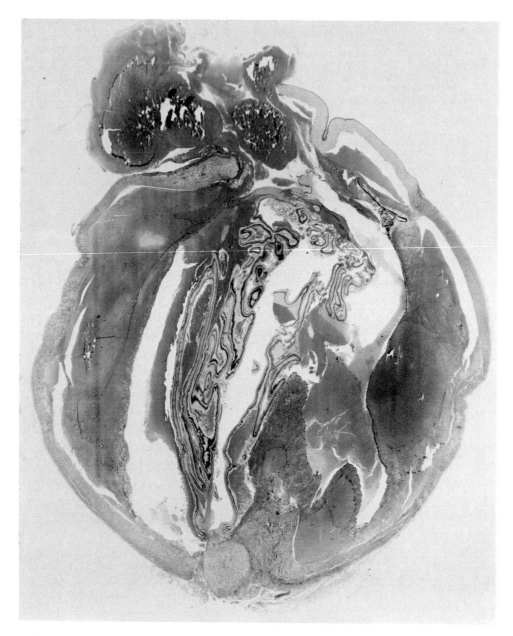

Fig. 21-11. Expulsive hemorrhage after penetrating wound at limbus on upper left. (AFIP No. 98147.) (From Hogan, M. J., and Zimmerman, L. E.: Ophthalmic pathology, Philadelphia, 1962, W. B. Saunders Co.)

ranged in age from 4 months to 21 years. François and co-workers[54] also observed expulsive hemorrhage in four young subjects whose vascular system appeared good. Thus arterial hypertension and arteriosclerosis cannot be important factors in all cases.

Local factors within the eye may be important and include high myopia, observed in five of six eyes with expulsive hemorrhage in one series,[54] choroidal sclerosis, and perhaps congenital and familial weakness of choroidal vessels.

The mode of anesthesia has also been implicated. However, this implication is doubtful, since it occurs with both local and general anesthesia and regardless of whether epinephrine is added to the anesthetic solution used for retrobulbar injection.

A sudden precipitous fall in intraocular pressure, resulting from surgical decompression of the globe, may be a factor in some patients, especially in those with fragile vessel walls. Expulsive hemorrhage was encountered with greater frequency in eyes undergoing glaucoma surgery while the intraocular pressure was markedly elevated.[56] The intraocular pressure falls to atmospheric pressure in all eyes as soon as the globe is exteriorized. Therefore, the condition of hypotonia itself may not be the factor but rather the magnitude and rapidity of the fall in pressure. This is less likely to be an important consideration today because most globes are massaged after the retrobulbar injection, many patients are given a preoperative hyperosmotic agent, and the incision is usually not made until the intraocular pressure measures 4 mm Hg or less on the operating table. In these eyes, it is unusual to encounter a prolapse of the iris or gaping of the wound as the incision is made.

Theoretically, the condition of hypotonia should predispose more to a rupture of a posterior ciliary or a choroidal artery, since the difference between the intravascular and extravascular pressure is greater. However, a significant number of expulsive hemorrhages occur several days after surgery when extreme hypotension is usually not a factor.

Jain[43] has postulated some association between expulsive hemorrhage and the presence of a black cataract (cataracta nigra), the latter being in his opinion an indicator of the degree of arteriosclerosis present in the patient. Furthermore, Das[57] also felt that this relationship was significant and that eyes with high myopia and brown or black cataracts are particularly vulnerable. However, the occurrence of expulsive hemorrhage in eyes with immature cataracts, neither dark brown nor black, casts some doubt on this hypothesis.

Müller[49] states that the clinical picture of expulsive hemorrhage occurs sometimes on the basis of inflammatory, proliferative, degenerative, and obliterative processes. Since most patients are elderly, general senile deterioration must be a factor that may cause acute fibrinous vascular necrosis. However, local ocular causes may be important. They include severe chronic vascular damage, as a rule degenerative, sometimes inflammatory, that may result from chronic glaucoma, high myopia, and other conditions.

Müller further felt that in view of the clinical and histologic aspects one must presume that a special event such as a vascular crisis must occur in addition to predisposing factors. If acute fibrinous vascular necrosis occurs during or immediately after cataract extraction, the instillation or retrobulbar injection of drugs preparatory to the operation or the operation itself may be suspected to be responsible. An interesting fact is that expulsive hemorrhage may occur hours or even days later, even when the cataract extraction and the postoperative course have been uneventful. Müller suggests that the operation causes a change in the vascular reactivity over a period of several days. The reactivity of the other eye is likewise changed, as becomes apparent when this eye is operated on within a few days of the first intervention. Müller states that there is more marked hyperemia and a more marked hemorrhagic tendency in the second eye.

Admitting our ignorance of the pathogenesis of expulsive hemorrhage associated with cataract surgery, the following factors may be important in some cases but not in others:

1. Arterial hypertension
2. Generalized arteriosclerosis
3. Elevated intraocular pressure
4. Necrosis of intraocular arterioles
5. Local vascular sclerosis
6. High myopia
7. Vascular fragility
8. Polycythemia
9. Precipitous fall in intraocular pressure as a result of surgical decompression
10. Operative loss of vitreous
11. Congestion of the choroid
12. Hypotension

The tendency for expulsive hemorrhage to recur in the fellow eye has been established. This recurrence indicates that predisposing factors must exist in both eyes of the same individual.

Clinical findings

Expulsive hemorrhage may occur at the time of cataract surgery or sometime later. Pau[36] reviewed 53 cases from the world literature and reported that one third occurred during the surgery, one third between 3 and 6 hours later, and one third between 7 hours and 9 days. However, Newby[45] found that 19 of 22 cases at Wilmer Institute occurred during the cataract surgery.

If it occurs at the operating table, a gaping of the wound may occur, with a forward displacement of the lens and iris. It may occur slowly, so that the increase in forward thrust of the inner ocular contents is observed during the enlargement of the incision. If the lens has not yet been removed, it will deliver itself, followed by vitreous and perhaps uveal tissue. Finally, bright red blood appears. If the process occurs gradually, a dark mass may be observed through the pupil after the lens is removed. The patient, if awake, may complain of pain, although it is not constant. The pain is probably caused by the stretching of the ciliary nerves by the hemorrhagic mass.

Several years ago I had an unfortunate experience with an expulsive hemorrhage. The patient, an 80-year-old man, had bilateral, dense, nuclear cataracts. At surgery it took an unusually long time to lower the intraocular pressure to a satisfactory level, despite the use of preoperative glycerin administered orally and a retrobulbar injection of the anesthetic mixture followed by 5 minutes of digital pressure. The intraocular pressure was finally lowered to 8 mm Hg. Two preplaced sutures were inserted into previously prepared grooves. After an ab externo incision was made at 12 o'clock between these two sutures, the cornea did not collapse. Instead the iris and lens appeared to move forward against the cornea. After the incision was enlarged with scissors, the wound began to gape and the iris prolapsed through it. A sector iridectomy was performed, after which the cataract was ejected from the eye by the bulging vitreous. An attempt was made to close the wound, but formed vitreous bulged through it and finally ruptured. This was immediately followed by bright red blood. An 18-gauge needle was thrust into the posterior part of the vitreous cavity to aspirate fluid in the hope that it would be possible to close the wound. However, 3 ml of bright red blood was aspirated. The vitreous and iris moved posteriorly for 3 to 4 seconds, but the bulge reappeared. After three additional aspirations of approximately 5 ml of blood, an incision was made through the sclera in the inferior temporal quadrant. Bright red blood gushed through this opening. After 10 minutes the hemorrhage ceased. An estimated total of 30 ml of blood was lost. The wound gape disappeared. An anterior vitrectomy was performed, and the incision was closed with 10 silk sutures. To my pleasant surprise, the patient's final vision was 20/80.

Since the vision in the patient's opposite eye was reduced to the ability to count fingers at 5 feet, cataract surgery was performed on this eye 6 months later. The same difficulty was encountered in lowering the intraocular pressure. The patient's preoperative pressure was normal. However, an uneventful lens extraction was performed. To my disappointment, a vitreous hemorrhage was observed 4 days after surgery. It remained confined to the vitreous. After 2 weeks the vitreous cleared sufficiently to permit an examination of the posterior pole. A degenerative macular lesion that prevented the patient from achieving a visual acuity of better than 20/400 was present.

The large amount of blood lost from the first eye was about the same as that in a case reported by Duehr and Hogenson[58] in 1947. In their patient, 30 ml of blood was released from the eye after 6 reinsertions of the knife into the scleral wound. The ultimate visual acuity was 20/200.

At least half the instances of expulsive hemorrhage occur within the first few days after surgery. The patient usually complains of severe pain. Blood may come out from under the ocular dressing. Usually, however, the hemorrhage is first observed when the dressing is removed. A bloody mass, consisting of clotted blood, vitreous, uveal tissue, and perhaps the retina, is seen to extrude from the operative wound.

Treatment

In most instances the question of how to treat the eye rests on whether to perform an enucleation or an evisceration. Some favor the latter, since a violent hemorrhage may occur after the former.[59]

Prophylaxis. It is difficult to discuss the prophylactic therapy of a disorder whose pathogenesis is so unsettled. Some special attention should be given those patients with extensive vascular disease. Hypotensive (vascular) agents, vasodilators, ascorbic acid, and rutin have been recommended but are probably of little value. Maximal ocular hypotension achieved by hyperosmotic agents and digital pressure is probably of value. The patient should be relieved of excess anxiety as much as possible.

If an expulsive hemorrhage occurs in the first eye, it should be expected and anticipated in the second eye. At surgery the intraocular pressure should be reduced as close as possible to zero. The delivery of the lens should be slowed down. The wound should be closed with extra sutures. A preparatory trephine or scleral incision in the inferior temporal quadrant may be performed at the outset of the surgery.

Treatment on the operating table. Since Verhoeff[35] first recommended the successful treatment of an expulsive hemorrhage, a number of similar reports[42,58-62] have appeared. However, despite the optimistic tone of some of these reports, such an eye is rarely saved. Most successes are obtained during the cataract surgery when the surgeon has an opportunity to recognize the complication and act without delay.

The principles of surgical management consist of immediate posterior sclerotomy to release the subchoroidal blood and firm closure of the incision by multiple sutures. Forced injection of fluid such as saline or balanced salt solution into the anterior segment of the eye through an inferior limbal incision helps to push the retina and choroid backward and favors evacuation of the subchoroidal hemorrhage.

It probably matters little which quadrant is chosen for the posterior sclerotomy. The blood will escape from any opening made in the sclera. By externalizing the bleeding, the inner ocular structures are able to retain their contact with sclera.

Once the bleeding has ceased, reopening the wound and removing as much formed vitreous as possible from the anterior chamber may be advisable, lest the eye succumb to the fibroplastic reactions incited by the disturbed vitreous and blood within the eye. Once the iris falls posteriorly, the anterior vitrectomy is complete. The wound is then resutured.

The postoperative management consists of combatting inflammation by topical, subconjunctival, sub–Tenon's capsule, and systemic administration of steroids.

REFERENCES

1. Swan, K. C.: Hyphema due to wound vascularization after cataract extraction, Arch. Ophthalmol. **89:**87-90, 1973.
2. Watzke, R. C.: Intraocular hemorrhage from wound vascularization following cataract surgery, Trans. Am. Ophthalmol. Soc. **72:**242-252, 1974.
3. Irvine, A. R., Jr.: Corneal changes before and after cataract surgery. In Transactions of the New Orleans Academy of Ophthalmology, Symposium on Cataracts, St. Louis, 1965, The C. V. Mosby Co., pp. 238-249.
4. Duke-Elder, W. S.: System of ophthalmology. Vol. IX. Diseases of the uveal tract, St. Louis, 1966, The C. V. Mosby Co., p. 23.
5. Fenton, R. H., and Zimmerman, L. E.: Hemolytic glaucoma. An unusual cause of acute open-angle secondary glaucoma, Arch. Ophthalmol. **70:**236-239, 1963.
6. Eyb, Ch.: Ein Fall von beiderseitiger Randektasie der Hornhaut, Wein. Klin. Wschr. **61:**606, 1949.
7. Appelmans, M., and Michiels, J.: Xanthochromic aqueous humour. Acta XVI Int. Congr. Ophthalmol. London **1:** 702-706, 1950.
8. Klien, B. A.: Chronic posttraumatic syndromes leading to enucleation, Am. J. Ophthalmol. **28:**1193-1203, 1945.
9. Cibis, P. A.: Vitreoretinal pathology and surgery in retinal detachment, St. Louis, 1965, The C. V. Mosby Co., p. 72.
10. Jaffe, N. S.: Complications of acute posterior vitreous detachment, Arch. Ophthalmol. **79:**568-571, 1968.
11. Tasman, W. S.: Posterior vitreous detachment and peripheral retinal breaks, Ophthalmology (Rochester) **72:** 217-224, 1968.
12. Linder, B.: Acute posterior vitreous detachment and its retinal complication. A clinical biomicroscopic study, Acta Ophthalmol. Suppl. **87:**29-30, 1966.
13. Vogt, A.: Die operative Therapie und die Pathogenese der Netzhautablösung, Stuttgart, 1936, Ferdinand Enke Verlag.
14. Galli, L., and Nagy, M.: Intravitreal hemolysis, Szemeszet **100:**76-84, 1963.
15. Ballantyne, A. J., and Michaelson, I. C.: Textbook of the fundus of the eye, Baltimore, 1962, The Williams & Wilkins Co., p. 107.
16. Busacca, A.: Un nouveau phénomène observé dans le corps vitré antérieur au cours des uvéites, Ophthalmologica **126:**355-360, 1953.
17. Duke-Elder, W. S.: Textbook of ophthalmology. Vol. VI. Injuries, St. Louis, 1954, The C. V. Mosby Co., pp. 6198-6214.
18. Cibis, P. A., Yamashita, T., and Rodriguez, F.: Clinical aspects of ocular siderosis and hemosiderosis, Arch. Ophthalmol. **62:**180-187, 1959.
19. Makiuchi, S., and Oyamada, K.: Prophylaxis and therapy of siderosis retinae by medicines (ATP and Ca-EDTA), Jpn. J. Ophthalmol. **5:**149-154, 1961.
20. Racker, E., and Krimsky, I.: Inhibition of coupled phosphorylation in brain homogenates by ferrous sulfate, J. Biol. Chem. **1773:**519-533, 1948.
21. Wise, J. B.: Treatment of experimental siderosis bulbi,

vitreous hemorrhage, and corneal bloodstaining with deferoxamine, Arch. Ophthalmol. **75:**698-707, 1966.

22. Cibis, P. A., Brown, E. B., and Hong, S. M.: Ocular effects of systemic siderosis. II. Am. J. Ophthalmol. **44:**158-172, 1957.

23. Flocks, M., Littwin, S., and Zimmerman, L. E.: Phacolytic glaucoma, Arch. Ophthalmol. **54:**37-45, 1955.

24. Fenton, R. H., Johnson, F. B., and Zimmerman, L. E.: The combined use of microincineration and the Prussian blue reaction for a more sensitive histochemical demonstration of iron, J. Histochem. Cytochem. **12:**153-155, 1964.

25. Dugmore, W. N., and Raichand, M.: Intravitreal urokinase in the treatment of vitreous hemorrhage, Am. J. Ophthalmol. **75:**779-781, 1973.

26. Forrester, J., and Williamson, J.: Resolution of intravitreal clots by urokinase, Lancet **2:**179-181, 1973.

27. Machemer, R.: A new concept for vitreous surgery. II. Surgical technique and complications, Am. J. Ophthalmol. **74:**1022-1033, 1972.

28. Machemer, R.: A new concept for vitreous surgery. VI. Anesthesia and improvements in surgical techniques, Arch. Ophthalmol. **92:**402-406, 1974.

29. Machemer, R.: A new concept for vitreous surgery. Two instrument techniques in pars plana vitrectomy, Arch. Ophthalmol. **92:**407-412, 1974.

30. Parel, J.-M., Machemer, R., and Aumayr, W.: A new concept for vitreous surgery. IV. Improvements in instrumentation and illumination, Am. J. Ophthalmol. **77:**6-12, 1974.

31. Vail, D.: Posterior sclerotomy as a form of treatment in subchoroidal expulsive hemorrhage, Am. J. Ophthalmol. **21:**256-260, 1938.

32. de Wenzel, M. J. B.: Traité de la cataracte, Paris, 1786, P.-J. Duplain.

33. Münchow, W.: Die expulsive Blutung. Eine Betrachtung über die Erstbeschreibung, Klin. Mbl. Augenheilk. **143:**757-763, 1963.

34. Hellmann, J. C.: Der Graue Staar und dessen Herausnehmung, nebst einigen Boebachtungen, Magdeburg, 1774.

35. Verhoeff, F. H.: Scleral puncture for expulsive subchoroidal hemorrhage following sclerostomy-scleral puncture for post-operative separation of the choroid, Ophthal. Rec. **24:**55-59, 1915.

36. Pau, H.: Der Zeitfaktor bei der expulsiven Blutung, Klin. Mbl. Augenheilk. **132:**865-869, 1958.

37. Gasteiger, H.: Zur Frage der expulsiver Blutung nach Staroperation, Klin. Mbl. Augenheilk. **140:**497-503, 1962.

38. Owens, W. C., and Hughes, W. F.: Intra-ocular hemorrhage in cataract extraction, Arch. Ophthalmol. **37:**561-571, 1947.

39. Pfingst, A. O.: Expulsive choroidal hemorrhage complicating cataract extraction, South. Med. J. **29:**325-328, 1936.

40. Melanowski, W. H.: Rare but disastrous complications in the modern cataract extraction, Acta XIX Concilium Ophthalmol. New Delhi **1:**759-762, 1962.

41. Goren, S. B.: Expulsive subchoroidal hemorrhage, Am. J. Ophthalmol. **62:**536-537, 1966.

42. Vail, D.: After-results of vitreous loss, Am. J. Ophthalmol. **59:**573-586, 1965.

43. Jain, I. S.: Expulsive hemorrhage and black cataract, Orient, Arch. Ophthalmol. **3:**141-143, 1965.

44. Jaffe, N. S.: Expulsive hemorrhage. In Welsh, R. C., and Welsh, J., editors: The second report on cataract surgery, Miami, 1971, Miami Educational Press, pp. 119-121.

45. Newby, W. E.: Surgical treatment of expulsive choroidal hemorrhage, Audio-Digest Foundation, vol. 8, no. 19, 1970. Presented at the 1970 Clinical Conference celebrating the sesquicentennial of the New York Eye and Ear Infirmary, May 6, 1970.

46. DeVoe, G.: Hemorrhage after cataract extraction. Clinical and experimental investigation of its cause and treatment, Arch. Ophthalmol. **28:**1069-1096, 1942.

47. Wolff, E.: Anatomy of the eye and orbit, ed. 6, revised by R. J. Last, Philadelphia, 1968, W. B. Saunders Co., p. 90.

48. Manschot, W. A.: The pathology of expulsive hemorrhage, Am. J. Ophthalmol. **40:**15-24, 1955.

49. Müller, H.: Expulsive hemorrhage, Trans. Ophthalmol. Soc. U.K. **79:**621-634, 1959.

50. Best, C. H., and Taylor, N. B.: The physiological basis of medical practice, ed. 3, Baltimore, 1943, The Williams & Wilkins Co., p. 195.

51. Lange, F.: Studien zur Pathologie der Arterien insbesondere zur Lehre von der Arteriosklerose, Virchow Arch. Path. Anat. **248:**463-604, 1924.

52. Varella, H.: Expulsive hemorrhage at cataract surgery. Unsuspected choroidal melanoma, Arch. Ophthalmol. **71:**209-210, 1964.

53. Miller, J.: Ueber spontane Berstung des Augapfels, Klin. Mbl. Augenheilk. **60:**458-467, 1918.

54. François, P., Wannebroucq, C., and Guilbert-Legrand: Les hémorrhagies expulsives. A propos de 6 cas, Bull. Soc. Ophthalmol. **66:**579-585, 1966.

55. Cordes, F. C.: Linear extraction in congenital cataract surgery, Am. J. Ophthalmol. **52:**355-360, 1961.

56. van der Hoeve, J.: Der Vorgang bei der expulsiven Blutung, Graefe Arch. Ophthalmol. **140:**655-661, 1939.

57. Das, T.: Personal communication to Jain, I. S.: Expulsive hemorrhage and black cataract, Orient. Arch. Ophthalmol. **3:**141-143, 1965.

58. Duehr, P. A., and Hogenson, C. D.: Treatment of subchoroidal hemorrhage by posterior sclerotomy, Arch. Ophthalmol. **38:**365-367, 1947.

59. Cahn, P. H., and Havener, W. H.: Spontaneous massive choroidal hemorrhage with preservation of the eye by sclerotomy, Am. J. Ophthalmol. **56:**568-571, 1963.

60. Bair, H. L.: Expulsive hemorrhage at cataract operation. Report of a case and an additional recommendation for its management, Am. J. Ophthalmol. **61:**992-994, 1966.

61. Shaffer, R. N.: Posterior sclerotomy with scleral cautery in the treatment of expulsive hemorrhage, Am. J. Ophthalmol. **61:**1307-1311, 1966.

62. Vail, D.: Subchoroidal expulsive hemorrhage occurring during thiopental sodium (sodium Pentothal) anesthesia. Its treatment by sclerotomy, Arch. Ophthalmol. **42:**562-566, 1949.

CHAPTER 22

Endophthalmitis

Although the incidence of intraocular infection after cataract surgery has sharply declined over the past 30 years, it still is one of the most serious causes of anxiety for the surgeon. Although newer antibiotic agents are available that combat heretofore highly resistant organisms, numerous instances of fulminating infections that defy all therapeutic efforts still occur.

INCIDENCE

On the surface, one is somewhat surprised that the incidence of postoperative intraocular infection is not greater than it is. The eye, of course, cannot be completely sterilized before surgery, and it is surrounded by the eyelids, cilia, and lacrimal apparatus and is contiguous with the nasopharynx and sinuses. In addition, there are numerous avascular structures within the eye that traditionally resist infection poorly. Despite these considerations, the incidence of postoperative infection has always been less than that encountered in other parts of the body.

At the beginning of the century the incidence of apparent infection occurring after intraocular surgery was about 10%.[1] After the popularization of aseptic techniques, a sharp decline occurred, so that up to 1950 the rate of postoperative bacterial endophthalmitis dropped to about 1% (Table 22-1).[2] From 1945 to the present a further decline to 0.35% has been reported (Table 22-2).

Reports on the incidence of postoperative bacterial infection are always clouded by several factors. Seldom are the laboratory data adequate. The offending organism is rarely identified or reported. As discussed later, this problem is frequently not the fault of the surgeon. Undoubted-ly numerous cases have been included that are really aseptic postoperative uveitis or lens-induced uveitis, since hypopyon may occur in these conditions as well. In most reports, suppuration or sepsis has been taken to indicate bacterial endophthalmitis. In addition, some reports attribute endophthalmitis to a specific infectious agent that may have been cultured from the conjunctiva but not confirmed by intraocular cultures. On the other hand, not every case of bacterial infection is recognized or reported. A low-grade infection that improves spontaneously may be mistaken for aseptic uveitis. One must also consider that there is a natural reluctance on the part of some surgeons to report postoperative infections. In addition, since the incidence of infection is so low, a series is meaningless unless it includes a great number of cases. A surgeon may perform several hundred cataract extractions without a single postoperative infection. However, because of contamination of a solution used during surgery, several disasters may occur in one day. This situation will cause a major change in the statistics. Thus a series such as reported in Table 22-2, where each surgeon reported at least 500 cases and most more than 2000, is more meaningful.

The ophthalmic surgeon must not be lulled into complacency by the decreasing incidence of postoperative bacterial infection. There is an increasing tendency to inject a variety of materials, any of which may be contaminated, into the anterior chamber during surgery. Moreover, certain infections such as fungus infections, penicillin-resistant *Staphylococcus aureus*, *Staphylococcus epidermidis*, and *Proteus* species may actually be on the rise.

429

Table 22-1. Incidence of cataract infections before 1950*

Author	Period	Operations	Infections	Rate per 1000
Ramsay[3]	1898-1921	2,146	68	31.6
Parker[4]	1905-1920	1,421	10	7.3
Davenport[5]	1919-1925	2,368	29	12.2
Giri[6]	1921-1922	384	6	15.6
Parker[7]	1920-1926	300	2	6.6
Slocum[8]	1929-1932	882	14	15.8
Parker[9]	1927-1933	450	3	6.7
Guyton and Woods[10]	1926-1944	1,144	12	10.5
Berens and Bogart[11]	1936-1937	1,004	1	1.1
Dunnington and Locatcher-Khorazo[12]	1937-1943	2,508	11	4.4
		730	13	17.8
Hughes and Owens[13]	1925-1945	3,286	23	7.0
Foster[14]	1942-1949	673	7	10.2
Duthie[15]	1937-1946	996	14	14.0
TOTAL		18,292	213	11.6

*From Allen, H. F., and Mangiaracine, A. B.: Arch. Ophthalmol. **72:**454-462, 1964.

Table 22-2. Incidence of cataract infections after 1945

Author	Period	Operations	Infections	Rate per 1000
Cosmettatos[16]	1959	3,000	5	1.67
Callahan[17]	1947-1952	1,653	5	3.0
Mullen[18]	1944-1951	4,000	6	1.5
Townes and co-workers[19]	1946-1952	565	0	0
Liehn and Schlagenhauff[20]	1952	1,000	2	2.0
Locatcher-Khorazo and Gutierrez[21]	1945-1955	7,662	6	0.79
Pearlman[22]	1948-1955	6,201	13	2.1
Neveu and Elliot[23]	1954-1958	1,047	7	7.0
Truhlsen[24]	1959	500	3	6.0
Luke[25]	1954-1960	2,300	12	5.1
Allen and Mangiaracine[26]	1950-1964	20,000	22	1.1
Allen and Mangiaracine[26]	1964-1973	16,000	9	0.56
Freeman and Gay[27]	1953-1964	8.277	40	4.8
Christy and Lall[28]	1957-1972	77,093	385	5.0
TOTAL		149,298	515	3.45

The decrease in the rate of postoperative bacterial infection from the early part of this century to the present is undoubtedly due to the advent of improved aseptic technique in ophthalmic surgery. In addition, the prophylactic and therapeutic role of antibiotics may be important. In some studies, endophthalmitis after cataract surgery shows a higher incidence when no antibiotics are used than when preoperative topical antibiotics and subconjunctival antibiotics are used (Table 22-3). However, even this is difficult to evaluate, since series that included the use of some type of antibiotic are more recent and are compared with less recent series in which no antibiotics were used.

The type of operation performed has some bearing on the incidence of postoperative bacterial infection. Probably operative loss of vitreous and excessive intraocular manipulation will increase the incidence. In addition, the risk of

Table 22-3. Incidence of endophthalmitis after cataract surgery

Author	No. of cases	Incidence (%)
Without antibacterial agents		
Dunnington and Locatcher-Khorazo (1945)[12]	2,508	0.49
Callahan (1953)[17]	6,137	0.57
Hughes and Owens (1947)[13]	2,096	1.01
Allen and Mangiaracine (1964)[2]	660	0.75
With preoperative topical antibiotics		
Allen and Mangiaracine (1964)[2]	19,340	0.96
Allen and Mangiaracine (1974)[26]	15,000	0.02
Pearlman (1956)[22]	1,773	0.51
Locatcher-Khorazo and Gutierrez (1956)[21]	7,662	0.08
Hughes and Owens (1947)[13]	1,200	0.17
Christy and Lall (1973)[28]	26,630	0.63
Whiston (1968)[29]	1,754	0.57
With subconjunctival antibiotics		
Pearlman (1956)[22]	3,226	0
Cassady (1967)[30]	1,212	0
Chalkley and Shoch (1967)[31]	571	0.35
Kolker and co-workers (1967)[32]	1,960	0.15
Christy and Lall (1973)[28]	50,463	0.42
Jaffe and co-workers (1978)[33]	4,321	0.07

Table 22-4. Type of operation and postoperative infection

Author	Rate of infection (intracapsular:extracapsular)
Guyton and Woods[10]	1:2
Dellaporta and co-workers[34]	1:5
Locatcher-Khorazo and Gutierrez[21]	1:7
Allen and Mangiaracine[2]	1:4
Christy and Lall[28]	1:3

infection may be greater after extracapsular extraction than after intracapsular extraction. This risk is shown in Table 22-4. This refers to unplanned extracapsular cataract extraction and probably is unrelated to current methods. However, I repeat that reports making these claims may be discussing aseptic uveitis and not bacterial endophthalmitis.

SOURCE OF INFECTION

There are numerous possible sources of infection after cataract surgery. These sources have been summarized as follows by Allen and Mangiaracine[2]:

1. Airborne contaminants
   Respiratory origin
   Surface origin (skin, clothing, and so on)
   Air conditioning system
2. Solutions and medications
   Saline for irrigation and other purposes
   Collyria
   Ointments
   Instruments disinfectants
   Skin antiseptics
   Alpha-chymotrypsin
3. Tissues
   Skin of hands
   Skin of operative field
   Lid margins and lashes
   Conjunctival sac
   Lacrimal sac
   Nasal mucosa
   Corneal grafts
   Vitreous implants
   Fellow eyes
4. Objects and materials
   Optical instruments
   Surgical instruments
   Tonometers
   Magnets
   Hypodermic needle, blood lancets
   Cotton balls, swabs, drapes, dressings, masks, and gowns
   Rubber gloves, bulbs, droppers
   Glass syringes, bottles, irrigating tips
   Plastic tubing, sheeting, retractors
   Contact lenses
   Orbital implants
   Intraocular lenses
   Sutures
5. Miscellaneous

Airborne contamination

There are numerous airborne routes that microorganisms may follow to enter the eye undergoing surgery. These organisms generally arise from the respiratory tracts of the surgeons, the nursing personnel, the orderlies, and the patient; from the unsterilized skin of the patient;

from clothing and sheets; and from the cooling and ventilation apparatus.

No one with a respiratory infection, including the patient, should be permitted to enter the operating room. The wearing of a face mask does not afford full protection even though both the nose and mouth are covered. There is no completely satisfactory mask. Most cotton fabric masks are ineffective. The use of impermeable material deflects air out the sides and is therefore of limited value. The ideal mask permits air to pass through but captures droplets expelled during speaking. Excessive talking during the surgery, the presence of numerous visitors, and the failure to change masks between cases greatly increase the risk of airborne contamination. However, the magnitude of these violations is small compared to the presence of an upper respiratory infection, which increases the contamination rate 1000 times.[35] There is still a place for routine nose and throat cultures of all operating room personnel, including the surgeons. Surgeons who encounter more than one infection within several days or weeks may be carriers of a pathogen that causes no personal discomfort. It is commendable practice to insist that all talking be done by the surgeon, that even this be kept to a necessary minimum, and that laughter and boisterous remarks be forbidden.

Since clothing may be a source of contamination, the standard practice is to require all operating room personnel to remove street clothes and wear freshly laundered scrub suits or gowns covered by sterile garments. Unfortunately, circulating nurses and orderlies do not wear sterile garments. The spreading use of sterile disposable gowns and drape sheets is to be encouraged, since they greatly minimize the problem of lint and dust. The patient's blankets and bedding should be in place before he enters the operating room, since a considerable amount of dust may be raised while they are handled. Street shoes should not be worn unless they are suitably covered. Some surgeons now wear special shoes in the operating room, and it is becoming mandatory to cover these in many hospitals.

There have been great improvements in the eye and drape sheets used during surgery. The older cotton drapes with a round hole in the center afforded little protection, since they became contaminated by capillary attraction when wet.

The numerous plastic face sheets and drapes now available are a definite improvement.

Operating room air may be a source of airborne contamination, as emphasized by Anderson,[36] who cultured *Pseudomonas aeruginosa* from air passing through a cooling unit. Williams and co-workers[37] emphasized that no material that will increase the risk of contamination should be used in the building of an operating room. Crompton[38] discovered that some plaster used to fill a hole in the ceiling of his operating room took origin in the soil and was strengthened by hemp prepared in India under unhygienic conditions. After encountering a case of postoperative panophthalmitis, he took samples from this plaster and grew colonies of *Clostridium welchii* and *C. tetani*. Such areas must be sealed by paint or tile so that the turbulence created by the ventilation system does not transport organisms to the open eye.

At present there is no entirely satisfactory method of ensuring that the air entering the operating room through air conditioning vents will be entirely free of organisms and other particulate debris. Increasing attention is being directed to this problem as a result of the space program. One may possibly utilize micropore filters such as those manufactured by the Millipore Corporation (Bedford, Mass.), which will filter out all bacteria, fungi, and particulate debris from air entering the operating room. These filters may be used to sterilize air (p. 449) used for intraocular injection.

An amazing amount of dust and organisms become airborne as a result of mopping and sweeping after surgery. There should be sufficient time between cases for the debris to settle.

Solutions and medications

The various solutions and medications used during intraocular surgery represent probably the most important source of intraocular infections. At least when infection does occur, contaminated solutions appear to be the most common and the most easily proved source of infection. If several intraocular infections are encountered in a single hospital, it is important to check the various solutions used during the surgery (including detergents for skin preparation), and cultures on various media should be made of the air that enters through air conditioning vents.

In 1951 Theodore[39] was the first to point out

the lack of any legal safeguards regarding the preparation of ophthalmic solutions. Working through the Council on Drugs of the American Medical Association, his watchdog activities resulted in a Food and Drug Administration regulation in 1953, requiring that all commercially prepared ophthalmic solutions must be sterile and contain suitable preservatives.[40] Later, in 1955, the U.S. Pharmacopeia, by stating that "ophthalmic solutions are sterile," implied that eye solutions other than those commercially prepared must also be sterile. However, this requirement has often been ignored by individual and hospital pharmacists. Ophthalmologists must never take for granted that any solution or medication prepared in the hospital pharmacy is sterile. Unless absolutely necessary, they should restrict themselves to sterile, one-dose medications contained in presterilized containers. Balanced salt solution for irrigation is available in such a package. The habit in many operating rooms is to use a large flask of saline solution for many operations on the same day and even for several weeks. The danger of this habit should be obvious. The possibility of introducing infection through contaminated ophthalmic ointments must also be considered, since they cannot be sterilized at this time.

There have been numerous reports in the past that prove conclusively that *P. aeruginosa* is the most common contaminant of ophthalmic solutions. The terrifying ocular pathogenicity of this organism, which is a common commensal of the gut, is discussed later. The frequency of this contaminant is probably related to its capacity to reproduce itself in the presence of little or no nutritional substrate other than water and sometimes a few salts. Moreover, it grows within a wide temperature range (4° to 42° C) and will live in 4% boric acid.[41] A recent outbreak of *P. aeruginosa* endophthalmitis occurred in a series of intraocular lens implantations as a result of contamination of the neutralizing solution (sodium bicarbonate) in which the lens implants were stored. A more serious outbreak of 12 cases of mycotic endophthalmitis resulted from the contamination of the neutralizing solutions of lens implants by *Paecilomyces lilacinus*.[42]

Elimination of contamination. The manufacturer of pharmaceuticals must ensure that ophthalmic solutions are not only void of mi-

croorganisms but free of particulate contamination as well.

During the past decade there has been an increasing tendency to inject a variety of materials into the eye in the performance of intraocular surgery. Although these materials have increased the effectiveness of intraocular surgical procedures and have reduced the incidence of certain complications, they may create other complications such as the introduction of particulate matter and microorganisms into the eye. The ophthalmic surgeon must rely on the manufacturer of pharmaceuticals for preparations that are not only free of microorganisms but also of particulate matter. The preparation itself may not be the only offender; the container that enclosed it may also be a significant source of contamination.

Although some attention to the elimination of contaminants from ophthalmic solutions used in irrigating the eye during intraocular surgery has been reported in the past,[43,44] it is insufficient and unemphatic given the trend toward placing more materials within the eye. These materials include salt solutions, enzymes, miotics, mydriatics, hemostatic agents, and air.

Common foreign matter found in these preparations used for intraocular irrigation include cotton, asbestos, glass, rubber, metal, resins, and sand. The presence of such contaminants points to inadequate filtration during packaging. The presence of fibers could be the result of using depth filters such as asbestos pads, which characteristically slough off fibers. Resinous particles could come from unfiltered deionized makeup water. In addition, any solution in a rubber-capped container will be contaminated with rubber particles, and when these solutions are aspirated into a syringe, thousands of pieces of rubber are scattered by the needle that penetrates the cap; then they are carried into the syringe for ultimate dispersal within the eye. When air is injected into the eye, it is usually from the operating room atmosphere, which contains a myriad of foreign particles and possibly some microorganisms.

It usually comes as no surprise to ophthalmologists to discover particles of lint, rubber, and plastic within the eye during a postoperative examination with the slit lamp. They have observed it before, and console themselves with the eye's usual lack of reaction to this foreign material.[45] However, reports, although few in number, have appeared that describe the intraocular response to foreign substances introduced during ophthalmic surgery.[46,47] The following description does not document the reaction of the intraocular structures to contamination by particulate matter but rather emphasizes the presence of such contamination in almost every ophthalmic solution intended for intraocular use and describes a simple technique to ensure its elimination (p. 446).

The most troublesome biologic contaminants in ophthalmic solutions are *P. aeruginosa*, *S. aureus*, *Proteus vulgaris*, and various streptococci.

Tissues

The preparation of the patient can never be entirely satisfactory. There are probably as many surgeons who cut the patient's eyelashes as those who do not. It is probably best to cut the cilia the night before the surgery, since cutting them just before surgery may disseminate more microorganisms than are removed. It is questionable whether cutting the patient's eyelashes reduces the possibility of infection, since microorganisms are most concentrated at the base of the cilia. The most practical advantage of cutting the cilia is that removing them from the surgical field improves visibility. Despite the most vigorous preparation, nearly half the patients will still have viable bacteria on their lashes, some of which are likely to be pathogenic.[48]

Although completely sterilizing the skin is virtually impossible, the number of microorganisms may be greatly reduced by careful skin preparation. Too often this important task is delegated to an unskilled person. The surgeon, or at least a trained assistant should oversee this procedure. Many combinations of soaps and disinfectants are satisfactory. Lid margins should not be neglected. These solutions should not be used for prolonged periods and should be subjected to culture methods from time to time. There have been numerous reports indicating a jar of contaminated preparation solution such as benzalkonium chloride (Zephiran) in a series of intraocular infections attributed to a pathogen such as *P. aeurginosa*.[35,38]

Theodore and Feinstein[40,49] gave an early warning regarding the use of cationic detergents.

For example, benzalkonium is a cationic detergent and is therefore incompatible with soap, an anionic detergent. They found that eyelids cleansed with aqueous Zephiran showed the presence of many more colonies of *Staphylococcus albus*, both immediately after its use and after the operation, than when iodine and alcohol were used. Moreover, they found that even alcoholic tinctures of benzalkonium, as well as of thimerosal (Merthiolate) and mitromersol (Metaphen) were less effective than the actual alcohol and acetone used in such tinctures. Considerations such as these should stimulate the ophthalmic surgeon to investigate the numerous disinfectant solutions available and to question their effectiveness in ophthalmic surgery.

Elimination of contamination. It would be impractical to describe all the patient skin preparation and surgeon scrub solutions available. Therefore, only three commonly used solutions are described here.

Benzalkonium chloride (Zephiran). Benzalkonium chloride, cationic detergent, has gained popularity in ophthalmology for cleansing of skin and mucous membranes. It is used in 1:750 dilution. Anionic detergents such as soap or pHisoHex *must* be thoroughly removed with water or alcohol before the Zephiran is applied to the skin surface.

pHisoHex. The anionic detergent pHisoHex has also gained popularity. It contains 80% sodium octylphenoxyethopyethyl ether sulfonate, 3% hexachlorophene, and lanolin esters. It is cautioned that the first ingredient may be extremely toxic to the cornea.[50] Thus whenever this agent is used, the eye should be thoroughly irrigated after the skin is cleansed.

Povidone-iodine (Betadine). An organic iodine and polyvinylpyrroliodone complex, Betadine slowly releases iodine. As a skin antiseptic it is considered somewhat less effective than aqueous and alcoholic solutions of elemental iodine, but it may be less irritating, less toxic, and nonsensitizing to the skin. As a surgical scrub it is used in a 0.75% solution (the percentage indicates the amount of available iodine).

•   •   •

The effectiveness of scrubbing the skin is not completely understood by many ophthalmic surgeons. One should not be deluded into thinking that mere scrubbing of the skin with soap or a detergent provides sterility. About half the original resident bacterial population always remains. Frequent scrubbing tends to reduce the residual organisms.

The variety of organisms present on the exposed skin depends to some extent on recent exposure. Apparently, virulent staphylococci are never resident in normal skin.[51] Price[52] has observed that skin of the cleanest human being rarely harbors less than 10,000 organisms per square centimeter. Crompton[38] stated that almost all the transient organisms are removed by routine scrubbing in the first 2 minutes. Such mechanical cleansing reduces the basic resident flora at a constant logarithmic rate of roughly one half each 6 minutes. Thus by this method it would take 2½ hours to sterilize the skin. Soap reduces the transient flora but slows the removal of the resident organisms. The latter are dislodged and removed by scrubbing with brushes. The temperature of the water or the use of unsterile tap water containing a few hundred bacteria per millimeter makes no difference in the rate of removal of bacteria. To reduce the resident bacteria to less than 2%, chemical sterilization is necessary.[53] Quaternary agents such as benzalkonium chloride (Zephiran) are cationic and are not effective detergents on the skin because they alter the electrostatic potential of the skin so as to attract bacteria to it. Other anionic detergents like entsufon (pHisoderm) are better but are less alkaline and therefore less effective than soap. Their main advantage lies in the ability to lower the resident bacterial population after use for several days prior to surgery. Otherwise a single scrub with such a product is no better than a routine scrub with soap. A very effective method is a 2-minute immersion of the hands in 70% isopropyl alcohol. The skin should then be dried by a sterile towel after the preparation to avoid subsequent dilution of the soaking solution.

It will surprise many ophthalmologists in the United States that most ophthalmic surgeons in other areas of the world do not wear gloves while operating. What may be even more surprising is that the incidence of infection encountered by them is probably no higher than that among surgeons who use gloves. The wearing of gloves does not ensure that bacterial contamination from the surgeon's hands will not spread to the patient's eye. Devenish and Miles[54] examined 6585 rubber gloves immediately after operations. In 24% of gloves worn repeatedly and 14% of gloves worn for the first time, there were holes. The holes occurred during surgery, since they were all tested before surgery. They demonstrated that even the tiniest hole is sufficient to let through numerous bacteria. Moreover, gloves introduce other problems such as powder and talc, which may cause granulomatous lesions within the eye. The glove powder is difficult to sterilize and may contain viable bacteria and fungi.

The new, thin, disposable surgical gloves, which are powdered only on the inside, have solved many of these problems. They are so thin that dexterity is not reduced. They are discarded after each use. Although the advantages of wearing surgical gloves are hard to prove, they are probably better than bare skin in contact with the patient's eye.

Objects and materials

Sterilization of surgical instruments is usually left to the hospital personnel, probably an unavoidable procedure. However, surgeons should become familiar with the procedure at the hospitals where they perform surgery, since in the final analysis they are responsible for the sterility.

Autoclaving is the most popular method of sterilization. In most hospitals the flash type of 3-minute autoclave, which employs a rapid rise of temperature to almost 300°, is used. This may damage some types of plastic instruments. This damage should not lead the surgeon to accept less efficient methods of sterilization. Since many rubber and some plastic materials cannot be steam autoclaved, they should be gas autoclaved. Too often, chemical sterilization, which inadequately sterilizes spores, is substituted. The bulb of the erisiphake is a notorious refuge for bacterial and fungal contamination.

For many years the tradition was to soak-sterilize sharp cutting instruments for fear of dulling the cutting edges in the autoclave. I have not found this to happen and prefer to autoclave all instruments. Many of these instruments are now disposable, a progressive step, in my view. Auto-clavable Schiφtz tonometers are also available.

Ethylene oxide has become a useful method of sterilization and may be substituted for autoclaving when the latter cannot be used. The gas is usually mixed with 81.25% Freon in the United States and 90% carbon dioxide in Europe. This makes the gas noninflammable and nonexplosive. Ethylene oxide, in concentration of 10 g per liter of space, will sterilize even resistant organisms and spores within 2 hours. The time required is a practical drawback.

The surgeon should insist that manufacturers use materials that will withstand the high temperature of autoclaves in general usage in the United States. It is meaningless to advertise that a plastic tubing can be autoclaved up to 250°, since most hospitals use autoclaves that drive the temperature levels higher than this. The surest way to get manufacturers to comply is to refrain from purchasing their equipment.

Certain instruments such as mirrors, lenses, electrical instruments, and various kinds of plastic tubing are damaged by autoclaving. They are not used with great frequency. They may be gas sterilized, stored in plastic containers covered by polyethylene bags, and opened as needed.

Miscellaneous

There are other possible sources of infection related to the patient, the hospital, and the surgeon. Patients with poor hygiene, health, or nutrition and those with an active periocular infection may run a higher risk of infection. The frequency of surgery on the patient's eye may also increase the risk. For example, complications arising from the initial cataract extraction that require one or more additional surgical procedures increase the possibility of septic endophthalmitis. Prolonged hospitalization and crowded wards may also increase the possibility of infection. Certain surgeons appear to encounter more infections than others. This may be related to prolonged duration of surgery, vitreous loss, or rough handling of tissues, along with other factors.

OCULAR MICROBIOLOGY

The eye demonstrates a character all its own regarding intraocular infections. The incidence of infection after intraocular surgery has always been less than that which occurs after surgical procedures in other parts of the body. However, when an infection does occur, it is frequently disastrous. Whether the eye is protected by the mechanical cleansing of the cornea and conjunctiva by the eyelids or tear film, or whether the latter possesses any potent antiseptic properties is not definitely known.

The reaction of the body to infection is based on the following conditions:

1. Virulence of the infecting microorganism
2. Immunity of the patient
3. Resistance of the organ to the microorganism
4. Resistance of the specific tissues of the organ
5. Change of the virulence of the microorganism for the tissue over a period

Although the eye shows a lower incidence of postoperative infection than most other organs, it may be rapidly destroyed by microorganisms that gain entry to its avascular structures. This avascularity is certainly partly responsible for this unusual propensity. There are many organisms that are considered commensals elsewhere in the body but that are highly pathogenic within the eye. Among these are *P. aeruginosa*, *Bacillus subtilis*, *Proteus* species, *Enterobacter aerogenes*, certain fungi, and herpes simplex virus.

There is probably no better example of this than *P. aeruginosa* (*Bacillus pyocyaneus*), which has long been considered an organism of limited general pathogenicity but which, through its affinity for contamination of solutions used in ophthalmology, has demonstrated its special virulence for ocular structures. As mentioned earlier, this organism can survive in the presence of little or no nutritional substrate and is the most common contaminant of ophthalmic solutions.[35,36] Whenever a number of postoperative intraocular infections occur in a single operating day or within a short period in the same hospital, more than likely *Pseudomonas* is the causative organism, and the source of the infection is one of the solutions used during surgery or in the preparation of the patient.

From the experimental point of view, investigators have shown that if only 50 of these organisms are injected into the anterior chamber of a rabbit's eye, a severe fulminating infection will result.[55]

It has been generally accepted that *Staphylococcus aureus* accounts for about one half of all the postoperative intraocular infections in the United States and Canada[2] and that 25% are due to gram-negative organisms. Partly responsible for this acceptance is a 1964 report by Allen and Mangiaracine.[2] In a 1973 report,[56] they found that two thirds of their most recent infections were due to gram-negative species. Forster[57] reported 31 eyes with postoperative endophthalmitis. The etiologic agent was a gram-positive species in 16, a gram-negative species in 12, and a fungus in three. Peyman and co-workers[58] reported 26 cases of culture-proved endophthalmitis. Eleven were caused by a gram-positive species, 10 by a gram-negative species, and five by a fungus. Eichenbaum and co-workers[59] performed vitrectomy in nine eyes with presumed bacterial endophthalmitis. A gram-positive organism was isolated from the vitreous in all nine eyes. The importance of these findings is that in any case of suspected postoperative endophthalmitis the etiologic agent is probably just as likely to be a gram-negative as a gram-positive species. The therapeutic implications of this are obvious. The eyelids and skin of the patient as well as the skin of the surgeon and assistants probably are the main source of postoperative infections with coagulase-positive *S. aureus*. Although not implicated as frequently as *Pseudomonas*, this organism has also been reported as a contaminant of ophthalmic solutions. The increasing frequency of *Staphylococcus* organisms in hospitals has become alarming in recent years, and the surgeon must become increasingly alert for its presence.

Staphylococcus epidermidis (albus), B. subtilis, B. proteus, and *E. aerogenes* are bacteria considered to be of limited pathogenicity, yet the eye appears particularly vulnerable to them. Forster[57] emphasized this in summarizing the results of 46 positive isolates from 45 culture-positive eyes in a series of 94 consecutive eyes with clinical endophthalmitis. Nine eyes were infected with *S. epidermidis,* the most frequent isolate, and two eyes were infected with *Propionibacterium acnes,* organisms likely to be found in the normal ocular flora and previously considered to be of low virulence and nonpathogenic. The increased recognition of *S. epidermidis* as an etiologic agent in endophthalmitis is supported by the work of Eichenbaum and co-workers[59] who isolated *S. epidermidis* from the vitreous in six of nine eyes with endophthalmitis treated by vitrectomy, and by Valenton and co-workers,[60] who reported two cases of *S. epidermidis* endophthalmitis. These findings are indirectly supported by the work of Abelson and Allansmith,[61] who reported an incidence of 29.5% *S. epidermidis* on four consecutive postoperative daily cultures in 50 patients, and that of Perkins and co-workers,[62] who noted that approximately 44% of normal conjunctiva, when cultured anaerobically, grew *P. acnes.*

Crompton and co-workers[55] studied various organisms experimentally in rabbit's eyes. *P. aeruginosa, P. vulgaris, Salmonella typhimurium,* and *Streptococcus viridans* proved to be the most virulent. As mentioned earlier, a dose as low as 50 organisms of *Pseudomonas* caused panophthalmitis, whereas a dose of 8 million *B. subtilis* organisms was required to produce the same end result. An intracameral injection of 1000 to 3000 coagulase-positive staphylococci phage-type 80/81 organisms resulted in panophthalmitis. On the other hand, Maylath and Leopold[63] performed similar experiments with *S. aureus, P. aeruginosa,* and *Escherichia coli* and found that the first was more virulent than the last two. However, there may be some question

Table 22-5. Bacteria responsible for infections after cataract surgery

Gram-positive	Gram-negative
Staphylococcus aureus	*Pseudomonas aeruginosa*
Staphylococcus epidermidis (albus)	(*B. pyocyaneus*)
Diplococcus pneumoniae (Pneumococcus)	*Proteus species*
	Klebsiella pneumoniae (Friedländer's bacillus)
Streptococcus hemolyticus	*Escherichia coli (B. coli)*
Streptococcus viridans	*Enterobacter aerogenes*
Bacillus subtilis	Other coliform bacteria
Bacillus megaterium	*Neisseria catarrhalis*
Clostridium perfringens (B. welchii)	

Modified from Theodore, F. H.: Int. Ophthalmol. Clin. **4:**839-859, 1964.

about the statistical significance of this comparison. Table 22-5 lists some of the bacteria responsible for infections after cataract surgery.[64]

Postoperative mycotic endophthalmitis appears to be increasing in frequency. Whether this is due to the increased use of steroids, antibiotics, or both, is not settled. Fungi in general, and saprophytic fungi in particular, were relatively ignored until 1958 when Foster and co-workers[65] reported three instances of fungus endophthalmitis after cataract extraction. In each, *Volutella* mold species was isolated late in the course of the infection. This fungus is related to *Cephlosporium* and is generally considered to be nonpathogenic. Many reports followed, but in some only a histopathologic study was performed, so that the specific fungus involved could be diagnosed only by morphologic characteristics. Fine and Zimmerman[66] performed such a study and demonstrated the presence of intraocular fungus infection in 10 patients who had lost their eyes because of undiagnosed endophthalmitis after cataract extraction. The fungi resembled species of *Aspergillus*, *Cephalosporium*, *Fusarium*, and *Volutella*. Theodore and co-workers[67] reported eight cases of presumed fungus endophthalmitis after cataract extraction. Three were proved by culture to be caused by so-called contaminant fungi (*Neurospora sitophila*, *Cephalosporium*, and *Volutella*). They made the interesting point that whenever the infecting fungi could be identified by culture methods, they were shown to be what are considered saprophytic contaminant organisms. Thus a major problem appears to be with the large group of soil and air contaminants rather than with recognized fungal pathogens. They concluded that, despite the opinion of mycologists that such fungi were nonpathogenic because elsewhere in the body they did not cause infection, as far as the eye was concerned, there was no such thing as a harmless fungus.[68,69]

Forster's[57] series of 45 culture-positive eyes with clinical endophthalmitis included two postoperative mycotic infections (*Fusarium episphaeria* and *Acromonium* species) and one after a filtering bleb (*Fusarium episphaeria*).

De Almeida[70] reported 13 instances of mycotic infections in 2076 cataract extractions, an unusually high percentage (0.62%).

Table 22-6 lists the responsible fungi reported in cases of mycotic endophthalmitis after cataract surgery.[71]

In recent years it has been recognized that any organism can cause endophthalmitis and probably enters the site by a diversity of routes, as

Table 22-6. Mycotic endophthalmitis after cataract extraction: responsible fungi[*]

Contaminant fungi (grown on culture)		Cases
Cephalosporium species	7	(Theodore,[71] de Almeida,[70] Crompton and co-workers,[55] Küper[72])
Volutella species	4	(Foster and co-workers,[67] Theodore[71])
Neurospora sitophila	1	(Theodore[71])
Hormodendrum	1	(François and co-workers[73])
Hyalosporus	1	(de Almeida[70])
Cephalosporium or *Penicillium*	1	(de Almeida[70])
Cephalosporium or *Hyphas*	1	(de Almeida[70])
Hyalopus bogolepofi	1	(Paiva and co-workers[74])
Fungal pathogens		
Actinomyces species		(morphology)
Sporotrichum schenkii		(François and co-workers,[73] Küper[72])
Candida species		
Fusarium species		(Forster[75])

NOTE: Fungus cultures should be done without cyclohexamide, which most mycologists put in culture media to kill the supposed saprophytic fungi such as *Fusarium* and *Cephalosporium* species, since recent reports suggest that these are important pathogens in ophthalmology.

[*]From Theodore, F. H.: Int. Ophthalmol. Clin. 4:861-881, 1964.

discussed on p. 431. The most common source is probably the patient's own indigenous flora of the eyelids and conjunctiva. In several cases investigated by Locatcher-Khorazo and Gutierrez,[21] the phage type of S. aureus in the case of endophthalmitis was the same as that present in the preoperative cultures in six of 13 cases.

DIAGNOSIS OF POSTOPERATIVE ENDOPHTHALMITIS
Clinical features

The characteristics of the immediate and subacute inflammatory response are probably the same regardless of the injurious agent. Physiologic and morphologic adjustments are evident, the purpose of which is to dilute, sequester, eliminate, or destroy the infecting agent. Despite this orderly process, the ultimate manifestations of clinical appearance and severity are necessarily modified by the specific agent and host response. The reparative process of inflammation, given our present inability to treat most cases of infectious endophthalmitis successfully, is superceded by destructive processes.

When the eye is invaded by a specific microbe, basic vascular alterations occur, which result in vasodilatation and increased capillary permeability, with its secondary anterior chamber and vitreous reaction. Injured cellular membranes account for exudation of plasma proteins and white blood cells. A rapid and dynamic process is called into play in response to the insulting agent, resulting in vascular changes, fluid exudation, and cellular infiltration as a combined event rather than in sequence.

Animal experimentation suggests that the anterior chamber and, to a lesser extent, the vitreous are able to handle a small number of inoculated organisms.[63] In such cases the initial inflammatory response presumably limits further organism reproduction, and the process becomes self-limited. This same defense mechanism probably exists in the human eye, and progressive infection with secondary manifestations occurs only when there is an adequate inoculum of organisms of sufficient virulence or a patient with a reduced, incompetent inflammatory response.

Clinical symptom appearance in suspected endophthalmitis depends on two factors: first, the severity of a new or postoperative inflammatory response and second, the ocular condition, that is, acute or late postoperative onset, metastatic, traumatic, or other. In the immediate postoperative period, the surgeon anticipates that the patient will experience mild discomfort, hyperemia, and protective guarding of the globe for the extent of the surgical procedure. Symptoms out of proportion to the expected inflammatory response such as increasing pain, hyperemia, chemosis, lid edema, and particularly anterior chamber and vitreous reaction make one suspect endophthalmitis. Therefore the patient's symptoms in postoperative and posttraumatic endophthalmitis may be of little help, and the clinician must rely on a change in diagnostic signs to denote infective endophthalmitis.

Just as the significance of the symptoms in endophthalmitis depends on the severity and ocular condition, the ocular signs vary according to the specific type of endophthalmitis. The earliest signs in the postoperative period can be appreciated only if observation is conducted with care and proper magnification. For instance, mild corneal edema and anterior chamber reaction can be appreciated by slit lamp microscopy but go undetected with a hand light at the bedside. Exaggeration of the usual inflammatory signs should alert one to suspect endophthalmitis in the postoperative period. Increasing protective hyperemia, undue corneal edema, and anterior chamber and vitreous reaction are the first signs of endophthalmitis, and to diagnose the inflammation promptly the physician should conduct regular evaluation of visual function, slit lamp biomicroscopy, and direct or indirect ophthalmoscopy rather than wait for loss of the red reflex or for complaints by the patient.

In most instances the symptoms and signs of postoperative bacterial infections manifest themselves to some degree in 24 to 48 hours. The patient may complain of an inordinate amount of pain. There is usually marked swelling and redness of the upper eyelid. The globe is intensely inflamed, and the bulbar conjunctiva may be chemotic. The cornea is usually hazy, and epithelial edema may be present. The anterior chamber appears turbid, and hypopyon may be apparent (Fig. 22-1). The red fundus reflex may be absent, and the patient may have difficulty perceiving light with this eye, with projection

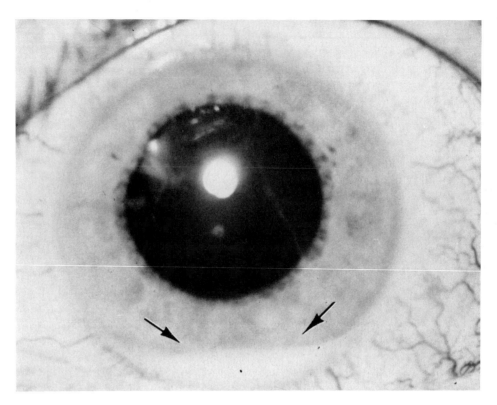

Fig. 22-1. Hypopyon *(arrows)* uveitis after extracapsular cataract extraction.

often being faulty. There may be marked photophobia, and the eyelids may be extremely sensitive to touch. Inspection of the area of incision may reveal suppuration, usually at a suture site. If the vitreous can be examined through a dilated pupil, it will appear diffusely infiltrated with inflammatory cells and membranes very early in the process.

If the process is manifested soon after surgery and the course is fulminating, *Pseudomonas* infection is the most likely cause. However, other gram-negative organisms as well as *S. aureus* may induce a similar response. There is little doubt that such infections are initiated at the time of surgery and represent some type of contamination from one of the many sources considered earlier. It is becoming increasingly apparent, however, that some infections related to the sugery do not manifest themselves early or commence in a benign manner, only to gain momentum later. The use of postoperative antibiotics, steroids, or both may possibly modify the

early course of the infection. It is also likely that certain less virulent organisms, which are usually overcome, may establish themselves as time elapses because of impairment of the defense mechanism, related or unrelated to the use of steroids.

It has become increasingly apparent that postoperative septic endophthalmitis may not give the classic clinical picture for weeks or months after surgery. There are at least four kinds of delayed clinical postoperative endophthalmitis. In the first two to be described, the organisms enter the eye at the time of surgery. In the last two, the eyes become infected sometime after the surgery.

The first form of delayed postoperative infection is mycotic. The early postoperative course is usually uneventful until 2 to 3 weeks, or even longer, after surgery. The onset is marked by redness of the eye and some pain. A mild hypopyon may appear, and whitish membranes may be observed in the anterior vitreous near the pupillary border. The membranes usually line the inner surface of the anterior hyaloid membrane. The hypopyon is usually transient, but the process within the vitreous continues unabated. Light perception may be retained for a long time. The anterior chamber becomes involved with whitish, stringy exudative strands, extending from the anterior vitreous across the iris to the bottom of the anterior chamber. The entire tempo of the process is usually low grade in contrast to the explosive course of bacterial endophthalmitis.

A second form of delayed postoperative infection is bacterial. As with mycotic endophthalmitis, the early postoperative course may be uneventful. However, some eyes show two to three plus cells in the anterior chamber without any of the other typical signs of bacterial endophthalmitis. After a variable period the inflammatory process rapidly increases in severity. Hypopyon, infiltration of the vitreous, loss of the fundus reflex, and toxic visual loss may occur within hours of the appearance of other classic signs and symptoms of bacterial endophthalmitis such as pain, swelling of the eyelids, redness of the bulbar conjunctiva, and chemosis. The organisms responsible for this clinical picture may be those of lesser or greater virulence. For example, *Staphylococcus epidermidis*, or *Propionibacterium acnes* may cause an indolent, inflammatory reaction in which diagnosis may be delayed 4 to 8 weeks postoperatively. Of course, these organisms are also able to cause clinical endophthalmitis 24 to 72 hours after surgery. The same delayed clinical picture may occur with more virulent organisms, with which inflammation is relatively little at first because of prophylactic treatment at surgery with periocular antibiotics.

The third later form of postoperative infection has been emphasized recently by Ruiz and Teeters[76] who termed it the "vitreous wick syndrome." The early course is benign. A postoperative rupture of the anterior hyaloid membrane with incarceration of strands of vitreous in the wound occurs. Necrosis at the site of a suture occurs, permitting vitreous to prolapse slightly. If a fornix-based flap has been used and has retracted posterior to the line of incision, the exposed vitreous acts as a wick for infection. The removal of deep sutures may occasionally cause a wound leak, which increases the risk of infection. In these situations, antibiotic coverage until the problem is corrected is probably of value.

A fourth form of late endophthalmitis is that associated with a postoperative filtering bleb. This was emphasized in a recent report by Kanski.[77] His series included 20 cases of endophthalmitis in eyes with filtration blebs, six after cataract extraction and 14 after antiglaucomatous filtering procedures. None of the patients were using prophylactic antibiotic eye drops at the time of involvement. Negative conjunctival cultures were obtained in most eyes, since most were being treated with antibiotics at the time of the author's examination. No intraocular cultures were taken. Predisposing factors consisted of type of bleb (thin-walled, cystic bleb, with a positive Seidel's test), contact lens wear, ocular hypotonia, and gonioscopic manipulation. In aphakic patients with blebs, the average interval between cataract extraction and infection was relatively short (11 months). Therefore early treatment of the bleb was recommended. The therapeutic results were outstanding, with 16 of the 20 responding with no loss of visual acuity. Treatment consisted of methicillin sodium 150 mg, gentamicin sulfate 20 mg, and betamethasone subconjunctivally; fusidate sodium (Fucidine) 500 mg orally three times daily (this is a strong bactericidal, antistaphylococcal agent), prednisolone 10 mg orally four times daily; and gentamicin and dexamethasone eye drops. Some doubt must be shed on the diagnosis of some of the cases, in view of the negative cultures and excellent response to therapy. Nevertheless, the potential danger of a thin-walled, cystic bleb after cataract extraction is worth emphasizing. Late infections in eyes with filtering blebs has been emphasized by others.[75,78,79]

A definitive etiologic diagnosis is often difficult. It is surprising that purulent material from the conjunctival sac, the margins of the wound, and the anterior chamber is often sterile on smear and culture. This sterility was emphasized by Maylath and Leopold.[63] It was suggested that this may be attributed to the surrounding iris cells and readily available circulation. Friedenwald and Pierce[80] injected inert particles such as India ink into the anterior chamber and found that they were readily absorbed by the iris endothelial cells. Bacteria introduced into the anterior chamber may be similarly removed by these same cells. Friedenwald and others[81] found that 1 hour after the injection of virulent staphylococci into the anterior chamber, cultures of the aqueous were sterile, and the iris epithelial cells were loaded with organisms.

The vitreous is said to resist infection much more poorly than does the anterior chamber. Spread of infection supposedly occurs much more rapidly from the vitreous to the anterior chamber than in the reverse direction. This is possibly caused by the lack of anti-infection properties of the vitreous and the flow of intraocular fluids from the posterior to the anterior chamber. This tendency may provide a possible explanation for producing negative anterior chamber cultures in the face of an actively infected vitreous.

Nonetheless, every effort should be made to establish an etiologic diagnosis. As discussed on p. 457, treatment should not be delayed pending the identification of the invading organism. Separate smears and cultures should be taken from the material in the conjunctival sac, from the anterior chamber, and from the vitreous. They may differ in their microorganismal content. Sample material from the anterior chamber and vitreous should be aspirated in the operating room, with appropriate patient sedation and retrobulbar anesthesia. A 25- or 27-gauge needle attached to a 1 ml tuberculin syringe is used to enter the anterior chamber, and 0.1 to 0.2 ml of fluid is collected. In aphakic patients a second tuberculin syringe fitted to a 22-gauge needle is passed through the first opening into the vitreous and manipulated until 0.2 to 0.3 ml of aspirate is obtained. If an inadequate vitreous sample is obtained or if one suspects a fungal etiology, the opening into the anterior chamber is enlarged, and a vitreous instrument is introduced to remove a sample of formed vitreous. Such a sample, diluted by the irrigating solution, is then passed through a disposable membrane filter system. After appropriate vacuum is applied, the system is disassembled, the filter is sterilely removed to a sterile Petri dish, and it is cut into pieces for appropriate inoculation onto the media[57] (Figs. 22-2 and 22-3).

Specimens aspirated from the anterior cham-

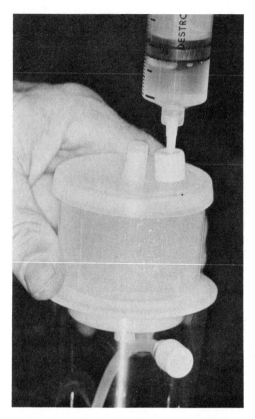

Fig. 22-2. Membrane filter culture technique. Vitreous sample is transferred into filter-vacuum system. (From Forster, R. K.: Ophthalmology [Rochester] **85:**320-326, 1978.)

ber and vitreous, or from sections of the membrane filter through which a vitreous sample is concentrated are inoculated onto blood agar and chocolate agar and into liquid brain-heart infusion and thioglycollate to be incubated at body temperature (37° C). Sabouraud agar and blood agar are likewise inoculated and maintained at room temperature (25° C) for fungal isolation. Careful application of the drops of aspirate away from the edges of the plate and flaming of the tubes of liquid media before and after inoculation will prevent or reduce contamination. Slides are routinely prepared for Gram and Giemsa stains and, more recently, for the modified Grocott's methenamine silver (GMS) stain for fungi.[82]

Theodore[64] recommends that a drop of the collected aqueous be placed in the center of the

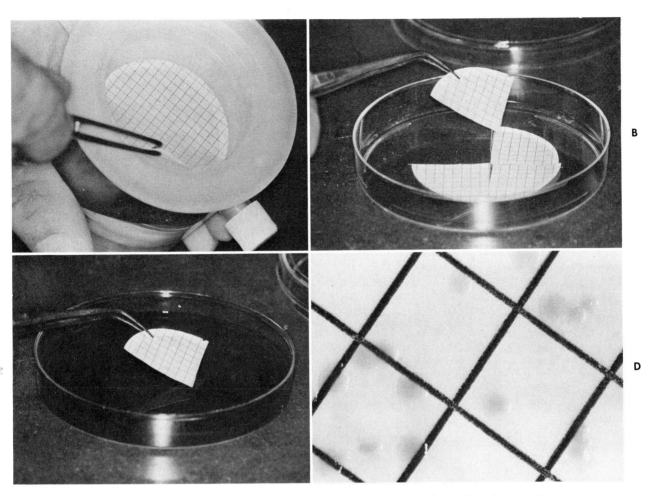

Fig. 22-3. A, Membrane filter (45 μm/pore size) is removed and transferred to sterile Petri dish. **B,** Filter is cut into four or more sections. **C,** Sections of filter are placed on agar media (top surface up). **D,** Growth after 24 hours of alpha-streptococcus on membrane filter. (From Forster, R. K.: Ophthalmology [Rochester] **85:**320-326, 1978.)

plate rather than that the entire plate be streaked. Thus if a contaminant should fall elsewhere onto the plate while the test is performed, it will be readily recognized. Sabouraud's agar slants without cyclohexamide should be used so that, as discussed earlier, so-called saprophytic fungi such as *Fusarium* and *Cephalosporium* species, now known to be ocular pathogens, will not be excluded. Smears are often very important, since they are rapid and, if positive, may save valuable time. In addition, the organism may not grow in the culture media. Many smears should be prepared for diagnosis by Gram stain and others. Forster[57] has established culture criteria to con-

firm the etiology in endophthalmitis more accurately. A positive culture is defined as growth of the same organism on two or more media or semiconfluence on one or more solid media at the inoculation site (Fig. 22-4). An equivocal culture is defined as growth in one liquid medium or scant growth on one solid medium only.

I emphasize again that negative smears and cultures do not rule out an intraocular infection. Cultures possibly will be more rewarding if the aspirates are collected prior to starting treatment. Treatment should be determined by the clinical picture.

The importance of obtaining samples of vitre-

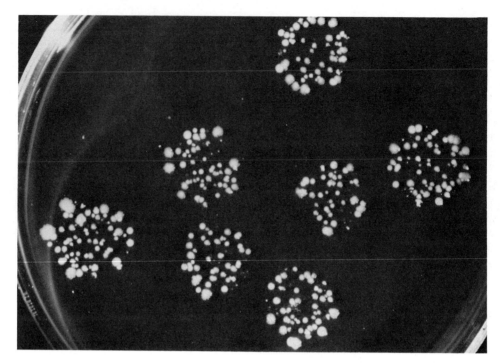

Fig. 22-4. Culture-positive *P. acnes* on chocolate agar. Each cluster of colonies represents growth from one drop of vitreous fluid. (From Forster, R. K.: Ophthalmology [Rochester] **85**:320-326, 1978.)

ous to establish an etiologic diagnosis is increasingly emphasized. Although paracentesis of the anterior chamber is a rational and often rewarding diagnostic approach in suspected infectious endophthalmitis, Forster and co-workers[83] has shown that aspiration of the vitreous proves more specific. He reviewed 58 eyes with clinical postoperative endophthalmitis, which were cultured at the Bascom Palmer Eye Institute in Miami from July 1969 to July 1977. Of these, 44 eyes with suspected infectious endophthalmitis were seen in patients who had recently undergone intraocular surgery (39 after cataract surgery, one after keratoplasty, and four after elective vitrectomy). There were 14 eyes with inadvertent postcataract and postglaucoma surgical filtering blebs with endophthalmitis that occurred months or years after surgery. Thirty-one positive microbial isolates were cultured from the 58 eyes, including 23 of 44 eyes recently having undergone surgery and eight of 14 eyes with delayed onset. Isolates were considered quivocal in five, since growth was present in only one liquid

medium or scant on one solid medium. Cultures were negative in 22 eyes, 18 recent and four delayed postoperative. There were 13 eyes in which the vitreous culture was positive but the concomitant anterior chamber culture was negative. Eight of the 13 eyes were aphakic, including three with intraocular lenses. In no case was there a negative culture from the vitreous and a positive culture from the anterior chamber. These findings strongly support the recommendation to aspirate vitreous in all cases of suspected endophthalmitis and confirm the observation that a negative anterior chamber aspiration does not rule out an intraocular infection.

In some cases, differentiation of an intraocular infection from a postoperative aseptic uveitis may be difficult. The latter usually commences later than a bacterial infection. However, this is not a reliable index. I have seen several cases of hypopyon commence 3 to 4 days after surgery and respond solely to steroids. The symptoms and signs are usually less intense. Swelling of the upper eyelid and pain are less frequent. The

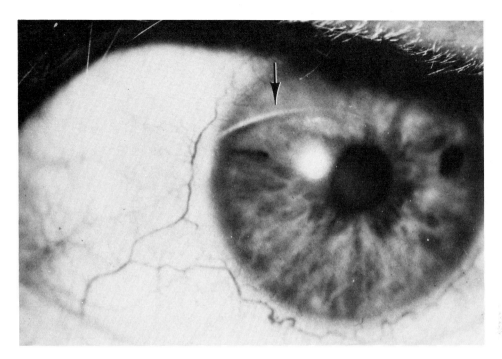

Fig. 22-5. Cilium *(arrow)* in anterior chamber after cataract extraction.

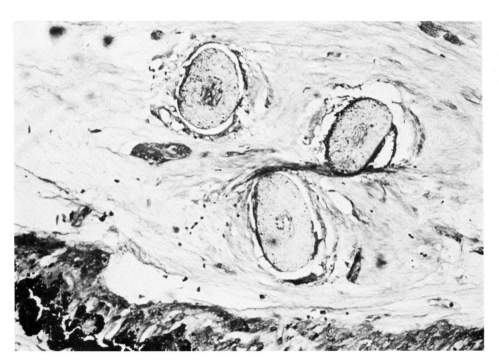

Fig. 22-6. Cross section of three cilia in midst of fibroplastic reaction just anterior to iris.

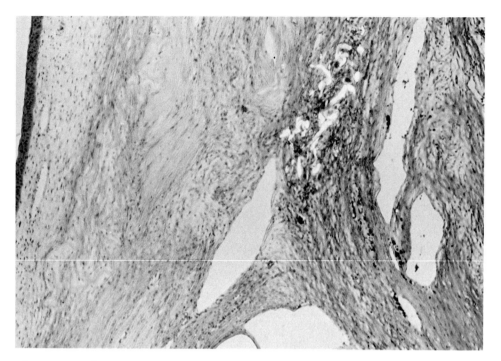

Fig. 22-7. Birefringent material (cotton) in middle of granulomatous reaction in anterior chamber.

fundus reflex may be lost because of involvement of the vitreous.

The introduction of particulate debris, irritating chemicals, and other foreign material (Figs. 22-5 and 22-6) may also cause a violent intraocular inflammation. Sections of such globes, if enucleated, may reveal evidence of particulate contamination in the middle of a granulomatous reaction (Figs. 22-6 and 22-7).

Phacoanaphylactic endophthalmitis may simulate a bacterial infection. However, one usually has no difficulty in making this diagnosis because of the presence of cottony and fluffy retained lens material. This entity is discussed on p. 490.

PROPHYLAXIS

The prevention of postoperative infection should include the elimination of those sources of infection discussed earlier. Further elaboration of these methods is not necessary. The treatment of postoperative filtering blebs is discussed on p. 441. However, the following will be discussed in greater detail:

1. Sterilization by micropore filtration
2. Preoperative examination
3. Preoperative antibiotics

Sterilization by micropore filtration

A very effective method of eliminating contamination, both particulate and microorganismal, from air and from all solutions intended for intraocular use is the use of a micropore filter.

The Millipore filter (Millipore Corporation, Bedford, Mass.) is a thin, porous structure composed of cellulose esters or similar polymeric materials. Its most significant characteristic is absolute surface retention of all particles and organisms larger than filter pore size. Table 22-7 shows four common biologic contaminants of ophthalmic solutions. It is evident that a Millipore filter whose pore size is 0.22 μm will screen out instantly and positively the smallest of these organisms.

These filters are integral structures and do not contain fibers that can work loose to contaminate the filtrate. They are only 150 μm thick. Each square centimeter of the filter surface contains millions of capillary pores of uniform size that

Table 22-7. Four microorganisms with minimum dimension of filter required for screening out each

Organism	Minimum dimension (μm)
P. aeruginosa	0.3 to 0.7
S. aureus	0.8 to 1.0
P. vulgaris	0.4 to 0.6
Streptococcus	0.6 to 1.0

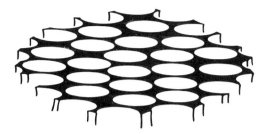

Fig. 22-8. Illustration approximates large open volume (80%) of Millipore filters in reaction to solid filter material (20%). Typical Millipore filter used for analysis contains close to a billion pores. (From Jaffe, N. S.: Ophthalmology [Rochester] **74**:406-416, 1970.)

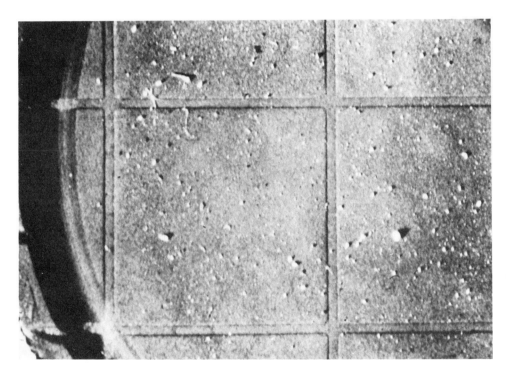

Fig. 22-9. Solution of alpha-chymotrypsin passed through Millipore filter. Note particulate matter distributed over entire filter. (×40.) (From Jaffe, N. S.: Ophthalmology [Rochester] **74**:406-416, 1970.)

occupy approximately 80% of the total filter volume, with 20% being solid (Fig. 22-8). This high porosity results in flow rates at least 40 times faster than those through conventional filters approaching the same particle size–retention capability.

The need for a method of elimination of particulate contamination is illustrated in Fig. 22-9. A sample of mixed alpha-chymotrypsin taken from the operating room medicine cabinet revealed contamination with particles of cotton, rubber, glass, sand, and metal when passed through a Millipore filter. To demonstrate the effectiveness of this filter, another solution of alpha-chymotrypsin was passed through a second filter. A similar particulate contamination of

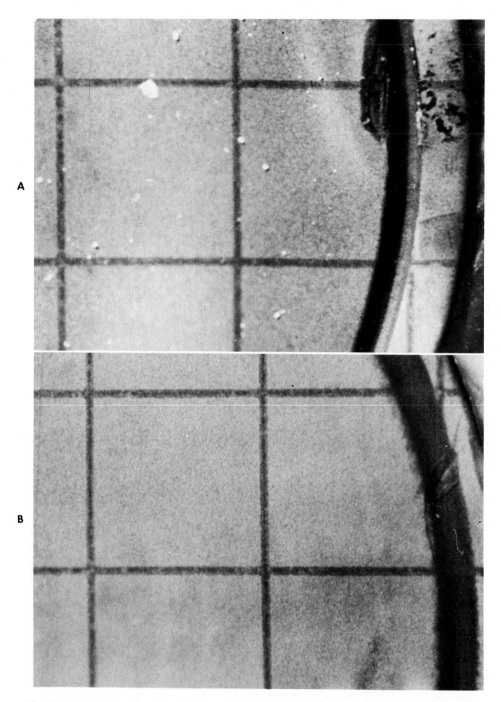

Fig. 22-10. A, Particulate matter contained on Millipore filter after passage of solution of alpha-chymotrypsin through it. **B,** Filtrate of enzyme solution in **A** passed through another Millipore filter with no particulate contamination. (×40.) (From Jaffe, N. S.: Ophthalmology [Rochester] **74:**406-416, 1970.)

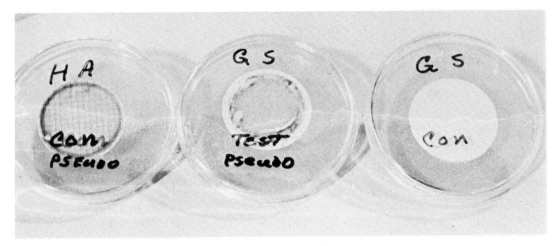

Fig. 22-11. Solution containing *Pseudomonas aeruginosa* was passed through left filter, *HA*, with pore size 0.45 μm. Filtrate was then passed through center filter, *GS*, with pore size 0.22 μm. Resulting filtrate was then passed through right filter, *GS*, with pore size 0.22 μm. Triphenyltetrazolium chloride (TPZ) stain 24 hours later demonstrated growth of organisms on left and center filters but lack of growth of organisms on right filter. This demonstrates effectiveness of 0.22 μm pore filter and ineffectiveness of 0.45 μm filter in screening out organisms. (From Jaffe, N. S.: Ophthalmology [Rochester] **74:**406-416, 1970.)

this filter was observed. The filtrate was passed through another filter. The latter showed no contamination (Fig. 22-10).

A solution containing *P. aeruginosa* organisms was passed through an HA Millipore filter with a pore size of 0.45 μm. The filtrate was then passed through a GS Millipore filter with a pore size of 0.22 μm; this filtrate was then passed through another GS 0.22 μm filter. The first two filters demonstrated abundant growth of organisms, but the final filter showed no growth (Fig. 22-11). This test demonstrates that a filter whose pore size is 0.22 μm can effectively screen out the *P. aeruginosa* organisms, whereas a filter whose pore size is 0.45 μm is ineffective.

To demonstrate the growth of the organisms, the three filters were stained after 24 hours with triphenyltetrazolium chloride (TPZ stain). The darkness of the two filters, left and center, indicates the positive growth of organisms; the third filter, right, was unstained.

These low-cost units are disposable. A sterile package (Figs. 22-12 and 22-13) is available for operating room use. Only one unit is used for all the solutions in the irrigation of the eye dur-

ing surgery (alpha-chymotrypsin, saline solution, acetylcholine, and so on). It is necessary to change only the syringe containing the medication. The flow rate is satisfactory for irrigation of blood from the anterior chamber, although the rate is reduced from the usual syringe-cannula system without a Millipore filter. When one presses on the plunger of the syringe, there is a slight lag before fluid comes through the cannula because the fluid must pass through the filter unit first. If air is placed in the anterior chamber, it should be done through a second dry unit, since an inordinate amount of pressure (which may rupture the filter) is required to push air through a wet filter because of capillary action.

Preoperative examination

It is axiomatic that any patient undergoing intraocular surgery should be in the best physical condition possible. Diabetics should be under control and respiratory and skin infections eliminated. The conjunctiva and lacrimal tract must be free of infection. If an infection has been present recently, it is wise to culture the area that was infected. However, this step should be done at

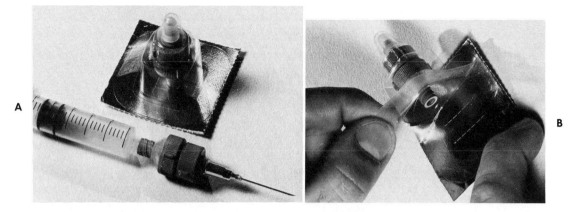

Fig. 22-12. A, Swinnex-13 filter unit (pore size 0.22 μm) in disposable sterile container and shown attached to syringe. **B,** Filter unit made ready for use by peeling open container. (From Jaffe, N. S.: Ophthalmology [Rochester] **74:**406-416, 1970.)

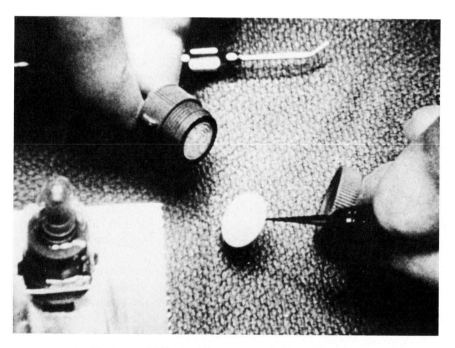

Fig. 22-13. Millipore filter removed from filter unit.

least 2 weeks before surgery to allow enough time for all bacteria and most fungi to grow out. If there is any possibility of dental sepsis, it should be eliminated well before the surgery. If there is a permanent obstruction of the nasolacrimal duct and no history of infection, I tend to leave the lacrimal sac as is. If there have been repeated infections in the past, a dacryocystorhinostomy may cure the problem.

One must always bear in mind that cataract surgery is usually an elective procedure, and there is sufficient time to eliminate many potential hazards before surgery. Because of some patients' advanced age and the hardship of a severe visual handicap, surgery will often be performed on patients who can never be brought to a satisfactory physical level. The use of preoperative systemic and local antibiotics should be considered in all patients who have had recent or repeated infections. If preoperative smears and cultures reveal one or more specific microorganisms, appropriate therapy can be prescribed. Otherwise the choice of antibiotics must be empirical, as discussed below.

Routine preoperative smears and cultures are advocated by some and ignored by others. I have found them of little value, especially when one considers that 12% to 25% of normal eyes harbor coagulase-positive S. aureus, and 1% to 4% harbor P. aeruginosa. In addition, pneumococcus, Streptococcus, and Proteus strains are found in normal eyes. Supporting this view are reports by Goodner,[84] who found 59% positive cultures, and McMeel,[85] who found 66% positive cultures at the time of surgery. The value of preoperative cultures is minimized by another report by Allansmith and co-workers.[86] They found S. aureus on the lid margins about one third of the time. They found at least a 20% chance S. aureus would be present on the lid margin on the day of surgery even if cultures were negative the day before.

Preoperative antibiotics

Strong sentiment for and against the routine use of prophylactic antibiotics exists. Except for cases where a history reveals frequent recurrences of sinusitis or some other infection, the routine use of systemic antibiotics is probably of little value. In addition, such use is not without risks such as sensitization, drug toxicity, and hypersensitivity reactions. In elderly patients, toxic reactions are likely to be high.

However, the routine use of topical antibiotics has been advocated by several investigators,[13, 21] who report a decreased incidence of postoperative infection after its use. Locatcher-Khorazo and Gutierrez[21] recommended several days of topical antibiotic therapy to eliminate persistent staphylococcal infections, but Allen and Mangiaracine[2] found that suppression of growth could be obtained in many cases within 24 hours before surgery. They suggested a schedule consisting of antibiotic eye drops four times daily for 2 days and antibiotic ointment at bedtime for 2 nights before intraocular surgery. The drops should be used right up to the time of operation. They do not state that such treatment is foolproof, but their statistics for 660 patients in whom topi-

cal antibiotics were omitted and 19,340 patients who were given topical antibiotics reveal that the rate of infection was 12 times greater (0.75% compared to 0.06%) in eyes that received no topical antibiotics. An update on this series by the same authors[26] reviewed 36,000 consecutive cataract extractions and reported that in the last 15,000 cases an incidence of bacterial endophthalmitis of 0.02% was found. This is the lowest incidence reported for any comparable series. They attributed these results to assiduous application of these principles: meticulous aseptic technique, minimally traumatic surgery, preoperative antibiotic prophylaxis with a combination of chloramphenicol–polymyxin B sulfate drops and erythromycin ointment, and anticipation of eyes and patients at special risk of infection, for example, alcoholics and diabetics.

Allen[87] more recently advocated the following regimen:

Day before hospital admission: Chloramphenicol drops three times daily and erythromycin ointment at bedtime.
Day of admission: Chloramphenicol drops morning and noon, gentamicin drops four times in the evening, and erythromycin ointment at bedtime.
Day of surgery: Gentamicin drops twice before surgery.

In the choice of topical antibiotics, I feel that a combination of bacitracin and gentamicin will probably cover a better spectrum and in a more effective manner than any other combination.

Certain factors support the use of preoperative topical antibiotics. These include the following: indigenous bacteria are frequently responsible for endophthalmitis, topical antibiotics reduce the number of organisms, there is no evidence that short-term use adversely alters the conjunctiva flora, and adverse reactions are probably infrequent.

Other factors are unfavorable to the use of preoperative topical antibiotics. These include the following: preoperative topical antibiotics rarely sterilize the external eye and do not provide significant intraocular concentration during surgery, evidence for reduction in the incidence of endophthalmitis after topical preoperative antibiotics is at best inconclusive, and this form of prophylactic therapy may be expensive, inconvenient, and possibly toxic.

Table 22-8. Incidence of postoperative endophthalmitis following cataract extractions[*]

Cases		Antibiotics used	Percent with endophthalmitis
Before 1964	22,832 (14.5% extracapsular)	Topical only	0.66
1964-1972	1. 3,798	Topical only	0.45
	2. 40,676	Chloramphenicol orally plus topical	0.40
	3. 1,812	Framycetin subconjunctivally at surgery plus topical	0.39
	4. 4,112	Chloramphenicol sodium succinate subconjunctivally at surgery plus topical	0.56
	5. 1,709	Gentamicin sulfate subconjunctivally at surgery plus topical	0.76
	6. 2,154	Penicillin subconjunctivally at surgery plus topical	0.37
TOTAL	77,093		0.50

[*]From Christy, N. E., and Lall, P.: Arch. Ophthalmol. **90**:361-366, 1973. Copyright 1973, American Medical Association.

The benefit of preoperative antibiotics is still unsettled, yet an increasing number of negligence suits have been directed against ophthalmologists who have not prescribed such therapy in patients who have suffered a bacterial endophthalmitis. Therefore, the following series, which is more than double the size of the preceding one, should be noted.

Christy and Lall[28] reviewed the incidence of postoperative endophthalmitis after cataract extractions in a series of 77,093 consecutive operations performed mainly by two surgeons in a village hospital in Pakistan over a period of 16 years (Table 22-8). A "no-touch" technique was strictly adhered to, gloves were not worn, the anterior chamber was not irrigated, and all instruments were steam sterilized in speed autoclaves.

In the 44,000 cases in which subconjunctival antibiotics were not used, the infection rate was 0.405%, and in the 10,000 cases in which they were used, the rate was 0.521%. Virtually all cases of postoperative endophthalmitis went on to loss of useful vision. When infection occurred, the onset did not seem to be delayed by the subconjunctival administration of antibiotics. From this mammoth series, the authors concluded that the most effective way to overcome postoperative endophthalmitis is to prevent it. The prophylactic use of antibiotics is no substitute for meticulous aseptic technique.

Short-term therapy is probably better for prophylaxis, since prolonged use of topical antibiotics might cause alteration of normal bacterial flora, with the subsequent appearance of microorganisms such as various fungi and *Pseudomonas*. The agents favored for topical prophylactis therapy include those antibiotics that cause a minimum of allergic reactions and that are not generally used systematically. These would include combinations of neomycin, bacitracin, and polymyxin B; chloramphenicol; gentamicin; and erythromycin in combination with other agents.

The routine use of subconjunctival antibiotics at the conclusion of surgery has been advocated.[22,30] However, infections have been reported after its use.[31] Nonetheless, there are probably instances when prophylactic subconjunctival antibiotics might be indicated, such as with extracapsular lens extraction, operative loss of vitreous, and excessive surgical manipulation. When indicated, the subconjunctival injection might be given at the outset rather than the conclusion of the surgery.

The rationale for using subconjunctival antibiotics at the time of surgery differs from that for topically administered preoperative antibiotics. The critical factor in endophthalmitis is probably the introduction of organisms at the time of surgery, by whatever means. Topical antibiotics probably do not gain significant anterior chamber levels, and they retard only organisms present at the time they are given, not those introduced at the time of surgery.

Barza and co-workers[88] found good aqueous and serum penetration of gentamicin after subconjunctival use. They found poor penetration of gentamicin after topical and parenteral administration. Several other antibiotics have been tried by the subconjunctival route, with good levels obtained. Supporting this is another recent report by Ultermann and co-workers,[89] who gave varied amounts of gentamicin to 135 patients before cataract extraction. Aqueous humor samples were withdrawn at the start of surgery to determine ocular penetration of the drug. After an intravenous injection of gentamicin 80 mg, an aqueous level of only 0.5 μg/ml was reached. This is not a therapeutic level for most bacteria. A subconjunctival injection of gentamicin 40 mg consistently gave aqueous concentration greater than 10 μg/ml within 15 minutes. This level was maintained for 12 hours and then fell between 12 and 24 hours after injection. A subconjunctival injection of 20 mg also achieved therapeutic aqueous concentration, but 10 mg did not. Topical application did not give therapeutic aqueous levels.

Most studies have confirmed that the more efficacious route is subconjunctival, the less the sub-Tenon route, either through the inferior culde-sac or through skin. Antibiotics given by subconjunctival injection at the time of surgery reach high levels of concentration in the anterior chamber for 3 to 5 hours postoperatively. In addition, there is little chance for the development of resistant organisms.

Opponents of this method of administration feel that it may simply delay the onset of infection, and several cases of endophthalmitis suggest that this is so. Also, Christy and Lall's[28] large study showed that this method does not reduce the rate of endophthalmitis, although the conditions under which their study was done differ significantly from those in modern Western experience.

I currently use gentamicin 20 to 40 mg subconjunctivally at the conclusion of surgery. Cephaloridine 100 mg may be added for better coverage.

Systemic antibiotic therapy is also in current use. It would be impractical to discuss all the available antibiotics. New ones regularly appear, and old ones become obsolete. Therefore those most commonly used are discussed with the understanding that some will be out-dated and new ones will be added within a relatively short time.

Gentamicin. Gentamicin is effective against *Pseudomonas aeruginosa* and many gram-negative organisms but is ineffective against *Neisseria*. It has limited activity against some gram-positive bacteria, for example, *Staphylococcus*. Resistant genera include *Clostridium, Pneumococcus,* and *Streptococcus*. It may be given in a dose of 0.8 mg/kg IM initially, followed by 0.4 mg/kg every 6 hours. However, since this agent can be nephrotoxic[90] and ototoxic,[91] a baseline blood urea nitrogen determination should be obtained first. Serum creatinine levels should be determined every 48 to 72 hours. Fatalities have resulted from this therapy. Ototoxicity is most likely to occur in patients with impaired renal function. To minimize this possibility, the interval between doses must be lengthened in proportion to the degree of renal failure, as estimated by creatinine clearance. Gentamicin should not be given with other ototoxic drugs, since the effects might be additive.

Gentamicin may produce neuromuscular blockade that enhances the action of other neuromuscular blocking drugs, general anesthetics, parenterally administered magnesium, or other agents with muscle relaxant properties. This drug is incompatible with heparin, with which it reacts to form a precipitate. It is inactivated when mixed with carbenicillin and allowed to stand.

Gentamicin has become popular because it is active against a wide variety of gram-negative and gram-positive organisms and is particularly useful because of its significant activity against *Pseudomonas, Proteus, Klebsiella,* and *Escherichia coli* and against staphylococci and streptococci that have developed resistance to combinations of neomycin, bacitracin, and polymyxin B.

When using gentamicin, it is useful to measure the serum level 1 hour after giving a dose and just before the next dose. The manufacturer (Schering) makes kits to monitor the serum level of gentamicin. As just stated, a serum creatinine level should be determined every 48 to 72 hours. If the patient has renal disease, an initial dose of 2.0 to 2.2 mg/kg followed by 0.8 mg/kg every half-life of serum gentamicin concentration should be given. The half-life is determined by multiplying the serum creatinine level by 3 or 4. Thus if the serum creatinine level is 4 mg/100 ml the dose is 0.8 mg/kg every 12 to 16 hours.

Preparation: Garamycin (Schering)
Topical:
    Ointment: 3 mg/g in ⅛ ounce containers
    Solution: 3 mg/ml in 5 ml containers
Injection:
    Solution: 40 mg/ml in 2 ml containers
    Intravenous: given over a period of 90 minutes

Cephaloridine. Cephaloridine is one of a group of cephalosporins that are semisynthetic antibacterial agents closely related chemically to the penicillins and, like them, contain a beta-lactam ring as part of the nucleus. They interfere with the synthesis of the bacterial cell wall by inactivating a transpeptidase, thereby preventing cross-linkage of peptidoglycan chains.

Cephaloridine is effective against most gram-positive cocci and against many gram-negative organisms, most prominently *Escherichia coli*, *Proteus mirabilis*, and *Klebsiella*. *Pseudomonas*, most species of indole-positive *Proteus*, and *Enterobacter* are resistant. Cross allergenicity between the cephalosporins and penicillins has occurred, but most patients sensitive to a penicillin can be safely treated with a cephalosporin. Cephaloridine penetrates the eye well after systemic administration.

The most dangerous adverse effect produced by cephaloridine is renal tubular necrosis, which may result in fatal uremia. Therefore assessment of renal function before and during treatment is essential. Cephaloridine should not be used with other potentially nephrotoxic drugs such as the aminoglycoside antibiotics, for example, gentamicin and kanamycin. It is also advisable to monitor hepatic and hematopoietic function when therapy is extended beyond 10 days, since elevated levels of serum glutamic-oxaloacetic transaminase (SGOT) and alkaline phosphatase as well as leukopenia have been reported.

Preparation: Loridine (Lilly)
Intravenous, intramuscular: 1 g every 6 hours for adults
Subconjunctival: 100 mg in 0.5 ml of isotonic sodium chloride or sterile water for injection

Carbenicillin disodium. Carbenicillin disodium is a semisynthetic penicillin for parenteral use; it is not absorbed by the oral route. It acts by interfering with the synthesis and cross-linkage of mucopeptides essential for the formation and integrity of the bacterial cell wall; this is the same for all penicillins. It is especially active against *Pseudomonas aeruginosa*, *Proteus* (particularly the indole-positive strains such as *P. vulgaris*), and susceptible strains of *Escherichia coli*. Most species of *Klebsiella* are resistant, and many strains of *Pseudomonas* develop resistance rapidly. It is said to have a synergistic action with gentamicin against *Pseudomonas*.

Carbenicillin is relatively well tolerated, but hypersensitivity reactions such as pruritus, rash, urticaria, and fever can occur. Serious anaphylactic reactions have occurred. As with other penicillins, blood abnormalities have been reported. Local pain at the site of the intramuscular or intravenous injection and phlebitis after intravenous administration are common.

Pain, chemosis, and conjunctival hyperemia occur after subconjunctival injection. This may persist for several days.

Preparations: Geopen (Roerig) and Pyopen (Beecham Labs)
Intravenous, intramuscular: adults 5 to 7 g every 4 hours
Subconjunctival: 250 mg in 0.5 ml of isotonic saline solution or sterile water for injection

Bacitracin. Bacitracin, a mixture of polypeptide antibiotics produced by a strain of *Bacillus subtilis*, and its zinc salt are bactericidal against gram-positive organisms and *Neisseria*. They are inactive against most other gram-negative organisms. Systemic use has been abandoned because of nephrotoxicity. Oral administration is ineffective because the drug is not absorbed from the gastrointestinal tract.

Its antibacterial spectrum is similar to that of penicillin for topical use; few strains of organisms are resistant to it, but allergy is less frequent, and future sensitization to penicillin is avoided.

Preparations: Baciguent (Upjohn); many manufacturers under generic name
Ointment: 500 units/g in ⅛ ounce containers
Solution: 10,000 units/ml

Cephalothin sodium. Cephalothin sodium is a broad-spectrum antibiotic of the cephalosporin group (like cephaloridine) that is active against penicillin-sensitive and penicillinase-producing *Staphylococcus aureus*, beta-hemolytic streptococci, pneumococci, clostridia, *Escherichia coli*, *Klebsiella*, *Proteus mirabilis*, *Neisseria gonorrheae*, and some species of *Salmonella* and *Shigella*. Most species of enterococci, for example, *Streptococcus fecalis*, and *Enterobacter* are resistant. It is ineffective against *Pseudomonas* and many species of indole-positive *Proteus*.

Hematologic studies and liver and renal function tests should be performed periodically during prolonged cephalothin therapy, and blood concentrations should be monitored, if possible, in patients with impaired renal function to avoid excessive accumulation of the drug.

Cephalothin is less toxic than cephaloridine and penetrates the eye less well perhaps in daily doses of 4 g/day. However, it can be given in doses of 8 to 12 g/day, divided, every 3 to 4 hours.

Preparation: Keflin (Lilly)
Intravenous, intramuscular: 8 to 12 g/day, divided, every 3 to 4 hours
Subconjunctival: 50 mg in 0.5 ml or 100 mg in 1.0 ml of isotonic sodium chloride or sterile water for injection

Oxacillin sodium. Oxacillin sodium is a semisynthetic penicillin with an action and efficacy close to those of methicillin. Its antibacterial spectrum is similar to that of penicillin G. It is two to four times as strong as methicillin against staphylococcus, streptococcus, and pneumococcus. In addition, it may induce a lower incidence of interstitial nephritis than methicillin, although this is not statistically proven. Oxacillin may be better than methicillin: since the minimal inhibitory concentration is 2 to 4 times less for oxacillin, on a weight basis it is 2 to 4 times as potent. This is partly offset by the fact that oxacillin binds to protein about twice as much as methicillin; protein-bound antibiotic is inactive.

Preparations: Bactocill (Beecham Labs)
Intravenous: 2 to 2.5 g every 4 hours, given over a period of 15 to 30 minutes by "piggyback" through an indwelling venous catheter; it deteriorates, as do other penicillins, in an intravenous bottle

Table 22-9 indicates the dosage of various subconjunctival antibiotics.[92]
Pseudomonas is very difficult to eradicate and is consistently sensitive to polymyxin B, colistin, gentamicin, and carbenicillin. In addition, these agents are bactericidal to nearly all gram-nega-

Table 22-9. Dosage of subconjunctival antibiotics[*]

Antibiotic	Dosage
Amphotericin B	1 to 3 mg
Ampicillin	50 to 100 mg
Bacitracin	10,000 units
Carbenicillin	100 mg
Cephaloridine	50 to 100 mg
Cephalothin	50 to 100 mg
Chloramphenicol (sodium succinate)	40 to 50 mg
Colistin (Coly-Mycin)	15 to 20 mg
Erythromycin	10 to 20 mg
Gentamicin	10 to 30 mg
Kanamycin	10 to 30 mg
Linocomycin	75 mg
Methicillin	50 to 100 mg
Neomycin	100 to 500 mg
Nystatin	10,000 units
Oxacillin	50 to 100 mg
Penicillin G	500,000 units
Polymyxin B	5 to 10 mg
Streptomycin	40 to 50 mg
Tetracyclines	2.5 to 5 mg
Vancomycin	15 to 25 mg

[*]From Ellis, P. P.: Ocular therapeutics and pharmacology, ed. 5, St. Louis, 1977, The C. V. Mosby Co.

tive organisms, with the exception of *P. vulgaris*. A combination of penicillin and streptomycin was popular for many years. However, colistimethate sodium (Coly-Mycin) 20 mg or gentamicin 3 mg (20 mg is the currently recommended dose) may be substituted for streptomycin, since both agents are effective against *Pseudomonas* as well as a wide spectrum of gram-negative organisms. Ampicillin 50 mg could replace penicillin G because of its wider antibacterial spectrum. To eliminate the possibility of resistant staphylococci, methicillin 50 to 100 mg, cephalothin 50 mg, or cephaloridine 50 mg may be used. Methicillin is unstable in acid solutions and therefore should be dissolved just before use.

The surgeon not infrequently encounters patients with cataracts who are receiving long-term steroid therapy for one of numerous disorders such as rheumatoid arthritis or one of the blood dyscrasias. Some patients indiscriminately use topical steroids for eyelid and conjunctival abnormalities. These agents may stimulate bacterial and viral growth. In addition, the incidence of fungi in the eye may rise sharply. Mitsui and Hanabusa[93] reported the incidence of fungi after topical steroid therapy to be 67%, whereas in control cases it was 18%. In a series of 18 patients whose eyes were free of fungi originally, fungus cultures became positive in nine patients after administration of topical steroids for 3 weeks. It would therefore appear prudent to perform fungus culture on such patients before surgery. This procedure requires at least 2 weeks.

Table 22-10. Systemic antibiotics available for treatment of bacterial endophthalmitis*

Effective against gram-positive and gram-negative organism (excluding *Pseudomonas*)

Antibiotic	Adult dosage
Cephalothin (Keflin)	2 g IV or IM every 6 hr
Cephaloridine (Loridine)	1 g IV or IM every 6 hr
Chloramphenicol (Chloromycetin, Mychel)	1 g IV every 8 hr or 2 g orally initial dose, then 1 g every 8 hr
Penicillin G with streptomycin	Penicillin: 8-12 million units over 16- to 20-hour period
	Streptomycin: 0.5 g IM every 8 hr or 1 g every 12 hr
Ampicillin (Polycillin, Penbritin, Amcill, Principen)	1 g IV or IM every 6 hr
Kanamycin (Kantrex)	500 mg IM every 8 hr or 1 g every 12 hr
Sulfadiazine-sulfamerazine mixture, or mixed sulfonamides	2 g initial dose orally; then 1 g every 6 hr

Effective against gram-positive organisms (including penicillin G–resistant staphylococci)

Antibiotic	Adult dosage
Semisynthetic penicillins	
Methicillin (Staphcillin, Dimocillin)	2 g IV or IM every 4 to 6 hr
Nafcillin (Unipen)	1 g IV, IM, or orally every 4 to 6 hr
Oxacillin (Prostaphlin)	1 g IV, IM, or orally every 4 to 6 hr
Dicloxacillin (Dynapen, Pathocil, Veracillin)	1 g IV, IM, or orally every 4 to 6 hr
Cephalothin (Keflin)	1 g IV or IM every 4 to 6 hr
Cephaloridine (Loridine)	1 g IV or IM every 4 to 6 hr
Lincomycin (Lincocin)	1 g orally every 6 hr: 600 mg IV or IM every 8 to 12 hr
Vancomycin (Vancocin)	1 g IV every 6 to 8 hr for 48 hr; then 1 g every 12 hr
Erythromycin estolate (Ilosone) Erythromycin stearate (Erythrocin stearate)	500 mg orally four times a day
Erythromycin ethyl succinate (Erythrocin-IM)	100 mg IM four times a day
Erythromycin lactobionate (Erythrocin lactobionate)	1 to 4 g IV daily

Effective against *Pseudomonas* infections

Agent	Systemic	Subconjunctival	Topical
Colistin (Coly-Mycin)	1.5-5 mg/kg/day IM in two to four divided doses	20 mg	1.5-3 mg/ml
Polymyxin B (Aerosporin)	4.5-2.5 mg/kg/day IV as single dose or divided into two doses	10 mg	10,000 units/ml
Gentamicin	0.8 mg/kg initially IM then 0.4 mg/kg every 6 hr	20 mg	3-10 mg/ml

*From Ellis, P.P.: Postoperative endophthalmitis. In Symposium on ocular pharmacology and therapeutics, Transactions of the New Orleans Academy of Ophthalmology, St. Louis, 1970, The C. V. Mosby Co.

TREATMENT OF POSTOPERATIVE BACTERIAL ENDOPHTHALMITIS
Antibiotics

New antibiotics appear with such regularity that one must expect any discussion of specific antibiotics for the treatment of postoperative intraocular infections to become obsolete within a relatively short period. For a complete listing and discussion of all available antibiotics for use in ophthalmology, the reader is referred to one of several books available on ocular pharmacology.

The systemic antibiotics available for treatment of bacterial endophthalmitis and their dosages are shown in Table 22-10.

In case of a severe intraocular infection, subconjunctival injections of an appropriate or empiric antibiotic should be performed every 24 hours. The solutions for injection are prepared by dissolving the antibiotic powder in 0.25 to 0.33 ml of sterile water. The subconjunctival dosage for several antibiotics is as follows:

Methicillin	100 mg
Cephalothin	100 mg
Cephaloridine	100 mg
Ampicillin	50 mg
Colistin	20 mg
Gentamicin	15 to 20 mg

Intravitreal injections of antibiotics (as well as steroids) are being reported more frequently. Although at this time the toxicity of these agents to the retina, optic nerve, and other intraocular structures is not definitely known, intravitreal administration may be justified in postoperative endophthalmitis.

Peyman and co-workers[94] recommended the following doses for intravitreal injection:

Gentamicin	400 μg/0.1 ml
Lincomycin	1.5 mg/0.1 ml
Dexamethasone	400 μg/0.1 ml
TOTAL DOSE TO BE INJECTED	0.1 to 0.2 ml

At the onset of a presumed intraocular infection, one may have a difficult time differentiating a true infection from an aseptic uveitis, even in the presence of hypopyon. If there is little ocular injection, lid edema, and pain and if light projection remains accurate, one may be permitted the luxury of treating the eye intensively with steroids on the presumption that the process is not infectious. If this diagnosis is correct, the clinical picture will show improvement, or at least there will be no deteriorating symptoms and signs. However, if there is reasonable suspicion that the process is infectious, efforts toward diagnosis and treatment must be undertaken simultaneously and without delay. Delaying treatment until the etiologic organism is isolated may result in unnecessary damage.

Certain options are available at the onset of a presumed infectious endophthalmitis. Although its management must be much more aggressive than what has been practiced in the past, there is as yet no correctly defined degree of aggressiveness. Considerably more clinical experience will be required before this is settled. The challenge is great because of the consistently poor results obtained by conventional therapy. More potent antibiotics are now available, yet the salvage rate is low. The low salvage rate is partly attributable to the poor penetration of topically, and more systematically administered, antibiotics into the anterior chamber and particularly into the vitreous, which is now considered the primary site of established infection.

Direct intraocular therapy

Ample experimental data now exist to justify direct intraocular therapy. Some of these date back to the 1940s when several reports[97-101] described the successful treatment of experimental endophthalmitis with intravitreal penicillin. More recently Peyman and co-workers[102-109] and Zachary and Forster[110] evaluated several antibiotics given intraocularly in animals, using retinal observations, electroretinography, and subsequently histopathology to determine dosage levels that are relatively safe and nontoxic to the retina. This work has been augmented by clinical experience.[83,94,111] Their work established that comparative bacteriocidal levels obtained in the vitreous by direct intravitreal injection far exceed the minimal bacteriocidal levels or concentration that can be achieved by systemic, periocular, or topical routes, and determined the relative safety of a number of antibiotics in both animals and humans. The clearance of gentamicin has been studied by Peyman and co-workers[103] and Forster,[57] who compared the clearance of gentamicin in aphakic and phakic rabbit eyes, both with and without intraocular infection, to determine the most reasonable time for repeated intraocular antibiotic injection.

Combined therapeutic vitrectomy and intraocular antibiotics

Some background justification now exists for combined therapeutic vitrectomy and intraocular antibiotics. Maylath and Leopold[63] demonstrated in experimental animals the ability of the anterior chamber, as opposed to the vitreous, to eliminate infection. Forster[57] confirmed this in his study of infectious endophthalmitis in humans. He obtained negative anterior chamber cultures from 13 eyes in which vitreous cultures were positive. In no case was there a negative culture from the vitreous but a positive culture from the anterior chamber. In a rabbit model of endophthalmitis, using *S. aureus* and *S. epidermidis*, Cottingham and Forster[112] demonstrated that either at 24 to 31 hours or at 40 to 49 hours after inoculation, eyes treated by combined vitrectomy and intraocular gentamicin had a significantly greater number of negative cultures 1 week later than those treated by intraocular antibiotics alone.

There is also some theoretical rationale for combined therapeutic vitrectomy and intraocular antibiotics. The combined approach treats the vitreous abscess by the conventional method of incision and drainage. It removes the culture medium and most of the infectious organisms. It eliminates sequestered and loculated infected pockets. It converts the vitreous cavity into a permeable chamber, allowing greater mobility of instilled antibiotics, possible anti-inflammatory agents, and natural defense mechanisms.

Suggested modern regimen

There are probably many approaches to the management of infectious endophthalmitis, depending on the aggressiveness of the surgeon. Forster[57] has recommended an approach. Since the dosage of antibiotic is critical to avoid retinal toxicity, this regimen is presented in detail.

The patient is hospitalized. Intraocular samples are taken from the anterior chamber and vitreous for smears and culture, as outlined on p. 442. This is done in the operating room so that the antibiotics for intraocular injection can be prepared and injected at the same time. The dilu-

tions of the antibiotics must be carefully checked to ensure accurate, consistent dosages. The following dilutional method for gentamicin and cephaloridine is recommended.

Intraocular gentamicin (Garamycin) 0.1 mg (100 μg)

1. Withdraw 0.1 ml (4 mg) from the vial containing gentamicin 40 mg/ml.
2. Add to 9.9 ml of nonbacteriostatic saline solution if final volume of 0.25 ml for injection is desired, *or* to 3.9 ml of nonbacteriostatic saline solution if final volume of 0.1 ml is desired.
3. Each 10 ml dose contains 4 mg gentamicin; 1 ml contains 0.4 mg; 0.25 ml contains 0.1 mg; *or* 4 ml contains 4 mg; 1 ml contains 1 mg; 0.1 ml contains 0.1 mg.
4. The surgeon injects either 0.25 ml containing 0.1 mg gentamicin or 0.1 ml containing 0.1 mg gentamicin into the anterior vitreous through the keratotomy or pars plana site from which samples were taken for smear and culture.

Intraocular cephaloridine (Loridine)

1. Reconstitute powder with 10 ml sterile sodium chloride (1000 mg in 10 ml).
2. Add 0.1 ml (10 mg) of suspension to 3.9 ml nonbacteriostatic saline solution; 10 mg in 4 ml contains 1 mg cephaloridine in 0.4 ml.
3. The surgeon injects 0.1 ml containing 0.25 mg cephaloridine.

There is some question about the acceptable dosage of gentamicin for intraocular injection. Peyman and co-workers[94] have recommended the injection of gentamicin 0.4 to 0.5 mg into the anterior vitreous, combined with intraocular corticosteroids. Based on laboratory and clinical experience with the human eye, this dosage is apparently satisfactorily tolerated.

After completing the intraocular antibiotic injections, gentamicin 40 mg and cephaloridine 100 mg or methicillin 100 mg is injected subconjunctivally. In cases of recent onset, or when a fungal etiology is not considered likely, triamcinolone (Aristocort) is injected infraorbitally.

The patient is immediately given topical antibiotic therapy consisting of gentamicin 9 mg/ml and bacitracin 5000 units/ml hourly. Patients are empirically given cephaloridine 1000 mg as a starting dose and 500 mg every 6 hours intravenously. It is convenient to have an intravenous drip solution maintained 24 hours daily. Antibiotics intended for intravenous use can be injected into the intravenous tubing. If the antibiotic must be given for a longer period, for example, for 15 to 90 minutes, it can drip in slowly through a piggyback unit. Serum creatinine or blood urea nitrogen level is measured. Combined therapy with these antibiotics provides rational coverage for most organisms for which the patient is at risk.

This diagnostic and therapeutic regimen takes place during the first 24 hours. If cultures are negative and the smears noncontributory, the patient is maintained on the same therapy topically and systemically. After 48 hours, by which time essentially all bacteria and fungi should be making initial appearance on culture media, if the cultures are still negative the management is as for a noninfectious sterile endophthalmitis. If the cultures are positive for a nonvirulent organism such as S. aureus or P. acnes, topical hourly treatment, daily repeated subconjunctival therapy, and systemic antibiotics are continued. If a virulent organism such as S. aureus, a streptococcal species, or a gram-negative organism is cultured, the intraocular antibiotics are repeated at the bedside or in a treatment room 48 and 96 hours after the original culture and intraocular treatment. With a previous keratotomy or pars plana entry site, this can be accomplished with relative ease by mild sedation, topical anesthesia, and the introduction of a needle through the site, using a lid speculum and fine forceps for stabilization. Approximately 0.1 ml of aqueous or liquid vitreous is withdrawn, and then a similar volume of both intraocular antibiotics is injected, depending on the anticipated or determined sensitivity of the cultured organism.

The role of vitrectomy is currently being evaluated clinically. If the approach just described appears aggressive, the following may appear to some to be unwarranted. This will be discussed later. In selected cases in which a virulent organism has been cultured and in which corneal clarity allows good visibility, a pars plana or anterior segment subtotal vitrectomy with repeat intraocular antibiotics may be considered. This procedure may also be used in eyes in which liquid vitreous cannot be aspirated at the time of the original culturing. The vitreous instrument is introduced for diagnostic purposes, and a subtotal vitrectomy is performed before instillation of intraocular antibiotics.

It may prove that immediate vitrectomy is indicated in all cases of presumed infectious endophthalmitis. In cases where it is most indicated, that is, where the etiologic organism is highly virulent, waiting for a positive culture may permit widespread intraocular destruction. The justification for immediate vitrectomy is the generally dismal outcome in cases not treated by vitrectomy, despite sporadic reports of the successful treatment of postoperative endophthalmitis[94] and despite an improved incidence of etiologic diagnosis.[75] For example, Forster and co-workers[83] reported the use of intraocular antibiotics in 26 eyes, 15 of which had positive cultures. Useful vision of 20/400 or better was achieved in six of 15 culture-positive cases. The etiologic organisms in these were S. epidermidis in five cases and P. acnes in one case. There are organisms of low virulence. Not a single eye with a culture-proven organism of known greater virulence attained useful vision. Contrast this with the report of Eichenbaum and co-workers,[59] who treated nine eyes with presumed postoperative infectious endophthalmitis by initial vitrectomy and instillation of intraocular antibiotics. An etiologic agent was cultured in every case: S. epidermidis in six, S. aureus in two, and Streptococcus faecalis in one (with late infection of postoperative filtering bleb).

Even if one does not attribute significance to the six eyes with S. epidermidis, the results obtained with the eyes infected with S. aureus and Streptococcus faecalis are highly impressive. All eyes had the same treatment. After removal of anterior chamber and vitreous samples for smears and cultures and pars plana vitrectomy, gentamicin 0.1 mg and cephaloridine 0.25 mg were instilled into the vitreous cavity. Cephaloridine 1000 mg was given intravenously four times daily. Gentamicin 20 mg and triamcinolone 40 mg sub-Tenon's capsule injections were given daily, and cephaloridine 100 mg was given daily subconjunctivally. Topical therapy included gentamicin, bacitracin (5000 units/ml), triamcinolone, and atropine.

More recently, Forster[57] reported four cases in which ambulatory vision was salvaged in eyes infected by more virulent organisms. In these cases the patients received not only intraocular antibiotics but in two instances repeat intraocular antibiotics and in two combined therapeutic vitrectomy and intraocular antibiotics. An eye infected with *Proteus mirabilis* was treated with three intraocular injections of gentamicin 48 hours apart and had a final visual result of 20/40 1 year later. A second eye infected with *Haemophilus influenzae* had a primary subtotal vitrectomy combined with three injections of gentamicin and cephaloridine 48 hours apart. A final visual acuity of 20/50 resulted. A third eye infected with *Pseudomonas multiphilia* achieved 4/200 vision after three intraocular injections of gentamicin and cephaloridine. The fourth eye was infected with alpha-streptococcus. The initial anterior chamber and vitreous cultures were negative, but intraocular antibiotics were injected at the time of diagnostic aspiration. A recrudescence of the inflammatory process occurred, and a therapeutic vitrectomy was performed with repeat intraocular injections. This time the culture from the vitreous material was positive when concentrated on a membrane filter. Three months later the visual acuity was 20/70.

Although an aggressive approach is justified for this highly serious complication, considerably more experience is necessary before one can recommend whether intraocular antibiotics alone or in combination with therapeutic vitrectomy is indicated. It must also be established whether immediate primary vitrectomy is justified, since some eyes are infected with relatively nonvirulent organisms that may respond to more conservative therapy. The results of vitrectomy in combination with intraocular antibiotics must be evaluated for safety in these cases, since if the results are favorable they would tend to justify a more radical approach than waiting for an etiologic diagnosis. The safety of intraocular antibiotics in the dosages used is being evaluated. Forster and co-workers[83] successfully performed electroretinograms on 12 of 14 eyes that had received intraocular antibiotics 1 to 4 months after treatment. Normal or slightly abnormal tracings were present in three cases, moderately abnormal tracings in eight cases, and a markedly abnormal electroretinogram was seen in one eye that achieved 20/60 vision after subtotal vitrectomy and instillation of gentamicin 0.1 mg and amphotericin B 0.005 mg. These findings do not necessarily reflect the safety or toxicity of the antibiotics, since the infectious process itself undoubtedly causes some if not most of the destruction.

TREATMENT OF POSTOPERATIVE FUNGAL ENDOPHTHALMITIS

The treatment of fungal endophthalmitis is difficult. Attempts should be made to determine the exact fungus responsible for the infection. Sensitivity tests to antifungal drugs should be obtained if possible. At the onset of endophthalmitis, if a fungal etiology is anticipated, as evidenced by time of onset and clinical appearance, Forster[57] recommends initial vitrectomy for both diagnostic and therapeutic purposes with intraocular injection of both gentamicin and amphotericin B, 0.005 to 0.01 mg (5 to 10 μg). This dose of amphotericin B (Fungizone) was established by Axelrod and co-workers,[113] since it did not cause any toxic changes in rabbits that could be detected clinically, microscopically, or by electroretinography. The injections must be performed slowly into the center of the vitreous. Injections of 25 g or more caused retinal necrosis and retinal detachment. The commercial preparation contains sodium deoxycholate as a solubilizing agent. An intravitreal injection of 0.1 ml of the latter caused no toxic changes.

The same investigators[114] injected 1000 *Candida* organisms into the vitreous of rabbits. Endophthalmitis was apparent within 24 hours. A single intravitreal injection of amphotericin B 5 mg was effective in reversing the course of the infection when administered up to 5 days after inoculation of the organisms. The successful treatment of postoperative *Candida parakrusei* endophthalmitis was reported by Rosen and Friedman.[115] Treatment consisted of sub-Tenon injections of amphotericin B 750 mg every second day for a total of eight doses. The usual recommended dose of the agent is 150 mg. The authors felt justified in greatly increasing the dosage in view of the usual outcome of this infection. The patient was rewarded with an eye that recovered 20/30 visual acuity.

Forster[57] recommends that if a yeast such as *Candida* is cultured 24 to 36 hours after aspiration, the patient should be given 5-fluorocytosine in a dosage of 100 to 150 mg/kg/day orally. Subconjunctival injection of nystatin 50,000 units/ml may also be administered. Nystatin (Mycostatin) is not well absorbed from the intestine. Therefore oral administration is ineffective in the treatment of fungal endophthalmitis. Amphotericin B is extremely nephrotoxic, and there is probably little rationale for using it systemically in cases of postoperative filamentary fungal endophthalmitis. Forster[57] recommends subconjunctival injections of 0.5 to 1.0 mg. Allen[116] used subconjunctival amphotericin B in a dose of 5 mg in two cases of suspected fungal endophthalmitis, and, although it was tolerated relatively well, he recommends a maximum dose of 2.5 mg.

Whether intraocular steroids should be used is still unsettled.

STEROIDS

The role of systemic steroids in the treatment of postoperative endophthalmitis is presumably to minimize the violent inflammatory reaction within the eye, since this in itself is destructive. Dosages of 8 to 12 tablets of a steroid may be given daily. The following preparations may be used:

Prednisone	40 to 60 mg
Prednisolone	40 to 60 mg
Triamcinolone	32 to 48 mg
Methylprednisolone	32 to 48 mg
Dexamethasone	6 to 9 mg
Betamethasone	4.8 to 7.2 mg

Appropriate precautions should be taken in patients with diabetes mellitus and those with a history of peptic ulcer. Steroid therapy is not without risk, especially when one considers that if the causative organism is not susceptible to the antibiotic therapy, the infection may be worsened. In addition, it may potentiate the spread of a fungus infection. One report indicates that adding steroids to the antibiotic therapy of a bacterial endophthalmitis does not improve the final results over those obtained with antibiotics alone.[27] However, because one may be dealing with a severe aseptic uveitis and because of the urgency of minimizing the destructive intraocular inflammation, the advantages appear to overshadow the disadvantages. If systemic steroids must be avoided, an injection under Tenon's capsule of 1 ml (40 mg) of triamcinolone (Kenalog) may be given every 5 to 7 days. The injection is given just above the junction of the middle and lateral

thirds of the floor of the orbit. The needle is directed as for a retrobulbar injection. A 0.5-inch 27-gauge disposable needle is used. This chemical will provide a surprisingly high degree of steroid effect within the eye. These injections may be used alone or with systemic steroids. As has already been mentioned,[94,95] steroids may be injected with antibiotics into the vitreous. The dosage for dexamethasone injected intravitreally is 400 μg in 0.1 ml of solution.[94]

As with aseptic uveitis, cycloplegics and mydriatics should be prescribed along with topical antibiotics and steroids. If secondary glaucoma develops, carbonic anhydrase inhibitors may be prescribed. In extreme cases a systemically administered hyperosmotic agent may be necessary.

REFERENCES

1. Axenfeld, T.: The bacteriology of the eye. Translated by A. Macnab, New York, 1908, Wood & Co., p. 95.
2. Allen, H. F., and Mangiaracine, A. B.: Bacterial endophthalmitis after cataract extraction, Arch. Ophthalmol. **72:**454-462, 1964.
3. Ramsay, A. M.: Discussion on the causes of infection after the extraction of senile cataract, Trans. Ophthalmol. Soc. U.K. **41:**387-391, 1921.
4. Parker, W. R.: Senile cataract extraction, a comparative study of results obtained in 1,421 operations, Trans. Sect. Ophthalmol. A.M.A. **72:**202-216, 1921.
5. Davenport, R. C.: The after results of cataract extraction, Br. J. Ophthalmol. **12:**85-93, 1928.
6. Giri, D. V.: Some observations on intra-capsular extraction of cataract, with description of a simple technique, Trans. Ophthalmol. Soc. U.K. **43:**248-262, 1923.
7. Parker, W. R.: Cataract extraction; comparative results obtained by the combined, simple and Knapp-Török methods of procedure, Trans. Sect. Ophthalmol. A.M.A. **78:**222-228, 1927.
8. Slocum, G.: Employment of a conjunctival bridge and suture in cataract extraction, Arch. Ophthalmol. **10:**329-341, 1933.
9. Parker, W. R.: Comparative results in the extraction of senile cataracts using the combined simple and Knapp-Török intracapsular methods, Arch. Ophthalmol. **11:**183-186, 1934.
10. Guyton, J. S., and Woods, A. C.: Oral use of prophylactic sulfadiazine for cataract extractions, Am. J. Ophthalmol. **26:**1278-1282, 1943.
11. Berens, C., and Bogart, D. W.: Certain postoperative complications of cataract extraction, Am. J. Surg. **42:**39-61, 1938.
12. Dunnington, J. H., and Locatcher-Khorazo, D.: Value of cultures before operation for cataract, Arch. Ophthalmol. **34:**215-219, 1945.
13. Hughes, W. F., Jr., and Owens, W. C.: Postoperative

complications of cataract extraction, Arch. Ophthalmol. **38:**577-595, 1947.

14. Foster, J.: Principles and practice of asepsis: the value of pre-operative cultures, Trans. Ophthalmol. Soc. U.K. **69:**389-390, 1949.

15. Duthie, O. M.: Discussion: The principles and practice of asepsis, Trans. Ophthalmol. Soc. U.K. **69:**365-374, 1949.

16. Cosmettatos, G. P.: Operative and postoperative complications of cataract, Bull. Soc. Hellén. Ophthalmol. **17:**233-244, 1950.

17. Callahan, A.: Effect of sulfonamides and antibiotics on panophthalmitis complicating cataract extraction, Arch. Ophthalmol. **49:**212-219, 1953.

18. Mullen, C.: Cited by Callahan, A.[17]

19. Townes, C. D., Moran, C. T., and Pfingst, H. A.: Complications of cataract surgery, Am. J. Ophthalmol. **35:**1311-1319, 1952.

20. Liehn, R., and Schlagenhauff, K.: 1000 intrakapsuläre Starextraktionen, ihre Ergebnisse und Kimplikationen, Wien. Klin. Wschr. **65:**988-992, 1952.

21. Locatcher-Khorazo, D., and Gutierrez, E.: Eye infections following cataract extraction, with special reference to the role of *Staphylococcus aureus,* Am. J. Ophthalmol. **41:**981-987, 1956.

22. Pearlman, M. D.: Prophylactic subconjunctival penicillin and streptomycin after cataract extraction, Arch. Ophthalmol. **55:**516-518, 1956.

23. Neveu, M., and Elliot, A. J.: Prophylaxis and treatment of endophthalmitis, Am. J. Ophthalmol. **48:**368-373, 1959.

24. Truhlsen, S. M.: Analysis of 500 cataract patients, Nebr. Med. J. **44:**230-235, 1959.

25. Luke, W. R. F.: Collected letters of the international correspondence society of ophthalmology and otology, series V, p. 37, March 15, 1960.

26. Allen, H. F., and Mangiaracine, A. B.: Bacterial endophthalmitis after cataract extraction, Arch. Ophthalmol. **91:**3-7, 1974.

27. Freeman, M. I., and Gay, A. J.: Systemic steroid therapy in postcataract endophthalmitis. In Becker, B., and Drews, R. C.: Current concepts in ophthalmology, St. Louis, 1967, The C. V. Mosby Co., pp. 163-177.

28. Christy, N. E., and Lall, P.: Postoperative endophthalmitis following cataract surgery: effects of subconjunctival antibiotics and other factors: Arch. Ophthalmol. **90:**361-366, 1973.

29. Whiston, G. J.: Review of postoperative endophthalmitis. Montreal General Hospital, 1955-1964, Can. J. Ophthalmol. **2:**63-69, 1967.

30. Cassady, J. R.: Prophylactic subconjunctival antibiotics following cataract extraction, Am. J. Ophthalmol. **74:**1081-1083, 1967.

31. Chalkley, T. H. F., and Shoch, D.: An evaluation of prophylactic subconjunctival antibiotic in cataract surgery, Am. J. Ophthalmol. **64:**1084-1087, 1967.

32. Kolker, A. E., Freeman, M. I., and Pettit, T. H.: Prophylactic antibiotics and post-operative endophthalmitis, Am. J. Ophthalmol. **63:**434-439, 1967.

33. Jaffe, N. S., Light, D. S., Clayman, H. S., and Eichenbaum, D. M.: Personal communication, 1978.

34. Dellaporta, A., Riemer, F., and Harmuth, E.: Eine vergleichende Untersuchung über die Infektionshäufigkeit nach Kataraktoperation in den Jahren 1936, 1941, 1946 und 1948 mit Berücksichtigung der Penicillinbehandlung, Klin. Mbl. Augenheilk. **115:**369-383, 1949.

35. Allen, H. F.: Aseptic techniques in ophthalmology, Trans. Am. Ophthalmol. Soc. **57:**377-472, 1959.

36. Anderson, K. F.: *Pseudomonas pyocyanea* disseminated from an air-cooling apparatus, Med. J. Aust. **1:**529, 1959.

37. Williams, R. E. O., Blowers, R., Garrod, L. B., and Shooter, R. A.: Hospital infection, causes and prevention, Chicago, 1960, Year Book Medical Publishers, Inc.

38. Crompton, D. O.: Personal observations on the prevention of sepsis following lens extraction, Int. Ophthalmol. Clin. **5:**183-205, 1965.

39. Theodore, F. H.: Contamination of eye solutions, Am. J. Ophthalmol. **34:**1764, 1951.

40. Theodore, F. H., and Feinstein, R. R.: Preparation and maintenance of sterile ophthalmic solutions, J.A.M.A. **152:**1631-1633, 1953.

41. Garretson, W. T., and Cosgrove, K. W.: Ulceration of the cornea due to *Bacillus pyocyaneus*, J.A.M.A. **88:**700-702, 1927.

42. Webster, R. G., et al.: Eye infections after plastic lens implantation, Morbidity Mortality **24:**437-443, 1976.

43. Drews, R. C.: Use of Millipore filters in ophthalmic surgery, Am. J. Ophthalmol. **50:**159-160, 1960.

44. Jaffe, N. S.: Safeguards in cataract surgery, South. Med. J. **61:**859-864, 1968.

45. Grant, W. M.: Toxicology of the eye, Springfield, Ill., 1962, Charles C Thomas, Publisher, pp. 151-152.

46. Brown, S. I.: Corneal edema from a cotton foreign body in the anterior chamber, Am. J. Ophthalmol. **65:**616-617, 1968.

47. Coles, R. S.: Uveal complications after cataract surgery, Int. Ophthalmol. Clin. **4:**895-912, 1964.

48. Anderson, K. F., Crompton, D. O., and Lillie, S.: Contaminated ophthalmic ointments, Trans. Ophthalmol. Soc. Aust. **23:**86-87, 1963.

49. Theodore, F. H., and Feinstein, R. R.: Practical suggestions for the preparation and maintenance of sterile ophthalmic solutions. I, Am. J. Ophthalmol. **35:**656-659, 1952.

50. Browning, C. W., and Lippas, J.: pHisoHex keratitis, Arch. Ophthalmol. **53:**817-824, 1955.

51. Elek, S. D.: *Staphylococcus pyogenes* and its relation to disease, Edinburgh, 1959, E. and S. Livingstone, Ltd.

52. Price, P. B.: The bacteriology of normal skin; a new quantitative test applied to a study of the bacterial flora and the disinfectant action of mechanical cleansing, J. Infect. Dis. **63:**301-318, 1938.

53. Price, P. B.: New studies in surgical bacteriology and surgical technic, with special reference to disinfection of the skin, **111:**1993-1996, 1938.

54. Devenish, E. A., and Miles, A. A.: Control of *Staphylococcus aureus* in an operating theater, Lancet **1:**1088-1094, 1939.

55. Crompton, D. O., Anderson, K. F., and Kennare, M. A.: Experimental infection of the rabbit anterior chamber, Trans. Ophthalmol. Soc. Aust. **22**:81-98, 1962.

56. Allen, H. F., and Mangiaracine, A. B.: Bacterial endophthalmitis after cataract extraction. II. Incidence in 36,000 consecutive operations with special reference to preoperative topical antibiotics, Ophthalmology (Rochester) **77**:581-588, 1973.

57. Forster, R. K.: Etiology and diagnosis of bacterial postoperative endophthalmitis, Ophthalmology (Rochester) **85**:320-326, 1978.

58. Peyman, G. A., Vastine, D. W., and Raichand, M.: Experimental aspects and their clinical applications, Ophthalmology (Rochester) **85**:374-385, 1978.

59. Eichenbaum, D. M., Jaffe, N. S., Clayman, H. M., and Light, D. S.: Pars plana vitrectomy as a primary treatment for acute bacterial endophthalmitis, Am. J. Ophthalmol. **86**:167-171, 1978.

60. Valenton, M. J., Brubaker, R. F., and Allen, H. F.: *Staphylococcus epidermidis (albus)* endophthalmitis, Arch. Ophthalmol. **89**:94-96, 1973.

61. Abelson, M. B., and Allansmith, M. R.: Normal conjunctival wound edge flora of patients undergoing uncomplicated cataract extraction, Am. J. Ophthalmol. **76**:561-565, 1973.

62. Perkins, R. E., et al.: Bacteriology of normal and infected conjunctiva, J. Clin. Microbiol. **1**:147-149, 1975.

63. Maylath, F. R., and Leopold, I. H.: Study of experimental intraocular infection, Am. J. Ophthalmol. **40**:86-101, 1955.

64. Theodore, F. H.: Bacterial endophthalmitis after cataract surgery, Int. Ophthalmol. Clin. **4**:839-859, 1964.

65. Foster, J. B. T., Almeda, E., Littman, M. L., and Wilson, M. E.: Some intraocular and conjunctival effects of amphotericin B in man and in the rabbit, Arch. Ophthalmol. **60**:555-564, 1958.

66. Fine, B. S., and Zimmerman, L. E.: Exogenous intraocular fungus infections with particular reference to complications of intra-ocular surgery, Am. J. Ophthalmol. **48**:151-165, 1959.

67. Theodore, F. H., Littman, M. L., and Almeda, E.: The diagnosis and management of fungus endophthalmitis following cataract extraction, Arch. Ophthalmol. **66**:163-175, 1961.

68. Theodore, F. H., Littman, M. L., and Almeda, E.: Endophthalmitis following cataract extraction due to *Neurospora sitophilia;* a so-called nonpathogenic fungus, Am. J. Ophthalmol. **53**:35-39, 1962.

69. Theodore, F. H.: The role of so-called saprophytic fungi in eye infections. In Dalldorf, G., editor: Fungi and fungus diseases, Springfield, Ill., 1962, Charles C Thomas, Publisher, Chapter 3.

70. de Almeida, A. A.: Infecção pós-operatória bacteriana e micótica, Rev. Bras. Oftalmol. **22**:53-64, 1963.

71. Theodore, F. H.: Mycotic endophthalmitis after cataract surgery, Int. Ophthalmol. Clin. **4**:861-881, 1964.

72. Küper, J.: Zur klinik postoperativer intraokularer Mykosen, Klin. Mbl. Augenheilk, **140**:827-834, 1962.

73. François, J., DeVos, E., Hanssens, M., and Elewant-

Rijsselaere, M.: Mycoses intra-oculaires, Ann. Oculist. **195**:97-119, 1962.

74. Paiva, C., Chaves Batista, A., and Gomez, A.: Endoftalmicótica pós-operatória por *Hyalopus bogolepofii*, Rev. Bras. Oftalmol. **19**:193-202, 1960.

75. Forster, R. K.: Endophthalmitis. Diagnostic cultures and visual results, Arch. Ophthalmol. **92**:387-392, 1974.

76. Ruiz, R. S., and Teeters, V. W.: The vitreous wick syndrome. A late complication following cataract extraction, Am. J. Ophthalmol. **70**:483-490, 1970.

77. Kanski, J. J.: Treatment of late endophthalmitis associated with filtering blebs, Arch. Ophthalmol. **91**:339-343, 1974.

78. Yannuzzi, L. A., and Theodore, F. H.: Cryotherapy of post-cataract blebs, Am. J. Ophthalmol. **76**:217-222, 1973.

79. Kirk, H. Q.: Treatment and prevention of filtering blebs following cataract extraction. In Emergy, J. M., and Paton, D., editors: Current concepts in cataract surgery, St. Louis, 1974, The C. V. Mosby Co., pp. 259-262.

80. Friedenwald, J. S., and Pierce, H. F.: Circulation of the aqueous. IV. Reabsorption of colloids, Arch. Ophthalmol. **14**:599-611, 1935.

81. Friedenwald, J. S., et al.: Ophthalmic pathology: an atlas and textbook, Philadelphia, 1952, W. B. Saunders Co.

82. Forster, R. K., Wirta, M. G., Solis, M., and Rebell, G.: Methenamine-silver-stained corneal scrapings in keratomycosis, Am. J. Ophthalmol. **82**:261-265, 1976.

83. Forster, R. K., Zachary, J. G., Cottingham, A. J., Jr., and Norton, E. W. D.: Further observations on the diagnosis, etiology, and treatment of endophthalmitis, Am. J. Ophthalmol. **81**:52-56, 1976.

84. Goodner, E. K.: Routine preoperative and postsurgical management of glaucoma, Int. Ophthalmol. Clin. **3**:119-132, 1963.

85. McMeel, J. W.: Infections and retina surgery. II. Incidence and significance of positive wound site cultures, Arch. Ophthalmol. **74**:45-47, 1965.

86. Allansmith, M. R., Anderson, R. P., and Butterworth, M.: The meaning of preoperative cultures in ophthalmology, Ophthalmology (Rochester) **73**:683-690, 1969.

87. Allen, H. F.: Prevention of postoperative endophthalmitis, Ophthalmology (Rochester) **85**:386-389, 1978.

88. Barza, M., Kane, A., and Baum, J.: Intraocular penetration of gentamicin after subconjunctival retrobulbar injection, Am. J. Ophthalmol. **85**:541-547, 1978.

89. Utermann, D., Matz, K., and Meyer, K.: Aqueous humor levels of gentamicin after parenteral, subconjunctival, and topical administration, Klin. Monatsbl. Augenheilkd. **171**:579-583, 1977.

90. Falco, F. G., Smith, H. M., and Arcieri, G. M.: Nephrotoxicity of aminoglycosides and gentamicin, J. Infect. Dis. **119**:406-409, 1969.

91. Wersäll, J., Lundquist, P. G., and Bjorkroth, B.: Ototoxicity of gentamicin, J. Invest. Dis. **119**:411-416, 1969.

92. Ellis, P. P.: Ocular therapeutics and pharmacology, ed. 5, St. Louis, 1977, The C. V. Mosby Co.

93. Mitsui, Y., and Hanabusa, J.: Corneal infections after cortisone therapy, Br. J. Ophthalmol. **39**:244-250, 1955.

94. Peyman, G. A., Vastine, D., Crouch, E., and Herbst, R.: Clinical trials with intravitreal injection of antibiotics in treatment of endophthalmitis, Ophthalmology (Rochester) **78:**862-875, 1974.

95. Peyman, G. A.: Bacterial endophthalmitis. Treatment with intraocular injection of gentamicin and dexamesone, Arch. Ophthalmol. **91:**416-418, 1974.

96. Daily, M. J., Peyman, G. A., and Fishman, G.: Intravitreal injection of methicillin for treatment of endophthalmitis, Am. J. Ophthalmol. **76:**343-350, 1973.

97. von Sallman, L., Meyer, K., and DiGrandi, J.: Experimental study on penicillin treatment of ectogenous infection of vitreous, Arch. Ophthalmol. **32:**179, 1944.

98. Leopold, I. H.: Intravitreal penetration of penicillin and penicillin therapy of infections of the vitreous, Arch. Ophthalmol. **33:**211, 1945.

99. Mann, I.: The intraocular use of penicillin, Br. J. Ophthalmol. **30:**134, 1946.

100. Duguid, J. P. et al.: Experimental observations on intravitreous use of penicillin and other drugs, Br. J. Ophthalmol. **31:**193, 1947.

101. Sorsby, A. and Ungar, J.: Intravitreal injection of penicillin: study on the levels of concentration reached and therapeutic efficacy, Br. J. Ophthalmol. **32:**857, 1948.

102. May, D. R., Ericson, E. S., Peyman, G. A., and Axelrod, A. J.: Intraocular injection of gentamicin: single injection therapy of experimental bacterial endophthalmitis, Arch. Ophthalmol. **91:**487, 1974.

103. Peyman, G. A., May, D. R., Ericson, E. S., and Apple, D.: Intraocular injection of gentamicin: toxic effects and clearance, Arch. Ophthalmol. **92:**42, 1974.

104. Axelrod, A. J., Peyman, G. A., and Apple, D. J.: Toxicity of intravitreal injection of amphotericin B. Am. J. Ophthalmol. **76:**578, 1973.

105. Peyman, G. A., Nelson, P., and Bennett, T. O.: Intravitreal injection of kanamycin in experimental induced endophthalmitis, Can. J. Ophthalmol. **9:**322, 1974.

106. Nelson, P., Peyman, G. A., and Bennett, T. O.: BB-K8: a new aminoglycoside for intravitreal injection in bacterial endophthalmitis, Am. J. Ophthalmol. **78:**82, 1974.

107. Bennett, T. O., and Peyman, G. A.: Use of tobramycin in eradicating experimental endophthalmitis, Albrecht von Graefes Arch. Klin. Ophthalmol. **191:**93, 1974.

108. Schenk, A. G., Peyman, G. A.: Lincomycin by direct intravitreal injection in the treatment of bacterial endophthalmitis, Albrecht von Graefes Arch. Klin. Ophthalmol. **190:**281, 1974.

109. Pague, J. T., and Peyman, G. A.: Intravitreal clindamycin phosphate in the treatment of vitreous infection, Ophthalmic. Surg. **5:**34, 1974.

110. Zachary, I. G., and Forster, R. K.: Experimental intravitreal gentamicin, Am. J. Ophthalmol. **82:**604, 1976.

111. Peyman, G. A., Herbst, R.: Treatment of bacterial endophthalmitis with intraocular injection of gentamicin dexamethasone: a case report, Arch. Ophthalmol. **91:**416, 1974.

112. Cottingham, A. J., and Forster, R. K.: Vitrectomy in endophthalmitis, Arch. Ophthalmol. **94:**2078, 1976.

113. Axelrod, A. J., Peyman, G. A., and Apple, D. J.: Intravitreal injection of amphotericin B. I. Evaluation of toxicity, Am. J. Ophthalmol. **76:**578-583, 1973.

114. Axelrod, A. J., and Peyman, G. A.: Intravitreal injection of amphotericin B. III. Treatment of experimental fungal endophthalmitis, Am. J. Ophthalmol. **76:**584-588, 1973.

115. Rosen, R., and Friedman, A. H.: Successfully treated postoperative *Candida parakrusei* endophthalmitis, Am. J. Ophthalmol. **76:**574-577, 1973.

116. Allen, H. F.: Amphotericin B and exogenous mycotic endophthalmitis after cataract extraction, Arch. Ophthalmol. **88:**640-644, 1972.

CHAPTER 23

Uveitis

Postoperative uveitis may be considered a normal accompaniment of cataract surgery. It is also associated with other postoperative complications such as retained lens material, epithelial invasion of the anterior chamber, operative loss of vitreous, iris prolapse and so on. To avoid lengthy repetition, refer to those chapters where the role played by inflammation is considered.

After cataract extraction, the causes of uveitis may be any of the following:

1. Surgical trauma
2. Foreign material introduced during surgery
   Cilia
   Lint
   Cellulose and cotton sponge
   Talc
   Rubber
   Glass
   Ointment
   Suture material
   Plastic lens implant
3. Chemical and physical agents
   Skin preparation solutions
   Instrument disinfectants
   Alpha-chymotrypsin
   Acetylcholine
   Cryogenics
4. Wound incarcerations
   Iris
   Lens
   Vitreous
   Zonules
5. Ocular conditions
   Preexisting uveitis
   Heterochromic cyclitis
6. Systemic conditions
   Rheumatoid arthritis
   Diabetes
7. Other postoperative complications
   Epithelial invasion of the anterior chamber
   Fibrous ingrowth
   Hyphema
   Vitreous hemorrhage
   Retained lens material (lens-induced uveitis)
   Operative loss of vitreous
   Retinal detachment
   Infection
8. Sympathetic ophthalmitis

SURGICAL TRAUMA

Cataract surgery, which requires decompression of the globe, manipulation of the iris, lysis of zonules, irrigation of the anterior chamber, and placement of sutures, would reasonably be expected to result in a transitory uveitis. This reaction subsides rapidly and usually leaves no permanent sequelae. However, a small but significant number of patients are troubled by a more persistent uveitis for which there is no apparent cause. Although the cause of this kind of reaction remains unknown, it is reasonable to assume that the tissues of some patients are sufficiently sensitive to respond to the manipulation of surgery by remaining chronically inflamed.

The changes induced in the anatomy and physiology of the eye by cataract surgery have been summarized by Gillman as follows[1]:

1. Changes induced at the site of surgical manipulation
   a. Local tissue necrosis
   b. Axon-reflex vascular reaction
   c. Liberation of intracellular metabolites, enzyme systems, and chemotactic substances
   d. Surgical exposure permitting fortuitous airborne

and instrument-borne contamination with pathogenic organisms and agents

2. Changes induced by anterior chamber decompression
   a. Loss of the anatomic limits of the anterior chamber, exteriorization of the anterior chamber
   b. Incisional hypotension
   c. Early wound incarcerations
3. Changes induced by posterior decompression
   a. Vasocongestion, edema, and hemorrhage in the retina and choroid
   b. Serous and hemorrhagic separation of the retina
   c. Perichoroidal serous and hemorrhagic separations with extension to the periciliary space, with the implicit threat of inhibitional hyposecretion hypotension
   d. Foward displacement of vitreous, loss of fluid or formed vitreous, and anterior and posterior vitreous separations

The inflammatory response to surgical manipulation is still little understood but evidently is essential for normal healing. It is the stimulus for the initial phase of wound repair, which is usually referred to as the "lag phase." We now know that this phase is in reality a period of intense biochemical activity. The cells in the area of repair become reorganized and develop their enzyme machinery preparatory to the synthesis of new connective tissue, which occurs in the "fibroblastic phase" of healing. If the response is excessive or if other postoperative complications arise, the usually innocuous surgical inflammatory response may cause a troublesome postoperative uveitis.

Although the recovery from surgical trauma varies according to the tissue sensitivities in different individuals, the following characterizes the early healing process: There is little bleeding because of the relative avascularity of the tissues involved. Endowed with an intense axon-reflex activity, these tissues respond to cutting capillaries and some of the larger vessels by an immediate localized vasoconstriction and vessel retraction. These axon reflexes are mediated through the sympathetics and constitute a mechanism of defense against mechanical injury. The cut vessel tends to contract over a considerable length, often to complete obliteration. In a few seconds, the contraction subsides, but a clot has already formed and bleeding is prevented. The short-lived phase of localized vasoconstriction and

vessel retraction results in immediate blanching in the adjacent sclera. However, the reactions in the iris vessels are probably of longer duration. This is followed by a phase of hyperemia, vasocongestion, vasodilation, and increased capillary permeability. This reaction is more prolonged and is characterized by edema, localized bleeding, tissue swelling, and increased aqueous turbidity.

The effects of surgical decompression on the posterior portion of the globe are even more dramatic and profound than the response of the anterior segment to surgical manipulation. These effects are described on p. 293. The sudden release of intraocular pressure initiates profound changes in the capillary beds of the ciliary body, choroid, and retina. This results in capillary dilatation, congestion, edema, and hemorrhage. Marked changes in the vitreous also occur, exemplified by vitreous turbidity, anterior ectasia of the vitreous, and increased vitreous mobility. In most eyes these changes are well tolerated, with the cells in the aqueous and vitreous disappearing after several days as the global integrity is restored. However, more serious distant sequelae may arise that may not be recognized in the early postoperative period. Among these may be included decreased endothelial cell density (p. 333), cystoid macular edema (p. 367), or a macular hole.

Prostaglandins. It is becoming more apparent that prostaglandins help mediate the response of the eye to acute trauma. This irritative response is characterized by hyperemia of the conjunctiva, miosis, disruption of the blood-aqueous barrier, and a transient increase in intraocular pressure followed by relative hypotonia. This can be produced by a variety of stimuli, including anterior chamber paracentesis and stroking of the iris. Evidence is accumulating that prostaglandins are found in the aqueous humor of eyes with experimentally induced, as well as clinical, uveitis. The source of the prostaglandins in uveitis may be the leukocytes. A current view is that the prostaglandins play a role in the development of ocular inflammation, which may be associated with the effect on ocular permeability.

Like the steroids, prostaglandins are lipids, and like the steroid family, the prostaglandin family is a large one. The two members that have attracted most attention from research workers and clinicians are prostaglandin E_2 (PGE_2) and prostaglandin F_2 alpha (PGF_2 alpha).

Prostaglandins are virtually ubiquitous in animal tissues and have been found in most human organs. Unlike the classic hormones, prostaglandins are neither synthesized by special types of cells nor stored in the tissues that form them. The prostaglandins that can be extracted from an organ probably represent material recently synthesized but not yet metabolized. Although not yet certain, it appears likely that prostaglandins act as local mediators or modulators at the site of release rather than as circulating hormones, since their half-life is very short.

As just stated, prostaglandins are not stored in cells, and their presence in the aqueous is the result of de novo synthesis. Since the eye does not contain the enzyme 15-prostaglandin dehydrogenase to deactivate prostaglandins, their removal depends on an active transport pump located in the ciliary epithelium. Bitot and Salvado[2] have shown that his pump is inoperable for at least 3 weeks after ocular trauma.

Two significant findings are worthy of note. The first is that the prostaglandins are manufactured enzymatically in the cell from unsaturated fatty acids such as arachidonic acid. This precursor is itself formed from linoleic acid, an essential constituent of human and animal diet. The second is that the enzymatic conversion of arachidonic acid to PGE_2 and PGF_2 alpha is blocked by aspirin. This raised the possibility that prostaglandins might have an essential role in the genesis of fever, pain, and inflammation. It also made aspirin-like drugs significant as research tools in elucidating the biologic role of prostaglandins. Thus inhibition of prostaglandin synthesis has been suggested as the mechanism of action of many nonsteroidal anti-inflammatory drugs such as aspirin and indomethacin.

A modulator role of PGE_2 at peripheral nerve endings seems well established. On sensory fibers subserving pain, PGE_2 enhances and prolongs the action of pain-producing substances sucy as bradykinin and 5-hydroxytryptamine. This type of PGE_2 production is found clinically in inflammatory disorders such as uveitis, burns (including sunburn), rheumatoid arthritis, as well as in experimentally produced inflammatory. By blocking PGE_2 production peripherally, aspirin is able to exert its analgesic action.

The role of prostaglandins in ocular inflammation will be clarified in the future.

Aseptic uveitis may be severe enough to result in hypopyon and haziness of the vitreous. As stated on p. 444, postoperative aseptic uveitis may occasionally be difficult to differentiate from an intraocular infection. Aseptic uveitis is generally observed slightly later than an infection, usually 3 to 4 days after surgery. The external appearance of the globe may be unremarkable, the upper eyelid is not swollen, the eye is relatively white, and pain may not be severe. However, the intraocular findings are much more severe. Hypopyon may be present, and there is usually an intense infiltration of cells into the vitreous. The fundus reflex may be absent.

Early postoperative sterile hypopyons may be more common than expected if searched for as reported by Hunter.[3] Two hundred sixty-six eyes were examined by slit lamp 24 hours after uncomplicated intracapsular cataract extraction. An unexpectedly high incidence of 15% macroscopic hypopyons was found, with a further 13% showing a trace. This was found only in the first and second days postoperatively and largely disappeared by the third and fourth days. The hypopyons require slit lamp viewing to bring them out, and the cellular settling is enhanced by the patient being in a sitting position. My suggested explanation of hypopyon production is that operative plasmoid aqueous production, inflammatory reaction, and hyphema, coupled with early mobilization, allow gravitational sedimenting out of blood constituents, so that white cells will fall late, forming a layer above other blood constituents.

Attention to early postoperative sterile hypopyon in association with intraocular lens implantation was directed by Binkhorst[4] as long ago as 1962. He stated:

Though there are individual variations in intensity, there is usually a very sharp and extensive cellular reaction of the anterior uvea with deposits of cell-clumps in the anterior chamber, on the lens surfaces, sometimes in the anterior vitreous, frequently accompanied by a hypopyon of varying height. These exudative changes usually reach their maximum within two or three days. The hypopyon always disappears rapidly within 24 or 48 hours, but the cellular deposits elsewhere can interfere with visual acuity for a much longer period.*

Treatment consists of intensive steroid therapy. The clinical picture is sufficiently characteristic that antibiotics may be withheld pending the initial response to therapy. An immediate sub-Tenon's injection of 1 ml of a repository steroid should be given. I prefer triamcinolone (Kenalog). This is highly effective. I usually combine this with hourly instillations of steroid eye drops and topically administered atropine (three or four times daily). Unless medically contraindicated, orally administered steroids may be prescribed in an initial dosage of 8 to 10 tablets daily. The hypopyon usually disappears rapidly (within 1 to 2 days), but clearing of the vitreous is more prolonged. The prognosis is usually favorable.

FOREIGN MATTER INTRODUCED DURING SURGERY

An enormous amount of foreign material is introduced into the eye during a cataract extraction. In most instances, this material is well tolerated, since the inflammatory response to particulate debris is usually small. Particles of lint, rubber, cilia (Figs. 22-5 and 22-6), cotton (Fig. 22-7), and suture material are occasionally found in the anterior chamber resting on the iris or the anterior vitreous face. They remain unchanged for long periods of time and rarely cause significant intraocular inflammation.

It is difficult to prevent particulate debris from the operating room atmosphere from entering the eye while it is open. Moreover, an increasing tendency to inject a variety of materials into the eye during cataract surgery has occurred. These materials include saline solution, balanced salt solution, alpha-chymotrypsin, acetylcholine, epinephrine, pilocarpine, and air. One would be shocked at the particulate contamination of some of these materials. This is discussed on p. 433. Although documenting the intraocular inflammatory response to these foreign substances is difficult, one can reasonably assume that they play a

---

*From Binkhorst, C. D.: An. Instituto Barraquer 3(4):562, 1962.

role in some cases of unexplained postoperative uveitis. An effective method of eliminating particulate debris from air and all ophthalmic solutions intended for intraocular use has been described.[5] It involves using a presterilized, disposable Millipore filter (p. 446). Laminar airflow systems are being employed increasingly in operating rooms through the United States to prevent particulate atmospheric debris from entering the eye.

CHEMICAL AND PHYSICAL AGENTS

Various chemicals may be responsible for postoperative uveitis. Disinfectants used during preparation of the operative field may enter the eye and cause intraocular inflammation. "Soak" disinfectant solutions are still used by some surgeons to sterilize certain instruments such as knives, keratomes, scissors, and plastic tubing used in cryoextraction machinery. If they are inadequately rinsed, they represent another source of irritating chemicals. Solutions such as alpha-chymotrypsin and acetylcholine may cause uveitis in some patients.

I have the distinct impression that the method of cryoextraction of cataracts has increased the frequency and severity of postoperative aseptic uveitis. Over a period of approximately 14 years, I observed only two cases of postoperative hypopyon, both occurring on the same operating day and attributed to a contaminated instrument disinfectant solution. During the past 15 years, I have personally observed more than 20 instances of postoperative hypopyon uveitis. This coincided with the introduction of cryoextraction as my routine method of cataract extraction. In each instance the same clinical picture presented. After an uneventful cataract extraction the eyes healed well until the third to sixth postoperative day, when the patient complained of pain that ranged from moderate to severe in the operated eye. Examination revealed a hypopyon level in the anterior chamber and involvement of the vitreous. White membranous sheets were visible in the pupillary area and appeared to extend downward from the superior vitreous base. The fundus reflex was either dull or completely absent. Visual acuity with an appropriate cataract lens was in many cases reduced to hand motion or light perception. Despite this ominous intraocular situation, the degree of bulbar redness, chemosis, and edema of the upper eyelid was relatively little. There were several eyes that were practically white externally. Initially the patients were treated with antibiotics and steroids in high dosage, both systemically and locally, as if these were cases of postoperative bacterial endophthalmitis. Several anterior chamber paracenteses revealed no growth. Because the fact became apparent that these were cases of aseptic uveitis, since all eyes recovered, treatment more recently has included steroids without antibiotics. The results have been the same. The earlier the inception of treatment, the more rapid has been the resolution of the inflammation.

After eliminating what we thought were possible causes without altering the occurrence of this complication, my associate, David Light, and I embarked on a program whereby one group of cataract extractions was performed with the use of forceps and alpha-chymotrypsin and the other with only the cryoextraction method. The following results were obtained:

Technique	Number of cases	Hypopyon uveitis
Forceps	124	0
Cryoprobe	172	8

Other ophthalmologists have told me that their incidence of postoperative uveitis has risen greatly since changing from forceps to lens cryoextraction delivery. With the aid of the microscope, tiny ice particles can be observed darting all over the anterior chamber as soon as the cryoprobe makes contact with the lens capsule. In some cases the freezing vapor is copious. The more prolonged the extraction, the greater the exposure to the subfreezing temperature. Instruments that freeze to lower temperatures are likely to cause more uveitis. It has also been suggested that if the cryoprobe is applied too close to the superior equator, the zonular lamella may be frozen (Fig. 3-69). This freezing may cause undue traction on the ciliary body, which favors uveitis. However, I feel at this time that this has little to do with the higher incidence of uveitis. I feel more strongly that the method of iris retraction may be related to postoperative uveitis. The curved portion of some retractors is so large that massaging the ciliary body is almost impossible

to avoid. When we abandoned the use of one of these large retractors and changed to a Hoskins No. 19 forceps, not a single instance of hypopyon uveitis was observed in more than 700 cataract extractions. Therefore I would suggest a change in the method of iris retraction for those who encounter excessive uveitis after cryoextraction.

As discussed on p. 162, intraocular lens implant surgery carries with it a greater risk of uveitis caused by chemical and physical agents. This is attributable to problems associated with sterilizing and packaging a plastic implant. Ethylene oxide sterilization increases the possibility of uveitis resulting from residual gas sterilant on the implant at the time of implantation. Monitoring residual ethylene oxide has become a significant problem for the manufacturer, for the Food and Drug Administration, and for the surgeon. The use of gamma radiation as a physical sterilant of implants in 1976 also brought forth a higher incidence of inflammation. This practice has been discontinued in the United States.

I am aware of disagreement with the conclusions just discussed, but nonetheless, they reflect my observations in several thousand cataract extractions.

WOUND INCARCERATIONS

The incarceration of ocular structures in the operative wound often leads to an irritable eye associated with uveitis. Iris and vitreous are most frequently involved. The causes of iris incarceration are discussed on p. 500. Aside from other complications that this might cause, such as epithelial invasion of the anterior chamber, fibrous ingrowth, and sympathetic ophthalmitis, the stretched and structurally altered iris may become chronically inflamed. Vitreous may become incarcerated as a result of operative loss of vitreous or postoperative rupture of the anterior hyaloid membrane. Such incarceration is discussed on p. 255. Chronic intraocular inflammation may result from the fibroplastic changes associated with adherence of vitreous to the wound. Such changes are caused by the traction created on the iris and ciliary body. The presence of lens capsule in the wound is more serious than lens cortex, since it fails to absorb. It may cause interference with wound healing and provide a framework for epithelial and fibrous ingrowth (Fig.

27-9). Zonular fragments in the operative wound are not easily diagnosed clinically but are occasionally found in excised globes that demonstrate wound defects. The significance of these structures in the wound is underscored by the fact that this contamination is largely preventible by careful toilet of the wound. Whether a sector iridectomy or peripheral iris openings are performed, the would should be inspected for the presence of iris. If vitreous is lost during surgery, residual strands will likely adhere to the operative wound no matter how meticulous the wound closure is, unless an anterior vitrectomy is performed.

OCULAR CONDITIONS

Preexisting uveitis is not likely to cause much difficulty postoperatively if the cataract surgery is performed while the uveitis is inactive. There are times, however, when one must operate on eyes with active uveitis, including both the juvenile (Still's and rheumatoid types) and the chronic adult forms. Decreasing the inflammatory process in these eyes is very difficult and sometimes impossible. Surgery cannot be delayed when vision drops markedly. Steroids should be prescribed preoperatively, both systemically and locally, a subconjunctival injection of a long-acting steroid should be given during surgery, and steroids should be continued postoperatively. An inflammatory membrane frequently occludes the pupil, and the pupil is often updrawn after surgery. It is therefore advantageous to perform a sector iridectomy and an inferior sphincterotomy in such cases.

In my experience, heterochromic cyclitis responds well to cataract extraction, despite some reports to the contrary. It is not unusual to observe a diminution or even complete disappearance of the typically white keratic precipitates after cataract extraction. The iris is usually atrophic and should be handled gently during surgery. I do not treat these eyes any differently from other eyes after cataract surgery. I have found no tendency for them to develop an inflammatory pupillary membrane. In fact, it is likely that this is not an inflammatory process at all but may be the result of trophic changes in the ocular tissues produced by a disturbance in sympathetic innervation. The changes in the iris appear to be of degenerative, rather than inflammatory, origin (Fig. 23-1).

This optimistic view concerning the results of surgery in this condition is supported by a retrospective study[6] of the outcome of surgery in 29 patients with Fuchs' heterochromic cyclitis. Glaucoma was the only significant complication occurring in six of the 29 patients. However, since glaucoma is frequently encountered in the

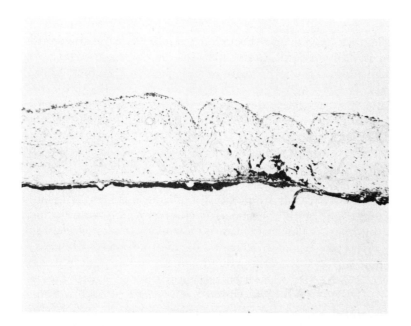

Fig. 23-1. Heterochromic iridocyclitis. Iris contains minute focal areas of necrosis involving pigment epithelium, but there is virtually no inflammatory reaction. (×80.) (AFIP No. 751122.) (From Hogan, M. J., and Zimmerman, L. E.: Ophthalmic pathology, Philadelphia, 1962, W. B. Saunders Co.)

late course of Fuchs' syndrome whether surgery is performed or not, its detection was not considered remarkable. In general, it was felt that the results of cataract extraction in patients with heterochromic cyclitis were as favorable as those in the general population.

SYSTEMIC CONDITIONS

Despite a report by Algan and LeGrand[7] that incriminates chronic polyarticular rheumatoid arthritis as a cause of postoperative uveitis, I have not been impressed by this conclusion. These authors reported a violent nongranulomatous uveitis that occurred between the third and twentieth days after cataract surgery. They observed adhesions between the iris and the anterior hyaloid membrane, hypotonia, and loss of the anterior chamber. The patients had had rheumatoid arthritis for 15 to 27 years and were in remission at the time of surgery. In my experience, postoperative uveitis is a very rare complication of cataract surgery in a patient with chronic rheumatoid arthritis.

Based on equally flimsy evidence is the consideration that diabetes mellitus is a cause of increased incidence of postoperative uveitis.[8] Although it is true that diabetics frequently show loss of uveal pigment during the cataract operation, I have not been aware of a higher incidence of uveitis.

OTHER POSTOPERATIVE COMPLICATIONS

One would expect postoperative uveitis to accompany other postoperative cataract complications. These complications are epithelial invasion of the anterior chamber, fibrous ingrowth, hyphema, retained lens material, operative loss of vitreous, retinal detachment, and infection.

SYMPATHETIC OPHTHALMITIS

Sympathetic ophthalmitis is a rare bilateral inflammation involving the entire uveal tract. Although it almost invariably occurs after a perforating wound involving uveal tissue, it is of unknown etiology. The disease commences in the injured eye (exciting eye) sometime after injury, closely followed by involvement of the uninjured eye (sympathizing eye). The clinical and pathologic pictures found in the two eyes are similar.

Historical background

The possibility of involvement of an uninjured eye after perforation of the opposite eye was recorded in the eighteenth century by Duddell[9] and LeDran.[10] However, a century elapsed before Mackenzie,[11] in 1830, presented an orderly clinical description of the disease and provided the name "sympathetic ophthalmia." Although Wardrop,[12] in 1818, drew attention to the fact that veterinarians practiced destruction of the injured eye of a horse to save the good one, credit for the first to practice enucleation therapeutically belonged to Pritchard.[13] A short time later, Critchett[14] demonstrated that enucleation was ineffective once the inflammation commenced and thus advocated prophylactic removal of the injured eye. Although much has since been written about this entity, the etiology is still unknown.

Incidence

It is difficult to determine an accurate incidence of a rare disease, since one is compelled to accept the data of numerous observers to accumulate a large number of cases. Moreover, there is a definite proportion of error in the clinical diagnosis of sympathetic ophthalmitis, and this error is magnified by the variability of opinions regarding its diagnosis.

Apparently this disease is becoming increasingly rare because of improvements in surgical techniques for injuries, as well as for cataracts and other ocular disorders. Nonetheless, perforating wounds account for about 65% of cases in the literature and operative wounds for 25%. The remaining 10% include cases that follow nonperforating contusions with subconjunctival scleral rupture, perforating corneal ulcers, and intraocular malignant tumors.[15] The proportions have been changing more recently. Winter[16] reported 257 histologically proved cases gathered from the files of the American Registry of Pathology, Armed Forces Institute of Pathology, and the Wilmer Institute. Traumatic wounds accounted for 54% of the cases, and 43% were associated with operative wounds. Roper-Hall[17] reported that sympathetic ophthalmitis is more frequent after planned surgery than after industrial accidents.

Cataract extraction accounts for approximately

60% of cases of sympathetic ophthalmitis after all types of ocular surgery. Coles[18] ascribes this high percentage to the frequency of cataract surgery compared to other operations, to the potentiating effect of inflammatory cortical lens matter after extracapsular cataract extraction, to tugging on the uvea associated with rupturing zonules, and to trauma to the iris and ciliary body during the manipulation of making a section and delivering the lens. He considers retained lens matter the most important factor and attributes the decreasing incidence of sympathetic ophthalmitis after cataract surgery to the popularization of the intracapsular method. This viewpoint supports to some degree the contention of Blodi[19] that there is an association between phacoanaphylactic endophthalmitis and sympathetic ophthalmitis such that low degrees of the former predispose the eye to develop the latter.

Pathogenesis

Researchers have been thwarted for well over 100 years in their attempts to determine the etiology of sympathetic ophthalmitis. The bilaterality of lesions in this disorder might appear unique except that bilateral symmetry of lesions involving paired organs has been recorded in many endogenous infections such as renal tuberculosis and mumps orchitis. However, what is unusual in sympathetic ophthalmitis is the bilaterality of the lesion in paired organs after an injury to only one of the pair.[20] This has not been noted in other paired organs.

Of the numerous etiologic theories that have been offered, only two remain and the evidence for them is far from overwhelming.

Infection. Although the clinical behavior and pathologic appearance of the disease strongly suggest an infective origin, bacteriologic confirmation has not been forthcoming. Research purportedly demonstrating a causative organism has run the gamut from bacterial, viral, and fungal to rickettsial. However, in most instances the organism isolated appeared fortuitous and animal inoculations never produced the typical lesions of sympathetic ophthalmitis.

Allergy. The possibility has been suggested that sympathetic ophthalmitis is connected with allergy to some autogenous substance. The basis of the theory indicting a hypersensitive autoim-

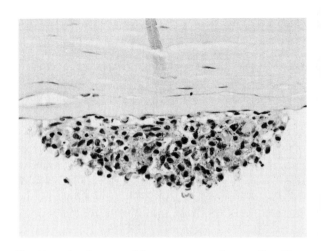

Fig. 23-2. Agglutinated large mononuclear cells adherent to corneal endothelium (mutton fat keratic precipitates). (×305.) (AFIP No. 273515.) (From Hogan, M. J., and Zimmerman, L. E.: Ophthalmic pathology, Philadelphia, 1962, W. B. Saunders Co.)

mune reaction is that uveal pigment is capable of acting as an antigen. This theory was put forth by Elschnig,[21] who termed this concept "horror autotoxicus." A considerable amount of evidence exists supporting the formation of circulating autoantibodies to uveal tissue that can react specifically with normal ocular tissues. In this sense, sympathetic ophthalmitis shows a close parallel to lens-induced uveitis.[19,22-24] The two conditions occasionally coexist. If this joint occurrence proves to be more than coincidental, it would lend support to the allergic theory. Blodi[19] reviewed the development and present status of the allergic theory of sympathetic ophthalmitis and concluded that allergy to uveal pigment by itself does not precipitate the disease but sets the stage for a second, perhaps infectious, factor.

Clinical findings

The clinical picture of sympathetic ophthalmitis is so varied that one cannot predict a sympathetic involvement in the second eye by the findings in the operated or injured eye. However, the most typical sequence is the appearance in the operated eye of a granulomatous anterior uveitis, characterized by a heavy aqueous cellular flare, mutton-fat keratic precipitates (Fig. 23-2), a thickened iris that dilates poorly, nodules on the iris surface and at its margins (Fig. 23-3), adhe-

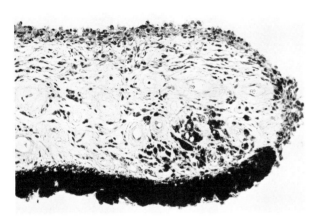

Fig. 23-3. Cells similar to those in Fig. 23-2 adherent to anterior surface and pupillary margin of iris. (×200.) (AFIP No. 273515.) (From Hogan, M. J., and Zimmerman, L. E.: Ophthalmic pathology, Philadelphia, 1962, W. B. Saunders Co.)

sions of the iris to the anterior vitreous surface, hypotension, and eventually a tendency to phthisis bulbi. The cataract surgery and initial healing may be uneventful, but usually there is a complication such as incarceration of iris, capsule, or vitreous in the wound or iris prolapse. The eye does not clear up rapidly and develops a persistent, indolent, low-grade uveitis with intermittent exacerbations and remissions. The most ominous sign is the appearance of lardaceous keratic precipitates. The vitreous becomes turbid. If the fundus can be adequately visualized, peripheral choroiditis, blurring of the disc margins, macular edema, and perhaps generalized retinal edema may be observed. Small, white, drusenlike spots may appear because of changes in the pigment epithelium (Dalén-Fuchs nodules).

The involvement of the sympathizing eye parallels that in the operated (exciting) eye. The signs just described, along with capsular clouding of the lens and early visual failure, appear.

The clinical course of sympathetic ophthalmitis is variable, since even in the years before steroids were used, cases were observed that ran a short, mild, bilateral course with eventual recovery. However, the course is most typically chronic with ultimate blindness and phthisis bulbi. The introduction of steroids has drastically changed the clinical course and improved the ultimate prognosis (p. 478).

The interval between surgery (or injury) and the onset of inflammation is of great importance. Although cases have been reported before the second week after injury or after several years, Duke-Elder[15] stated that cases occur exceptionally before an interval of 2 weeks, 65% occur before 2 months, 80% before 3 months, and 90% before 1 year. The most dangerous time lies between the fourth and eighth weeks. Although one may assume that there is little chance of its development after 3 months, a definite possibility of its occurrence exists.

Frequently, one may be alerted to the imminence of sympathetic ophthalmitis by the appearance in the unoperated eye of prodromal symptoms such as photophobia, transient obscurations of vision because of accommodative failure, or the development of transient myopia as seen in early cyclitis. These symptoms may be associated with lacrimation, ciliary injection, and ocular tenderness.

Pathology

The pathologic description of sympathetic ophthalmitis by Fuchs[25] in 1905 represents a truly classic study; therefore little has since been added to our knowledge of the morphologic characteristics of the disease.

In general the pathologic changes in the exciting and the sympathizing eye are identical, aside from changes in the exciting eye directly related to surgery or injury (Fig. 23-4). The inflammation is granulomatous in character, consisting of a massive round cell infiltration of the entire uveal tract, especially the choroid, with an abundance of epithelioid cells, some giant cells, and a tendency toward the formation of nodular aggregations. Examination of the cells involved reveals a diffuse lymphocytic infiltration of the uveal tissues. Nodular areas of epithelioid cells with giant cells scattered among them are superimposed on the lymphocytic infiltrate . Caseation or necrosis is rare (Fig. 23-5). Initially the epithelioid cell nests are widely scattered, but later they grow and coalesce so that the uveal tract takes on a mottled appearance in which pale-staining epithelioid infiltrates alternate with darker-staining areas of lymphocytic infiltration. Uniform in-

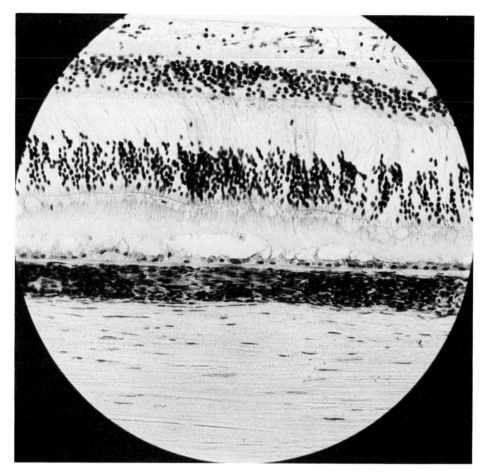

Fig. 23-4. Choroidal infiltrate in sympathizing eye is similar to that seen in exciting eye. (×400.) (AFIP No. 195025.) (From Hogan, M. J., and Zimmerman, L. E.: Ophthalmic pathology, Philadelphia, 1962, W. B. Saunders Co.)

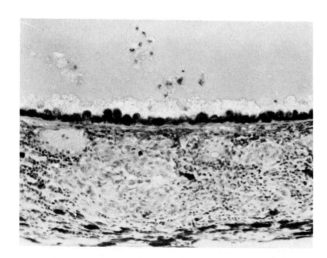

Fig. 23-5. Sympathetic ophthalmitis. Noncaseating aggregations of epithelioid cells in choroid. Diffuse lymphocytic infiltration. Choriocapillaris involved only slightly, if at all. (×75.) (AFIP No. 329514.) (From Hogan, M. J., and Zimmerman, L. E.: Ophthalmic pathology, Philadelphia, 1962, W. B. Saunders Co.)

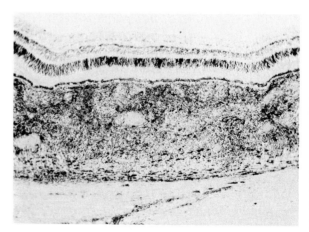

Fig. 23-6. Sympathetic ophthalmitis. Diffuse thickening of choroid by inflammatory cell infiltration. No involvement of retina. (×75.) (AFIP No. 37381.) (From Hogan, M. J., and Zimmerman, L. E.: Ophthalmic pathology, Philadelphia, 1962, W. B. Saunders Co.)

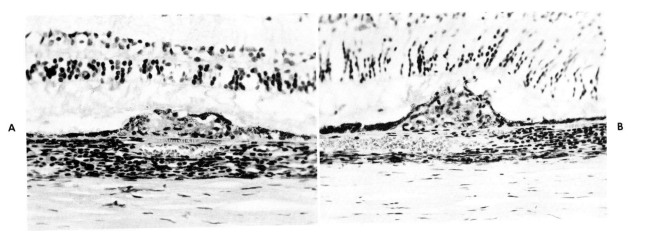

Fig. 23-7. Dalén-Fuchs nodule in sympathetic ophthalmitis. (**A,** ×305; **B,** ×265.) (AFIP No. 909319.) (From Hogan, M. J., and Zimmerman, L. E.: Ophthalmic pathology, Philadelphia, 1962, W. B. Saunders Co.)

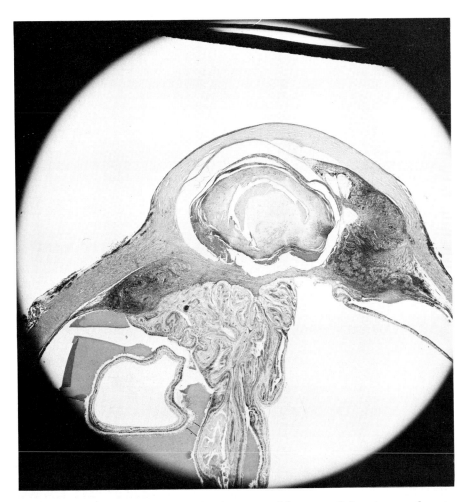

Fig. 23-8. Sympathetic ophthalmitis. Exuberant proliferation of chronic granulomatous inflammatory tissue has filled posterior chamber. Although often massive, these anterior segment lesions are less diagnostic of the disease than are posterior lesions. (×12.) (AFIP No. 891154.) (From Hogan, M. J., and Zimmerman, L. E.: Ophthalmic pathology, Philadelphia, 1962, W. B. Saunders Co.)

volvement is typical for the entire uveal tract, but this may vary. It is characteristic for the pigment epithelium and retina to be walled off from involvement by the underlying Bruch's membrane and choriocapillaris (Fig. 23-6), a feature that distinguishes sympathetic ophthalmitis from other forms of granulomatous uveitis such as tuberculosis and syphilis, which cause massive destruction of the overlying pigment epithelium and retina. Occasionally, small nodular lesions consisting of epithelioid cells and cells of the pigment epithelium are found in the pigment epithelium. These lesions are known as Dalén-Fuchs nodules[25,26] (Fig. 23-7).

Extension from the choroid into the sclera occurs along the sheaths of the perforating vessels and nerves, and episcleral nodules are found at the emergence of these channels.

In the ciliary body and iris, where the lamina vitrea is either absent or forms a poor boundary, destruction of epithelial layers is common, with a massive exudate of epithelioid cells and lymphocytes usually forming on the surface of the ciliary processes and in the posterior chamber (Fig. 23-8).

The differential between phacoanaphylactic uveitis and sympathetic ophthalmitis can be made pathologically by the choroidal changes in the latter. One frequently has difficulty distinguishing these entities clinically, especially if an extracapsular extraction has been done or if a penetrating ocular injury causes disruption of the

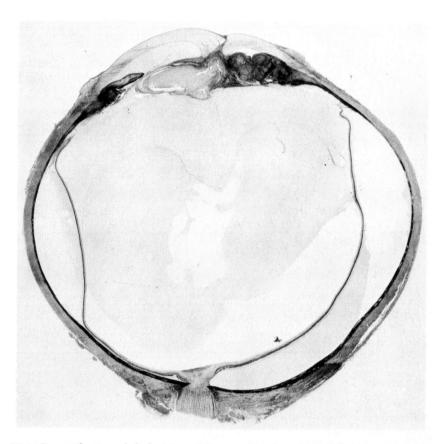

Fig. 23-9. Sympathetic ophthalmitis and lens-induced endophthalmitis after perforating wound of cornea and lens. In complicated case like this, diagnosis of sympathetic ophthalmitis is difficult to make from anterior segment alone; choroid, however, reveals diagnostic alterations. (×6.) (AFIP No. 28571.) (From Hogan, M. J., and Zimmerman, L. E.: Ophthalmic pathology, Philadelphia, 1962, W. B. Saunders Co.)

lens (Fig. 23-9). As has been mentioned earlier, it is not surprising that these conditions may coexist.

Fuchs[25] has demonstrated that the infiltrating epithelioid cells in the early stages of the disease often contain scattered melanin granules and show no tendency for necrosis (Fig. 23-10). This situation is in sharp contrast to other affections of the uvea wherein the melanin granules that are liberated by the death or injury of the melanocytes are usually phagocytosed by macrophages that become heavily laden with pigment and often show necrosis. This distinction is not absolute, for in tuberculous or syphilitic uveal lesions, melanin granules may be found in an occasional epithelioid cell.[20] Nevertheless, in sym-

pathetic ophthalmitis, the characteristic prominence of early pigment phagocytosis by epithelioid cells is a morphologic feature of the disease.

A review[27] of the clinical and histologic features of 252 patients with sympathetic ophthalmia revealed that the eyes of black patients demonstrated more numerous and larger nests of epithelioid cells in the choroid. Apparently, differences in the degree of racial pigmentation of the uvea are clearly associated with differences in the histopathologic features of sympathetic ophthalmia.

Treatment

The sharp reduction in the incidence of sympathetic ophthalmitis in recent years may be attributed to improvements in surgical techniques regarding the repair of penetrating ocular injuries and complications arising from intraocular surgery. Another cause is the recognition of the value of early enucleation of the injured eye in preventing the disease in the opposite eye. If an eye is hopelessly blinded by injury, enucleation performed within 2 weeks is usually considered to be a reliable preventive measure. Joy[28] emphasized that if enucleation is done 14 days or more after the initial injury, sympathetic uveitis may still develop in the second eye, even if there are no symptoms at the time of surgery. Supporting this view is a recent case report[29] that describes an enucleation performed on the fifteenth day after injury. The patient had been taking systemic corticosteroids (20 mg daily) from the time of initial injury, through enucleation, to 1 week prior to the development of symptoms in the sympathizing eye. When the sympathizing eye developed symptoms, treatment was started with local and systemic corticosteroids. The inflammation was successfully controlled. This suggested that systemic steroids prophylactically may not prevent the development of sympathetic ophthalmitis but may induce a milder form of the disease.

Once definite signs of the disease have commenced in the sympathizing eye, enucleation of the exciting eye is of no use. In fact, it may be contraindicated, since the injured or operated eye may prove ultimately to be the better eye. Such an opinion was offered by Winter,[16] who studied 257 histologically proved cases of sympa-

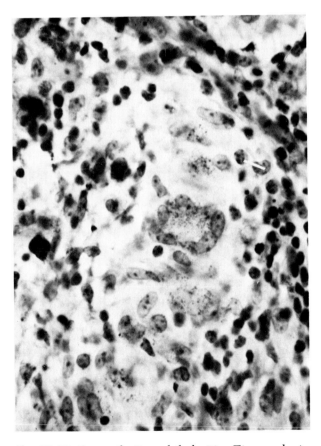

Fig. 23-10. Sympathetic ophthalmitis. Fine melanin granules in epithelioid and giant cells. (×655.) (AFIP No. 37381.) (From Hogan, M. J., and Zimmerman, L. E.: Ophthalmic pathology, Philadelphia, 1962, W. B. Saunders Co.)

thetic uveitis and concluded that "the principal lesson derived from the study emphasizes the fact that routine enucleation of the exciting eye should not be done coincident with the onset of symptoms in the sympathizing eye. The data indicate that this procedure does not materially improve the final visual result for the patient but for a number of other reasons may be detrimental." The diagnosis of sympathetic ophthalmitis is frequently in error. In addition, unless the health of the sound eye is definitely known, it is risky to assume the diagnosis.

Steroid therapy has drastically changed the clinical course and eventual prognosis of this disease. Many eyes are being saved. Shortly after the availability of steroids, a report (1952)[30] showed that in 72 patients with sympathetic uveitis a favorable result was observed in 64% under treatment with cortisone or adrenocorticotropic hormone. The results have improved further, since improved steroid preparations, which cause fewer side effects, are now available, and more effective methods of administration (injection under Tenon's capsule and under the conjunctiva of repository steroids) are being practiced.

I agree with Haik and co-workers' contention[30] that intraocular surgical procedures such as an iridectomy or a cataract extraction can be carried out under the protection of steroids without much risk of a flare-up of the sympathizing disease. In 1955 I performed a cataract extraction on the sympathizing eye of a patient whose other eye had histologically proved sympathetic ophthalmitis after an iridencleisis. The eye has remained useful ever since and requires only topical steroid application.

REFERENCES

1. Gillman, A. M.: Pathogenesis of complications following cataract surgery, Int. Ophthalmol. Clin. **5:**207-256, 1965.
2. Bitot, L. W., and Salvado, E. V., Intraocular fluid dynamics. 3. The site and mechanism of prostaglandin transfer across the blood intraocular fluid barriers, Exp. Eye Res. **14:**233-241, 1972.
3. Hunter, J. W.: Early postoperative sterile hypopyons, Br. J. Ophthalmol. **62:**470-473, 1978.
4. Binkhorst, C. D.: The pupillary lens (iris clip lens), An. Instituto Barraquer **3** (4):562, 1962.
5. Jaffe, N. S.: Elimination of contamination from ophthalmic solutions for intraocular surgery, Ophthalmology (Rochester) **74:**406-416, 1970.
6. Smith, R. E., and O'Connor, G. R.: Cataract extraction in Fuchs' syndrome, Arch. Ophthalmol. **91:**39-44, 1974.
7. Algan, B., and LeGrand, P.: L'uvéite rheumatismale post-operatoire de la cataracte. II. Bull. Soc. Belg. Ophthalmol. **115:**251-260, 1957.
8. Dhanda, R. P., and Kalevar, V. K.: Cataract surgery in diabetics, Antiseptic **59:**477-480, 1962.
9. Duddell, B.: A treatise of the diseases of the horny coat of the eye and the various types of cataract, London, 1972, J. Clark.
10. LeDran, H. F.: Traité ou réflexions tirées de la pratique sur les playes d'armes à feu, Paris, 1737.
11. MacKenzie, W.: A practical treatise on the diseases of the eye, London, 1830, Longman, Rees, Orme, Brown & Green.
12. Wardrop, J.: Essays on the morbid anatomy of the human eye, Edinburgh, 1818, G. Ramsay & Co., vol. 2, p. 139.
13. Pritchard, A.: Causes of affections of the nerves distributed to the eye and its appendages, Prov. Med. Surg. J. **15:**202-206, 1851.
14. Critchett: Ueber sympathische Ophthalmie, Klin. Mbl. Augenheilk. **1:**440-450, 1863.
15. Duke-Elder, S.: System of ophthalmology. Vol. IX. Diseases of the uveal tract, St. Louis, 1966, The C. V. Mosby Co., pp. 562, 566.
16. Winter, F. C.: Sympathetic uveitis. A clinical and pathologic study of the visual result, Am. J. Ophthalmol. **39:**340-347, 1955.
17. Roper-Hall, M. J.: Sympathetic ophthalmia, Trans. Ophthalmol. Soc. U.K. **82:**189-197, 1962.
18. Coles, R. S.: Uveal complications after cataract surgery, Int. Ophthalmol. Clin. **4:**895-912, 1964.
19. Blodi, F. C.: Sympathetic uveitis as an allergic phenomenon with a study of its association with phacoanaphylactic uveitis and a report on the pathologic findings in sympathizing eyes, Ophthalmology (Rochester) **63:**642-649, 1959.
20. Hogan, M. J., and Zimmerman, L. E.: Ophthalmic pathology; an atlas and textbook, ed. 2, Philadelphia, 1962, W. B. Saunders Co., p. 382.
21. Elschnig, A.: Studien zur sympathischen Ophthalmie. II. Die Antigene Wirkung des Augenpigmentes, Graefe Arch. Ophthalmol. **76:**509-546, 1910.
22. deVeer, J. A.: Endophthalmitis phacoanaphylactica and its relation to sympathetic ophthalmia, Arch. Ophthalmol. **23:**237-252, 1940.
23. Irvine, S. R., and Irvine, A. R., Jr.: Lens-induced uveitis and glaucoma. I. Endophthalmitis phacoanaphylactica, Am. J. Ophthalmol. **35:**177-186, 1952.
24. Scheffler, M. M.: Endophthalmitis phacoanaphylactica with granulomatous iritis, Am. J. Ophthalmol. **36:**1449-1453, 1953.
25. Fuchs, E.: Ueber sympathisierende Entzündung (nebst Bemerkungen über seröse traumatische Iritis), Graefe Arch. Ophthalmol. **61:**365-456, 1905.
26. Dalén, A.: Zur Kenntnis der sogenannten Chorioiditis sympathica, Mitt. Augenklinik Carolin. Med.-Chir. Inst. zu Stockholm, Jena, 1904, G. Fischer Verlag, no. 6, pp. 1-21.

27. Marak, G. E., Jr., Font, R. L., and Zimmerman, L. E.: Histologic variations related to race in sympathetic ophthalmia, Am. J. Ophthalmol. **78:**935-938, 1974.

28. Joy, H. H.: Survey of cases of sympathetic ophthalmia occurring in New York State, N.Y. State J. Med. **36:**85, 1936.

29. Kay, M. L., Yanoff, M., and Katowitz, J. A.: Development of sympathetic uveitis in spite of cortocosteroid therapy, Am. J. Ophthalmol. **78:**90-94, 1974.

30. Haik, G. M., Waugh, R. L., Jr., and Lyda, W.: Sympathetic ophthalmia. Similarity to bilateral endophthalmitis phacoanaphylactica. New therapeutic methods, Arch. Ophthalmol. **47:**437-453, 1952.

CHAPTER 24

Retained lens material

An extracapsular lens extraction, whether by design or mischance, usually provides an excellent functional result and leaves an eye whose anatomic integrity in some ways exceeds that seen after an intracapsular extraction. There is a far lower incidence of postoperative rupture of the anterior hyaloid membrane, with vitreous in contact with the cornea and the operative wound. On a theoretical basis a good case can be argued for the choice of an extracapsular extraction in special situations, such as in eyes with cornea guttata and in the prevention of certain postoperative complications such as cystoid macular edema and retinal detachment. The location of the anterior vitreous face at or behind the level of the iris and its protection by a transparent posterior lens capsule should provide the eye with anatomic relationships better suited to protection against physical abuse than those available after an intracapsular lens extraction. It was for these reasons, along with the lesser hazards of the surgery, that many of the older clinicians persisted in performing extracapsular extractions, even after the techniques and safety of the intracapsular procedure were well established.

Because of a number of impracticalities associated with its choice and the overall higher incidence of postoperative complications, the extracapsular lens extraction has given way to the intracapsular operation. Younger ophthalmologists, however, have formulated their opinions relative to the merits of both techniques on the basis of their observations of the extracapsular lens extraction as an accidental occurrence during the course of an attempted intracapsular delivery of the lens. The planned extracapsular lens extraction, is followed by far fewer complications than

the mishap of a ruptured capsule of an immature cataract. Modern extracapsular lens extraction techniques, including phacoemulsification, usually leave relatively little residual lens material in the eye.

With the advent of modern techniques in cataract surgery, such as induced hypotension, enzymatic zonulysis, and cryosurgical extraction, discussion of retained lens material as a complication of a routine intracapsular cataract extraction may not be worthwhile. However, as any ocular pathologist will attest, this complication still occurs and is responsible for many specimens that are the subject of histologic examination.

As to terminology, the remnants of the lens retained in the eye after an extracapsular extraction, a discission, or traumatic destruction of the lens have been referred to as "aftercataract" or "secondary cataract." The latter term is somewhat erroneous, since it is more suited to the description of a cataract secondary to ocular disease.

CLASSIFICATION OF LENS REMNANTS

Duke-Elder[1] has classified lens remnants as follows:
1. Capsular remains
2. Capsulolenticular remains
3. Pigmentary, hemorrhagic, or inflammatory fibrous elements

Capsular remains usually consist of the posterior capsule, which is thin and transparent. It may be entirely invisible with the ophthalmoscope and may not interfere at all with vision. However, it can always be detected with the slit lamp. Whenever an aphakic eye shows a spacious posterior chamber with an intact anterior vitreous face, one should suspect the presence of a posterior capsule or a lens extraction complicated by postoperative iridocyclitis or hyphema.

The posterior capsular remnant is usually not of uniform thickness. It may appear as a glistening sheet with lines of traction in one area and folds in another. Usually this veillike curtain is flat and prevents any bulge of vitreous through the pupil. The anterior hyaloid membrane can be detected through the posterior capsule and may be separated from it by a clear space or may be adherent. The posterior capsule may be responsible for the beautiful polychromatic luster that is occasionally evident on slit lamp examination. As stated previously, the persistence of the posterior capsule usually prevents the vitreous from herniating into the anterior chamber to reach the cornea or the operative wound so frequently seen after an intracapsular lens extraction. However, the posterior capsular remnant may be so diaphanous and thin that a localized bulge of vitreous with an intact vitreous face may occur, or the anterior hyaloid membrane may actually rupture, and the anterior chamber may become invaded by loose vitreous fibrils and membranes.

Associated with the capsule is the subcapsular epithelium, which may be responsible, as a result of proliferation, for a later decline in the patient's vision. Although the proliferative activity of the epithelium is more vigorous in younger individuals, it is by no means limited to them. It is this activity that represents the main disadvantage of a planned extracapsular lens extraction.

The changes in the subcapsular epithelium are interesting to follow with the slit lamp. They are highly variable, with some eyes showing extensive proliferation to make it appear as if the lens has regenerated, whereas in others this activity is attenuated. Frequently the epithelium will line the entire posterior capsule in a uniform distribution. It may, however, proliferate to such a degree that it may line the anterior and posterior surfaces of remnants of the anterior capsule. Another interesting development is the deposition of hyaline material, which resembles lens capsule. This may be laid down in irregular sheets, or it may be interspersed between layers of proliferating subcapsular epithelium.

The individual subcapsular epithelial cells enlarge and swell to such a degree that they give

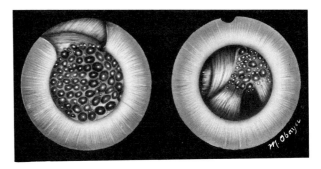

Fig. 24-1. Elschnig's pearls.

the appearance of soap bubbles. It has been suggested that this represents aberrant attempts of the epithelium to form new lens fibers.[1] Although noted earlier by Hirschberg,[2] they are usually referred to as Elschnig's pearls[3] (Fig. 24-1). These may be distributed over the posterior capsule in a uniform manner, or they may accumulate in clusters like a bunch of grapes. Particularly in young subjects, this activity may occlude the entire pupillary space. A single epithelial cell may swell to a considerable size and reach a diameter of 2 mm.[4] These pearls may appear shortly after cataract surgery and continue to accumulate. In some eyes, they disappear over a period of years, probably because of rupture of their thin walls.

In addition to the formation of new capsular material, the epithelium may be responsible for another type of lenticular remains—free lentoid bodies, which are small and consist of parallel, closely packed lenticular fibers that run in the same direction. They may adhere to the iris and cornea and may even be found in the vitreous.[5]

At surgery a variable amount of lens cortex may remain in the eye along with the capsular remnants described earlier (Fig. 24-2). They usually undergo lysis by the aqueous, but they may persist. When they do persist, they are usually amassed in the periphery, where they become incorporated in a ringlike structure first described by Soemmering[6] (Figs. 24-3 and 24-4). This formation occurs when the residual anterior capsule retracts and its central torn edge folds inward to reach the posterior capsule. This results in a folded capsular structure shaped like the ring of a doughnut and containing within its walls large numbers of lenticular fibers and pro-

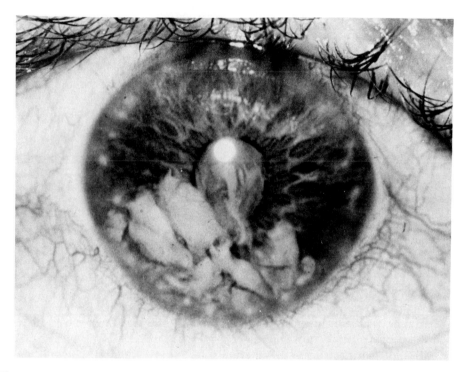

Fig. 24-2. Lens cortex and capsule remnants retained in eye after unplanned extracapsular cataract extraction.

liferated epithelial cells. The ring may increase in size because of the regenerative activity within its walls, with the new fibers being protected from the lytic action of the aqueous by the capsule. The center of the ring consists of the posterior capsule, and it may be all that is seen with the slit lamp, since the opaque ring may be obstructed from view by the iris unless a sector iridectomy has been performed or the pupil has been widely dilated. The ring may be complete or incomplete, but it is usually segmented like a string of sausages.

Microscopic examination of Soemmering's ring reveals that it consists of anterior and posterior capsule lined by proliferated epithelium (Fig. 24-5). Products of the latter, such as hyaline material and new lens fibers, may cause a considerable increase in the size of the ring. Also enclosed within are degenerative changes, resulting in the formation of amorphous debris, morgagnian globules, and calcareous degeneration.[1]

The fate of this ring structure has also excited considerable interest. It usually remains fixed in its position behind the iris, to which it may be adherent in some places, and anterior to the anterior hyaloid membrane, to which it may likewise be attached. If it remains in situ, it generally causes no visual impairment, since its axial portion usually remains relatively clear. However, occasionally, as the result of trauma or at other times spontaneously, the ring may tear loose from its moorings. It may obstruct the pupillary aperture, enter the vitreous cavity, or lodge itself in the anterior chamber. In the last situation, it may incite a considerable inflammatory response and perhaps an elevation of intraocular pressure.

Superimposed on the capsular and capsulolenticular remnants are often found other depositions such as pigment, organized hemorrhage, and inflammatory exudate. Pigment may be derived from the posterior surface of the iris and from the ciliary body to which the retained lens material may be attached. Occasionally, because of proliferation, large pigmented formations occur and become interspersed with the lenticular remnants. This condition is probably more evident in diabetics. A more serious occurrence, because it obstructs vision, is the organization of

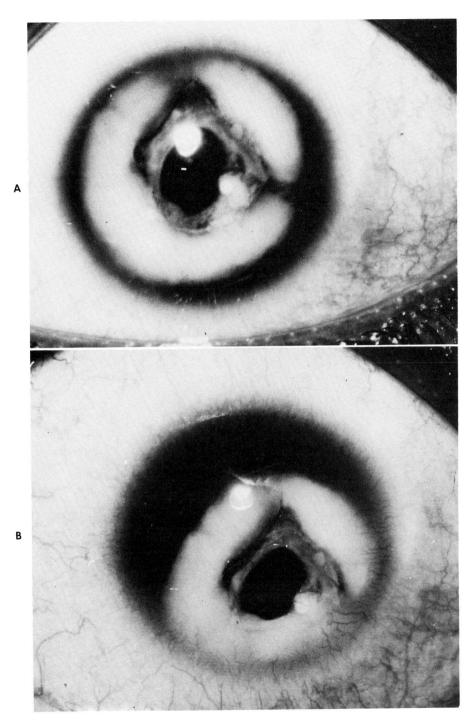

Fig. 24-3. A, Unusual photograph of Soemmering's ring in eye with aniridia. **B,** Change in position of ring several months later.

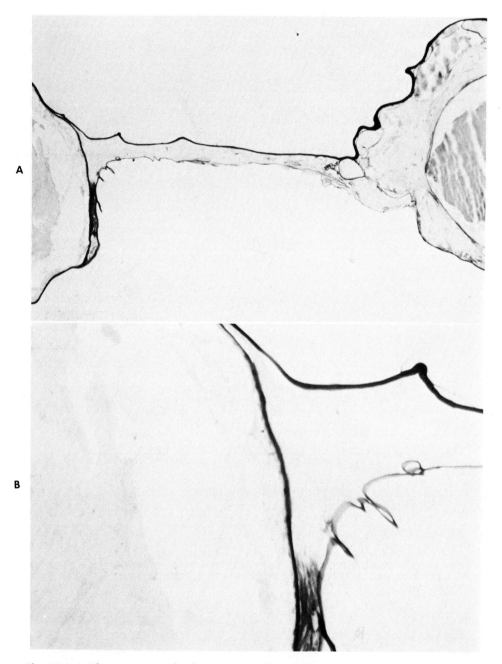

Fig. 24-4. A, Photomicrograph of Soemmering's ring. **B,** High-power view of left portion of **A.** Note union of capsule remnant in center with capsule surrounding lens material.

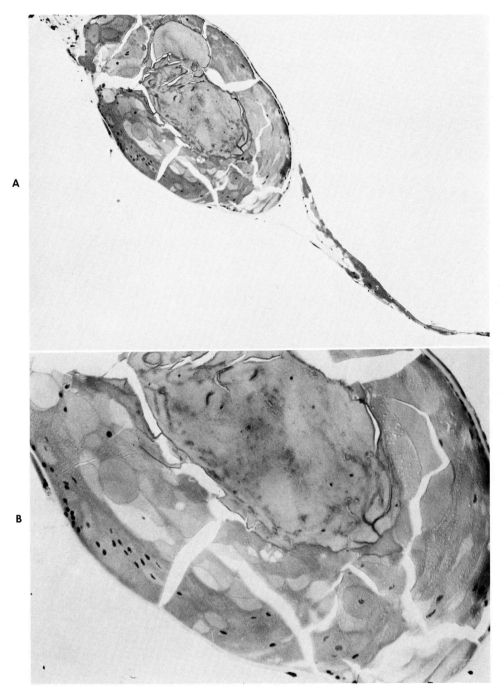

Fig. 24-5. A, Photomicrograph of Soemmering's ring showing anterior and posterior lens capsule lined by proliferated epithelium. **B,** High-power view of **A,** showing degenerative changes consisting of amorphous debris and morgagnian globules.

a postoperative hemorrhage or an inflammatory exudate. Cellular invasion followed by fibroblastic proliferation and cicatrization may give rise to a thick, opaque, tenaceous pupillary membrane. If such an exudate becomes extensive, it may become periciliary in distribution, the globe ultimately suffering disintegration in the form of phthisis bulbi.

TREATMENT OF AFTERCATARACT

The very best prevention of an aftercataract, of course, is an uncomplicated intracapsular lens extraction. In a planned extracapsular extraction, it is important to remove as much of the anterior capsule as possible without rupturing the posterior capsule. This is discussed on p. 73. In an unintended extracapsular extraction, if suitable measures, such as induced hypotension and enzymatic zonulysis, have been instituted prior to the delivery of the lens, it is possible to remove ruptured capsular remains without damaging the anterior face of the vitreous. The very best modality available to prevent capsule rupture is the use of a cryoextraction method of lens delivery. It is not unusual to proceed through a series of several hundred cryoextractions without a single capsule rupture. Its performance in this regard cannot be matched by any other method.

The treatment of an aftercataract is usually undertaken for optical reasons. The incision of a thin posterior capsule is one of the simplest procedures in ophthalmic surgery, but the creation of an adequate opening in a dense, fibrotic, capsulolenticular membrane may severely test the ingenuity and skill of the ophthalmic surgeon.

In general the surgical approaches to the creation of an adequate pupillary opening may be divided into four categories:
1. Simple discission for a relatively thin membrane
2. Scissors section or two-knife section for thicker membranes
3. Removal of a portion of the membrane through a larger limbal incision for the thickest membranes
4. Pars plana membranectomy

There are certain basic principles to be observed. Surgery should be delayed until all postoperative reaction has subsided, lest the opening created be closed by continuing inflammation. The maneuvers inside the anterior chamber should not be too forceful because it is possible to create a vicious plastic exudative response or a retinal detachment by stretching membranes that are attached to the ciliary body or the retina.

It is important to perform a careful slit lamp examination with full mydriasis, if possible, before surgery to determine the direction of the fibers of the membrane so that the discission can be made perpendicular to them to ensure that the margins of the incised membrane will separate as widely as possible. In the case of very dense membranes, it will be possible to determine the points of densest anchorage.

The operating microscope is particularly advantageous in the surgery of aftercataract. The surgeon can be very precise in accurately incising the membrane. It is invaluable for the aspiration of Elschnig's pearls as well as for the careful insertion of scissors blades when excising the membrane.

Techniques are discussed below. In some patients with very thick membranes, it may be best to perform a membranectomy through the pars plana.

Discission

There are numerous satisfactory methods of incising an aftercataract membrane. One favorite is the method of Wheeler.[7] The patient is prepared as for a cataract extraction. The pupil is widely dilated. Any one of the many discission knives or knife needles are used. With secure fixation of the globe, the knife enters the anterior chamber through a limbal stab wound at a point perpendicular to the principal direction of the fibers of the membrane. When the knife reaches the margin of the pupil farthest from the point of entry, the blade is rotated so that the cutting surface is perpendicular to the membrane. One smooth stroke is made by using the limbal stab wound as a fulcrum. Through the microscope, one can readily observe whether the blade is separating the fibers. If so, the incision is made, and the knife is withdrawn from the eye in one single motion. If the membrane does not split, a slower sawing motion may be made.

A variation of these techniques may be used if the membrane does not separate. The anterior

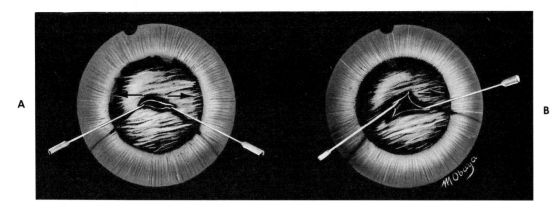

Fig. 24-6. A, Double-knife method of discission of aftercataract membrane. Tips of knives meet in center of membrane, and slow sawing motion is used to incise it, both instruments cutting in direction toward their original point of entry into anterior chamber. **B,** Aftercataract membrane is engaged with tip of one knife near one pupillary margin. Second knife then incises membrane in sawing motion directed away from first knife, while tip of first knife holds membrane taut.

chamber is permitted to re-form. A second knife needle is introduced into the anterior chamber through a limbal stab incision 180 degrees from the first wound. The first knife needle enters the anterior chamber through the original incision. One of two methods may be used: The tips of the knives meet in the center of the membrane, and a slow, sawing motion is used to incise it, with both instruments cutting in a direction toward their original point of entry into the anterior chamber (Fig. 24-6, *A*). An alternate technique is to enlarge the membrane with the tip of one knife near one pupillary margin. The second knife then proceeds to incise the membrane in a sawing motion directed away from the first knife, while the tip of the first knife holds the membrane taut (Fig. 24-6).

The most satisfactory method involves the use of a disposable 25- or 27-gauge needle, the tip of which has been bent to create a sharp hook (p. 167). The needle is attached to an elevated bottle of irrigating solution. A limbal stab wound is made temporally. The needle enters the anterior chamber through this opening, engaging the membrane at the most convenient location, and the membrane is torn. This is a simple technique that can be performed with a formed anterior chamber (Fig. 24-7).

Occasionally, a thin membrane may be adherent to the iris, which has been drawn upward into a hammock pupil. The techniques just described may be applied to this situation except that a radial inferior sphincterotomy is performed at the same time. However, often the membrane is too thick to be incised and a scissors method may be necessary.

A small incision is made under a conjunctival flap because of the possibility of loss of vitreous, in which case the flap is an added protection against infection. It should be made just large enough to admit the blades of the scissors of de Wecker, Vannas, or Barraquer. One blade is placed behind the membrane and the inferior border of the iris. The membrane and iris are cut together. The wound is sutured after a partial bubble of air is left in the anterior chamber. Mydriatics and local steroid therapy are prescribed. A subconjunctival injection of a steroid may be helpful.

Aspiration of Elschnig's pearls and polishing of the posterior capsule may be performed in those eyes that might benefit from the preservation of an intact posterior capsule. Examples are eyes where the risk of retinal detachment is high or where the possibility of cystoid macular edema is greater because of its occurrence in the first eye after cataract surgery. This is best performed with the nonultrasonic aspirator handpiece and tip of the phacoemulifier. A 0.2 mm tip is safest. The posterior capsule is then polished with a

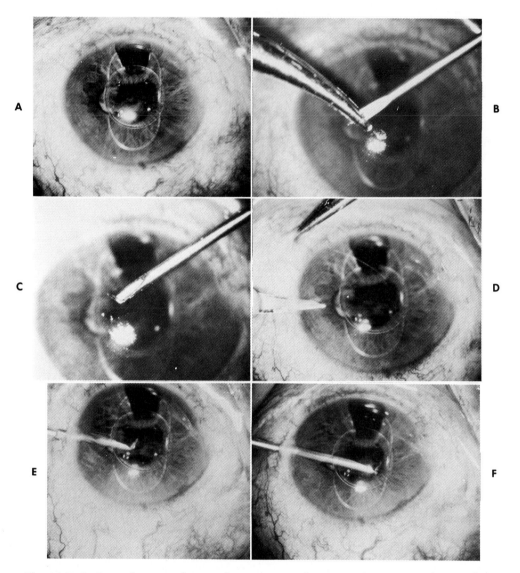

Fig. 24-7. **A,** Secondary membrane after extracapsular cataract extraction (12 weeks) with implantation of a Binkhorst iris-clip lens. Maximum mydriasis shown. (Visual acuity = 20/400.) **B,** Hook created at tip of 25-gauge disposable needle using needle holder. **C,** Bent tip shown. **D,** Limbal stab wound made with No. 75 Beaver blade. **E,** Needle is attached to irrigating solution and enters anterior chamber, passing behind implant. **F,** Tip of needle engages membrane as irrigating flow is stopped. **G,** Hole in membrane is created as irrigating flow resumes. **H,** Membrane is drawn toward limbal wound. **I,** Opening in membrane is enlarged still further. **J,** Final result. Visual acuity improved to 20/25 3 months later. (From Jaffe, N. S.: Pseudophakos, St. Louis, 1978, The C. V. Mosby Co.)

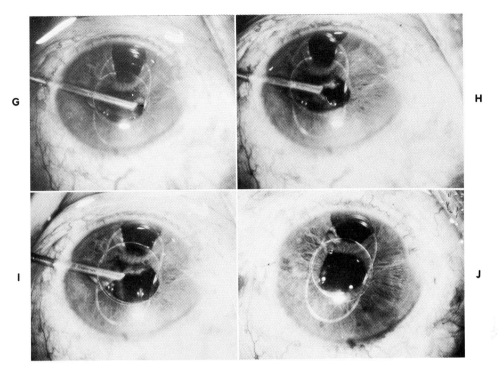

Fig. 24-7, cont'd. For legend see opposite page.

sandblasted irrigating device such as the Kratz scratcher (p. 76).

Thick aftercataract membranes

Thick aftercataract membranes are much more difficult to treat because they are irregular in thickness and the fibers may run in several directions with multiple points of anchorage, which create traction in different directions. A simple discission will usually be ineffective because if the membrane can be incised at all, the opening will usually close.

Since one must make a larger incision and since more maneuvers in the anterior chamber are contemplated, it is extremely important to dehydrate the vitreous by using a systemically administered hyperosmotic agent and digital message. The pupil is dilated as widely as possible. A Flieringa ring may be a useful adjunct, particularly in young patients. A 5 mm limbal incision is made under a conjunctival flap. A solution of alpha-chymotrypsin may be irrigated behind the iris after posterior synechias are separated. If the aftercataract membrane occupies the entire pupillary space, it may be grasped near the upper

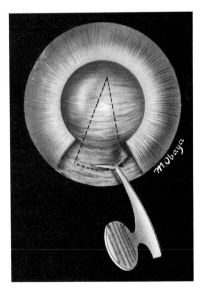

Fig. 24-8. Surgery of thick aftercataract membrane. Membrane is grasped near upper pupillary border with forceps and buttonholed with scissors. Horizontal section is completed. From each extremity of incision, oblique cuts that meet at inferior pupillary border are made. In this way, triangular piece of membrane is removed.

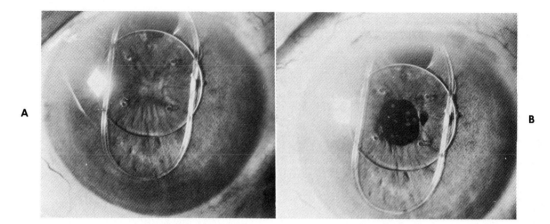

Fig. 24-9. **A,** Dense retrolental membrane in eye of patient who suffered hypopyon uveitis 3 days after intracapsular cataract extraction and implantation of Binkhorst iris-clip lens. (Visual acuity = hand motion at 1 foot.) **B,** Membrane and anterior vitreous removed with Douvas Roto-Extractor. Pupil reshaped. Visual acuity 4 months later was 20/40. (From Jaffe, N. S.: Pseudophakos, St. Louis, 1978, The C. V. Mosby Co.)

pupillary border with fine forceps and buttonholed with de Wecker, Vannas, or Barraquer scissors. A horizontal section is then completed (Fig. 24-8). From each extremity of this incision, oblique cuts that meet at the inferior pupillary border are made. In this way a triangular piece of membrane may be removed.

An alternate method is to grasp the membrane with a cryoprobe and remove it completely. Alpha-chymotrypsin may be very helpful in this situation. A larger incision is necessary, and a 1 mm diameter tip is recommended.

This type of surgery is simpler to describe than to perform. The surgeon must be alert and the maneuvers deftly and gently performed, since the membrane may be attached to the vitreous or other vital structures. A careful preoperative examination will usually guide the surgeon to the most effective approach. The operating microscope is invaluable in these situations.

Thick membranes are much more difficult and often impossible to manage by the techniques just described. These membranes may be so extensive as to adhere to the ciliary processes, and it would be dangerous to pull on such a membrane. Another approach is recommended in this situation. One of the various types of automated vitrectomy instruments may be used. In these cases the iris on all sides of the pupil is often pulled centrally, except at the origin posts of the

posterior loops of an iris-supported lens implant or at the apices of a Copeland implant. The pupil may have the shape of a vertical and horizontal hourglass. The cutting instrument is usually passed through a pars plana incision until it appears in the pupillary space. If the membrane is confined to the posterior capsule or the anterior vitreous, fiber optics illumination is not required. The dense membrane is removed. The pulled-in portions of iris may also be resected. This will usually not result in undue mydriasis. The iris is resected until a square-shaped pupil is fashioned (Fig. 24-9). The surgeon may elect to create a V-shaped notch in the inferior border of the pupil. The surgery is concluded when a clear fundus reflex is visible through the surgical microscope. Some surgeons prefer to perform the surgery through the anterior chamber via a limbal incision. The advantage of avoiding an incision through the pars plana is somewhat offset by the increased possibility of dislocating an implant and the lessened freedom of maneuvers behind an implant. When properly performed, this technique rarely damages or dislocates an implant.

PHACOANAPHYLACTIC UVEITIS

That complications from retained lens material are not limited to optical considerations is evidenced by the intraocular inflammatory response

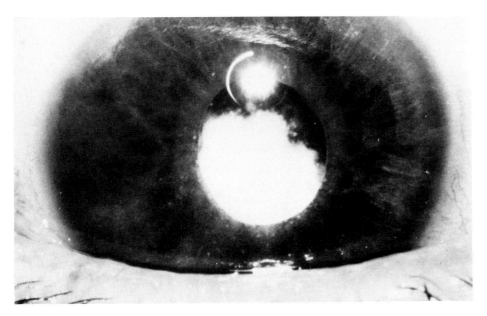

Fig. 24-10. Phacoanaphylactic uveitis occurring after spontaneous rupture of lens. Keratic precipitates appear along with posterior synechias on left.

to this material. This form of lens-induced uveitis is referred to as phacoanaphylactic uveitis. This is an acute uveal tract inflammation that occurs when the eye is exposed to lens proteins liberated within it after an extracapsular cataract extraction, a discission, trauma to the lens, or a spontaneous rupture of its capsule (Fig. 24-10).

Historical background

Schirmer[8] (1899) was the first to emphasize the intraocular response to lens proteins remaining in the eye after an extracapsular cataract extraction. Twenty years later, Straub[9] described an entity that he differentiated from sympathetic ophthalmia, that is, the occurrence of an inflammation in the unoperated or untraumatized eye after the extracapsular extraction of a cataract in the opposite eye. Straub attributed the uveitis to a toxicity to lens proteins. A similar view was expressed by Elschnig[10] (1922), Gifford and Steinberg[11] (1925), and Gifford[12] (1927), so that an entity known as phacotoxic uveitis evolved.

Considerably earlier, Uhlenhuth[13] (1903) observed that the serum of cattle immunized to heterologous lens proteins contained antigens that reacted not only to the lenticular proteins of cattle but also to those of other species. This finding

of organ specificity of the lens proteins, in contrast to species specificity, has been subsequently supported. Verhoeff and Lemoine[14] (1922), although contending that some of these inflammatory problems were toxic in origin, proposed that others represented an anaphylactic reaction. They termed this latter response "endophthalmitis phacoanaphylactica." The choice of terminology is probably unfortunate if one accepts the concept that anaphylaxis is the result of antigen-antibody complexes that release pharmacologically active compounds such as histamine and serotonin from tissues.[15]

Considerable controversy raged in the literature over these mechanisms and other types of lens-induced inflammation. The Irvines[16] (1952) attempted to subdivide them into the following separate pathologic entities, although they recognized that considerable overlapping existed: (1) endophthalmitis phacoanaphylactica, (2) phacotoxic reaction, and (3) phacolytic glaucoma. The last, a peculiar type of glaucoma occurring in some eyes with a hypermature cataract, was termed "phacogenic glaucoma" by Zeeman[17] (1943) and "phacolytic glaucoma" by Flocks and co-workers[18] (1955) (Fig. 24-11). Its pathogenesis is related to clogging of the trabecular meshwork

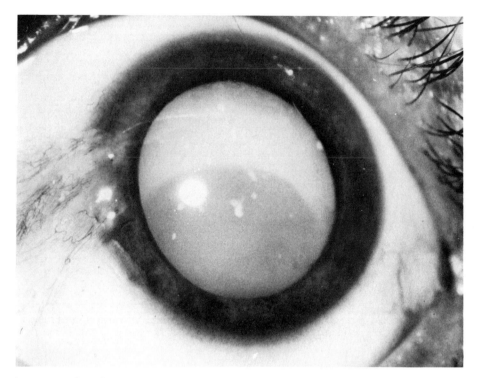

Fig. 24-11. Phacolytic glaucoma in eye with morgagnian cataract. Note dark nucleus sunken downward in liquefied cataract.

by macrophages swollen from phagocytized liberated lens material.

This concept has recently been challenged by Epstein and co-workers,[19] who found quantities of heavy molecular weight (greater than 150×10^6) soluble lens protein sufficient to obstruct aqueous outflow in the aqueous humor of patients with phacolytic glaucoma. None were found in control eyes. They reported that the concentration of this protein in hypermature cortical samples is roughly 14 times greater than that found for cortical samples from immature cataractous lenses. The role of macrophages as key factors in inducing phacolytic glaucoma is, as a consequence of this investigation, possibly deemphasized.

Allergic nature of phacoanaphylactic reaction

Although many seeming contradictions arise in the theory supporting the allergic nature of the phacoanaphylactic reaction, considerable circumstantial evidence that strongly compels one to accept this concept has accumulated.

During embryonic development and early life the lens proteins are probably shielded from exposure to immunologically active cells by the lens capsule. The body therefore does not "get to know" its own tissue.[20] However, disruption of the lens capsule at any stage in later life will present to the body previously unexposed lens material that is treated as foreign by antibody production. It has been shown that vertebrate lens material has at least five or six antigenic components to which antibodies can be produced. This provides a sound theoretical basis for the concept of autoimmune disease involving the lens.

Circulating antibodies against lens protein have been demonstrated in serum,[21] vitreous, or aqueous[22,23] of patients. The passive transfer of the hypersensitivity state can be accomplished by the passage of whole leukocytes from patients with active phacoanaphylactic uveitis.[24] Immunoelectrophoretic studies have also shown the presence of soluble lens antigen in the aqueous of involved eyes.[22] Witmer[25-27] has devised a method that is based on the comparative determination of circulating antilens antibodies in blood serum and aqueous humor. Using a method of indirect hemagglutination, he reported a significantly positive result in 10 of 15 patients with the clinical signs of phacoantigenic uveitis.[27] Blood-borne antibodies can be demonstrated by skin test exposure to lens antigens, as shown by Verhoeff and Lemoine,[14] and these eyes, when given a desensitizing course of intramuscular injections of lens protein, rapidly show an amelioration of their symptoms.

Apparently the phacoanaphylactic reaction does not occur without perforation of the lens capsule and exposure of lens substance. When the reaction occurs in both eyes, there is obvious exposure of lens substance in the first eye. Not many microscopic studies have been performed on the second eye but, when done, they have revealed lens capsule breaks.[28] In addition, local antibody formation in the iris of the second eye has been demonstrated by the fluorescent antibody-staining technique.[27]

Luntz and Wright[24] recently demonstrated circulating antibodies to lens in a patient who developed a severe uveitis in the second eye after bilateral extracapsular lens extraction. The patient's lymphocytes transferred hypersensitivity to the lens of the guinea pig.

Another recent confirmatory report was that of Wirostko and Spalter,[29] which demonstrated that autologous sensitization to lens protein occurs in humans after disruption of the lens capsule. The antilens antibodies were not found in normal controls and in the serum of only two of 64 patients at the time of surgery. Patients who had had intracapsular cataract extraction and presumably no remaining lens matter within the eye failed to demonstrate antibodies. Not all patients who had extracapsular cataract extractions developed serum antilens antibodies. The authors believed that a minimal amount of antigenic material (lens material) had to be present before sensitization could occur or that the patients varied in their responsiveness to this antigenic stimulus. Of the 64 patients in this group of unplanned extracapsular cataract extractions, 28 developed signs and symptoms that fulfilled the criteria for lens-induced uveitis. Newly developed antibodies appeared in 14 patients post-operatively, and 13 of them suffered from uveitis. A second group of patients examined after the onset of a uveitis suggestive of being lens induced were similarly studied for the presence of antilens antibodies. Of 13 in this group, seven demonstrated significant titers by hemagglutination.

This report is highly significant, since it is the first documented finding of the development of antilens antibodies after extracapsular cataract extraction in a patient known to have no antilens antibodies on the day of surgery.

Despite the compelling evidence just mentioned, the relationship of antilens antibodies to lens-induced uveitis is not clear. One must bear in mind that extensive manipulation within the eye during an unplanned extracapsular extraction may be sufficient cause for the uveitis. In addition, low-grade infection might be present, and as observed in animal experiments, this may cause a particularly severe uveitis.

Although this evidence compels one to accept a mechanism of hypersensitivity, there are several findings that appear contradictory. Some of the earlier investigators[30-32] failed to reproduce the sensitivity experimentally in animals. Attempts to induce a uveitus by treating animals with homologous lens protein and adjuvants, but without touching the eye itself, have failed.[33,34] There appears to be a weak antigenicity of lens protein, with the alpha-crystalline component being the organ-specific element.[35] This antigenicity can be increased by physical or chemical denaturation[36] and by microbes.[37] Thus the intermediary action of a strongly antigenic adjuvant such as staphylococcus toxin together with lens protein will effectively increase antigenicity. This is emphasized further by injecting lens protein and herpes simplex virus intravitreally in animals, causing a severe uveitis and significant antibodies against the homologous lens. Control eyes, however, contacted either with lens protein or the virus showed less uveitis and no antibodies.[38] Hackett and Thompson[39] reported serum antibodies to lens in 50% of healthy humans and animals; therefore the significance of the finding of circulating antilens antibodies in disease states is placed in doubt. The finding of positive skin tests by Verhoeff and Lemoine[14] must be accepted with reservation, since their controls were not chosen. Halbert and Manski[40] were not able to detect differences between patients with suspected lens-induced uveitis and controls.

Despite some seeming discrepancies, it appears safe to accept phacoantigenic uveitis as a well-defined disease associated with the autoimmune process.

Clinical findings

When phacoanaphylactic uveitis is associated with cataract surgery, it usually occurs after an extracapsular extraction, whether by design or mischance. Rarely, after what appears to be an intracapsular extraction, an intense postoperative uveitis alerts one to search for and find a small amount of residual lens material attributable to an unrecognized rupture of the capsule.

The uveitis usually occurs 2 to 4 weeks after what seemed like an uneventful postoperative course. However, the reaction may appear within 48 hours. The duration of the latent period bears no relationship to the severity of the ensuing process, nor is there any relationship between the quantity of liberated lens material and the degree of uveitis. An intense ciliary injection

associated with large mutton-fat keratic precipitates arises. These precipitates are irregular and appear to be mixed with lens material. The aqueous is filled with cells and floating lens debris. Posterior synechia formation is common. Hypopyon may occur in severe cases.

The intraocular pressure may become elevated as lens material and lens-laden macrophages clog the trabecular meshwork. The chamber angle is open. The cornea may become edematous.

Generally, the symptoms abate as the lens material absorbs, but if healing is prolonged, peripheral anterior synechias and a pupillary membrane formed as a result of continued inflammation may aggravate the glaucoma. Cystic degeneration of the macula, retinal detachment, and permanent corneal edema are late findings in neglected cases.

The presence of keratic precipitates in phacoanaphylactic uveitis is often used to differentiate this entity from phacolytic glaucoma. Flocks and co-workers[18] emphasize that the macrophages engorged with lens material are not sticky and therefore do not adhere to the back of the cornea. However, this point of differentiation has

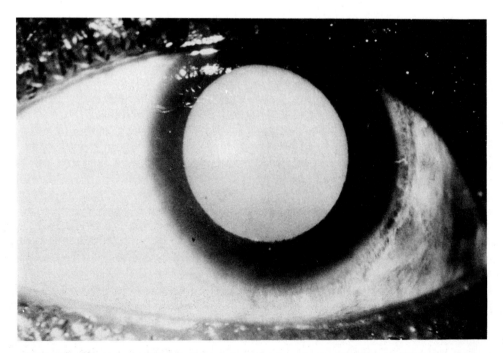

Fig. 24-12. Hypermature cataract in eye with phacolytic glaucoma and uveitis. Note absence of posterior synechias.

been refuted by others[41-43] who have noted keratic precipitates in phacolytic glaucoma.

A more reliable differentiating point may be the presence of posterior synechias in phacoanaphylactic uveitis (Fig. 24-10) and their absence in phacolytic glaucoma (Figs. 24-11 and 24-12). Irvine and Irvine[16] attributed this to the lack of fibrinogen in the latter condition.

There is still no accepted explanation of why some patients with leakage of lens material develop phacolytic glaucoma instead of phacoanaphylactic uveitis.

Pathology

The reaction of phacoanaphylaxis is mainly restricted to the anterior segment of the eye and is marked by several characteristic features.

The inflammatory response centers on retained lens debris, which is found in varying stages of degeneration. The central zone of the activity includes the lens material surrounded principally by polymorphonuclear leukocytes and a smattering of lymphocytes, plasma cells, and eosinophils (Fig. 24-13). This is surrounded by a zone of chronic granulomatous inflammatory cells, including phagocytic epithelioid and giant cells.

Between the uvea and adjacent retained lens material, a fibrovascular proliferation results in widespread adhesions characterized by pupillary and periciliary membranes. These adhesions often involve the operative wound.

Chronic nodular inflammatory foci may be found in the iris and ciliary body, and macrophages may aggregate posteriorly on the surface of the retina.

The bilateral implications of phacoanaphylactic uveitis have played a strong role in establishing the allergic etiology of this disorder, as discussed earlier. Although the inflammation in the operated eye is granulomatous in character, the second eye usually shows a nongranulomatous reaction. This differentiates the condition from sympathetic ophthalmia, as well as the fact that the removal of lens debris from the first eye often results in rapid resolution of the inflammation in both eyes. On the rare occasion when the second eye exhibits a granulomatous inflammation the lens is frequently cataractous, and the capsule may be slightly ruptured. Under these circumstances the differentiation from sympathetic ophthalmia may be very difficult.

Treatment

Phacoanaphylactic uveitis is a surgical condition that should be suspected in any eye after an extracapsular cataract extraction complicated by a granulomatous intraocular inflammation. Although the temptation to temporize by using steroids in these highly inflamed eyes is very strong, this practice must be resisted to the extent that permanent structural deformities are prevented. The prompt removal of the residual lens matter from the anterior chamber usually restores the normal state of the eye in dramatic fashion.

The surgery is probably best performed under general anesthesia, since local anesthesia tends to be less effective in a highly inflamed eye. A hyperosmotic agent administered intravenously is of value. A paracentesis wide enough to permit evacuation of all the lens debris by irrigation is performed. After the anterior chamber lavage the wound is tightly sutured, and steroids are administered during the postoperative course. Irrigation alone is sometimes inadequate. One may need to enlarge the incision and extract the lens remnants with forceps. Alpha-chymotrypsin may be helpful in this situation.

PHACOTOXIC UVEITIS

Although phacotoxic uveitis has been described by Schirmer[8] (1899) and later supported by Straub[9] (1919) and numerous others thereafter, there appears to be some doubt that this represents a clear-cut clinical entity differing from phacoanaphylactic uveitis. As stated previously, Verhoeff and Lemoine[14] considered that although some of the ocular reactions to retained lens material were anaphylactic, others represented a purely toxic reaction to lens protein. Shedding some suspicion on the etiology of this condition are the findings indicating that morgagnian lens material (Knapp,[44] 1927) and lenticular proteins, whether normal, cataractous, or hypermature (Burky and Woods,[45] 1931; Muller,[46] 1963) are not primarily toxic. This fact has prompted Zimmerman[47] to suggest that this condition to be called "phacogenic chronic nongranulomatous uveitis."

The literature states that the clinical findings

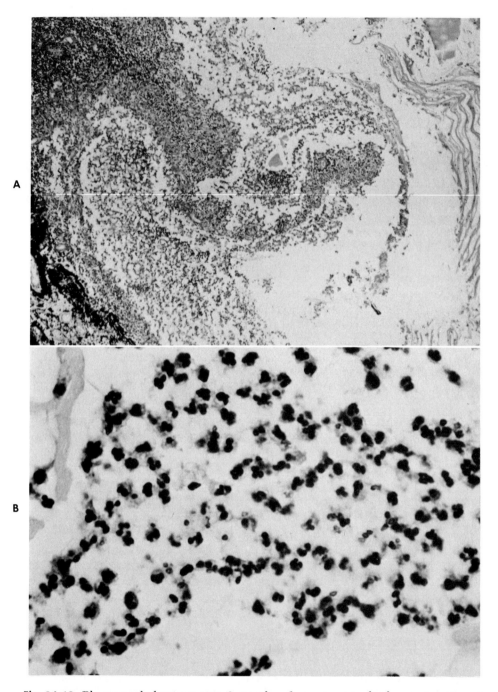

Fig. 24-13. Phacoanaphylactic uveitis 6 months after extracapsular lens extraction. **A,** Severe inflammatory reaction around retained lens debris on right. Iris lower left. **B,** Central zone of activity includes lens material surrounded principally by polymorphonuclear leukocytes.

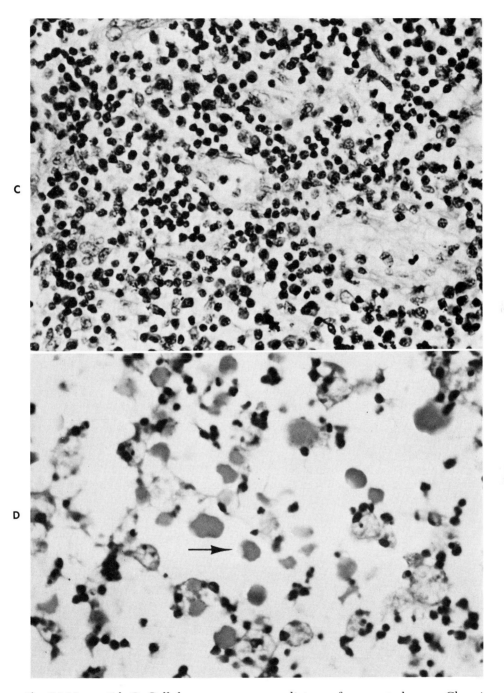

Fig. 24-13, cont'd. C, Cellular response some distance from central zone. Chronic granulomatous inflammatory cells including lymphocytes, epithelioid, and plasma cells. **D,** Macrophages containing lens debris and amorphous Russell bodies *(arrow)* (end stage degeneration of plasma cells).

do not differ from those of phacoanaphylactic uveitis, and the histologic picture is similar, with one exception. The cellular response is primarily an infiltration of lymphocytes and plasma cells. The absence of giant cells and polymorphonuclear leukocytes is said to differentiate the condition.

REFERENCES

1. Duke-Elder, W. S.: System of ophthalmology. Vol. XI. Diseases of the lens and vitreous, glaucoma and hypotony, St. Louis, 1969, The C. V. Mosby Co., pp. 234-236.
2. Hirschberg, J.: Einführung in die Augenheilkunde. II. Hälfte. I. Abt., Leipzig, 1901, G. Thieme Verlag, p. 159.
3. Elschnig, A.: Klinisch-anatomischer Beitrag zur Kenntnis des Nachstares, Klin. Mbl. Augenheilk. 49:444-451, 1911.
4. Cowan, A., and Fry, W. E.: Secondary cataract, with particular reference to transparent globular bodies, Arch. Ophthalmol. 18:12-22, 1937.
5. Thiel, R.: Ein Beitrag zur Spaltlampenmikroskopie des Auges im ultravioletten Licht, Z. Augenheilk. 58:86-91, 1926.
6. Soemmering, D. W.: Beobachtungen über die organischen Veränderungen im Auge nach Staaroperationen, Frankfurt, 1828, W. L. Wesché.
7. Wheeler, J. M.: Secondary cataract opening by single straight incision; iridotomy by same method, Ophthalmology (Rochester) 29:149-158, 1924.
8. Schirmer, O.: Ueber benigne postoperative Cyklitis auf infektiöser Basis. IX Int. Ophthal. Congr., Utrecht, 1899. Abstract in Z. Augenheilk. 2(suppl.):25-26, 1899.
9. Straub, M.: Over ontstekingen van het oog veroorzaaht door oplossing van lensmassa in de oog lymphe, Amsterdam, 1919, Uitgeverij J. H. de Bussy.
10. Elschnig, A.: Spezielle Indikationen zur Staroperation. In Graefe-Saemisch Handbuch der gesamten Augenheilkunde, eds. 2 and 3, Augenärztliche Operationslehre, Berlin, 2:1191, 1922, Springer Verlag.
11. Gifford, S. R., and Steinberg, A. A.: Allergic and toxic properties of lens protein. I. Immune reactions to lens protein, Trans. Sect. Ophthalmol. A.M.A. 76:82-101, 1925.
12. Gifford, H.: The cause of the glaucoma of hypermature cataract, Arch. Ophthalmol. 56:457-459, 1927.
13. Uhlenhuth, P.: Zur Lehre von der Unterscheidung verschiedener Eiweissarten mit Hilfe spezifischer Sera, Festschr, zum 60. Geburtst. v. Robert Koch, Jena, 1903, G. Fischer Verlag, pp. 49-74.
14. Verhoeff, F. H., and Lemoine, A. N.: Endophthalmitis phacoanaphylactica, Int. Congr. Ophthalmol. Washington D.C. 1:234-284, 1922.
15. Raffel, S.: Immunity, ed. 2, New York, 1961, Appleton-Century-Crofts.
16. Irvine, S. R., and Irvine, A. R., Jr.: Lens-induced uveitis and glaucoma. I. Endophthalmitis phaco-anaphylactica, Am. J. Ophthalmol. 35:177-186, 1952.
17. Zeeman, W. P. C.: Zwei Fälle von Glaucoma phacogeneticum mit anatomischem Bufund, Ophthalmologica 106:136-142, 1943.
18. Flocks, M., Littwin, C. S., and Zimmerman, L. E.: Phacolytic glaucoma, Arch. Ophthalmol. 54:37-45, 1955.
19. Epstein, D. L., Jadziniak, J. A., and Grant, W. M.: Identification of heavy–molecular-weight soluble protein in aqueous humor in human phacolytic glaucoma, Invest. Ophthalmol. 17:398-401, 1978.
20. Berg, E. F.: Lens-induced inflammation. In Becker, B., and Burde, R. M.: Current concepts in ophthalmology, St. Louis, 1969, The C. V. Mosby Co., vol. 2, pp. 123-129.
21. Miescher, A.: Experimentelle Untersuchungen zur Pathogenese der sympathischen Ophthalmie, Ophthalmologica 130:128-150, 1955.
22. Ehrlich, G., Halbert, S. P., and Menski, W.: Cytotoxicity of antitissue antibodies. II. Effects of antilens sera in tissue culture, J. Immunol. 89:391-399, 1962.
23. Cooper, S. N.: Immunological study of lens proteins, J. All India Ophthalmol. Soc. 5:23-50, 1957.
24. Luntz, M. H., and Wright, R.: Lens-induced uveitis, Exp. Eye Res. 1:317-323, 1962.
25. Witmer, R.: Phakogene uveitis, Ophthalmologica 133:326-329, 1957.
26. Witmer, R. H.: Phaco-antigenic uveitis, Docum. Ophthalmol. 16:271-276, 1962.
27. Witmer, R. H.: Zur Frage der Auto-Immunerkrankung des Auges: Die phako-antigene Uveitis, Int. Arch. Allergy 24(suppl.):58-64, 1964.
28. de Veer, J. A.: Bilateral endophthalmitis phacoanaphylactica. Pathologic study of the lesion in the eye first involved and, in one instance, the secondarily implicated, or "sympathizing," eye, Arch. Ophthalmol. 49:607-632, 1953.
29. Wirostko, E., and Spalter, H. F.: Lens-induced uveitis, Arch. Ophthalmol. 78:1-7, 1967.
30. Hektoen, L.: Immune reactions of the lens, Am. J. Ophthalmol. 6:276-279, 1923.
31. Rötth, A.: On the question of phacoanaphylactic endophthalmitis, Arch. Ophthalmol. 55:103-112, 1926.
32. Braun, R.: Ueber eine primäre Giftwirkung der Linsensubstanz und ihren Einfluss auf anaphylaktische Experimente, Arch. Augenheilk. 106:99-144, 1932.
33. Goodner, E. K.: Experimental lens-induced uveitis in rabbits. In Maumenee, A. E., and Silverstein, A. M., editors: Immunopathology of uveitis, Third Alfred P. Sloan Symposium, 1963, Baltimore, 1964, The Williams & Wilkins Co., pp. 233-242.
34. Halbert, S. P., Locatcher-Khorazo, D., Swick, L., Witmer, R., Seegal, B., and Fitzgerald, P.: Homologous immunological studies of ocular lens. II. Biological aspects, J. Exp. Med. 105:453-461, 1957.
35. Burgy, E. L., Woods, A. C., and Woodhall, M. B.: Organ specific properties and antigenic power in homologous species of alpha crystallin, Arch. Ophthalmol. 9:446-449, 1933.
36. Makino, M.: Beitrag zu den Linsenantigen. Okayama Igakkai Zasshi 42:1819-1840, 1930. (Abstract in Zbl. Ges. Ophthalmol. 24:215-216, 1931.)
37. Burky, E. L.: Production of lens sensitivity in rabbits by

the action of staphylococcus toxin, Proc. Soc. Exp. Biol. Med. **31:**445-447, 1934.

38. Witmer, R., and Martenet, A. C.: Experimentelle phako-antigene Uveitis, Ber. Deutsche Ophthalmol. Ges. **66:**59-62, 1964.

39. Hackett, E., and Thompson, A.: Anti-lens antibody in human sera, Lancet **2:**663-666, 1964.

40. Halbert, S., and Manski, W.: Symposium on the lens: biological aspects of auto-immune reactions in the lens, Invest. Ophthalmol. **4:**516-530, 1965.

41. Gupta, J. S., and Dhawan, S. K.: A clinical study of phacolytic glaucoma, Eye Ear Nose Throat Mon. **49:**35-40, 1970.

42. Chandler, P. A.: Problems in the diagnosis and treatment of lens-induced uveitis and glaucoma, Arch. Ophthalmol. **60:**828-841, 1958.

43. Brini, A., and Fritz, B. V.: Glaucome phakolytique, Bull. Soc. Ophthalmol. France **64:**70-75, 1964.

44. Knapp, A.: Observations on glaucoma in morgagnian cataract, Arch. Ophthalmol. **56:**124-127, 1927.

45. Burky, E. L., and Woods, A. C.: Lens extract: its preparation and clinical use, Arch. Ophthalmol. **6:**548-553, 1931.

46. Muller, H.: Phacolytic glaucoma and phacogenic ophthalmia (lens-induced uveitis), Trans. Ophthalmol. Soc. U.K. **83:**687-702, 1963.

47. Zimmerman, L. E.: Lens-induced inflammation in human eyes. In Maumenee, A. E., and Silverstein, A. M., editors: Immunopathology of uveitis. Third Alfred P. Sloan Symposium, 1963, Baltimore, 1964, The Williams & Wilkins Co., pp. 221-232.

CHAPTER 25

Iris prolapse

Separation of the healing cataract incision with incarceration or prolapse of uveal tissue through its margins is a serious postoperative complication that is encountered far less frequently than formerly. Improved methods of wound closure and better suture material have reduced its incidence to a virtually insignificant level.

On a clinical basis, it appears proper to divide the inclusion of iris in the lips of the wound into a true prolapse whereby the appearance of a dark blue mass appears under the conjunctival flap or becomes truly externalized and an incarceration wherein the iris merely lines the wound margins. Therefore iris prolapse may be divided into complete and incomplete types.

A complete iris prolapse most frequently occurs within the first few postoperative days and is often associated with a sudden increase in intraocular pressure from restlessness and squeezing of the lids, direct trauma to the eye, coughing, or sneezing. The amount of iris involved depends on the rapidity of onset and the degree of wound rupture. The sudden increase in intraocular pressure and the subsequent wound separation, escape of aqueous, and prolapse of iris usually are accompanied by a sudden pain in the eye.

A delayed form of prolapse may occur weeks or months after surgery. Unlike the complete type, it is gradual in onset and may appear as a small bluish spot or discoloration at the incision line, which slowly enlarges. This is usually an incarceration or incomplete iris prolapse, since the involved iris rarely becomes exteriorized. Because of the continued thrust of the intraocular pressure, a small anterior synechia or incarceration gradually extends over a larger portion of the wound.

In both forms, there is usually a distortion of the pupil, which becomes pear shaped with the apex pointing toward the area of prolapse. In a wide incarceration the wound may appear staphylomatous because of thinning of its posterior layers, which are lined with iris (Fig. 25-1). A filtering bleb may occasionally be found over the prolapse (Fig. 25-2), but usually the iris tissue securely plugs the wound defect so that aqueous does not escape from the eye. The eye usually remains irritable and iritis is frequent.

CAUSES OF IRIS PROLAPSE

1. Poorly executed incision
2. Inadequate wound closure
   a. Insufficient number of sutures
   b. Inadequate placement of sutures
   c. Too rapid absorption of catgut sutures
   d. Too tightly tied nonabsorbable sutures, favoring tissue necrosis
3. Vomiting, coughing, and wheezing
4. Accidental trauma
5. Pupillary block
6. Inadequate iridectomy opening

CONSEQUENCES OF IRIS PROLAPSE

An iris prolapse is never to be regarded lightly. It is much simpler to repair earlier than later, although not every prolapse requires surgical repair. They are always larger than they look, and they tend to worsen with time. If unattended, an iris prolapse may initiate the following variety of serious consequences:

1. *Defective wound healing.* The presence of iris tissue between margins of the wound disturbs the normal pattern of wound healing. The wound may remain weak.

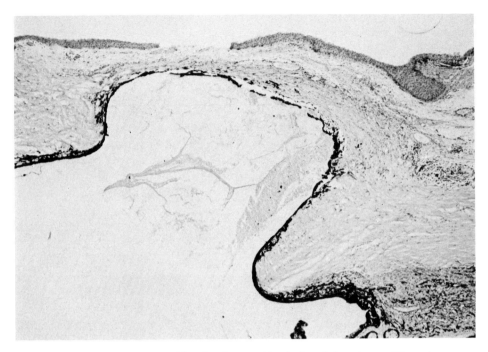

Fig. 25-1. Iris prolapse covered by thin layer of limbal and flap tissue. Wound appears staphylomatous because of thinning of its posterior layers, which are lined with iris.

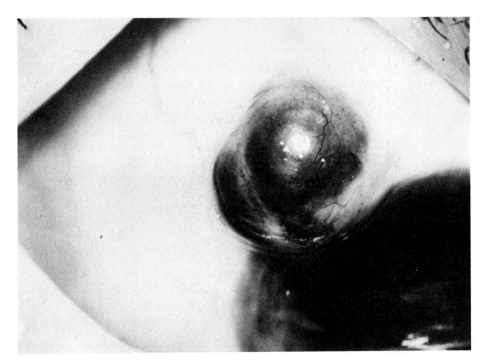

Fig. 25-2. Large iris prolapse with filtering bleb over it.

2. *Cystoid cicatrix.* The prolapsed or incarcerated uveal tissue may act as a wick, allowing aqueous to escape under the conjunctival flap if it is present. Thus a permanent filtering bleb results.
3. *Excessive astigmatism.* Excessive astigmatism invariably results when reasonable wound apposition is prevented and more so when the incision is relatively anterior. When excessive, it may prevent binocular vision.
4. *Flat anterior chamber.*
5. *Hypotension.* Hypotension is usually not serious, but if excessive may cause reduced vision attributable to posterior pole changes.
6. *Corneal complications.* Striate keratopathy or corneal edema may result from defective wound healing hypotension, glaucoma, or iritis.
7. *Iridocyclitis.* Iridocyclitis may result from tugging on the ciliary body because of the stretched iris. Cystoid macular edema may also result.
8. *Endophthalmitis.* This disaster may occur, particularly if the prolapse is uncovered by conjunctiva. However, a thinly covered prolapse is also vulnerable in the same manner as after a filtering operation.
9. *Secondary glaucoma.*
10. *Epithelial downgrowth.* Defective wound healing associated with uveal tissue favors the ingrowth and survival of epithelial cells.
11. *Fibrous ingrowth.* An excessive stromal overgrowth of fibrous elements may result from the same mechanism.
12. *Sympathetic ophthalmitis.* This complication becomes a possibility when uveal tissue accidentally prolapses through the lips of a cataract incision.

PROPHYLAXIS

An iris prolapse, now a rare complication, is usually preventable if the surgeon communicates the preferred postoperative regimen to the patient. The eye should be protected with a plastic shield or shatterproof glasses during the day and with a plastic shield for at least 3 weeks at night. Some patients seem to have an uncontrollable desire to rub their eyes. This rubbing often occurs during sleep. Coughing should be controlled as well as possible with medication. Asthmatics should be treated. Antiemetics should be prescribed when indicated. Tranquilizers and sedatives are often of value.

During surgery, careful attention to the incision and its closure is of paramount importance. An adequate iridectomy opening is necessary to prevent pupillary block. In the case of preservation of a round pupil, multiple peripheral iris openings are better than one.

TREATMENT

The surgical treatment of iris prolapse is never as simple as the appearance of the eye would indicate. It must be approached with caution and a variety of complications must be anticipated. A recent iris prolapse should be treated promptly. An older prolapse that does not appear to be increasing in size and that is not causing significant ocular inflammation is probably best left alone.

There are four general approaches to the treatment of an iris prolapse:
1. Surgical excision or reposition
2. Photocoagulation
3. Cryothermy coagulation
4. Chemical cautery

Surgical excision is best performed under general anesthesia, since local anesthesia is usually difficult to accomplish if the eye is inflamed and the lids are swollen. Also, a retrobulbar injection may cause a greater prolapse of iris along with vitreous. Maximum hypotension is obtained by administering a hyperosmotic agent intravenously (mannitol or urea). If the prolapse is small and less than 48 hours old, an attempt may be made to reposit it. I prefer to make a small limbal stab wound approximately 4 mm from the prolapse. Acetylcholine solution is irrigated into the anterior chamber through this opening. If the pupil constricts and the prolapse retracts into the anterior chamber, the defective area of the wound should be resutured. If not, a very fine iris spatula may be inserted through the limbal wound and the iris reposited in this manner. Although this route appears more devious than repositing the iris directly from without at the site of the prolapse, I have found it more effective. Approximately two thirds of the anterior chamber is filled

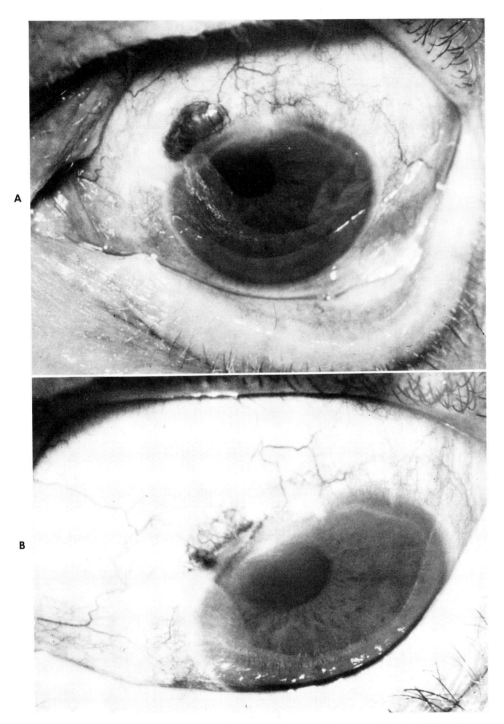

Fig. 25-3. A, Iris prolapse. B, After photocoagulation. (Courtesy Dr. E. W. D. Norton, Miami, Fla.)

with air. This keeps the iris back and tends to seal the defective wound.

In most instances, it is more prudent to excise the prolapsed iris. This is performed by dissecting the conjunctiva from the prolapse and the neighboring limbus. The wound is slightly enlarged on both sides. The margins of the prolapsed iris are freed, and the protruding iris is excised after drawing it slightly from the anterior chamber. The pillars of the sector iridectomy are reposited. The wound is then tightly secured by several sutures in this relatively small area. A subconjunctival injection of a long-acting steroid is used in both of these procedures.

These surgical maneuvers are usually very effective if the anterior hyaloid membrane is intact and if it remains intact during the surgery. However, more often than not, the anterior hyaloid membrane is ruptured, and formed vitreous lines the prolapsed iris. This makes it difficult to reposit the iris, and if it is excised, there is difficulty in preventing the margins of the iridectomy from becoming incarcerated in the wound. The repair is best done under the operating microscope. If the iris can be reposited, as just described, and if the pupil remains centric, nothing further need be done. However, when it appears obvious that this will be impossible because of the presence of considerable vitreous in the anterior chamber, I prefer to open the entire cataract incision, excise the prolapsed portion of iris, and perform a partial anterior vitrectomy, as described on p. 268.

Photocoagulation is occasionally useful in reducing the size of an iris prolapse (Fig. 25-3). It should be reserved for those covered by conjunctiva. A considerable degree of astigmatism will likely remain even if the prolapsed uveal tissue becomes atrophic. I have had no personal experience with this technique.

Cryothermy coagulation of iris prolapse has gained some acceptance in recent years. It does not yield constantly good results. In some instances where the prolapse is well covered by conjunctiva, one may possibly create sufficient iris atrophy so that wound repair is unnecessary. However, I have observed the following results: One or 2 days after treatment, a cystoid bleb occasionally appears at the site of the prolapse and is undoubtedly caused by persistence of the wound defect, which is no longer plugged by iris. This is probably of little significance but could be a source of difficulty if persistent hypotension results or if vitreous prolapses into the bleb. In one instance I treated a 2 mm iris prolapse with a 30-second cryothermy application and observed an enlargement of the prolapse with rupture of the wound and loss of vitreous. One should keep in mind that water expands when frozen, and if aqueous fills the prolapse, it may cause the prolapse to enlarge and rupture the poorly united wound. For this reason, photocoagulation is probably a better technique than cryothermy coagulation.

Cauterization of an iris prolapse by chemical agents such as trichloracetic acid or silver nitrate is probably the least desirable method. Repeated light applications occasionally work, but they are time consuming, since many applications may be necessary. A violent inflammation may result from this method.

CHAPTER 26

Epithelial invasion of the anterior chamber

The invasion of the anterior chamber by epithelium after cataract surgery has been recognized since the nineteenth century, but its diagnosis and therapy continue to confront ophthalmic surgeons with one of their most severe challenges.

HISTORICAL BACKGROUND

Historically, most early reported cases of epithelial formations in the anterior chamber were associated with perforating injuries of the globe. MacKenzie[1] described a posttraumatic semitransparent cyst in the anterior chamber in 1830. In 1872 Rothmund,[2] provided a comprehensive study of epithelial cysts in the iris and anterior chamber, which included 37 cases. Most occurred after injury, but two occurred after cataract extraction. Collins and Cross[3] have often been cited as the first to emphasize epithelial implantation after cataract extraction, but one can see that the condition was known earlier. Many reports follows in the twentieth century. Perera,[4] in 1937, classified epithelial growths within the anterior chamber as (1) "pearl" tumors of the iris, (2) posttraumatic cysts of the iris, and (3) epithelialization of the anterior chamber. This division has been subsequently followed by later authors.

PEARL TUMORS

Epithelial pearl tumors of the iris are almost exclusively discovered after accidental trauma. They usually result from the implantation of a hair follicle or a piece of skin into the anterior chamber coincident with a perforating injury. These growths usually remain small and are confined to the iris. They appear as solid pearly tumors or opaque white cysts on the surface of the iris and are not connected with the wound of entry into the anterior chamber (Fig. 26-1). They usually grow slowly and only rarely exceed 2 to 3 mm in diameter, although exceptions exist. They are fairly firm in consistency and round or oval in shape. They are usually lodged at the anterior surface of the iris. Histologically, they are encapsulated and consist of layers of stratified or cuboidal epithelium sometimes closely resembling that of the cornea or conjunctiva. The central core is composed of either concentric layers of keratinized cells or a necrotic, amorphous mass of keratinized epithelium and cholesterol crystals. Occasionally, hair follicles or foreign bodies are found in the tumor. The lumen of the cyst forms as a result of degeneration of the centrally located cells, which lose their structure, as evidenced by the disappearance of nuclei and the deposition of globules of fat or cholesterol crystals.[5] Since they have only a remote relationship to cataract surgery, they will not be considered further.

EPITHELIAL CYSTS

Although postoperative epithelial cysts and epithelial downgrowths undoubtedly have a similar pathogenesis, separating them is practical, since they show a difference in course, symptomatology, treatment, and prognosis. These differentiating factors are in force only after the anterior chamber has been invaded.

Epithelial cysts appear as translucent or grayish cysts connected with the area of penetration into the anterior chamber. They are caused by invasion of a double continuous layer of epithelium into the anterior chamber that forms a closed cyst. Although they are usually in contact with

505

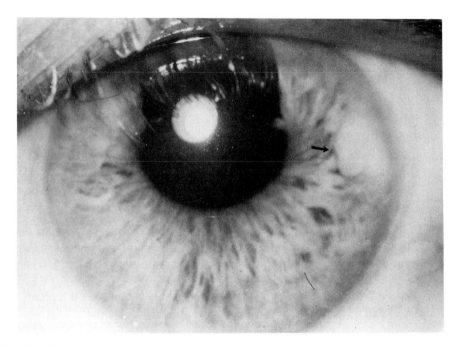

Fig. 26-1. Pearl tumor of iris *(arrow)*. (Courtesy Dr. P. Robb McDonald, Philadelphia.)

the wound of entry or the cataract incision, this continuity may be broken by the interposition of scar tissue.

Pathogenesis

The pathogenesis of these cysts appears to be related primarily to faulty technique at the time of cataract surgery. There is often a history of delayed formation of the anterior chamber associated with defective wound closure. Iris, lens debris, vitreous, and particulate matter may become lodged in the wound. Experimentally, the survival of the transplanted epithelial cells apparently depends on their contact with the iris and a plasmoid aqueous environment (p. 514).[6,7] These conditions are usually met when there is delayed closure of the operative wound. An open path is provided for the entry of the rapidly proliferating epithelial cells of the wound edges. Although hypotension is usually not present at the time an epithelial cyst is clinically recognized, it is probably present for a time after surgery. Once hypotension disappears with final closure of the wound, the implanted cells must fight for survival in a normal aqueous. Possibly these cells, which have been in contact with iris

or angle structures and which have been bathed by a plasmoid aqueous for several weeks, have the potentiality for cyst formation or downgrowth as a sheet over the back of the cornea and anterior surface of the iris.

We do not know what factors determine the ultimate growth characteristics of the implanted epithelial cells. Hogan and Goodner[8] have postulated that a small mass of epithelial cells near a wound edge and in contact with iris or angle structures, which survives for a few weeks and then loses contact with the surface after final wound closure, would be deterred from growing as a sheet over the cornea and iris by the more normal aqueous present after wound closure. These cells probably derive sufficient nutrition from the iris or angle structures to permit multiplication of those cells on the surface of the mass, whereas those in the center become necrotic and are replaced by fluid derived from the aqueous, thus producing a cyst. The final survival and growth of the cyst results from a balance between the growth potential of the cells and the inhibiting effects of normal or nearly normal aqueous humor. If would closure is delayed for much longer periods of time — in the presence of a fistu-

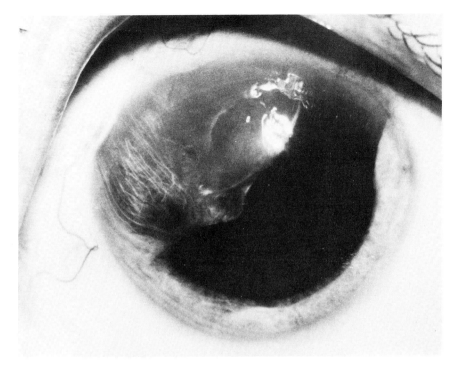

Fig. 26-2. Epithelial cyst after cataract extraction. Cyst is continuous with operative wound and is in contact with iris on left. (Courtesy Dr. E. Hersh, Hollywood, Fla.)

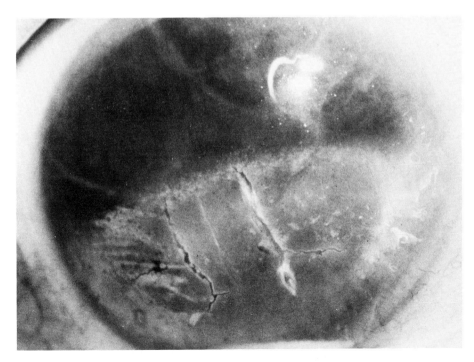

Fig. 26-3. Multiloculated epithelial cyst filling entire anterior chamber after cataract extraction. Extensive band keratopathy.

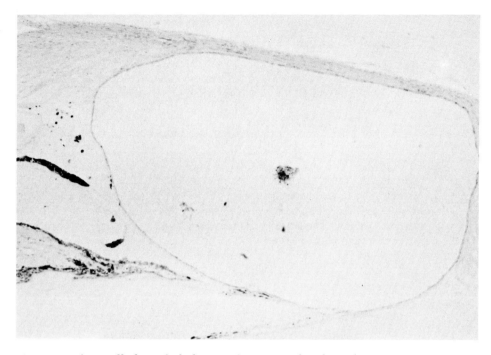

Fig. 26-4. Thin-walled epithelial cyst of anterior chamber after cataract extraction. (Hematoxylin and eosin, ×110.)

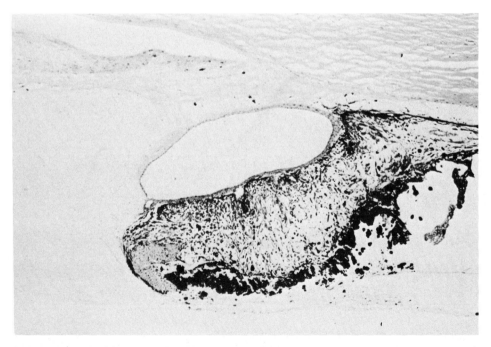

Fig. 26-5. Epithelial cyst in contact with iris after cataract extraction. Continuity with wound is broken. (Hematoxylin and eosin, ×125.)

la, for example—the presence of plasmoid aqueous supplies nourishment for the invading epithelium, which becomes adapted to its new environment and continues its relentless growth as a sheet over the back of the cornea and the iris.

Although it has been suspected for some time that epithelial cysts may result from implantation of epithelial cells at the time of surgery, little attention has been given to this possibility until recently. In such instances the cyst would not be connected with the point of entry into the anterior chamber. Ferry[9] observed two examples of a plaque of stratified squamous epithelium on the iris surface of two iridectomy specimens taken from eyes undergoing cataract extraction. He suggested that introduction of surface epithelium into the interior of the eye by contaminated instruments may be a pathogenetic factor in epithelial growths within the anterior chamber after intraocular surgery. Bennett and D'Amico[10] reached a similar conclusion after observing the development of an epithelial implantation cyst of the iris after a penetrating keratoplasty. The presence of good wound apposition throughout the postoperative course and the location of the cyst within the iris stroma suggested contamination with epithelial cells by instrumentation at the time of performing the peripheral iridectomies. They suggested a second set of instruments for intraocular manipulation.

Clinical findings

The early clinical findings may be a slight pupillary distortion or displacement of an iris pillar toward the site of the cyst. The signs and symptoms depend to some extent on the rate of growth of the cyst. This rate may be extremely variable. The cysts may be dormant for many years and cause no disturbance. When growth occurs, iridocyclitis and secondary glaucoma with its accompanying signs and symptoms often occur. These cysts may become huge, occupying almost the entire anterior chamber (Figs. 26-2 and 26-3). If the pupillary space is invaded, a decrease in vision results.

Pathology

Epithelial cysts are usually thin walled (Fig. 26-4), fairly transparent, and filled with a straw-colored fluid containing protein and some cho-

lesterol. They are circumscribed and localized and can be transilluminated. They may be in contact with the wound, but usually the continuity is broken by the time the cyst is recognized (Fig. 26-5). The posterior wall is often partially pigmented, especially when the cyst is in contact with the iris. The cyst may enter the posterior chamber through an iridotomy or even by eroding through the iris. It may then appear as a pigmented lesion and even be mistaken for a melanoma (Figs. 26-6 and 26-7).

Treatment

The treatment of epithelial cysts should be undertaken if the cyst is growing and if the eye is irritated. Many surgical techniques have been described, and new methods continue to be reported.

A recent method described by Ferry and Naghdi[11] employed a cryosurgical technique to treat an epithelial cyst that filled one third of the anterior chamber. The posterior wall of the cyst was adherent to iris stroma. The cyst was perforated with a fine needle. The needle was re-

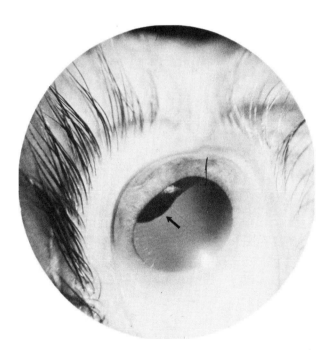

Fig. 26-6. Epithelial cyst entering posterior chamber through iridotomy and appearing as pigmented lesion that may be mistaken for melanoma. (Courtesy Dr. P. Robb McDonald, Philadelphia.)

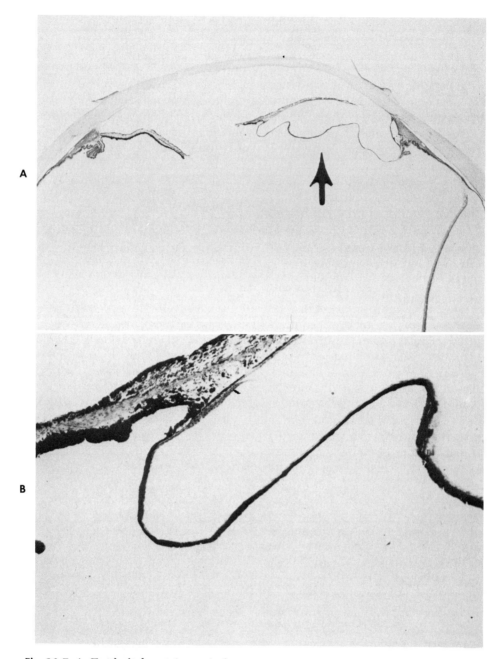

Fig. 26-7. A, Epithelial cyst *(arrow)* after cataract extraction in contact with wound. **B,** Same eye, showing pigmentation of posterior wall of cyst.

moved, and a cryostylet was placed within the sac. A temperature of 0 to −10° F was applied for 15 seconds. The sac of the cyst and the adherent iris were than exteriorized and excised. A safer modification of this method consists of aspiration of cyst contents followed by cryothermy over the chamber angle and photocoagulation to cyst remnants on the iris.[12]

Hogan and Goodner[8] described a relatively simple technique using diathermy coagulation. Diathermy coagulation was successfully used earlier by Vail[13] in three cases of traumatic im-

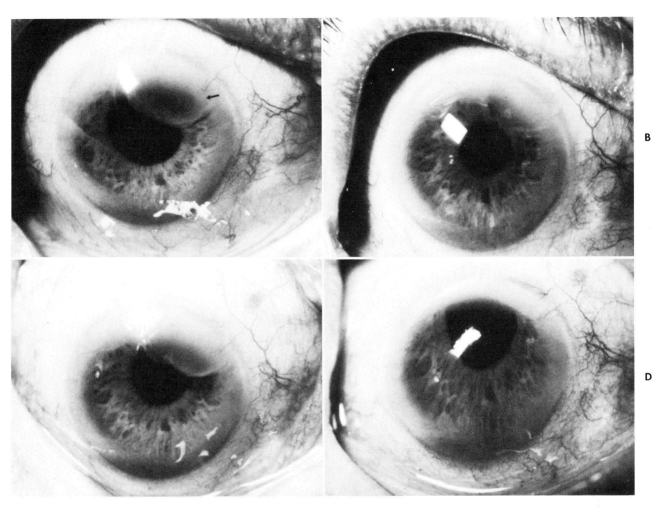

Fig. 26-8. **A,** Pretreatment epithelial implantation cyst *(arrow)*, September 11, 1972. **B,** Cyst showing marked reduction in size 1 month after initial photocoagulation treatment, October 24, 1972. **C,** Photograph showing recurrence of cyst prior to second photocoagulation treatment, November 29, 1972. **D,** Collapse of cyst 3 months after photocoagulation treatment, October 23, 1973. Note updrawn pupil. (From Okun, E., and Mandell, A.: Trans. Am. Ophthalmol. Soc. **72:**170-183, 1974.)

plantation cyst. This is by no means a new procedure because it has been reported by several authors, including Safar[14] in 1935.

Electrocoagulation or electrolysis has been used.[15,16] Radiotherapy has been used with uncertain success.[4,17] Aspirations have been performed with injections of material such as iodine,[18] radioisotopes,[19] and other sclerosing solutions such as 50% glucose,[20] carbolic acid, or trichloracetic acid. Sugar[21] reported posterior lamellar resection of the involved cornea togeth-

er with an excision of the involved iris. In addition to corneal edema and vitreous loss, in one instance this complicated surgical procedure was associated with an expulsive hemorrhage.[22]

Maumenee and Shannon[23] reported the subtotal removal or attempted total removal from the anterior chamber of 11 epithelial cysts. They recommend that large iridectomies in the area of the cyst and gentle denudation of the involved posterior corneal surface be part of the procedure. They emphasize early surgical removal if the cyst

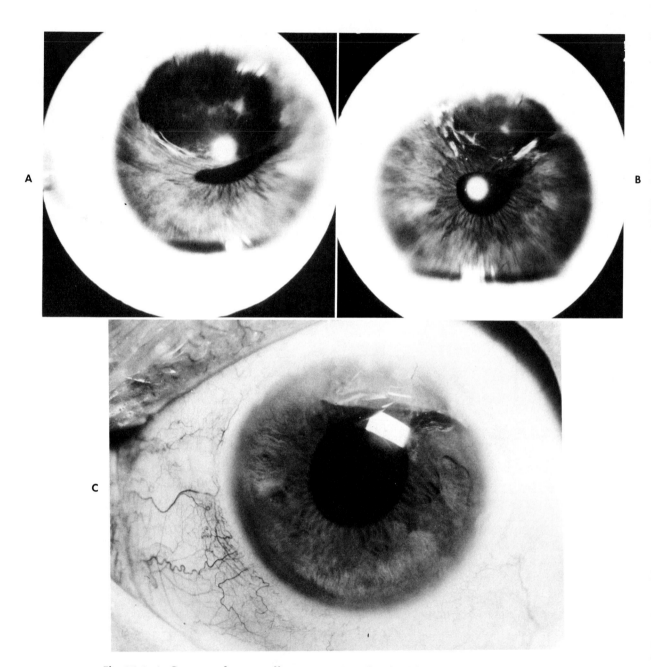

Fig. 26-9. A, Cyst invading pupillary space, March 25, 1971, prior to photocogulation treatment. **B,** Shrinkage of cyst approximately 1 month after initial treatment, April 27, 1971. **C,** Collapse of cyst 2 years following sixth photocoagulation treatment, May 6, 1974. (From Okun, E., and Mandell, A.: Trans. Am. Ophthalmol. Soc. **72:**170-183, 1974.)

is increasing in size or causes an iridocyclitis. There was no evidence of recurrence, complications, or epithelial downgrowth in any of these cases, which were followed for an average of 2 years and 9 months. This is undoubtedly a more hazardous procedure than the ones described previously but has produced good results in the hands of these authors. However, 19 years later, Harbin and Maumenee[24] emphasized the need for conservative management of epithelial cysts. Six patients had epithelial cysts converted into epithelial sheets or downgrowth after surgical intervention. Although surgical excision is effective in some cases, it presents, in addition to this complication, the possibility of corneal edema, glaucoma, and vitreous loss.

Okun and Mandell[25] successfully treated three epithelial implantation cysts following cataract surgery by employing xenon arc photocoagulation. This utilizes the principle of localized coagulation and convection of heat in a fluid-containing closed system. Using the surface coagulator of the Zeiss photocoagulator at a setting of 4.5° and G3 intensity, the spot was focused at the pigmented base of the iris cyst. The light was then delivered for approximately 1 to 3 seconds at a time, the end point being the production of very rapid movement of the fine particles within the cyst. If constriction of iris tissue is noted, this serves as an end point. Approximately 10 such applications are made over the entire cyst base at each session. One patient required six photocoagulation treatments (Fig. 26-8), the second, five treatments (Fig. 26-9), and the third, four treatments. In no case was an attempt made to turn the anterior cyst wall white for fear of corneal endothelial damage. The effect of photocoagulation is not often immediate and requires several weeks following treatment for shrinkage to occur. Photocoagulation does not completely eliminate the cyst wall but does appear to permanently damage and collapse it.

One should not lose sight of the fact these cysts can lie dormant for years and should not be treated until definite growth is seen.

EPITHELIAL DOWNGROWTH
Incidence

Epithelial downgrowth is a far more serious problem than epithelial cyst. Although it is a clin-

Table 26-1. Epithelial downgrowth in globes enucleated after cataract extraction

Author	Globes enucleated after cataract extraction	Epithelial downgrowth
Bernardino et al.[26]	181	13 or 7.2%
Perera[4]	35	4 or 11.4%
Theobold and Haas[7]	75	14 or 18.7%
Blodi[27] (senile)	251	63 or 25.1%
Dunnington[28]		
1929-1940	53	8 or 15.1%
1941-1954	118	54 or 45.7%
Shulze and Duke[29] (senile)	100	17 or 17.0%
Payne[30]		
1930-1955	333	60 or 18.0%
1955-1957	31	5 or 16.1%
Patz[31]	889	113 or 12.0%
Hervoüe[32]	163	27 or 16.6%
Allen[33]	50	13 or 26.0%
TOTAL	2279	391 or 17.2%

ically rare occurrence, it is present in 15% to 20% of globes enucleated after cataract extraction. Table 26-1 emphasizes this amount.

Theobold and Haas[7] reported an incidence of 1.1% of histologically verified cases of epithelial downgrowth after 8000 cataract extractions. Otradovec and Zicha[34] found seven cases (diagnosis made clinically) out of 3089 cataract extractions (0.2%). Christensen[35] observed eight cases out of 700 cataract extractions (1%) performed by the house staff at the University of Oregon Medical School from 1945 to 1951. After a change in surgical technique in 1961, no cases have been observed in over 4000 cataract extractions. These figures must be evaluated in the light of the fact that many eyes remain clinically undiagnosed until histologic examination is performed after enucleation.

The pathogenesis of epithelial downgrowth is not fully understood, since attempts to produce it experimentally have been largely unsuccessful. Regan[36] has provided an excellent review of the experimental attempts to produce epithelial invasion of the anterior chamber.

Experimental findings

Gundersen[37] transplanted free pieces of cornea including epithelium into the anterior chambers of cats and rabbits and concluded that the disappearance of corneal epithelium indicated that the aqueous humor was not a satisfactory medium. He pointed out that clinically, blood vessels were always found in proximity to epithelial ingrowths, whereas epithelial cysts probably derive nutritional support from iris or other uveal tissue.

Cogan[38] was able to produce several iris cysts within the iris stroma of rabbits after implantation of free pieces of conjunctiva in the anterior chamber. He found, however, that epithelium rapidly spread over the surface of the iris during the first few days but then ceased to grow. When the implant adhered to the cornea without an iris connection, the stroma was preserved, but the epithelium disappeared. The lack of mitotic activity in epithelial cells within the anterior chamber led Cogan to believe that epithelial extension is not an active growth process but a spread by sliding and that a vascular substrate is needed if the epithelial cells are to remain viable.

Corrado[39] introduced corneal flaps into the anterior chambers of rabbits and placed a celluloid strip between the edge of the wound and the flap for 15 days. Under these circumstances the corneal flap was preserved within the anterior chamber and became adherent to the iris. Moreover, if it was placed against the anterior surface of the lens, a spread of epithelium over the adjacent iris nearly always occurred. He concluded that hypotension resulting from an open wound was necessary for the viability of the corneal flap and that epithelial proliferation occurred when epithelial cells were in contact with a smooth surface.

Dunnington and Regan[40] observed growth of epithelium along the track of deeply placed silk sutures. It extended about 1 mm into the anterior chamber but produced neither the clinical nor the histologic appearance of true epithelial invasion.

Binder and Binder[41] and Bick[42] found that anticoagulants inhibited the formation of the fibrinous coagulum formed by the secondary aqueous. Binder and Binder also observed that in the presence of a serum prothrombin level less than 30% of normal early fibroblast formation was inhibited, and the epithelium was permitted to grow freely along the wound edges as far as the anterior chamber. In such eyes, epithelium soon completely lined both lips of a corneal incision, but in no instance did the epithelium invade the anterior chamber.

Regan[36] performed experiments in rhesus monkeys and produced growth of epithelium by various techniques. These growths resembled cysts of the iris and anterior chamber but in only two instances showed some of the histologic but not clinical characteristics of epithelialization of the anterior chamber. To have epithelial growth within the anterior chamber, the epithelial cells had to be in contact with iris stroma.

Thus experimental studies indicate that epithelium may invade the anterior chamber by implantation of free or attached epithelium or by spread along an irregular incision or smooth surface extending through the wound. For epithelium to proliferate in the anterior chamber, a more nutritious medium than aqueous appears to be required. This medium is supplied by the iris. Having established a supporting base on the iris, epithelium can spread by sliding over cornea, lens matter, and vitreous.

To supply an experimental model of epithelial growth in the anterior chamber, Smith and coworkers[43] performed reverse 4 mm corneal grafts in rabbits. The trephined corneal button was reversed and sutured in place. Epithelium-like tissue was found growing in the anterior chamber in more than 50% of the eye 4 weeks and longer postoperatively. Histologic examination suggested that this was in fact the same epithelium that was placed in the anterior chamber by the reverse corneal graft. The tissue consisted of cells indistinguishable from surface epithelial cells.

Pathogenesis

One would probably be fair in stating that most instances of epithelial downgrowth result from faulty surgical technique, although in some eyes the complication is unavoidable. The chief prerequisite is a cut proliferating edge of epithelium in contact with a fistula into the anterior chamber. Epithelial implantation of itself apparently is not sufficient to produce downgrowth. The wound must remain open for some time, and there must be some contact between the wound and adjacent uveal tissue. The wound may remain open because of some defect of wound healing, too deeply placed sutures, an imperfect incision, and incarceration of material such as lens remnants, uveal tissue, vitreous, or particulate debris between the lips of the wound. Allen[32] examined 20 eyes with epithelial downgrowth histologically and found iris tissue in 17 incarcerated in the incision or in contact with the incision. There is often a marked delay in restoration of the anterior chamber after surgery.

Dunnington[28] felt that the more widespread use of corneoscleral sutures in cataract surgery in the early 1950s probably was responsible for a higher incidence of epithelial downgrowth. However, just the opposite now appears to be true. A study by Allen and Duehr[44] of 5246 cataract operations revealed that multiple corneoscleral sutures do not cause an increase in epithelial downgrowths. It now appears that better methods of closing the incision, better suture material, better instrumentation, and a lessened frequency of operative loss of vitreous have lessened its incidence.

Although this complication is often preceded by an uneventful cataract extraction and an uneventful early postoperative course, it is more likely that the surgery and convalescent period are marked by some trauma, late loss of the anterior chamber, hyphema, iris incarceration or prolapse, late rupture of the anterior face of the vitreous with incarceration in the wound, or iridocyclitis.

For many years investigators[7,45] have stated that a limbus-based flap was superior to a fornix-based flap or to no flap at all in preventing epithelial downgrowth. My own personal experience of using a fornix-based flap for over 20 years refutes this statement. In addition, Maumenee and co-workers[46] examined 40 eyes with histologically proved epithelial downgrowth and stated, "We were unable to determine the often-quoted statement that epithelial downgrowth is more commonly found in eyes having had a fornix-based flap rather than a limbus-based flap at the time of cataract surgery." Before modern improvements were made in wound closure the limbus-based flap probably gave increased protection. However, this type of flap might actually be more hazardous if suture technique is faulty, since the conjunctiva may be incarcerated into the wound by the suture. Closing the wound under the flap is theoretically better. It is probably beneficial to keep the cut proliferating edge of the conjunctival flap well away from the operative incision, since epithelium at the edge can migrate through a fistulous tract and therefore into the eye. Christensen[35] observed that the epithelium, however, is incapable of eroding even the flimsiest obstructions, such as fibrin. In this respect, this migrating growth pattern differs from the truly invasive action of malignant tissue that is capable of eroding through an obstruction as well as migrating along surfaces. Intact basal epithelium also fills crevices, but it is incapable of the migratory action of the cut proliferating edge.

After Dunnington and Regan's[47] study of epithelial migration along the track of a silk suture and the apparent prevention of this migration along the track of a catgut suture, it appeared that the suture material itself might be important in pathogenesis. It has been shown subsequently that epithelium may grow down the track of a catgut suture, although it probably does this less readily than with silk. Whether the latter is caused by the smooth structure of silk, as Matsumoto[48] suggests, or by the difference in cellular response to the two substances is unknown. The truth may be that silk favors epithelial growth along its track because it does not have a tendency to swell and mechanically inhibit epithelial downgrowth, as does catgut.

Paufique and Hervouët[32] have found a high incidence of epithelial downgrowth in young patients, highly myopic people, and diabetics. When linear cataract extractions were performed in infants and young children, downgrowths were favored by the difficulties in suturing the thin tissues of the young eye. The same might apply to the eye with a high degree of myopia. The tendency for some diabetics to show poor wound healing might contribute to the role of this disease in favoring epithelial downgrowth.

Clinical findings

There are a number of signs and symptoms that should lead the surgeon to suspect the possibility of epithelial downgrowth. The patient may com-

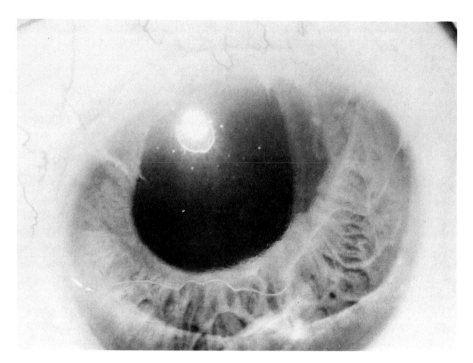

Fig. 26-10. Epithelial downgrowth after cataract extraction. Gray line retouched. Overlying cornea slightly edematous.

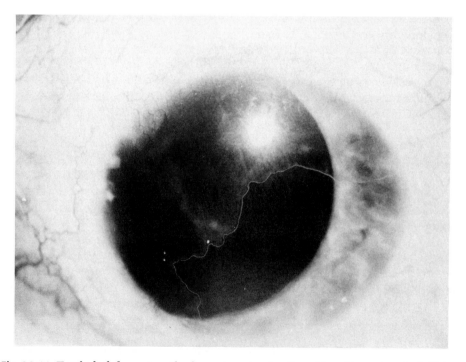

Fig. 26-11. Epithelial downgrowth after cataract extraction. Gray line retouched. Triangular epithelial involvement of vitreous plainly visible.

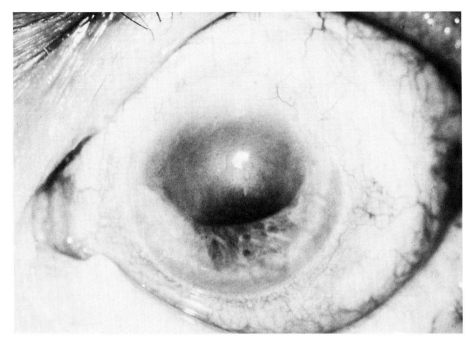

Fig. 26-12. Epithelial downgrowth after cataract extraction. Overlying cornea markedly edematous.

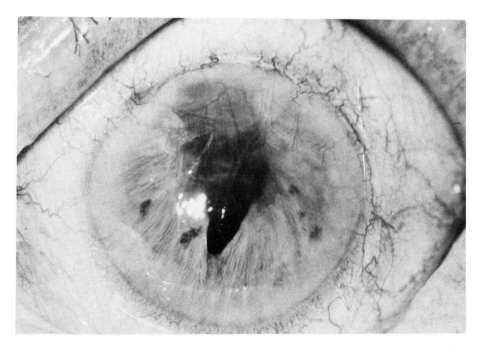

Fig. 26-13. Epithelial downgrowth after cataract extraction. Vascularization of deep layers of stroma.

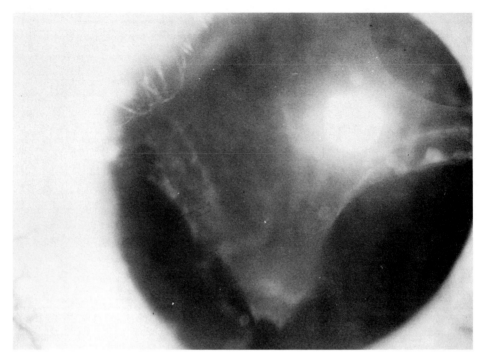

Fig. 26-14. Same eye as in Fig. 26-11. Epithelial sheet over anterior face of vitreous.

plain of tearing, photophobia, and pain after a relatively normal early postoperative course. Hypotonia may be present, and this should lead one to make a careful search for a fistula. An inordinate amount of Descemet's folds may be present, and there may be an associated iridocyclitis. The symptoms and signs often show great variation in intensity, especially if the patient shows a temporary improvement with steroid therapy.

Before long, the typical picture of the advancing border of the epithelial downgrowth on the back of the cornea is observed. This consists of a fine gray line that marks the advancing border of the thin, translucent membrane on the posterior surface of the cornea (Figs. 26-10 and 26-11). The cornea overlying the downgrowth is occasionally edematous (Fig. 26-12), and newly formed vessels may or may not be present in the deep layers of the stroma (Fig. 26-13). The iris may show loss of markings and may be drawn up toward the incision. A sheet of epithelium may be found on the vitreous (Fig. 26-14), especially where a sector iridectomy has been done. Significant corneal edema may be present. As the invasion proceeds over the angle structures, an in-

tractable secondary glaucoma usually results. Given sufficient time, the outcome in the untreated eye is invariably unfavorable. However, in some eyes the course may be very gradual and is of some significance in an elderly patient.

Pathology

In most pathologic specimens, surface epithelium is observed to extend some distance into the surgical wound. Occasionally, its continuity to the anterior chamber can be demonstrated. Vascularization in the cornea is often found, especially in the deep stroma near the surgical wound.

The most typical findings depend on the extent and character of the epithelialization. This consists of stratified squamous epithelium of the conjunctival or corneal type extending down over the back of the cornea (Fig. 26-15). It rarely passes more than one third the way down the cornea. Its advancing edge is usually irregular and wavy (Fig. 26-16). The layer is usually thin, being one cell or only a few cells thick. At the margin of the lesion, there is usually a piling up of cells, which probably accounts for the gray

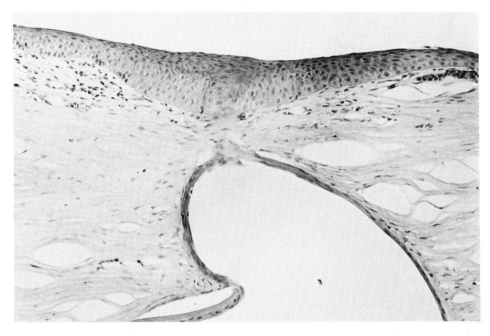

Fig. 26-15. Epithelial downgrowth after cataract extraction. Section adjacent to fistula, showing stratified squamous epithelium lining wound dehiscence. (Courtesy P. H. Y. Chee, Honolulu.)

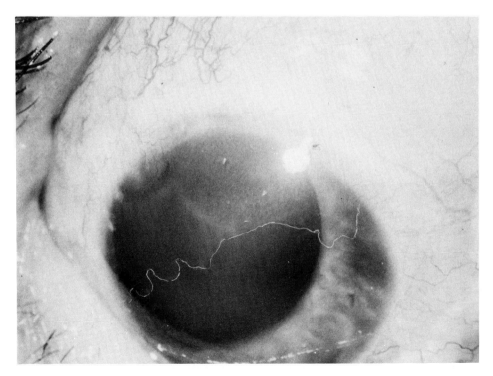

Fig. 26-16. Epithelial downgrowth after cataract extraction. Typically irregular and wavy gray line on back of cornea. (Retouched.)

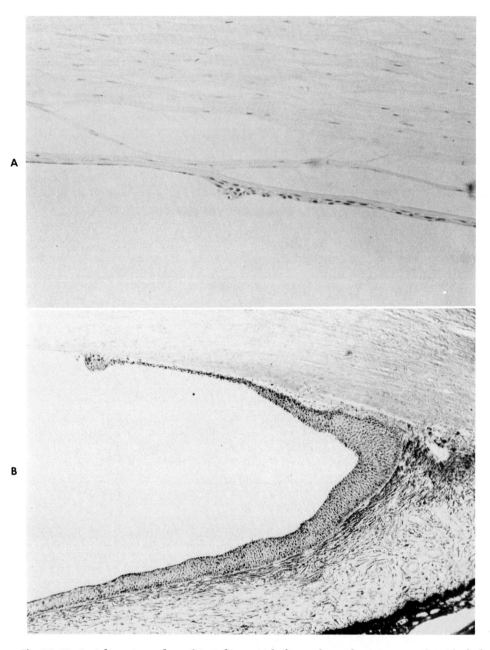

Fig. 26-17. A, Advancing edge of invading epithelium shows heaping up of epithelial cells to account for gray line seen clinically. **B,** Experimental production of epithelialization of anterior chamber in monkey eye 7 months after implantation of free conjunctiva. Note heaping up of epithelium at advancing edge of growth on back or cornea. (**A** courtesy P. H. Y. Chee, Honolulu; **B** from Regan, E. F.: Arch. Ophthalmol. **60:**907-927, 1958.)

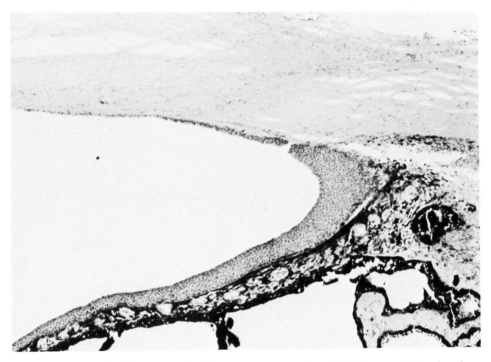

Fig. 26-18. Epithelial downgrowth after cataract extraction. Cellular growth in chamber angle and on anterior surface of iris is more luxuriant, exceeding that on back of cornea. (Trichrome, ×110.)

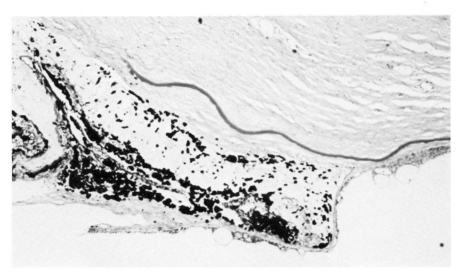

Fig. 26-19. Epithelial downgrowth after cataract extraction. Cellular growth over back of cornea and iris stump and onto ciliary body. (Periodic acid–Schiff, ×125.)

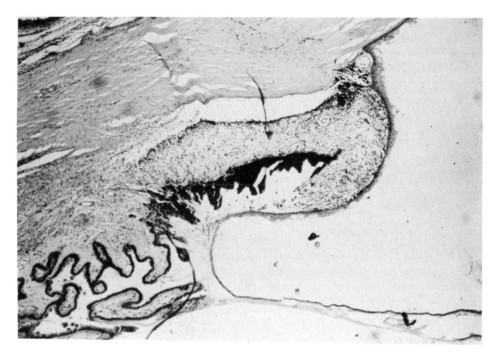

Fig. 26-20. Epithelial downgrowth after cataract extraction. Cellular growth causes inversion of iris and extends over anterior face of vitreous. (Trichrome, ×125.)

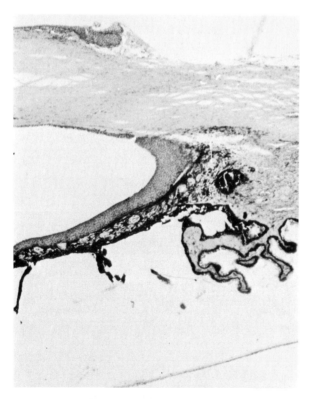

Fig. 26-21. Epithelial downgrowth after cataract extraction. Same eye as in Fig. 26-18. Epithelial growth over anterior face of vitreous resembles that on back of cornea, with membrane being one cell thick or, at best, a few cells thick. (Trichrome.)

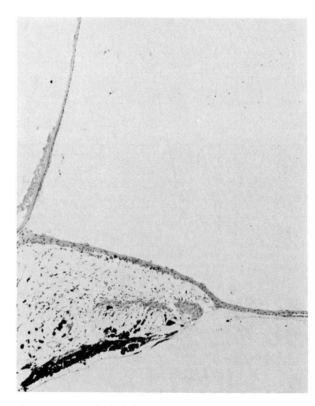

Fig. 26-22. Epithelial downgrowth after cataract extraction. Epithelium extends from anterior surface of iris to anterior face of vitreous. (Periodic acid–Schiff, ×125.)

line seen clinically (Fig. 26-17). Cellular growth in the chamber angle and on the anterior surface of the iris is more luxuriant and exceeds that found on the back of the cornea (Fig. 26-18) in almost every case. This may be attributable to the nourishing bed supplied by the uveal tissue. The epithelium extends over the anterior surface of the iris, through the pupil, over the posterior surface of the iris, and on to the ciliary body (Fig. 26-19). The coating of epithelium may cause an ectropion uveae, or the iris may show an inversion (Fig. 26-20). Extension of epithelium over the anterior face of the vitreous occurs frequently. The involvement here resembles that over the

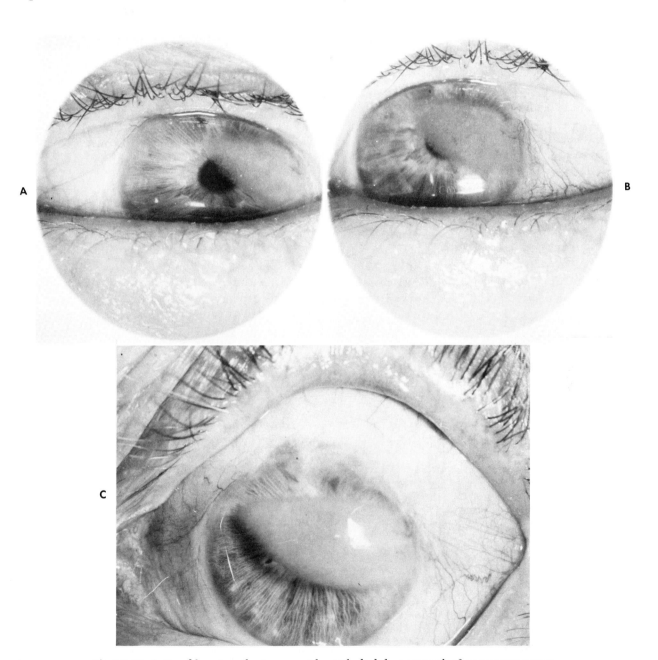

Fig. 26-23. A, Band keratopathy in eye with epithelial downgrowth after cataract extraction. **B,** Same eye 6 months later. **C,** Same eye 16 months after **A.**

back of the cornea, with the membrane being only one or, at best, a few cells thick (Figs. 26-21 and 26-22).

Glaucoma occurs frequently, although surprisingly, its mechanism may be varied. It occurs with a high incidence in those eyes that are ultimately enucleated. The glaucoma may result from epithelium lining the angle structures. However, some authors have observed that the chamber angle was usually closed by synechias when glaucoma was present.[49] Bernardino and co-workers[26] observed that dense anterior synechias occluded the angles, whereas the epithelium could be seen to line the false angle created by these adhesions in nine of their 12 patients with glaucoma. Anterior synechia formation is probably secondary to a wound leak occurring immediately or shortly after the cataract surgery. As suggested by Chandler and Grant,[50] pupillary block glaucoma may result from an epithelial occlusion membrane from downgrowth over the anterior surface of the vitreous. Terry and co-workers[49] also observed obstruction of the trabecular meshwork by "desquamating epithelium in the form of particulate matter," and this may cause glaucoma, a mechanism resembling that seen in phacolytic glaucoma where macrophages plug the angle meshwork.

Band keratopathy may be present,[26,51,52] although it is not a common finding (Fig. 26-23).

The occurrence of epithelial downgrowth in both eyes of the same individual after cataract extraction is very rare, but it has been reported.[26,51]

Diagnosis

The diagnosis may be made by considering the history and the signs just described. In addition, three useful procedures may be performed.

Seidel's test. A drop or two of 2% fluorescein is placed into the eye. A careful search is made for an aqueous leak. It is better to use such a fluorescein preparation instead of paper fluorescein strips because of the greater concentration obtained. The globe may be stroked gently to aid in finding the leak. Although a wound leak is probably present in every case at some time during the progress of the downgrowth, it is found in only 25% to 35% of eyes when searched for at the slit lamp, using a cobalt blue filter. A search for a leak in the operating room is often more productive.

Photocoagulation of the surface of the iris. Maumenee[53] has recommended the use of the photocoagulator to diagnose the presence of epithelium over the face of the iris, since it is sometimes difficult to determine this with the slit lamp. If epithelium is present, a white cotton-fluff ball forms immediately on the iris. This may also be used to determine the extent of iris involvement. Maumenee has found that this technique never fails to indicate the presence of epithelium on the iris when it is present.

Scraping of the back of the cornea. Scraping of the back of the cornea and microscopic examina-

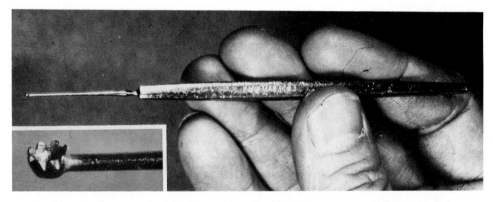

Fig. 26-24. One-millimeter serrated corneal foreign body curette used to engage suspected downgrowth material from back of cornea. (From Calhoun, F. P., Jr.: Am. J. Ophthalmol. **61** [pt. 2]:115-119, 1966.)

tion of the curetted material can often make the distinction between epithelium and endothelium. Calhoun[54] passes a 1 mm serrated corneal foreign-body curette (E. V. Mueller and Company, Chicago, Ill.) through a stab wound just inside the limbus (Fig. 26-24). The edges of the curette then gently engage the suspected downgrowth material, which clings to the teeth of the instrument like a cobweb, allowing a portion of it to be withdrawn from the eye. The operating microscope is of considerable help in this procedure. Using extremely fine pointed jeweler's forceps, the surgeon removes and spreads out the material engaged in the curette over a microscopic slide that has been coated with egg albumin. This adheres the tiny specimen to the slide, which should then be placed in a Coplin jar containing equal parts of alcohol and ether to fix the tissue and to prevent drying until staining. A hematoxylin and eosin stain is performed. It is not difficult to differentiate the evenly spaced cells and round nuclei of endothelium from squamous epithelial cells, which are more closely packed together and whose cytoplasm is denser and nuclei more rod shaped (Figs. 26-25 and 26-26).

Biopsy. A small biopsy taken from the suspected area close to the limbus will also help make the diagnosis (Fig. 26-27).

Specular microscopy. Specular microscopy may assist in the clinical diagnosis of epithelial downgrowth.[55] Although the technique requires a very cooperative patient and a great deal of patience on the part of the specular microscopist to bring the proper posterior corneal area into focus, the finding of a pattern of cell borders in suspected cases suggests that this method may be useful in diagnosing epithelial downgrowth. The pattern consists of a sharply defined border between normal corneal endothelial cells and the area of the epithelial downgrowth (Figs. 26-28 and 26-29). The border is observed with the endothelium in focus. The downgrowth itself appears devoid of structure at this focus. By adjusting the focus to a deeper plane in the area of the downgrowth, a pattern of interlacing borders

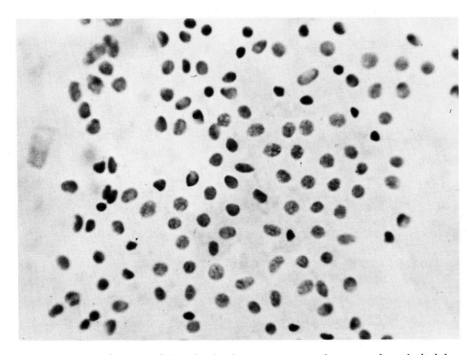

Fig. 26-25. Material removed from back of cornea in case of suspected epithelial downgrowth after cataract extraction. Note evenly spaced cells and round nuclei typical of endothelium. (Hematoxylin and eosin.) (From Calhoun, F. P., Jr.: Am. J. Ophthalmol. **61**[pt. 2]:115-119, 1966.)

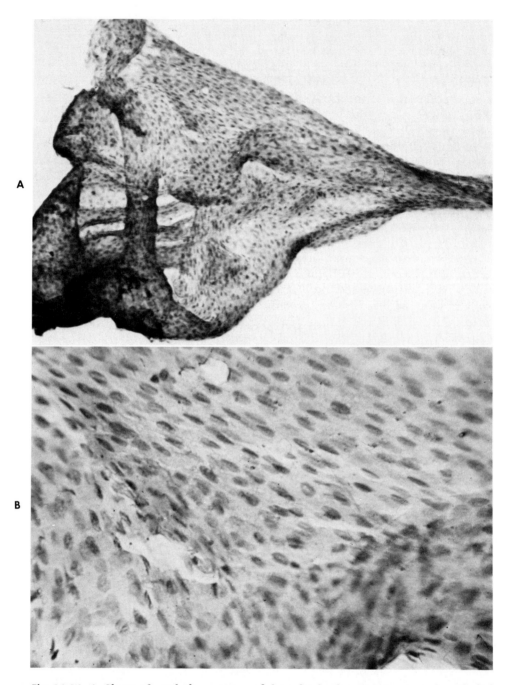

Fig. 26-26. A, Sheet of epithelium removed from back of cornea in case of epithelial downgrowth after cataract extraction. **B,** High-power view of epithelial cells. (Hematoxylin and eosin.) (From Calhoun, F. P., Jr.: Am. J. Ophthalmol. **61**[pt. 2]:115-119, 1966.)

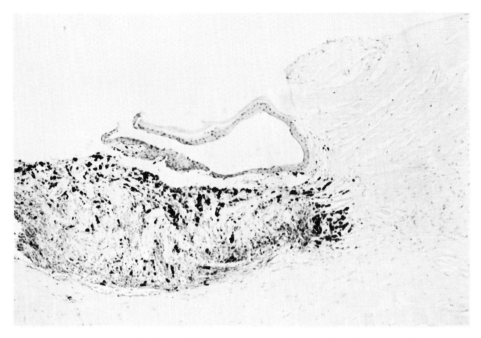

Fig. 26-27. Positive epithelial cell biopsy in case of epithelial downgrowth after cataract extraction.

appears that probably represents the cell margins of the epithelial cells. This noninvasive test may prove useful in making a clinical diagnosis of epithelial downgrowth.

Differential diagnosis

In considering the diagnosis of epithelial downgrowth, one must differentiate it from the following other conditions:

1. *Glassy membrane on the back of the cornea, anterior surface of the iris, and anterior surface of the vitreous.* These membranes usually occur in eyes that have undergone a prolonged iridocyclitis. The membrane consists of a reduplication of Descemet's membrane on the posterior surface of the cornea and its extension from above over the anterior surface of the iris.[23]

2. *Fibrous ingrowth.* Fibrous ingrowth occasionally results when the wound opens and connective tissue stroma enters the anterior chamber. It does not show a strong tendency to grow and may be highly vascular.

3. *Vitreocorneal adherence.* A gray condensation on the back of the cornea may be seen where vitreous is adherent to it. Particularly if it occurs

at the superior periphery of the cornea, it may be mistaken for an epithelial downgrowth. It usually does not advance and is easily differentiated by observing the relationship between the vitreous and the cornea at the slit lamp examination.

4. *Shelving corneal section.*
5. *Detachment of Descemet's membrane.*
6. *Peripheral corneal edema.*

Treatment

Treatment for epithelial downgrowth is usually unfavorable. However, techniques that may restore visual acuity to 20/50 or better in about 25% of cases have been devised. Maumenee and co-workers[46] have recommended the following procedure once the diagnosis has been made.

The photocoagulator is used immediately before surgery to map out the area of iris involvement that indicates the extent of iridectomy to be required. The intraocular pressure is lowered with a systemically administered hyperosmotic agent. A Flieringa ring is sutured to the episclera. The lower border of the epithelial downgrowth is marked on the anterior surface of the cornea by making an epithelium-deep scratch with the tip

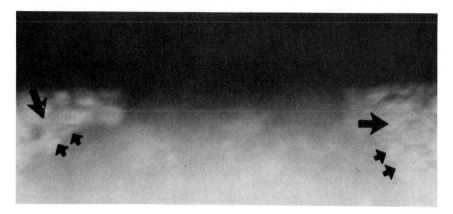

Fig. 26-28. Specular microscopy across area of scalloped margin of epithelial down-growth reveals normal endothelium *(large single arrows)* with sharp demarcation line noted at area of epithelial downgrowth *(double arrows).* (×400.) (From Smith, R. E., and Parrett, C.: Arch. Ophthalmol. **96:**1222, 1978. Copyright 1978, American Medical Association.)

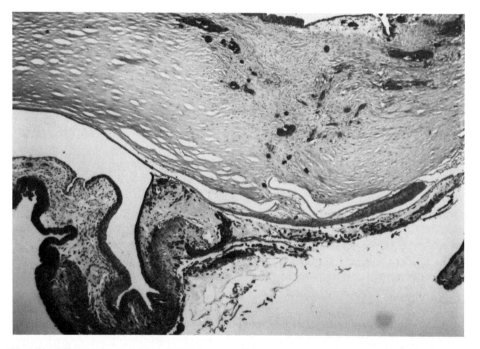

Fig. 26-29. Epithelium is seen lining iris and cornea in eye shown in Fig. 26-28. This confirms the diagnosis of epithelial downgrowth. (×10.) (From Smith, R. E., and Parrett, C.: Arch. Ophthalmol. **96:**1222, 1978. Copyright 1978, American Medical Association.)

of a knife blade. A search is then made for a fistula as follows: Fluorescein, 2%, is instilled on the eye, and gentle pressure is applied with a cotton stick applicator to demonstrate the site. If a fistula is present, a Smith-Green knife is introduced through the fistula into the anterior chamber, thereby laying open the fistula, which is subsequently excised by very small elliptical incisions on the corneal and scleral lips of the wound at this site. If no fistula is found, the anterior chamber is entered through an incision posterior to the original cataract incision so that as much of the angle structure as possible is exposed. Liquid vitreous is aspirated with a blunt No. 18 needle on a 2 ml syringe. Retrovitreal fluid may also be aspirated through a pars plana opening before the anterior chamber is entered.

The iris involved by epithelial downgrowth is excised by cutting it free from the ciliary body and performing as extensive an iridectomy as necessary to include all the involved tissue. If the epithelium covers the vitreous face, it is wiped free by using a plastic sponge. Maumenee now excises portions of the ciliary body where it is covered by epithelium. To ensure that no vitreous adheres to the already damaged cornea, an anterior vitrectomy may be required.

With the cornea retracted, a cryoprobe is applied to the already marked-off area of involvement on the cornea. It is left in place only long enough for an ice ball to form. It is then removed by allowing it to thaw, thus reducing the risk of peeling off Descemet's membrane. The corneal wound is then closed and the anterior chamber re-formed with balanced saline solution.

Earlier techniques consisted of curetting the epithelium from the back of the cornea or touching the epithelium with a cotton swab soaked in 70% ethyl alcohol.

X-ray irradiation has been used with very uncertain results. Perera[4] used five doses of 150 roentgens each at weekly intervals for 6 weeks. In Pincus'[45] series there was one case of definite recession and two of retardation of epithelial growth. Reese has reported 50% success in a series of 24 cases, the best of all reported series.

The surgical approach to epithelial downgrowth is radical but justified, even in an eye with good vision, in view of the otherwise completely unfavorable prognosis.

The results obtained by Maumenee and co-workers[46] in 40 consecutive, unselected cases of epithelial downgrowth, all histologically proved, bear out the gloomy prognosis that faces these patients. These eyes were treated with various combinations of surgical techniques, including cryotherapy of the cornea, photocoagulation of the involved iris, surgical excision of the involved iris, ciliary body, and vitreous, and methods of scraping, peeling, curettage, alcohol swabbing, and cotton applicator swabbing of the posterior corneal surface. The authors used the criterion of a 20/50 or better visual acuity postoperatively, regardless of preoperative acuity, as a surgical success. Also if glaucoma is present, it must be readily controlled. Eleven patients satisfied these stringent criteria, an incidence of 27.5%.

No single means of treating the downgrowth on the cornea could be singled out, in that this group included three cases with cryotherapy, three in which the involved area of the cornea was curetted, and two in which the area of downgrowth was touched with a cotton swab soaked in 70% ethyl alcohol. Of the remaining 29 eyes, there were a number with good postoperative vision but less than 20/50 and some in which the postoperative acuity was considerably improved over the preoperative acuity, although still markedly impaired.

Maumenee and co-workers[46] do not hesitate to point out that many undesirable findings were present after surgery in the 40 eyes of their series. These findings are as follows:

Complication	Number of eyes
Persistent corneal edema of clinical significance	20
Glaucoma	17
Hypotension	5
Hypotension advancing to phthisis bulbi	3
Vitreous haze or opacity	3
Retinal detachment	1
Hyphema	1
Ciliary body detachment	1
Vitreous hemorrhage	1
Residual fistula	1
Gaping wound	1
Eye enucleated	7

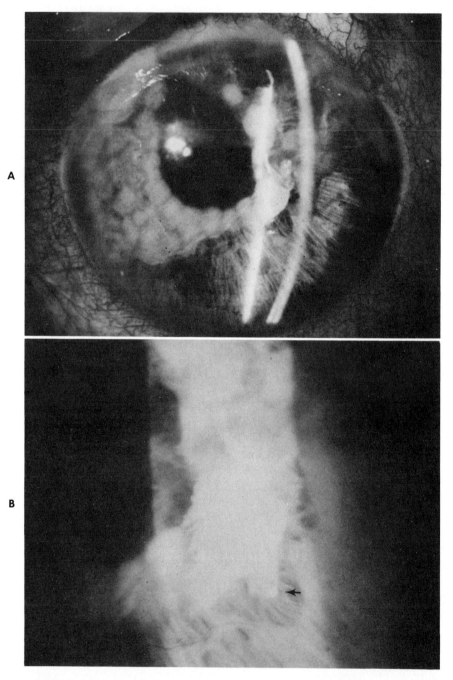

Fig. 26-30. A, Argon laser treatment to delineate extent of epithelial growth on anterior surface of iris. Photocoagulation caused epithelium to turn white and noninvolved iris tissue turned brown. **B,** Higher magnification of junction between epithelium (*arrow*) and adjacent noninvolved iris. (From Stark, W. J., Michels, R. G., Maumenee, A. E., and Cupples, H.: Am. J. Ophthalmol. **85:**772-780, 1978.)

Stark and co-workers[56] reported 10 consecutive cases of epithelial downgrowth operated on during a 33-month period. Photocoagulation of the iris followed by excision of the involved iris and vitrectomy were performed. The epithelium remaining on the posterior surface of the cornea, the ciliary body, and in the anterior chamber was destroyed by controlled transcorneal and transscleral cryotherapy. An intraocular air bubble was used to provide an insulating effect and a more effective, controllable freeze. All patients except two had improved vision postoperatively, and four of the 10 had 20/40 or better (Figs. 26-30 to 26-32).

Brown[57] employed a technique of deep lamellar resection described earlier by Sugar.[21] The technique is also a modification of Maumenee's technique just described. A groove is made at the surgical limbus and deepened to at least three fourths the depth of the limbic tissue. The groove is then extended around the limbus to just beyond the furthest progression of the downgrowth, whether this was on the iris or the posterior surface of the cornea. The sclera is dissected posteriorly as shown in Fig. 26-33, *top*. The extension of the downgrowth on the back of the cornea is delineated by a scratch through the epithelium with the back of a knife blade as recommended by Maumenee. The anterior chamber is entered through the most anterior portion of the groove (Fig. 26-33, *center*). The epithelial downgrowth on the back of the cornea is frozen and then allowed to thaw three times. The involved iris and posterior scleral flap, which includes the chamber angle, is excised en bloc (Fig. 26-33, *bottom*). Perfect approximation is difficult because the scleral wound edge is rather flaccid as a result of excision of its deepest layers. The cornea is then sutured, with both direct and running sutures, to the scleral edge of the wound.

Brown employed this technique in three eyes with advanced epithelial downgrowth. There were no observable recurrences. The histologic presence of epithelium to the edge of the excised tissue indicates that complete excision of the epithelium may not be necessary for the maintenance of the vital structures and function of the eye. The technique differs from that of Maumenee's only in exposing and excising of the chamber angle tissues, which may be a source for

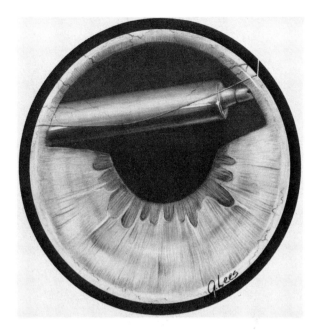

Fig. 26-31. Area of iris and vitreous involved by epithelial ingrowth is excised with vitrectomy instrument except for peripheral iris. (From Stark, W. J., Michels, R. G., Maumenee, A. E., and Cupples, H.: Am. J. Ophthalmol. **85:**772-780, 1978.)

recurrence of the downgrowth. One of these eyes that ultimately required a penetrating keratoplasty is illustrated in Figs. 26-34 and 26-35.

Brown[58] has recently expanded his series to 14 cases. In the first nine cases the technique just described was used. In six of these eyes the surgery resulted in a destruction of the downgrowth on the back of the cornea. Antiglaucoma medication was required to control elevation of intraocular pressure. Four of these six eyes required penetrating keratoplasty, which resulted in clear corneas. The epithelium could not be destroyed and continued to grow in the other three cases. Because of the inconsistent results with cryodestruction of the epithelium on the back of the cornea, Brown changed his technique to blunt dissection of the downgrowth from Descemet's membrane. At surgery, it was observed that in four of the 14 eyes, the downgrowth covered more of the inferior posterior iris than was apparent on the anterior surface. In six eyes the downgrowth covered the entire posterior surface of the iris and extended around the majority of the circumference of the ciliary body. Six of the nine

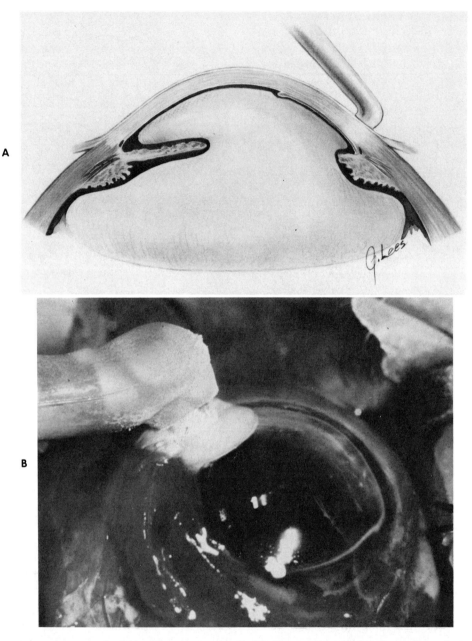

Fig. 26-32. A, Air bubble fills anterior one half of eye and provides thermal insulating effect to enhance cryotherapy applied in transcorneal and transscleral fashion. **B,** Full-thickness freeze can be advanced onto cornea with considerable precision to treat area of epithelial involvement and minimize damage to adjacent noninvolved tissue. **C,** Areas of ciliary body involvement by epithelial ingrowth are treated with transscleral cryotherapy. Ice is visible on ciliary processes *(arrow).* (From Stark, W. J., Michels, R. G., Maumenee, A. E., and Cupples, H.: Am. J. Ophthalmol. **85:**772-780, 1978.)

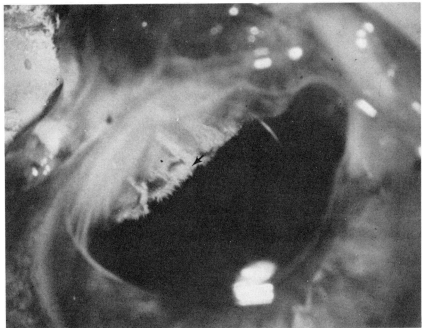

Fig. 26-32, cont'd. For legend see opposite page.

Fig. 26-33. *Top,* Groove is made at surgical limbus and deepened to at least three fourths the depth of limbic tissue. Groove is then extended around limbus to just beyond furthest progression of downgrowth. *Center,* Anterior chamber is entered through most anterior portion of groove. *Bottom,* Epithelial downgrowth on back of cornea is frozen and then allowed to thaw three times. Involved iris and posterior scleral flap, which includes chamber angle, is excised en bloc. (From Brown, S. I.: Ophthalmology [Rochester] **77:**OP 618-622, 1973.)

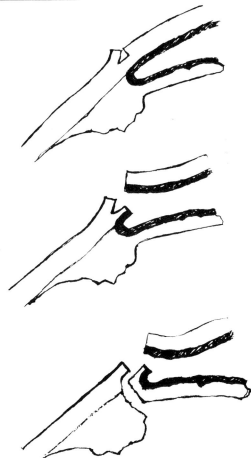

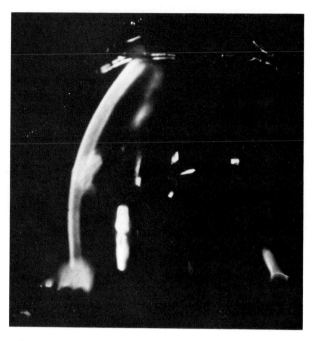

Fig. 26-34. Edge of epithelial downgrowth seen on back of cornea. (From Brown, S. I.: Ophthalmology [Rochester] **77:**OP 618-622, 1973.)

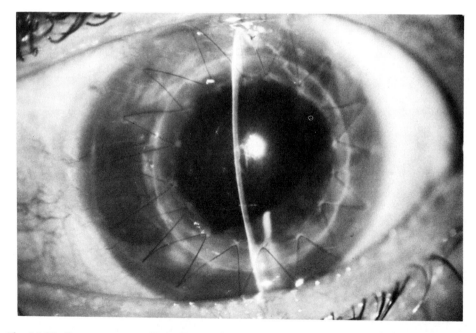

Fig. 26-35. Same eye as in Fig. 26-34. Clear cornea 6 months after penetrating keratoplasty and 42 months after excision of epithelial downgrowth. (From Brown, S. I.: Ophthalmology [Rochester] **77:**OP 618-622, 1973.)

initial cases eventually required cyclocryothermy to maintain normal intraocular pressure. Six eyes required penetrating keratoplasty, all resulting in clear corneas and all but one with improved vision.

REFERENCES

1. MacKenzie, W.: A practical treatise on the diseases of the eye, London, 1830, Longman, Rees, Orme, Brown & Green.
2. Rothmund, A.: Ueber Cysten der Regenbogenhaut, Klin. Mbl. Augenheilk. **10:**189-223, 1872.
3. Collins, E. T., and Cross, F. R.: Two cases of epithelial implantation cyst in the anterior chamber after extraction of cataract, Trans. Ophthalmol. Soc. U.K. **12:**175-180, 1892.
4. Perera, C. A.: Epithelium in the anterior chamber of the eye after operation and injury, Ophthalmology (Rochester) **42:**142-164, 1937.
5. Sitchevska, O., and Payne, B. F.: Pearl cysts of the iris, Am. J. Ophthalmol. **34:**833-839, 1951.
6. Vail, D.: Discussion of Perera, C. A.: Epithelium in the anterior chamber of the eye after operation and injury, Ophthalmology (Rochester) **42:**163, 1937.
7. Theobald, G. D., and Haas, J. S.: Epithelial invasion of the anterior chamber following cataract extraction, Ophthalmology (Rochester) **52:**470-482, 1948.
8. Hogan, M. J., and Goodner, E. K.: Surgical treatment of epithelial cysts of the anterior chamber, Arch. Ophthalmol. **64:**286-291, 1960.
9. Ferry, A. P.: The possible role of epithelial-bearing surgical instruments in pathogenesis of epithelialization of the anterior chamber, Ann. Ophthalmol. **3:**1089-1093, 1971.
10. Bennett, T., and D'Amico, R. A.: Epithelial inclusion cyst of iris after keratoplasty, Am. J. Ophthalmol. **77:**87-89, 1971.
11. Ferry, A. P., and Naghdi, M. R.: Cryosurgical removal of epithelial cyst of iris and anterior chamber, Arch. Ophthalmol. **77:**86-87, 1967.
12. Maumenee, A. E.: In Emery, J. M., and Paton, D., editors: Current concepts in cataract surgery. Selected Proceedings of the Third Biennial Cataract Surgical Congress, St. Louis, 1974, The C. V. Mosby Co., p. 312.
13. Vail, D.: Treatment of cysts of the iris with diathermy coagulation, Trans. Am. Ophthalmol. Soc. **51:**371-383, 1953.
14. Meller, J.: Ophthalmic surgery, ed. 6, New York, 1953, Blakiston Division, McGraw-Hill Book Co., pp. 390-391.
15. Thilliez: Traitement des kystes de l'iris par l'électrolyse, Bull. Soc. Franc. Ophthalmol. **25:**490-494, 1908.
16. Chailous, M. J.: Traitement par l'électrolyse des kystes transparents de la chambre antérieure, Bull. Soc. Franc. Ophthalmol. **31:**450-451, 1914.
17. Kubena, K.: Epithelial cysts in the anterior chamber. Cesk. Oftalmol. **15:**87-90, 1959.
18. Fralick, F. B.: Management of complications after cataract extraction, Trans. Pac. Coast Otoophthalmol. Soc. **32:**42-53, 1951.
19. Shaffer, R. N.: Alpha irradiation. Effect of astatine on the anterior segment and on an epithelial cyst. Trans. Am. Ophthalmol. Soc. **50:**607-627, 1952.
20. Esposito, A. C.: Personal communication. In Callahan, A., editor,: Surgery of the eye; diseases. Springfield, Ill., 1956, Charles C Thomas, Publisher, p. 226.
21. Sugar, H. S.: Resection of cornea for epithelial implantation cyst of the anterior chamber, Am. J. Ophthalmol. **54:**800-803, 1962.
22. Sugar, H. S.: Further experience with posterior lamellar resection of the cornea for epithelial implantation cyst, Am. J. Ophthalmol. **64:**291-299, 1967.
23. Maumenee, A. E., and Shannon, C. R.: Epithelial invasion of the anterior chamber, Trans. Pac. Coast Otoophthalmol. Soc. **36:**107-135, 1955.
24. Harbin, T. S., Jr., and Maumenee, A. E.: Epithelial downgrowth after surgery for epithelial cyst, Am. J. Ophthalmol. **78:**1-4, 1974.
25. Okun, E., and Mandell, A.: Photocoagulation treatment of epithelial implantation cysts following cataract surgery, Trans. Am. Ophthalmol. Soc. **72:**170-183, 1974.
26. Bernardino, V. B., Kim, J. C., and Smith, T. R.: Epithelialization of the anterior chamber after cataract extraction, Arch. Ophthalmol. **82:**742-750, 1969.
27. Blodi, F. C.: Failures of cataract extractions and their pathologic explanation, J. Iowa Med. Soc. **44:**514-516, 1954.
28. Dunnington, J. H.: Ocular wound healing with particular reference to the cataract incision, Arch. Ophthalmol. **56:**639-659, 1956.
29. Schulze, R. R., and Duke, J. R.: Causes of enucleation following cataract extraction, Arch. Ophthalmol. **73:**74-79, 1965.
30. Payne, B. F.: Epithelization of the anterior segment. II, Am. J. Ophthalmol. **45:**182-184, 1958.
31. Patz, A.: Personal communication. In Maumenee, A. E., editor: Symposium: postoperative cataract complications. III. Epithelial invasion of the anterior chamber, retinal detachment, corneal edema, anterior chamber hemorrhages, changes in the macula, **61:**51-68, 1957.
32. Paufique, L., and Hervouët, F.: L'invasion épithéliale de la chambre antérieure après opération de cataracte, Ann. Oculist. **197:**105-129, 1964.
33. Allen, J. C.: Epithelial and stromal ingrowths, Am. J. Ophthalmol. **65:**179-182, 1968.
34. Otradovec, J., and Zicha, Z.: Epithelial invasion into the anterior chamber after cataract extraction, Cesk. Oftalmol. **16:**131-139, 1960.
35. Christensen, L.: Epithelization of the anterior chamber. In Transactions of the New Orleans Academy of Ophthalmology, Symposium on cataracts, St. Louis, 1965, The C. V. Mosby Co. pp. 219-225.
36. Regan, E. F.: Epithelial invasion of the anterior chamber, Arch. Ophthalmol. **60:**907-927, 1958.
37. Gundersen, T.: Results of autotransplantation of cornea into the anterior chamber: their significance regarding corneal nutrition, Trans. Am. Ophthalmol. Soc. **36:**207-213, 1938.
38. Cogan, D. G.: Experimental implants of conjunctiva into the anterior chamber. II, Am. J. Ophthalmol. **39:**165-172, 1955.

39. Corrado, M.: Glaucoma secondario a penetrazione e proliferazione di epitelio in c. a. in occhio operato di catarratta, Ann. Ottal. **59:**706-717, 1931.

40. Dunnington, J. H., and Regan, E. F.: The effect of sutures and of thrombin upon ocular wound healing, Ophthalmology (Rochester) **55:**761-772, 1951.

41. Binder, R., and Binder, H.: Experimentelle Untersuchungen über den Einfluss von Anticoagulantien auf die Heilung von Hornhautschnittwunden, Graefe Arch. Ophthalmol. **155:**337-344, 1954.

42. Bick, M. N.: Heparinization of the eye, Am. J. Ophthalmol. **32:**663-670, 1949.

43. Smith, D. R., Somerville, G. M., and Shew, M.: An experimental model of epithelialization of the anterior chamber, Can. J. Ophthalmol. **2:**158-162, 1967.

44. Allen, J. C., and Duehr, P. A.: Sutures and epithelial downgrowth, Am. J. Ophthalmol. **66:**293-294, 1968.

45. Pincus, M. H.: Epithelial invasion of the anterior chamber following cataract extraction: effect of radiation therapy, Arch. Ophthalmol. **43:**509-519, 1950.

46. Maumenee, A. E., Paton, D., Morse, P. H., and Butner, R.: Review of 40 histologically proven cases of epithelial downgrowth following cataract extraction and suggested surgical management. Am. J. Ophthalmol. **69:**598-603, 1970.

47. Dunnington, J. H., and Regan, E. F.: Absorbable sutures in cataract surgery, Arch. Ophthalmol. **50:**545-556, 153.

48. Matsumoto, S.: Contribution to the study of epithelial movement: the corneal epithelium of the frog in tissue culture, J. Exp. Zool. **26:**545-564, 1918.

49. Terry, T. L., Chisholm, A. R., Jr, and Schonberg, A. L.: Studies on surface-epithelium invasion of the anterior segment of the eye, Am. J. Ophthalmol. **22:**1083-1110, 1939.

50. Chandler, P. A., and Grant, W. M.: Lectures on glaucoma, Philadelphia, 1965, Lea & Febiger, p. 243.

51. Calhoun, F. P., Jr.: The clinical recognition and treatment of epithelialization of the anterior chamber following cataract extraction, Trans. Am. Ophthalmol. Soc. **47:**498-553, 1949.

52. Thomas, C. I.: The cornea, Springfield, Ill., 1955, Charles C Thomas, Publisher, pp. 180-181.

53. Maumenee, A. E.: Complications of cataract surgery, Highlights Ophthalmol. **11:**120-132, 1968.

54. Calhoun, F. P., Jr.: An aid to the clinical diagnosis of epithelial downgrowth into the anterior chamber following cataract extraction, Am. J. Ophthalmol. **61:**1055-1059, 1966.

55. Smith, R. E., and Parrett, C.: Specular microscopy of epithelial downgrowth, Arch. Ophthalmol. **96:**1222-1224, 1978.

56. Stark, W. J., Michels, R. G., Maumenee, A. E., and Cupples, H.: Surgical management of epithelial ingrowth, Am. J. Ophthalmol. **85:**772-780, 1978.

57. Brown, S. I.: Treatment of advanced epithelial downgrowth, Ophthalmology (Rochester) **77:**OP 618-622, 1973.

58. Brown, S. I.: Results of excision of advanced epithelial downgrowth, Ophthalmology **86:**321-328, 1979.

CHAPTER 27

Fibrous ingrowth

Fibrous ingrowth is often confused with epithelial downgrowth, occurs at least as frequently, and is usually diagnosed by the pathologist. It is characterized by an ingrowth of connective tissue elements into the anterior chamber and aided and abetted by poor wound healing and incarceration of tissue such as vitreous, iris, or lens remnants into the surgical incision. It has also been referred to as stromal ingrowth,[1] stromal overgrowth,[2] fibroblastic ingrowth,[3] fibrocytic ingrowth,[4] and fibrous metaplasia.

HISTORICAL BACKGROUND

There has been much less written about this entity than epithelial downgrowth. Henderson[5] (1914) suggested that incarcerated iris or lens capsule might act as a bridge for subconjunctival tissue to grow into the anterior chamber through the edges of the wound. In the same year Collins[6] stated that such proliferation of connective tissue within the eyeball occurred only in the presence of infective material. Although Wood[7] (1932) observed this complication after a cataract extraction, it largely escaped attention until Levkoieva[8] (1947) and Tikhomirov[9] (1948) reported that it occurs to some extent in 25% of all eyes enucleated after a penetrating wound.

PATHOPHYSIOLOGY

Since this complication is related to wound healing, some of the principles associated with the repair of the corneoscleral incision (p. 19) are repeated here in brief. The cataract section may be corneal, limbal, or scleral, and there are differences in the healing of each.

Immediately after the completion of a corneal incision, the wound edges swell because of imbibition of fluid (presumably aqueous) by the corneal lamellae. Anterior and posterior triangles result because of retraction of the superficial and deep parts of the wound. The apices of these triangles point toward each other. The anterior triangle becomes filled with epithelial cells within 2 days (p. 16). The filling of the posterior triangle occurs more slowly. A posterior plug of fibrin results presumably from the secondary aqueous. Within a few days the endothelial cells cover this posterior plug and in time produce a new Descemet's membrane. Stromal tissue is reconstituted by migration of cells from the limbal area and transformation of existing stromal cells. These cells turn into keratocytes[10] that in turn become fibroblasts. The source of the fibroblasts is still controversial, but Weimar[11] estimated that 35% are derived from corneal stromal cells either by transformation alone or with accompanying mitoses and about 65% from the transformation and division of migrating monocytes. Wound healing requires the deposition of new collagen from the fibroblasts. A soluble procollagen is secreted by the fibroblast, and this polymerizes at the cell surface to form the true collagen.[12] The collagen that is formed in this manner differs from normal corneal collagen in that the fibrils show variable width and are not layered in an orderly fashion. Vitamin C appears to be necessary for the laying down of the initial substance into which the collagen fibrils later are deposited.

The healing of a scleral wound differs in some important respects from the healing of a corneal wound (p. 25). Unlike the corneal stroma, scleral fibers do not swell readily. In fact, the edges of a penetrating scleral incision may tend to retract.

There are no epithelial or endothelial surfaces to bridge across the gap, and the stromal cells of the sclera participate little, if at all, in the healing of a wound. As Swan[3] pointed out, healing by primary intention, as in a corneal wound, does not occur. Instead, the defect is filled in by the proliferation of mesenchymal tissue from the episclera and uvea. Repair of a scleral laceration is therefore comparable to healing of the dermis of the skin by secondary intention. There is an initial filling of the defect by fibroblastic tissue and, later, the laying down of collagen. The sclera itself plays a more or less passive role.

The usual incision for a cataract extraction is limbal or corneal and heals rapidly by primary intention. In a deep cataract section the incision is behind the limbus and enters the anterior chamber deep in the angle. The repair of such a wound acquires the characteristics of scleral, rather than corneal, healing.

Because of factors outlined on p. 543, an overabundance of fibroblastic repair may occur, leading to a fibrous ingrowth into the anterior chamber. As stated earlier, the source of the fibroblasts responsible for fibrous ingrowth is still controversial. The most likely sources are the following:

1. Subepithelial connective tissue
2. Corneal or limbal stroma
3. Metaplastic endothelium

Swan[13] favors subepithelial connective tissue as the primary source. Normally, bridging of the inner wound by endothelium seems to confine fibroplasia to the stromal defect, even when there is gaping of its inner edges. A defect in the endothelium predisposes to a fibroblastic retrocorneal membrane that may be difficult to differentiate from epithelial downgrowth. The extent of fibroplasia is variable. As in epithelial invasion, the structures of the anterior segment, such as the iris, angle, and vitreous face, may become involved.

Many consider the fibrous ingrowth to arise from the stromal keratocytes, which convert to fibroblasts. If such be the case, the stroma itself would be the source of the fibroplasia of the anterior segment of the eye. It is extremely difficult to determine the source by histologic examination. Most specimens make it appear as if the fibrous tissue in the anterior chamber is continuous with

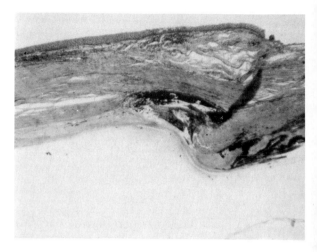

Fig. 27-1. Fibrous ingrowth extending over posterior surface of cataract incision and cornea. Uveal tissue incarcerated in wound. Descemet's membrane shown anterior to fibrous membrane. (Hematoxylin and eosin.) (From Allen, J. C., and DeVanecia, G.: Indian J. Ocul. Pathol. **1:**40-41, 1967.)

the corneal stroma on both sides of the wound. However, one can also implicate the subepithelial connective tissue in these same histologic specimens.

The third possibility, which is discussed more fully in the next chapter, involves fibrous metaplasia. In some cases, regeneration of incised or injured corneal endothelium is not normal but is characterized by an excessive amount of Descemet's membrane production. This is accomplished by conversion of endothelial cells into a fibroblast-like cell that produces fibrous tissue in addition to basement membrane.[14] Corneal endothelium is really a mesothelium that is the surface lining of a serous cavity. It is mesodermally derived (as are fibroblasts) and can undergo fibroblastic metaplasia. This is in contrast to a true endothelium, which is the lining of a vascular channel and usually does not convert to a fibroblast.[15] Strictly speaking, the anterior chamber is a serous cavity lined anteriorly by mesothelium.[16,17]

This ingrowth may assume many of the characteristics of epithelial downgrowth. The connective tissue invasion may clothe the back of the cornea (Figs. 27-1 and 27-2), the chamber angle (Fig. 27-3), the surface of the iris (Figs. 27-4 to

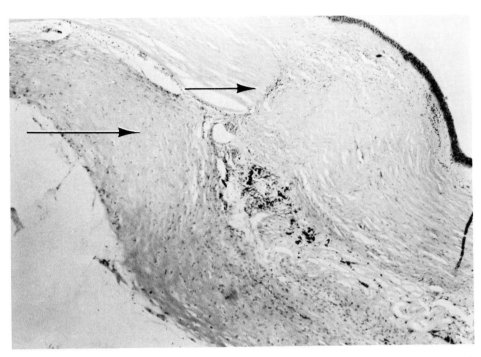

Fig. 27-2. Exuberant fibrous ingrowth *(long arrow)* from cataract incision *(short arrow)*, extending over back of cornea. Hemosiderosis present. (Hematoxylin and eosin.)

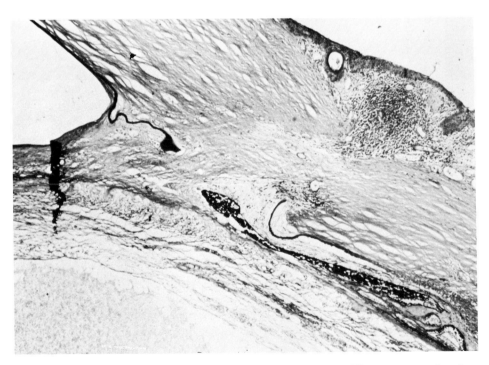

Fig. 27-3. Exuberant fibrous ingrowth from cataract incision filling anterior chamber and extending into chamber angle in eye that suffered iris prolapse after cataract surgery. Proplase was treated by cryothermy.

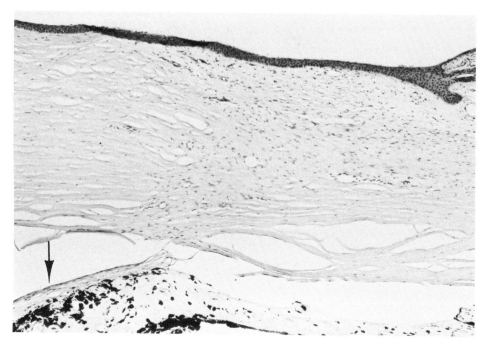

Fig. 27-4. Fibrous ingrowth extending from cataract incision onto anterior surface of iris *(arrow).* (Courtesy P. Henkind, Bronx, N.Y.)

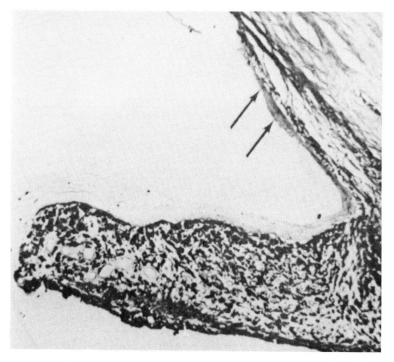

Fig. 27-5. Fibrous tissue *(arrows)* growing posteriorly in incarcerated strands of vitreous, across peripheral anterior synechia, along anterior surface of iris, and through pupil in eye with absolute glaucoma enucleated 3 months after intracapsular cataract extraction. (Periodic acid–Schiff, ×50.) (AFIP Neg. 69-240.) (From Bettman, J. W., Jr.: Am. J. Ophthalmol. **68:**1037-1050, 1969.)

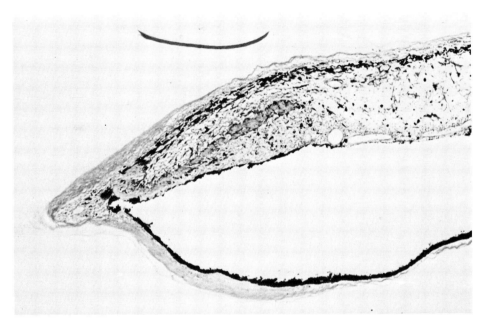

Fig. 27-6. Fibrous tissue growing over anterior and posterior surfaces of iris after cataract extraction. Artifactitious separation of pigment epithelium of iris.

27-6), and the anterior face of the vitreous (Fig. 27-7) and may go so far as to adhere to the retina. The process is not unlike that seen after traumatic perforation of the cornea with fibrous ingrowth (Fig. 27-8).

This problem may follow a penetrating keratoplasty.[18] A retrocorneal membrane consisting of fibrous tissue may cover the back of the cornea. The fibrous elements, consisting of collagen fibers and fibroblasts, pass through the poorly united margins of the host-graft tissue. The endothelium and Descemet's membrane of the graft may be intact, and a second or pseudo-Descemet's membrane may actually form behind it, presumably by secretion, on the side of the postgraft membrane adjacent to the aqueous.[12]

The cellular origin of the postgraft membrane after a penetrating keratoplasty is as controversial as the source of the fibrous tissue invasion of the anterior chamber following cataract extraction. There are many similarities between the two conditions.

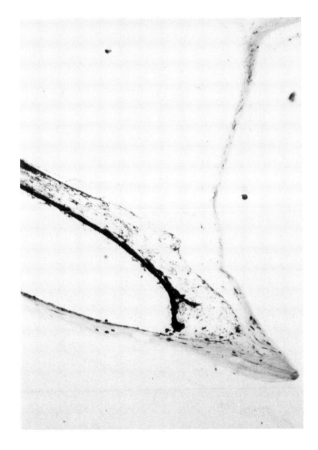

Fig. 27-7. Fibrous ingrowth extending down from cornea *(upper right)*, around pupillary border of iris, and over anterior hyaloid membrane posterior to iris. (Hematoxylin and eosin.) (From Allen, J. C., and DeVenecia, G.: Indian J. Ocul. Pathol. **1:**40-41, 1967.)

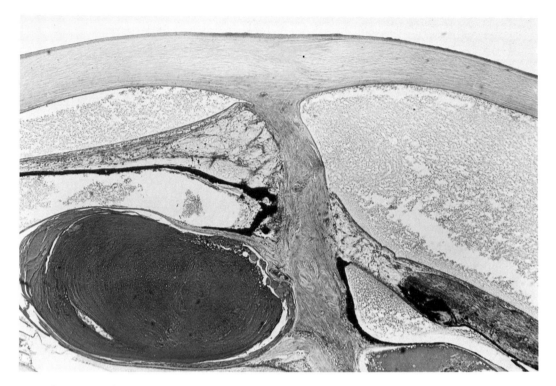

Fig. 27-8. Fibrous ingrowth from traumatic perforation of cornea. (Hematoxylin and eosin, ×35.) (From Allen, J. C.: Am. J. Ophthalmol. **65:**179-182, 1968.)

Waring and co-workers[14] have emphasized that retrocorneal fibrous membranes occur in two distinct settings: (1) after chemical or inflammatory insult to the cornea where Descemet's membrane remains intact and (2) after surgical or accidental perforating corneal wounds where Descemet's membrane is broken. In the former instance the retrocorneal membrane most likely results from fibroblast-like metaplasia of the endothelium, whereas in the latter the cell of origin may be either the fibroblast-like endothelial cell or the stromal keratocyte.

A retrocorneal fibrous membrane may form over an intact Descemet's membrane after chemical burns[17,19-21] following repeated focal freezing of the cornea[22] or after herpetic keratitis.[23] Matsuda and Smelser[19] demonstrated the endothelium's ability to form retrocorneal membranes. They burned the central area of rabbit corneas with alkali, leaving Descemet's membrane intact, and after 7 days noted that a multilayered sheet of fibroblast-like cells covered the burned area. They concluded that the endothelial cell of

the cornea was capable of differentiating into a fibroblast-like cell but that it retained enough regenerative potential to ultimately cover the posterior cornea with normal endothelium. The fibroblast-like cell from the angle apparently did not have the capacity to redifferentiate into a new endothelial cell.

It has been observed that although retrocorneal membranes with a break in Descemet's membrane occur most commonly after penetrating keratoplasty,[24-27] they also appear after cataract extraction[28] (34% of 84 enucleated aphakic globes),[29] accidental perforating corneal trauma,[30] and goniotomy and filtering surgery.[31] Other names for this phenomenon are postgraft membranes,[32] fibrous tissue plugs,[33] laminated membranes,[34] fusiform scars,[35] stromal overgrowth,[28] and fibroblastic ingrowth.[36] They are present in 50% to 80% of cloudy penetrating keratoplasties[34,37-39] but are often unrecognized clinically.[24,38] Careful inspection 2 to 3 weeks after a penetrating keratoplasty may reveal a narrow thickening on the posterior surface of the host-graft junction, which later may grow across the donor button to form a small crescent or to cover the entire posterior surface. Sometimes it appears as a fenestrated membrane suspended in the anterior chamber. The membrane connects to the stroma directly through the break in Descemet's membrane. It is usually thicker and more extensive over the donor button and it may be vascularized.[19,25,40]

The cells producing the retrocorneal membrane after penetrating keratoplasty are thought to be from the host,[37] but it is uncertain whether they are stromal keratocytes or endothelial cell derivatives.[17,22,34] The stromal keratocyte may convert to a fibroblast, migrate through the break in Descemet's membrane, and elaborate a connective tissue membrane across the posterior corneal surface where endothelial cells are absent. They proliferate until inhibited by the presence of healthy endothelium.[24-26,32,41] Following wounds at the limbus, the subconjunctival fibroblasts also have access to the anterior chamber.[13] Descemet's membrane and the endothelium play a key mechanical role in this theory, since a well-approximated Descemet's membrane wound that is rapidly sealed by endothelium will prevent fibroblastic ingrowth. Alternatively, the endothelial cells may be induced to fibroblast-like metaplasia by trauma, inflammation, and immunologic insult, and form the fibrous membrane.[22,40,42,43]

Another pertinent situation is external fibrous proliferation following a penetrating keratoplasty.[44] It has been referred to as corneal stromal outgrowth. This is a proliferation of corneal stroma from a corneal incision onto the surface of Bowman's membrane beneath the corneal epithelium. It is thought to arise from an anterior gaping of the wound. It may occur after a corneal cataract incision but is more common after a penetrating keratoplasty. This entity supports those who favor the corneal stroma as the source of fibroplasia in the anterior chamber after cataract extraction or penetrating keratoplasty but does not eliminate endothelial metaplasia as a possible cause.

PATHOGENESIS

1. Malapproximation of the wound edges characterized by posterior gaping or overriding of the wound may cause persistent irritation and slow recovery. In some patients, this alone is sufficient stimulus for an exuberant, reparative overgrowth. The greater the extent of the wound gape facing the anterior chamber, the greater the likelihood of fibrous ingrowth in the favorable milieu provided within the eye. In a study of a large series of enucleated eyes covering a wide time range, Dunnington[45] has concluded, as one would expect, that the incidence of fibrous ingrowth has decreased greatly since the advent of corneoscleral sutures in cataract surgery.

2. Incarceration of vitreous, iris (Figs. 27-1 and 27-3), or lens matter (Fig. 27-9) in the wound increases the possibility of fibrous ingrowth. In many of these cases there is a history of operative loss of vitreous. The inevitable protuberance of vitreous strands between the lips of the wound or, at the least, lining the posterior portion of the wound, provides a framework for downward growth of fibrous tissue elements. It is this fibroplastic response that results in many of the unfavorable sequelae after the loss of formed vitreous during cataract surgery. They are discussed more fully on p. 255. However, when this occurs, the wound must be scrupulously managed to ensure against incarceration of vitreous and other structures. I know of no better way to accomplish this than to excise all the formed vitreous from the anterior chamber (anterior vitrectomy) according to the method suggested by Kasner (p. 268). All previously recommended techniques, such as aspiration of retrovitreal aqueous, sweeping the iris out of the wound with a spatula, air in the anterior chamber, and so on, have at least in my hands failed to achieve this end. If the wound is not entirely free of formed vitreous, the pupil will be updrawn and misshapened, and ectropion uveae will result. The fibroplastic reactions that cause this are well developed within 48 hours of the surgery. If the vitreous is totally liquefied and if it escapes during cataract surgery, the aforementioned fibroplasia does not result. Thus, as Christensen[4] emphasized, it is not the reduction of bulk of the vitreous that is to be feared as much as the derangement created by its disruption and the fibrocytic reaction incited by its contact with the iris and the surgical wound. Therefore the previously mentioned sequelae of vitreous loss are related more to the physical state of the vitreous and its abnormal intraocular

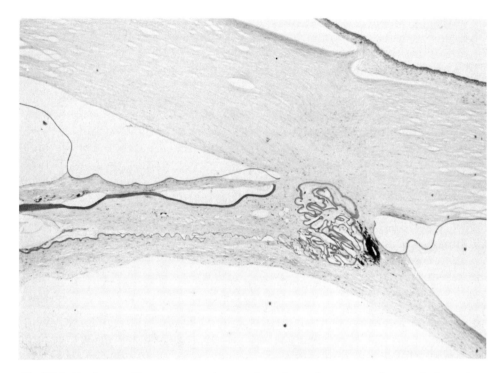

Fig. 27-9. Exuberant fibrous ingrowth extending down from corneal wound. Convoluted portion of lens capsule enmeshed within fibrous tissue. (Periodic acid–Schiff.)

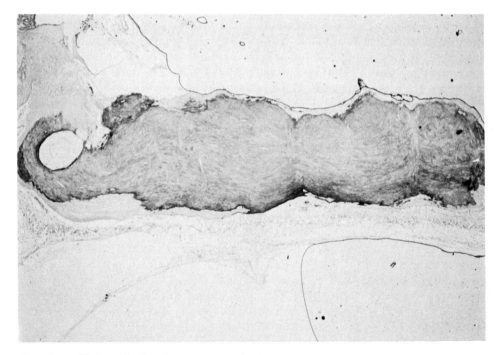

Fig. 27-10. Phthisis bulbi after extracapsular lens extraction. Lens remnant attached to inflammatory fibroproliferative tissue. (Periodic acid-Schiff.)

position than to the loss of vitreous per se.

If wound closure is also defective, the proper climate for abundant fibrous ingrowth is present. In my experience, it is far more likely for vitreous to adhere to a corneal wound than a limbal or scleral incision. When this occurs, it is not necessarily attributable to a rupture of the anterior hyaloid membrane. Because of the location of the corneal incision well within the limbus (when a prior filtering operation has been performed), the intact anterior surface of the vitreous may adhere to it. If fibrous ingrowth occurs to any appreciable extent, it may close the surgical fistula.

Iris may become incarcerated between the lips of the wound or adherent to its posterior surface. It may or may not be accompanied by vitreous. Also possible is for lens capsule and cortical remnants to become wedged into the wound in similar fashion (Fig. 27-9). In addition to interfering with proper coaptation of the lips of the wound, it causes enough irritation to create the proper climate for fibrous ingrowth. Therefore the likelihood of fibrous ingrowth increases after an unplanned extracapsular lens extraction (Fig. 27-10).

3. Intraocular inflammation, if prolonged and of low intensity, may give rise to an excessive reparative response. In fact, Christensen[4] felt that fibroplasia represents the end product of an inflammatory reaction, since its presence within the eye automatically signifies a preexisting inflammation. He concluded that inflammation must be the common denominator in the genesis of these sequelae, and it must be induced or enhanced in some manner by surgical error. Excessive repair can seriously disable the eye because the limitations of space in the eye do not permit an overabundance of any tissue without interfering with ocular physiology.

4. Excessive bleeding into the anterior chamber may occasionally cause a fibroplastic response in the anterior chamber. It remains questionable whether this bleeding encourages a fibrous ingrowth.

CLINICAL FINDINGS

Although there are some similarities in the pathogenesis and clinical features of epithelial downgrowth and fibrous ingrowth, the latter tends to be self-limiting in many cases, and the

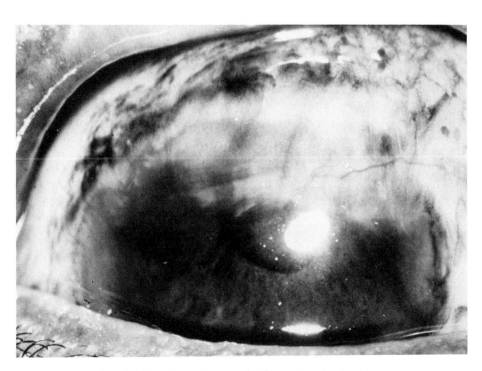

Fig. 27-11. Fibrous ingrowth after cataract extraction.

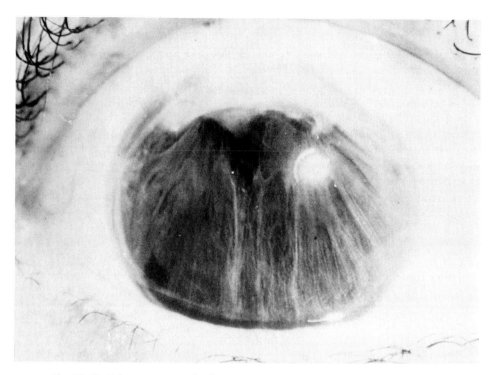

Fig. 27-12. Fibrous ingrowth after cataract extraction. Note updrawn pupil.

appearance of the membrane is different. In epithelial downgrowth the membrane on the back of the cornea shows a well-defined border (because of a heaping up of epithelial cells, p. 518), but the advancing edge of the fibrous membrane appears frayed, with irregular tonguelike strands running ahead (Figs. 27-11 and 27-12). The surface of the fibrous membrane is gray or white, and the appearance of the interlacing meshwork of fine fibers has been described as that of woven cloth.[3]

Fibrous ingrowth is easy to recognize when the membrane arises from the surgical wound and thickly envelops the iris and anterior surface of the vitreous. However, perhaps even more frequently, the membrane is thin and may appear as a fine gray sheet over the vitreous face. It will resemble the membrane usually seen after a postoperative iridocyclitis or a hyphema.

The presence of a detached Descemet's membrane should lead one to suspect fibrous ingrowth. Bettman[46] (p. 568) found this association in his series of 122 eyes enucleated after all kinds of intraocular surgery.

Bullous keratopathy or corneal edema often

occurs in these eyes, as it does with epithelial downgrowth. The entire cornea may be involved, but usually it is limited to that area of the cornea with the fibrous tissue backing.

Glaucoma is a frequent finding, as one would expect, since the fibrous tissue elements usually invade and cover the angle structures. The incidence of glaucoma is high, especially in eyes with fibrous ingrowth that have come to enucleation.

If the fibrous tissue invasion is extensive, the ingrowth may reach the posterior segment of the eye and cause a retinal detachment[4,46] (Fig. 27-13). Of interest is the fact that many enucleated eyes that suffered phthisis bulbi after an intraocular operation are found to harbor a fibrous ingrowth (Figs. 27-14 and 27-15). Of 12 phthisical eyes in Bettman's[46] series, seven (58%) revealed this ingrowth, whereas among 92 postsurgically enucleated eyes without fibrous ingrowth there were only five phthisical eyes.

The clinical course will vary with the virulence of the factors that encourage the fibrous ingrowth. Frequently the course will be insidi-

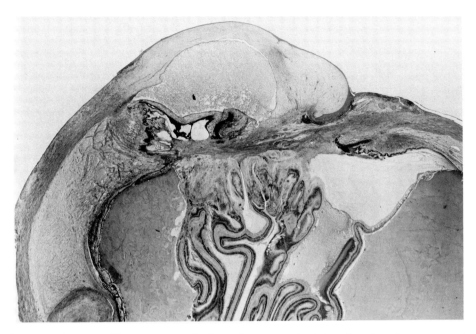

Fig. 27-13. Massive fibrous ingrowth through cataract incision, forming dense secondary membrane and causing retinal detachment. (Hematoxylin and eosin, ×10.) (From Allen, J. C.: Am. J. Ophthalmol. **65:**179-182, 1968.)

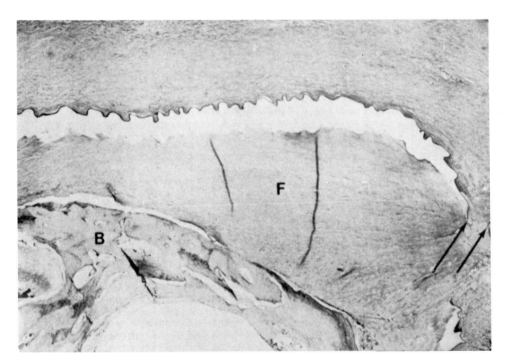

Fig. 27-14. Massive fibrous ingrowth, *F,* that has emanated through gap in Descemet's membrane *(arrows)* in phthisic eye enucleated 10 years after surgery for congenital cataract. Note bone, *B.* (Periodic acid–Schiff, ×21.) (AFIP Neg. 69-239.) (From Bettman, J. W., Jr.: Am. J. Ophthalmol. **68:**1037-1050, 1969.)

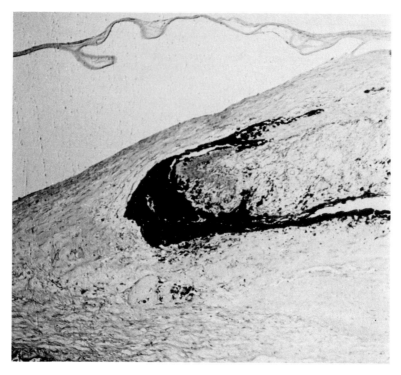

Fig. 27-15. Massive fibrous ingrowth in phthisic eye. Note fibrous tissue surrounding iris.

ous, with the patient complaining of little discomfort. As pointed out by Duke-Elder,[2] violent inflammatory and exudative changes are usually absent from the uveal tissues, for the iris and ciliary body, encased in the mass of regenerative tissue, remain relatively passive and suffer slow atrophy. However, chronic irritative changes eventually ensue, and the contraction of the newly formed tissue pulls on the corneal scar, flattening and depressing it and deforming the globe until the eye becomes atrophic or is removed in fear of sympathetic ophthalmia or because of the onset of a recalcitrant secondary glaucoma caused by the embarrassment of its drainage channels.

INCIDENCE

Estimating the incidence of fibrous ingrowth is difficult, since many of these cases remain unrecognized until the globe is enucleated.

Dunnington[45] examined 171 eyes histologically and observed fibrous ingrowth in 56 (32.8%). This number was compared to epithelial down-

growth, which occurred in 62 eyes (36.2%). To emphasize the relatively similar frequency of fibrous ingrowth and epithelial downgrowth in eyes enucleated after cataract extraction, Allen[1] observed 18 eyes (36%) with the former and 13 (26%) with the latter out of 50 such eyes. It is remarkable that Bettman[46] found 25 (34%) eyes with fibrous ingrowth out of 74 eyes enucleated after adult cataract extraction.

TREATMENT

There has been a great deal less written about the treatment of fibrous ingrowth than about epithelial downgrowth. Since many of these eyes remain quiescent for several years, treatment is often directed to a particular consequence of the fibrous ingrowth rather than the preservation of the globe. For example, a thin fibrous membrane covering the pupillary aperture may be incised with a discission knife. Secondary glaucoma may be treated by cyclodialysis if there is little evidence of intraocular inflammation, or else a cyclocryothermy may be useful. If the fibrous ingrowth reaches the posterior segment of the globe and causes retinal detachment by direct traction, the prognosis is gloomy, but an effort should be made to save these globes by severing the fibroplastic bands and performing some type of buckling procedure.

For many years I have recommended performing an inferior sphincterotomy when extracting a cataract via a corneal incision from an eye that has had a prior filtering procedure. These eyes frequently show an updrawing of the pupil over a period of months or years because of fibrous ingrowth from the corneal stroma. As mentioned previously, this updrawing occurs with a very high frequency if the vitreous face becomes incarcerated in the corneal wound. Performing the sphincterotomy combats the tendency for the pupil to migrate just behind the corneal scar. An inferior extraction may avoid such an occurrence.

REFERENCES

1. Allen, J. C.: Epithelial and stromal ingrowths, Am. J. Ophthalmol. **65:**179-182, 1968.
2. Duke-Elder, S.: Textbook of ophthalmology. Vol. VI. Injuries, St. Louis, 1954, The C. V. Mosby Co., p. 6012.
3. Swan, K. C.: Some contemporary concepts of scleral disease, Arch. Ophthalmol. **45:**630-644, 1951.
4. Christensen, L.: Pathogenesis of surgical complications—the role of fibroplasia. In Transactions of the New Orleans Academy of Ophthalmology, Symposium on cataracts, St. Louis, 1965, The C. V. Mosby Co., pp. 196-211.
5. Henderson, T.: Postoperative complications of cataract extraction, Trans. Ophthalmol. Soc. U.K. **34:**88-91, 1914.
6. Collins, E. T.: Discussion on postoperative complications of cataract extraction, Trans. Ophthalmol. Soc. U.K. **34:**18-44, 1914.
7. Wood, D. J.: An unusual result following traumatic iridocyclitis, Br. J. Ophthalmol. **16:**546-548, 1932.
8. Levkoieva, E.: The regeneration of wounds of external membrane of the eye in the light of new pathologicoanatomical results, Br. J. Ophthalmol. **31:**336-361, 1947.
9. Tikhomirov, P. E.: Atrofia glaza posle pronikayushchykh ranienii i popytki lechenyz yeyo [Atrophy of eye following penetrating injuries, and their therapy], Vestn. Oftalmol. **27**(No. 1):22-25, 1948.
10. Leopold, I.: Medical therapy of corneal diseases. In King, J. H., Jr., and McTigue, J. W., editors: The Cornea World Congress, London, 1965, Butterworth & Co. (Publishers), Ltd., pp. 235-255.
11. Weimar, V. L.: The sources of fibroblasts in corneal wound repair, Arch. Ophthalmol. **60:**93-109, 1958.
12. Harris, J. E.: Corneal wound healing. In King, J. H., Jr., and McTigue, J. W., editors: The Cornea World Congress, London, 1965, Butterworth & Co. (Publishers), Ltd., pp. 73-79.
13. Swan, K. C.: Fibroblastic ingrowth following cataract extraction, Arch. Ophthalmol. **89:**445-449, 1973.
14. Waring, G. O., Laibson, P. R., and Rodrigues, M.: Clinical and pathological alterations of Descemet's membrane: with emphasis on endothelial metaplasia, Surv. Ophthalmol. **18:**325-368, 1974.
15. Bloom, W., and Fawcett, D. W.: A textbook of histology, ed. 9, Philadelphia, 1968, W. B. Saunders Co.
16. Fine, B. S., and Yanoff, M.: Ocular histology. A text and atlas, New York, 1972, Harper & Row Publishers, pp. 150-162.
17. Klouček, F.: The corneal endothelium, Acta Univ. Carol. Med. **13:**321-373, 1967.
18. Sherrard, E. S., and Rycroft, P. V.: Retrocorneal membranes. I. Their origin and structure, Br. J. Ophthalmol. **51:**379-386, 1967.
19. Matsuda, H., and Smelser, G. K.: Endothelial cells in akali-burned corneas. Ultrastructural alterations, Arch. Ophthalmol. **89:**402-409, 1973.
20. Mochizuki, K., Murakami, M., and Kitano, S.: Experimental studies on burns of the cornea. Report I. Histological findings on burns of the cornea with NaOH and HCl, Acta Soc. Ophthalmol. Jap. **71:**1112-1122, 1967.
21. Voino-Yaseneisky, V. V.: About new formation of glass membranes due to Descemet's endothelium and multilaminary fibrilous tissue, (Russian-English summary) Oftalmolmol. Zh. **25:**551-556, 1970.
22. Michels, R. G., Kenyon, K. R., and Maumenee, A. E.: Retrocorneal fibrous membrane, Invest. Ophthalmol. **11:**822-831, 1972.
23. Townsend, W. M., and Kaufman, H. E.: Pathogenesis of glaucoma and endothelial changes in herpetic keratouveitis in rabbits, Am. J. Ophthalmol. **71:**904-910, 1971.
24. Kurz, G. H., and D'Amico, R. A.: Histopathology of corneal graft failures, Am. J. Ophthalmol. **66:**184-199, 1968.
25. Sherrard, E. S., and Rycroft, P. V.: Retrocorneal membranes. I. Their origin and structure, Br. J. Ophthalmol. **51:**379-386, 1967.
26. Sherrard, E. S., and Rycroft, P. V.: Retrocorneal membrane. II. Factors influencing their growth, Br. J. Ophthalmol. **51:**387-393, 1967.
27. Werb, A.: The postgraft membrane, Internat. Ophthalmol. Clin. **2:**771-780, 1962.
28. Friedman, A. H., and Henkind, P.: Corneal stroma overgrowth after cataract extraction, Br. J. Ophthalmol. **54:**528-534, 1970.
29. Bettman, J. W., Jr.: Pathology of complications of intraocular surgery, Am. J. Ophthalmol. **68:**1037-1050, 1969.
30. Bresnick, G. H.: Eyes containing anterior chamber acrylic implants. Pathological complications, Arch. Ophthalmol. **82:**726-737, 1969.
31. Contreras, C. F.: Retrocorneal membranes. In Polack, F. M.: Corneal and external diseases of the eye, Springfield, Ill., 1970, Charles C Thomas, Publisher, pp. 135-145.
32. Werb, A.: The postgraft membrane, Int. Ophthalmol. Clin. **2:**771-780, 1962.
33. Stocker, F. W.: The endothelium of the cornea and its clinical implications, ed. 2, Springfield, Ill., 1971, Charles C Thomas, Publisher.

34. Chi, H. H., Teng, C. C., and Katzin, H. M.: Histopathology of corneal endothelium. A study of 176 pathologic discs removed at keratoplasty, Am. J. Ophthalmol. **53:** 215-235, 1962.

35. Rodrigues, M. D., Valdes-Dapena, M., and Kistenmacher, M.: Ocular pathology in a case of 13 trisomy, J. Pediatr. Ophthalmol. **10:**54-60, 1973.

36. Samuels, B.: Methods of formation of the posterior abscess in ulcus serpens, Arch. Ophthalmol. **7:**31-39, 1932.

37. Brown, S. I., and Kitano, S.: Pathogenesis of the retrocorneal membrane, Arch. Ophthalmol. **75:**518-525, 1966.

38. Hales, R. H., and Spencer, W. H.: Unsuccessful penetrating keratoplasties. Correlation of clinical and histologic findings, Arch. Ophthalmol. **70:**805-810, 1963.

39. Rycroft, P. V.: Corneal graft membranes, Trans. Ophthalmol. Soc. U.K. **85:**317-326, 1965.

40. Polack, F. M., and Kanai, A.: Electron microscopic studies of graft endothelium in corneal graft rejection, Am. J. Ophthalmol. **73:**711-717, 1972.

41. Sherrard, E. S.: Further studies on the retrocorneal membrane-endothelium relationship, Br. J. Ophthalmol. **53:** 808-818, 1969.

42. Maumenee, A. E.: Clinical patterns of corneal graft failure. In Corneal graft failure, New York, 1973, Excerpta Medica, pp. 5-23.

43. Polack, F. M.: Clinical and pathologic aspects of the corneal graft reaction. Ophthalmology (Rochester) **77:**418-431, 1973.

44. Girard, L. J., Caldwell, D. R., Spak, K. E., and Hawkins, R. S.: Corneal stromal outgrowth, Am. J. Ophthalmol. **76:** 445-450, 1973.

45. Dunnington, J. H.: Complications of wound healing after cataract surgery. In Haik, G. M.: Symposium on diseases and surgery of the lens, St. Louis, 1957, The C. V. Mosby Co., pp. 158-165.

46. Bettman, J. W., Jr.: Pathology of complications of intraocular surgery, Am. J. Ophthalmol. **68:**1037-1050, 1969.

CHAPTER 28

Corneal endothelial proliferation

Proliferation of corneal endothelium in the anterior chamber is less well known than epithelial invasion of the anterior chamber and fibrous ingrowth. We have already considered the proliferation of these two elements of the cornea—epithelium (Chapter 26) and stroma (Chapter 27)—within the anterior chamber, and now a third component, the endothelium, is considered.

HISTORICAL BACKGROUND

Wagenmann[1] (1892) was the first to have seen and understood the significance of a glass membrane over the anterior iris surface in an eye with extensive anterior synechias. He correctly explained his observations as a proliferation of corneal endothelium onto the iris and a new formation of a glass membrane by secretion. Earlier, Donders[2] (1857) had observed this in two eyes but did not recognize its significance. Parsons[3] (1904) stated that such membranes over the surface of the iris were common and usually seen in glaucomatous eyes with peripheral anterior synechias. However, surprisingly little attention was paid to this entity until recent years. Herbert[4] (1927) described glass membrane formation in eyes with long-standing chronic iridocyclitis. He suggested changing the name from hyaline membrane to glass membrane, since the latter signified a definite structure that stained with orcein (an elastic tissue stain). More recently, Donaldson and Smith[5] (1966) and Kroll[6] (1969) have described such formations around vitreous strands, and Wolter[7] (1969) has described them around zonular fibers. These were referred to as Descemet's membrane tubes, although Vogt[8] (1930) called them glassy cones. Thus, although

the basic process described in this chapter is the same, this entity has been referred to as hyaline membranes, glass membranes, corneal endothelial proliferation, glassy cones, glass tubes, and Descemet's tubes.

PATHOPHYSIOLOGY

As noted in the preceding chapter, corneal endothelium differs in many respects from that of a true endothelium. It is really a mesothelium, which is the surface lining of a serous cavity, and strictly speaking, the anterior chamber is a serous cavity lined anteriorly by mesothelium.[9,10] Corneal endothelium is mesodermally derived (as are fibroblasts) and can undergo fibroblastic metaplasia. This is in contrast to a true endothelium, which is the lining of a vascular channel and usually does not convert to a fibroblast.[11]

When Descemet's membrane and corneal endothelium are incised or injured, repair occurs rapidly. Because of its elasticity, Descemet's membrane retracts and curls into a spiral directed forward; thus an area of the posterior surface of the stroma is exposed. Within 24 hours the first evidence of endothelial regeneration appears, and by 48 hours there is a well-defined endothelial layer migrating over the defect from the cut and retracted Descemet's membrane.[12] Generally the growth of endothelium is prolific. It does not stop when the defective area is filled but continues to proliferate until a fusiform scar of cellular tissue is produced over the area of trauma. Mitotic and amitotic cell divisions in all phases can be seen. The number of mitoses are greatest during the 24- to 36-hour period. Whereas mitosis practically disappears from the injured area after 5 days, amitoses are still present after 2 weeks, although the denuded area is covered in the first few days.[13] Cogan[14] stated that mitoses are never seen in normal endothelium. Amitosis appears to be the method of regeneration of the corneal endothelium under normal conditions, whereas mitotic cell divisions occur under unusual circumstances.[13] Others have shown that whereas in childhood mitoses can be demonstrated, cell division by amitosis accounts for endothelial regeneration in the adult.[13,15,16] Thus the process is first marked by a migration of neighboring endothelial cells over the denuded area, with the cells increasing in size up to twice their diameter. The presence of mitotic division indicates a proliferation of the cells. Regeneration of endothelium is slower than that seen with epithelium. If the wound is widespread, repair may be permanently incomplete, leaving unprotected an area of stroma that shows persistent swelling and edema.[17] If a large gape in Descemet's membrane is caused by the wound, stromal fibroblasts may participate in the healing process. This forms a plug in the gape that shows no continuity with the curled Descemet's membrane and the endothelial cell layer. This plug has been discussed on p. 17. Descemet's membrane is eventually secreted by the endothelium in uncomplicated wounds. Fuchs[18] first suggested that the endothelium produces Descemet's membrane, and there is ample evidence to support this. The endothelial cells contain intracytoplasmic vacuoles of electron-dense material that are released into the region of Descemet's membrane.[19-22] They can lay down a basement membrane similar to Descemet's in tissue culture[22-24] and in ectopic intraocular locations. The chemical composition and structural organization of Descemet's membrane are similar to those of other

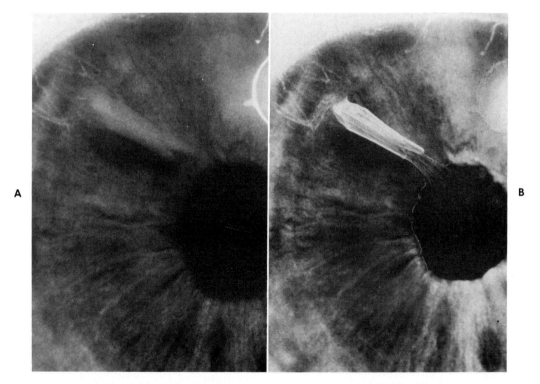

Fig. 28-1. Descemet's membrane tube in eye of older man who had multiple needlings for congenital cataracts about 60 years previously. Dense tubulelike structure extends about two thirds of way to pupil and is attached to cornea at old scar, and vitreous can be seen extending from posterior end of tube into pupil. **A,** Original photograph. **B,** Retouched photograph. (**A** courtesy Dr. D. D. Donaldson, Boston; **B** from Donaldson, D. D., and Smith, T. R.: Trans Am. Ophthalmol. Soc. **64:**89, 1966.)

mammalian basement membranes.[25,26] The formation of a new Descemet's membrane is a relatively slow process. A new Descemet's membrane probably does not begin to appear for several weeks. It may never reach its original thickness, although it is comparable in some respects to the old membrane. The regeneration of Descemet's membrane may not reach its peak for many months.

Regeneration function appears to decline with age but does not disappear. Stimuli to endothelial regeneration in childhood may provoke marked proliferation of endothelial cells and Descemet's membrane, whereas an identical stimulus in the adult may produce barely enough response to maintain corneal integrity.[27-29] For some reason, proliferation of endothelium is rare after intraocular surgery. One may consider that the smaller degree of inflammation produced by

surgery in comparison with that produced by accidental trauma and the fact that accidental trauma is more common in children and surgical trauma is more common in adults may account for this difference. In some cases an abnormal response occurs, characterized by an excessive amount of Descemet's membrane production. It does this by conversion of endothelial cells into a fibroblast-like cell (fibroblastic metaplasia) that produces fibrous tissue in addition to Descemet's membrane. This fibrous tissue becomes incorporated into Descemet's membrane, resulting in a thickened multilaminar "regenerated Descemet's membrane."[3] This differs from the typical Descemet's membrane, which has been described as a glass membrane because of its structureless appearance. However, early histologists detected a lamellar pattern by light microscopy and electron microscopy that has demonstrated

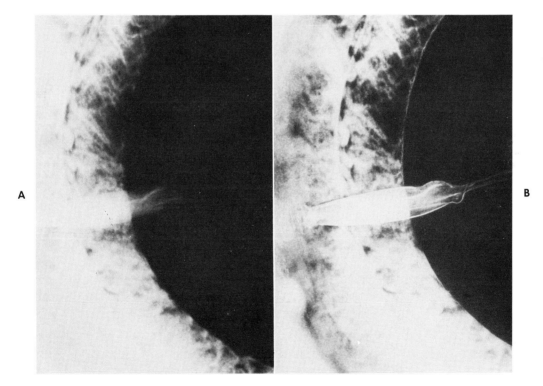

Fig. 28-2. Descemet's membrane tube in eye of older man who had needlings performed as child for congenital cataracts. Tube is attached to cornea and extends almost to vitreous face where fine strands of vitreous can be seen attaching to its posterior end. **A,** Original photograph. **B,** Retouched photograph. (**A** courtesy Dr. D. D. Donaldson, Boston; **B** from Donaldson, D. D., and Smith, T. R.: Trans. Am. Ophthalmol. Soc. **64:**89, 1966.)

two distinct regions: the anterior one third, which is 1 to 4 μm thick and displays a vertically banded pattern, and the posterior two thirds, which is 5 to 15 μm thick and appears amorphous and granular. This posterior portion contains smaller, less regularly arranged fibrils than the anterior one third, and the transition between the anterior and posterior zones is indistinct. Waring and co-workers[30] point out that terminology is a little confusing, since some authors restrict the use of "Descemet's membrane" to the original endothelial basement membrane, whereas others use the term in reference to the entire multilaminar structure. Some regard only the nonfibrillar basement membranelike substance as Descemet's membrane. It is also common to call the laminated structure a "reduplicated Descemet's membrane," an inaccurate term based on early light microscopic observations. They feel that

communication is best served by referring to the entire membrane as a multilaminar Descemet's membrane.

In addition to the process of repair of wounded endothelium and Descemet's membrane, we know that corneal endothelium has a tendency to proliferate in an attempt to cover free surfaces and to surround and enclose anything in contact with it.[11] This includes foreign bodies, calcified lens remnants, and rolled up portions of Descemet's membrane. It extends onto the iris, anterior synechias, scars in the anterior chamber, ciliary body, and anterior vitreous and may even reach the retina. It may grow along zonular fibers and vitreous strands, in which cases it forms tubular structures. New Descemet's membrane is laid down with time wherever the endothelium extends. Thus, depending on the circumstances involved, a variety of clinical and pathologic enti-

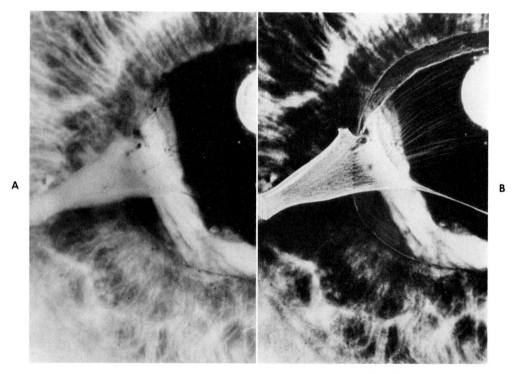

Fig. 28-3. Descemet's membrane tube in eye of old man who had multiple needlings for congenital cataracts approximately 63 years previously. Transparent tubular structure is seen to extend from old corneal scar down to vitreous face to which it is attached. **A,** Original photograph. **B,** Retouched photograph. (**A** courtesy Dr. D. D. Donaldson, Boston; **B** from Donaldson, D. D., and Smith, T. R.: Trans. Am. Ophthalmol. Soc. **64:**89, 1966.)

ties that involve a proliferation of corneal endo-thelium may be encountered.

Descemet's tubes

Donaldson and Smith[5] reported in a superbly illustrated clinical paper 18 tubule-appearing structures in patients who previously had needling operations for congenital cataracts or perforating corneal injuries. The tubes were glassy in appearance and extended from the corneal wound toward the pupillary area. They postulated that the endothelium proliferates on the surface of a strand of vitreous adherent to a corneal wound, followed by an elaboration of hyaline tubular structure by the endothelium. They raised the possibility that structures other than the vitreous could act as a framework for the formation of a Descemet's membrane tube, but they found no evidence for this in any of their cases.

The tube usually develops some years after the original surgery or injury. Apparently in some cases the proliferated endothelium produces Descemet's membrane for a relatively short time, and then the process stops, leaving a tube that reaches only part way to the vitreous face (Figs. 28-1 to 28-6).

In most instances of Descemet's tubes the surgery or injury occurs in childhood. This fact leads one to suspect that the young endothelium proliferates and produces Descemet's membrane more actively. However, Descemet's membrane tubes are seen after cataract surgery in adults (Fig. 28-17).

There has been some histologic verification of the nature of the fibers on which the endothelial proliferation occurs. Kroll[6] described a solid cylinder in a 19-year-old patient's eye enucleated 18 months after a perforating injury. It had a connec-

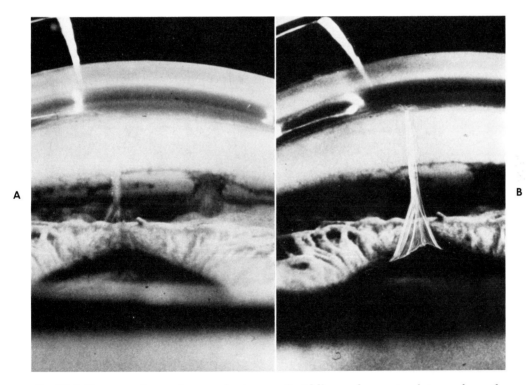

Fig. 28-4. Descemet's membrane tube in eye of middle-aged man struck in eye by nail 12 years previously. Gonioscopically, transparent tubular structure can be seen extending almost directly down from central position of cornea to pupillary margin and attaching to vitreous face. **A,** Original photograph. **B,** Retouched photograph. (**A** courtesy Dr. D. D. Donaldson, Boston; **B** from Donaldson, D. D., and Smith, T. R.: Trans. Am. Ophthalmol. Soc. **64:**89, 1966.)

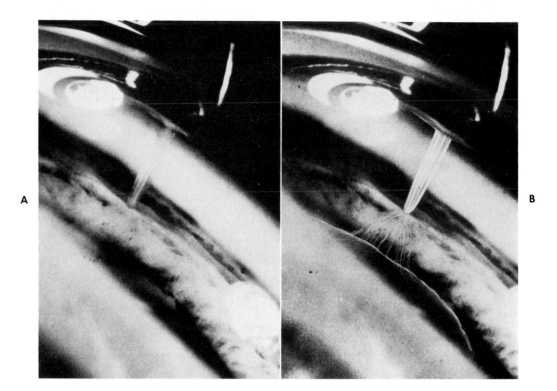

Fig. 28-5. Gonioscopic view of Descemet's membrane tube. Attachment of tube to cornea is easily visible, and vitreous strands to other end can be seen. **A,** Original photograph. **B,** Retouched photograph. (**A** courtesy Dr. D. D. Donaldson, Boston; **B** from Donaldson, D. D., and Smith, T. R.: Trans. Am. Ophthalmol. Soc. **64:**89, 1966.)

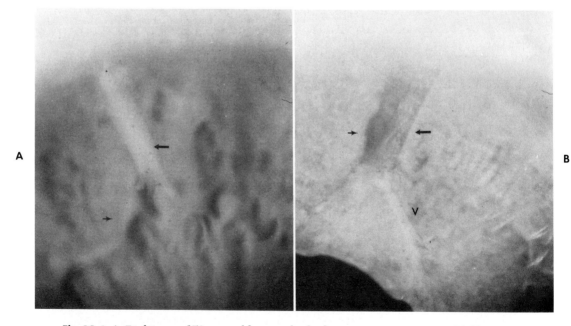

Fig. 28-6. A, Right eye of 72-year-old man who had cataract surgery at age 14. Note typical Descemet's tube *(large arrow)* with flaring out of vitreous *(small arrow)*. **B,** Left eye of same patient, which shows pigmented Descemet's tube *(large arrow)* that casts shadow *(small arrow)* on iris. Note flaring out of vitreous *(v)* below tube.

tive tissue core and was covered by endothelium continuous with the corneal endothelium and presumably identical to it (Figs. 28-7 and 28-8). The endothelium apparently elaborated Descemet's membranelike material that had identical staining characteristics to Descemet's membrane with periodic acid–Schiff and von Giesen staining techniques. This was the first histologic report of a Descemet's tube, but there was some variation from the usual clinical variety, since the cylindrical structure did not lead to a corneal perforation site anteriorly. In this case a subluxated lens occurred, and it is conceivable that at the time of injury a strand of vitreous reached the corneal endothelium and provided the scaffold for endothelial proliferation and subsequent glass membrane tube elaboration. However, the possibility that a strand of clotted blood or fibrin rather than a strand of vitreous formed the framework for endothelial proliferation cannot be excluded.

A similar case was reported by Wolter.[31] The histopathologic appearance of a typical Descemet's membrane tube extending from the ciliary body into the vitreous was described. The tube was found to be formed by corneal endothelium and a secondary Descemet's membrane surrounding a core of vitreous. The vitreous strand in this patient also did not arise from the corneal perforation site but originated from the ciliary body. The corneal endothelium had extended to its origin by proliferation across a false angle. It can be assumed, however, that Descemet's tubes inserting on the posterior cornea are histopathologically very similar or exactly like the Descemet's membrane tube of this patient. It presented an opportunity to view the vitreous strand typically surrounded by endothelium and newly secreted Descemet's membrane and a deeper portion of the strand not surrounded by endothelium (Figs. 28-9 to 28-12). It is of special interest that this Descemet's membrane tube had developed as part of extensive proliferation 30 years after a childhood trauma. Another case was described by Waring and co-workers[30] (Fig. 28-13).

That vitreous strands need not supply the scaffold was dramatically shown in another histologic description of a Descemet's membrane tube by

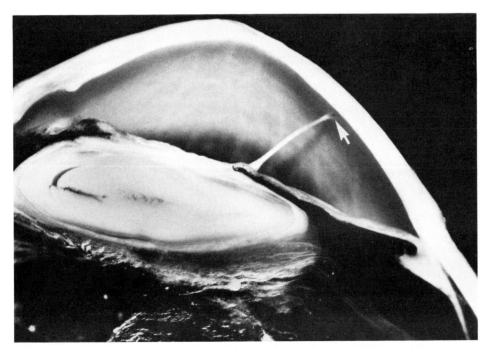

Fig. 28-7. Corneal attachment of cylindrical Descemet's membrane tube *(arrow)*. Upper half of anterior chamber after lower calotte was removed by horizontal meridional section. (From Kroll, A. J.: Arch. Ophthalmol. **82**:339-343, 1969.)

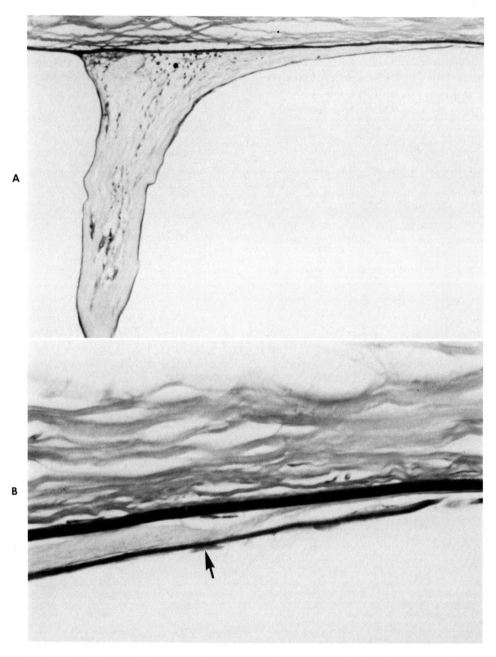

Fig. 28-8. A, Tangential section of corneal attachment of cylindrical structure that has flared anterior end and is attached to intact Descemet's membrane. It contains PAS-positive basement membrane continuous with branching from Descemet's membrane. **B,** Right side of **A,** showing PAS-positive basement membrane, itself covered by endothelium *(arrow)*, continuous with and presumably identical to corneal endothelium. (Periodic acid–Schiff and hematoxylin, slightly reduced from ×125, **A,** and from ×500, **B.**) (From Kroll, A. J.: Arch. Ophthalmol. **82:**339-343, 1969.)

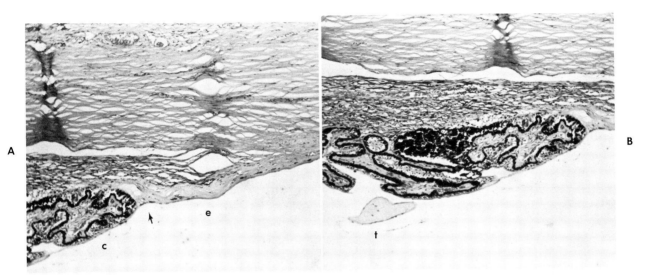

Fig. 28-9. A, Corneal endothelium *(e)*, false chamber angle *(arrow)*, and atrophic ciliary body *(c)* lined with corneal endothelium. **B,** Posterior extension of **A**, showing Descemet's tube *(t)*. (From Wolter, J. R.: J. Pediatr. Ophthalmol. **9:**39-42, 1972.)

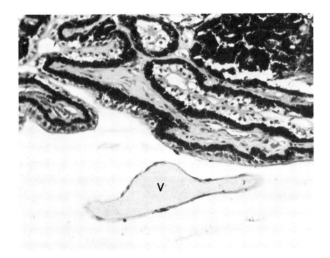

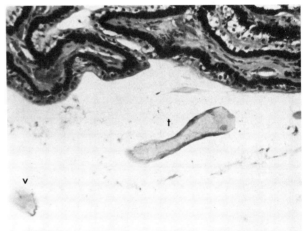

Fig. 28-10. Higher power view of Descemet's tube, exhibiting core of vitreous *(v)* and surrounding layer of corneal endothelium and newly formed Descemet's membrane. (×150.) (From Wolter, J. R.: J. Pediatr. Ophthalmol. **9:**39-42, 1972.)

Fig. 28-11. Same eye as in Figs. 28-9 and 28-10. Descemet's membrane tube *(t)* and basic vitreous strand without endothelium *(v)*. (×150.) (From Wolter, J. R.: J. Pediatr. Ophthalmol. **9:**39-42, 1972.)

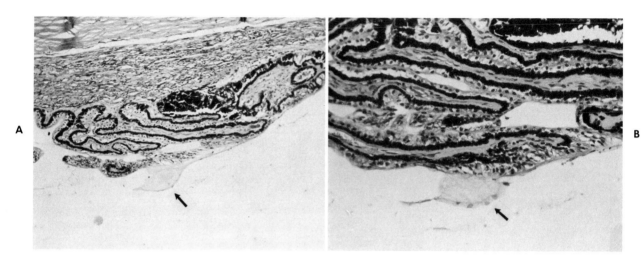

Fig. 28-12. A, Same eye as in Figs. 28-9 to 28-11. Origin of corneal endothelium at that part of ciliary body where it starts to extend onto vitreous strand *(arrow)*. B, Origin of vitreous strand with corneal endothelium extending from ciliary body onto it *(arrow)* at higher power (×150.) (From Wolter, J. R.: J. Pediatr. Ophthalmol. **9:**39-42, 1972.)

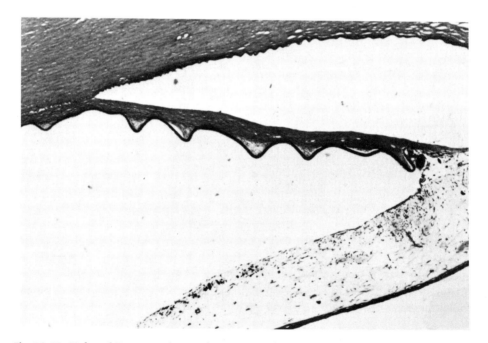

Fig. 28-13. Tube of Descemet's membrane extends from cornea to iris. Histopathology shows fibrous strand lined by regenerated Descemet's membrane. (×64.) (From Waring, G. O., Laibson, P. R., and Rodrigues, M.: Surv. Ophthalmol. **18:**325-368, 1974. Copyright © 1974, The Williams & Wilkins Co., Baltimore.)

Wolter.[7] An eye removed from a 22-year-old patient 19 years after an intraocular penetrating injury by a piece of glass demonstrated Descemet's tubes around zonular fibers of the lens. In this eye, corneal endothelium with a thick layer of newly formed Descemet's membrane extended onto the posterior surface of an iris stump involved in an anterior synechia and onto the atrophic ciliary body (Figs. 28-14 and 28-15). Corneal endothelium with its newly formed glass

membrane enclosed three fibers of the zonule of the lens (Figs. 28-15 and 28-16). The growth on the zonules progressed to half the distance between the ciliary body and the lens.

Aside from vitreous strands and zonular fibers just described, other structures may form the central core of Descemet's tubes. These include strands of iris, lens capsule, and persistent pupillary membrane after corneal birth trauma.

As observed previously, these glass tubes are found some time after discissions or corneal perforating injuries in young individuals. They are rare after cataract surgery in adults despite the fact that strands of vitreous not infrequently adhere to the cornea or the operative wound. One explanation has already been given, that is, that the young endothelium may proliferate and produce Descemet's membrane more actively. Another involves the site of the corneal perforation. Surgeons often make a beveled knife needle incision in performing a discission. The knife frequently enters the anterior chamber central to Schwalbe's line. Tubes may be seen after cataract surgery in adults if a markedly beveled corneal incision is made (Fig. 28-17). The corneal endothelium normally covers the posterior corneal surface as a delicate monolayer and ends peripherally at Schwalbe's line. Limbal incisions are unlikely to involve the corneal endothelium.

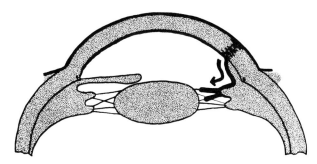

Fig. 28-14. Drawing of anterior segment of eye that suffered perforating injury. Iris stump is adherent to area of perforation. Endothelial proliferation and newly formed Descemet's membrane are shown on zonular fibers of lens. (From Wolter, J. R.: J. Pediatr. Ophthalmol. **6:**153-156, 1969.)

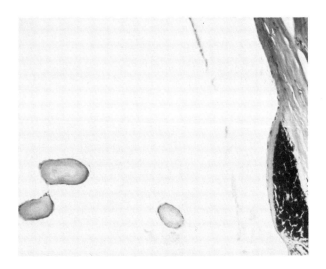

Fig. 28-15. Newly formed Descemet's membrane on stump of iris *(right)* and on zonular fibers *(left).* (Paraffin section, hematoxylin and eosin, ×148.) (From Wolter, J. R.: J. Pediatr. Ophthalmol. **6:**153-156, 1969.)

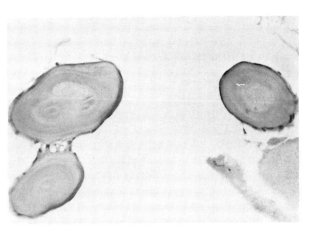

Fig. 28-16. High-power view of tubes, showing core of zonular fibers, newly formed Descemet's membrane, and proliferated endothelium on surface. (Paraffin section, hematoxylin and eosin, ×407.) (From Wolter, J. R.: J.Pediatr. Ophthalmol. **6:**153-156, 1969.)

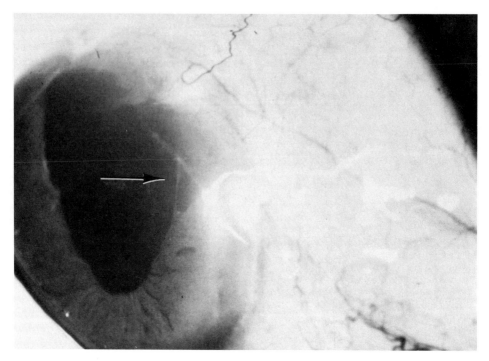

Fig. 28-17. Descemet's tube *(arrow)* extending from site of markedly beveled corneal incision, around border of iris, to vitreous in eye of 68-year-old man 7 years after intracapsular cataract extraction. Newly formed Descemet's membrane extends less than halfway down vitreous strand.

A strand of vitreous adherent to the cornea central to Schwalbe's line is more likely to be surrounded and enclosed by proliferating endothelium and a newly secreted Descemet's membrane.

Glass membranes on anterior surface of iris

In cases of glass membranes on the anterior surface of the iris the endothelial proliferation does not result in tube structures but instead forms a sheetlike membrane. This more closely resembles the anterior invasions associated with epithelium and stroma. The endothelium not only overgrows defects or rolled up pieces of Descemet's membrane on the posterior corneal surface after surgery or trauma (p. 17), but it may also grow onto the iris and form an extensive new glass membrane. Such membranes are seen in blunt trauma with angle recession,[28,32-34] after perforating injury,[29,35,36] in chronic iridocyclitis,[28,37] essential iris atrophy,[38,39] congenital glaucoma,[40] the anterior chamber cleavage syndrome,[10,40-42] retrolental fibroplasia,[30] after injection of staphylotoxin into the rabbit anterior chamber,[10] and in degenerated eyes with very extensive pathologic changes.[43] The normal structure of the angle seems to prevent this proliferation. It occurs only after the peripheral cornea has come in contact with iris or scar tissue overlying the iris. These eyes often show the unusual contrast of advanced atrophy of the endothelium proper with abundant proliferative extensions of the endothelium on the iris. Anterior adhesions of iris to the peripheral cornea form a "false angle" over which endothelial growth occurs more readily (Fig. 28-18). This usually occurs in advanced glaucomatous eyes and in some eyes with long-standing chronic iridocyclitis. There is one exception to the statement made earlier that peripheral anterior synechiae are a necessary scaffolding for endothelial proliferation lining the angle. Lauring[28] surveyed 136 eyes enucleated for glass membranes extending posterior to Schwalbe's line. Among 31 eyes

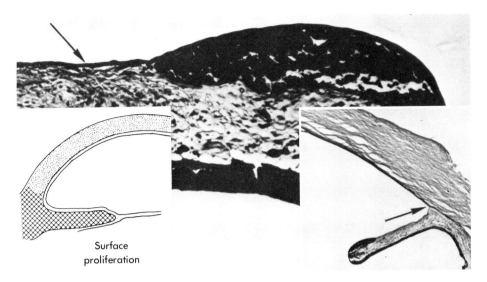

Surface
proliferation

Fig. 28-18. Ectopic proliferation of Descemet's membrane. Globe from eye of 32-year-old man who sustained blunt trauma to eye at age 8. Lower left insert shows angle closure with peripheral anterior synechia lined by downgrowth of Descemet's membrane (*arrow*, lower right insert), which extends over anterior and posterior surface of iris. (×4.) Major figure: Anterior iris surface is covered by prominent layer of Descemet's membrane (*arrow*). (×256) (From Waring, G. O., Laibson, P. R., and Rodrigues, M.: Surv. Ophthalmol. **18**:325-368, 1974. Copyright © 1974, The Williams & Wilkins Co., Baltimore.)

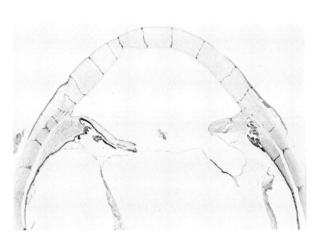

Fig. 28-19. Section of anterior segment showing scar in area of iridectomy *(right)*, aphakia, and dense membrane extending from scar on cornea to detached retina on opposite side. (Paraffin section, hematoxylin and eosin, ×10.) (From Wolter, J. R.: J. Pediatr. Ophthalmol. **7**:162-166, 1970.)

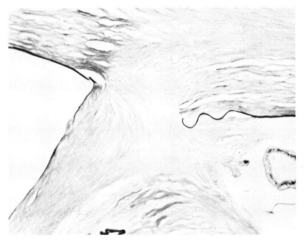

Fig. 28-20. Schiff stain showing peripheral end of interrupted Descemet's membrane within scar and newly formed glass membrane *(left)* extending from cornea onto scar. (Paraffin section, ×119.) (From Wolter, J. R.: J. Pediatr. Ophthalmol. **7**:162-166, 1970.)

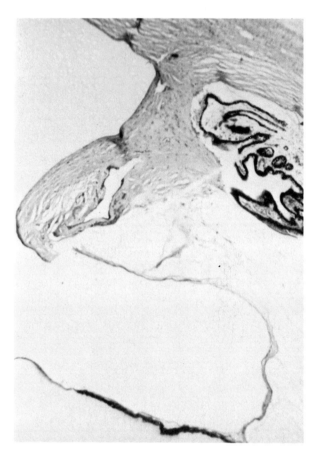

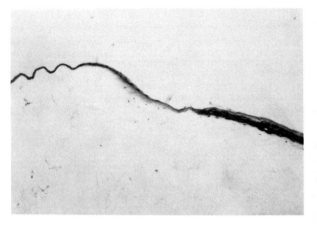

Fig. 28-22. Newly formed glass membrane over anterior vitreous. (Paraffin section, hematoxylin and eosin, ×70.) (From Wolter, J. R.: J. Pediatr. Ophthalmol. **7:** 162-166, 1970.)

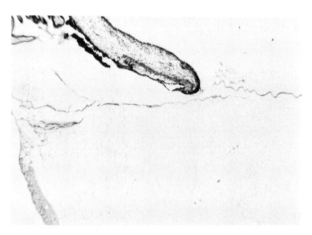

Fig. 28-21. Newly formed glass membrane can be followed from cornea over scar and into anterior vitreous *(bottom)*. (Paraffin section, hematoxylin and eosin, ×80.) (From Wolter, J. R.: J. Pediatr. Ophthalmol. **7:** 162-166, 1970.)

Fig. 28-23. Newly formed glass membrane in anterior vitreous extending to peripheral detached retina at left. (Paraffin section, hematoxylin and eosin, ×36.) (From Wolter, J. R.: J. Pediatr. Ophthalmol. **7:**162-166, 1970.)

with traumatic angle recession and glaucoma, ectopic Descemet's membrane lined the angle in 45% of cases. Approximately one half of these showed peripheral anterior synechiae, but significantly, one half did not. In contrast, only 4.9% of 41 eyes with contusion injury and glaucoma but without angle recession had ectopic Descemet's membranes. It is not clear why eyes with angle recession have a 10 times greater frequency of

ectopic Descemet's membrane. It has been suggested that these eyes received more severe trauma and had more inflammation as a stimulus to proliferation. For this reason, it is possible that this may not apply to cataract surgery but could apply to trauma and perforating injuries.

The extent to which a proliferating corneal endothelium can grow was demonstrated in a case reported by Wolter.[44] A young child suffered a perforating corneal injury and a traumatic cataract. An exuberant proliferation of corneal endothelium onto a retrocorneal scar (Figs. 28-19 and 28-20) through an iridectomy and into the anterior vitreous occurred (Figs. 28-21 and 28-22). In the vitreous, this membrane not only caused the extensive monolayer of endothelium with its glass membrane, but it also resulted in additional secondary vitreous bands. Both the endothelial membrane and the vitreous bands were found to extend to the peripheral retina and clearly exerted pull, probably causing the retinal detachment observed (Fig. 28-23).

Cases such as these should lead the surgeon to suspect and look for endothelial proliferation and newly formed glass membranes if trauma or surgery has involved the cornea central to Schwalbe's line and if a tissue bridge from the cornea to deeper ocular structures has remained. For some as yet unexplained reason the endothelium peripheral to Schwalbe's line also proliferates, but fortunately shows much less tendency to elaborate a glass membrane (as one would expect in the absence of metaplasia).

REFERENCES

1. Wagenmann, A.: Weitere Mittheilungen über Glashäutige Neubildungen an der Descemet'schen Membran und auf der Iris und über Veränderungen des Hornhautendothels, Graefe Arch. Ophthalmol. **38**:90-111, 1892.
2. Donders, F. C.: Beiträge zur pathologischen Anatomie des Auges. III. Neubildung von Glashäuten im Auge, Graefe Arch. Ophthalmol. **3**(pt. 1):150-165, 1857.
3. Parsons, J. H.: The pathology of the eye, London, 1904, Hodder & Stoughton.
4. Herbert, H.: Glass membrane formation in chronic iridocyclitis, Trans. Ophthalmol. Soc. U.K. **47**:155-164, 1927.
5. Donaldson, D. D., and Smith, T. R.: Descemet's membrane tubes, Trans. Am. Ophthalmol. Soc. **64**:89-109, 1966.
6. Kroll, A. J.: Proliferation of Descemet's membrane, Arch. Ophthalmol. **82**:339-343, 1969.
7. Wolter, J. R.: Descemet's membrane tubes on the zonular fibers of the lens, J. Pediatr. Ophthalmol. **6**:153-156, 1969.
8. Vogt, A.: Lehrbuch und Atlas der Spaltlampenmikroskopie des legenden Auges mit Anleitung zur Technik und Methodik der Untersuchung. Hornhaut und Vorderkammer, Berlin, 1930, Julius Springer Verlag, vol. 1, pp. 290-291.
9. Fine, B. S., and Yanoff, M.: Ocular histology. A text and atlas, New York, 1972, Harper & Row, Publishers, pp. 150-162.
10. Klouček, F.: The corneal endothelium, Acta Univ. Carol. Med. **13**:321-373, 1967.
11. Bloom, W., and Fawcett, D. W.: A textbook of histology, ed. 9, Philadelphia, 1968, W. B. Saunders Co.
12. Morton, P. L., Ormsby, H. L., and Basu, P. K.: Healing of endothelium and Descemet's membrane of rabbit cornea, Am. J. Ophthalmol. **6**:62-67, 1958.
13. Binder, R. F., and Binder, H. F.: Regenerative processes in the endothelium of the cornea, Arch. Ophthalmol. **57**:11-13, 1957.
14. Cogan, D. G.: Applied anatomy and physiology of the cornea, Ophthalmology (Rochester) **55**:329-359, 1951.
15. Chi, H. H., Teng, C. C., and Katzin, H. M.: Healing process in the mechanical denudation of the corneal endothelium, Am. J. Ophthalmol. **49**:693-703, 1960.
16. von Sallman, L., Caravaggio, L. L., and Grimes, P.: Studies on the corneal endothelium of the rabbit. I. Cell division and growth, Am. J. Ophthalmol. **51**:955-969, 1961.
17. Heydenreich, A.: Die Hornhautregeneration, Sammlung zwangloser Abhandlungen aus dem Gebiete der Augenheilkunde, suppl. 15, Halle, 1958, Carl Marhold Verlag.
18. Fuchs, E.: Erkrankung der hornhaut durch Schädigun von hinten, Arch. Ophthalmol. **92**:145-236, 1917.
19. Hogan, M. J., Alvarado, J. A., and Weddell, J. E.: Histology of the human eye, Philadelphia, 1971, W. B. Saunders Co.
20. Iwamoto, T., and DeVoe, A. G.: Electron microscopic studies on Fuchs' combined dystrophy. I. Posterior portion of the cornea, Invest. Ophthalmol. **10**:9-28, 1971.
21. Kuwabara, T., Quevedo, A. R., and Cogan, D. G.: An experimental study of dichloroethane poisoning, Arch. Ophthalmol. **79**:321-330, 1968.
22. Perlman, M., and Baum, J. L.: Collagen production in mass cultures of rabbit corneal endothelial cells. Presented at meeting of Assoc. Res. Vision Ophthalmol., Sarasota, Fla., May 3-7, 1973.
23. Kaye, G. I., Perlman, M., and Baum, J.: Fine structure and synthetic activity of rabbit corneal endothelium grown in vitro. Presented at meeting of Assoc. Res. Vision Ophthalmol., Sarasota, Fla., May 3-7, 1973.
24. Perlman, M., and Baum, J. L.: Synthesis of a collagenous basal membrane by rabbit corneal endothelial cells in vitro, Arch. Ophthalmol. **92**:238-239, 1974.
25. Kefalides, N. A.: The chemistry and structure of basement membranes, Arthritis Rheum. **12**:427-443, 1969.
26. Kefalides, N. A.: Isolation of a collagen from basement membranes containing three identical a-chains, Biochem. Biophys. Res. Commun. **45**:226-234, 1971.
27. Donaldson, D. D., and Smith, T. R.: Descemet's membrane tubes, Trans. Am. Ophthalmol. Soc. **64**:89-109, 1966.
28. Lauring, L.: Anterior chamber glass membranes, Am. J. Ophthalmol. **68**:308-312, 1969.
29. Wolter, J. R., and Fechner, P. U.: Glass membranes on the anterior iris surface, Am. J. Ophthalmol. **53**:235-243, 1962.
30. Waring, G. O., Laibson, P. R., and Rodrigues, M.: Clinical and pathological alterations of Descemet's membrane: with emphasis on endothelial metaplasia, Surv. Ophthalmol. **18**:325-368, 1974.

31. Wolter, J. R.: The histopathology of Descemet's membrane tubes, J. Pediatr. Ophthalmol. **9:**39-42, 1972.

32. Alper, M. G.: Contusion angle deformity and glaucoma, gonioscopic observations and clinical course, Arch. Ophthalmol. **69:**445-467, 1963.

33. Iwamoto, T., Witmer, R., and Landolt, E.: Light and electron microscopy in absolute glaucoma with pigment dispersion phenomena and contusion angle deformity, Am. J. Ophthalmol. **72:**420-434, 1971.

34. Wolff, S. M., and Zimmerman, L. E.: Chronic secondary glaucoma associated with retrodisplacement of iris root and deepening of the anterior chamber angle secondary to contusion, Am. J. Ophthalmol. **54:**547-563, 1962.

35. Redslob, E., and Brini, A.: Proliférations de l'-endothélium cornéen et de la membrane de Descemet, Ann. Ocul. **186:**969-986, 1953.

36. Wolter, J. R.: The histopathology of Descemet's membrane tubes, J. Pediatr. Ophthalmol. **9:**39-42, 1972.

37. Herbert, H.: Glass membrane formation in chronic iridocyclitis, Trans. Ophthalmol. Soc. U.K. **47:**155-164, 1927.

38. Günther, G.: Uber die verdoppelung der Descemet'schen membran. Beitrag sue anomalie der hinteren glashaut der cornea, Ophthalmologica **131:**410-416, 1956.

39. Oh, J. O.: Changes with age in the corneal endothelium of normal rabbits, Acta Ophthalmol. **41:**568-573, 1963.

40. Collins, E. T.: The anatomy and pathology of the eye, Lancet **1:**435-444, 1900.

41. Ballantyne, A. J.: Multiple congenital anomalies of the eyes, Proc. R. Soc. Med. **42:**756-762, 1949.

42. Reese, A. B., and Ellsworth, R. M.: The anterior chamber cleavage syndrome, Arch. Ophthalmol. **75:**307-318, 1966.

43. Wolter, J. R., and Fechner, P. U.: Glass membranes on the anterior iris surface, Am. J. Ophthalmol. **53:**235-243, 1962.

44. Wolter, J. R.: Proliferating corneal endothelium causing a vitreous membrane and incurable retinal detachment, J. Pediatr. Ophthalmol. **7:**162-166, 1970.

CHAPTER 29

Detachment of Descemet's membrane

Detachment of Descemet's membrane is a complication of cataract surgery that received little attention in the American ophthalmologic literature until recently. It represents another cause of postoperative corneal edema and opacification.

HISTORICAL BACKGROUND

The first attention to this complication in the American literature is attributed to Samuels[1] in 1928, who first became aware of it after being shown three cases by Adelbert Fuchs in the clinic of Josef Meller in Vienna. All three had shallow anterior chambers prior to glaucoma surgery. Shortly before, Sallmann[2] reported two similar cases. The first microscopic description of this entity is attributed to Böhm[3] in 1923 in an eye enucleated 11 weeks after an attack of secondary glaucoma. Numerous punctures and a cyclodialysis had been performed. Meller[4] describes the spatula passing forward between Descemet's membrane and the corneal stroma instead of tearing the fibers of the pectinate ligament as a frequent complication of cyclodialysis. Thus most early reports centered on detachment of Descemet's membrane as a complication of glaucoma surgery. However, Samuels stated that he saw cases of this type after cataract surgery in microscopic slides loaned to him by Ernst Fuchs. Extensive stripping of Descemet's membrane with cataract extraction was mentioned in the earlier literature only twice. Weve[5] reported two cases in 1927, and Wright[6] discussed this complication but reported no cases himself, referring to the earlier paper of Weve. After a virtual absence of this subect from the literature for almost 30 years, interest in it as a complication of cataract surgery

was awakened by Scheie[7] in 1965. There followed reports by Sugar[8] and Sparks,[9] both in 1967.

PATHOGENESIS

Detachment of Descemet's membrane may be seen in a variety of conditions. It may occur with birth trauma, contusions of the globe, buphthalmos, malignant melanoma of the ciliary body that grows forward between Descemet's membrane and stroma, exudate between these layers (serpiginous ulcer with hypopyon), organization of a heavy exudate in the anterior chamber that by contraction pulls away Descemet's membrane, lens adhesions, and intraocular surgery.

Samuels[1] mentioned detachments of Descemet's membrane caused by differences in elasticity between it and the stroma. In some atrophic globes the cornea may be half its normal size, yet the membrane remains smooth and accurately attached. Under other circumstances the cornea may be greatly distended, and Descemet's membrane accompanies it and remains well approximated. During intraocular surgery the cornea is folded back, and Descemet's membrane usually does not detach. This indicates a high degree of adhesiveness. However, in other cases this is not so, since a detachment may occur if there is rapid swelling or contraction of the stroma. That some eyes possess an anatomic predisposition for detachment, as suggested by Reese,[10] is emphatically supported by the occurrence of displacement of Descemet's membrane to a major or minor degree in both eyes of both patients reported by Sparks.[9] This is of practical significance in planning cataract surgery on the second eye of a patient who suffered this complication in the first eye.

In intraocular surgery the cause is probably a mechanical one related to faulty instrumentation or technique. A dull knife, keratome, or scissors, or inadvertent stripping by a spatula or anterior chamber irrigator are likely causes, but in these eyes there is the added possibility of an inherent predisposition. There is also the added consideration that one or more of the variety of solutions (alpha-chymotrypsin, acetylcholine, and so on) irrigated into the eye during surgery may be responsible. The possibility of this occurring during intraocular surgery is increased if difficulties are encountered. For example, in glaucomatous eyes with very shallow anterior chambers or anterior synechias, Descemet's membrane may be detached in making the incision. After the globe is decompressed in cataract surgery, there may be a forward displacement of the iris and vitreous so that enlargement with scissors becomes difficult and may cause stripping of Descemet's membrane. This may also occur with phacoemulsification or a planned extracapsular cataract extraction, in a closed system, during the performance of the anterior capsulotomy, during introduction of the ultrasonic or irrigation-aspiration handpiece through the 3 mm incision, or during the emulsification or aspiration parts of the procedure.

PATHOLOGY

Detachment of Descemet's membrane to a minor degree is not rare. It occurs more frequently with scissors-enlarged sections than with knife sections. These detachments appear as small transparent tags that curl inward from the corneal lip of the incision. Monroe[11] examined 120 eyes gonioscopically after cataract extraction and noted scrolls of detached Descemet's membrane in 11% of eyes and focal detachment of a ragged edge of this layer in 43%, with absence of clinically significant sequelae. Histologic study of eight of nine eyes after cataract extraction by Flaxel[12] showed fragmentation and dislocation of Descemet's membrane near the wound edge. These are usually of little consequence, since the endothelium covers these defects and slowly secretes a thin new Descemet's membrane. However, as previously mentioned (p. 546), detachment of Descemet's membrane may lead to more serious consequences by contributing to

fibrous ingrowth. Bettman[13] found this in 22% of adult and 10% of congenital cataract extractions in his series of 122 enucleated eyes after all kinds of intraocular surgery. Eighteen of 30 eyes (60%) with fibrous ingrowth had detached fragments of Descemet's membrane, whereas only five of 92 eyes (5.4%) without fibrous ingrowth had such an outcome. The portion of cornea denuded of Descemet's membrane becomes edematous and opaque. If the detachment is extensive, the edema may progress to bullous keratopathy. This is undoubtedly the result of exposure of the unprotected corneal stroma to aqueous. The cornea in this region becomes thicker than elsewhere. There is usually a sharp demarcation line between clear and edematous cornea (Fig. 29-1). This line may be highlighted by deposition of pigment in the trough formed by the detachment.[9] In other cases the edema is diffuse, and one has difficulty determining the extent of detachment without the slit lamp and without first reducing the edema with a topically administered hyperosmotic agent. Hecht[14] reported an interesting method of estimating the extent of planar Descemet's membrane detachment. After clearing the cornea with anhydrous glycerin, 10 ml of a 10% fluorescein solution is given intravenously. During the next 60 minutes the anterior chamber is observed. As the dye fills the anterior chamber, the patient's face may be directed downward or at any angle. The dye is thus able to concentrate behind Descemet's membrane, thereby outlining its posterior side (Fig. 29-2). The detached portion of Descemet's membrane may curl back into place, and the edema may subside. It may, however, become permanently adherent to the iris (Figs. 29-1 and 29-3). In addition, iris may adhere to the denuded portion of cornea in the form of anterior synechias. This is often associated with cellular infiltration of the posterior cornea and fibrous proliferation. It is surprising how large an area of denuded corneal stroma may be covered by newly regenerated Descemet's membrane (Fig. 29-4). Occasionally, Descemet's membrane may not curl inward as a sheet but may be detached from the stroma over a wide area, with only a narrow space between the two layers. In one such case, Sparks[9] observed that Descemet's membrane was detached from the posterior stroma by what looked like a dis-

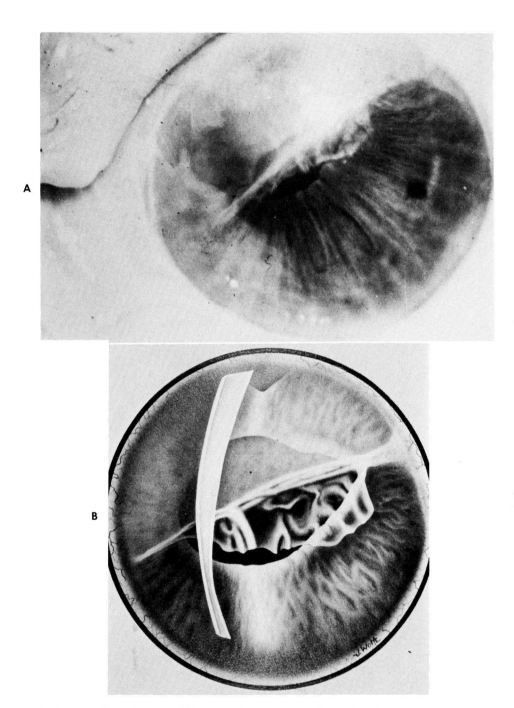

Fig. 29-1. A, Detachment of Descemet's membrane 8 months after cataract extraction, showing detached edge of Descemet's membrane in anterior chamber and attached to iris temporally. Hazy edematous portion of cornea sharply outlined at site of attachment of Descemet's membrane. **B,** Drawing of same eye through slit lamp microscope. (From Scheie, H. G.: Arch. Ophthalmol. **73:**311-314, 1965.)

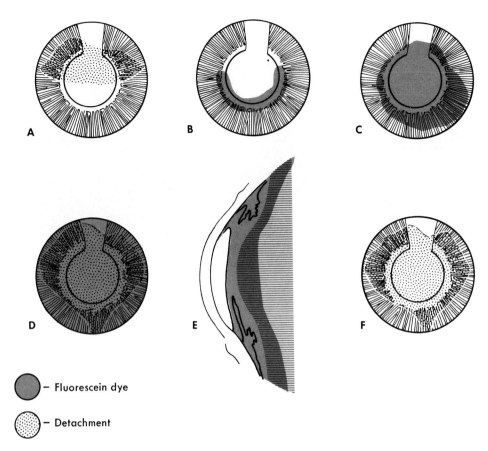

Fig. 29-2. **A,** First impression of extent of Descemet's membrane detachment after exhaustive darkroom examination. **B,** Dye beginning to appear after intravenous injection of fluorescein. Note that dye appears inferiorly first after production of sector iridectomy. **C,** Dye has now spread further into anterior chamber. **D,** Dye is seen to fill space behind detached Descemet's membrane in front view. **E,** In side view, one sees that dye has lined up behind Descemet's membrane detachment and also fills posterior chamber. It has not yet diffused into front compartment of anterior chamber. **F,** True extent of Descemet's membrane detachment, as proved by fluorescein. Note that there is detachment extending to cyclodialysis site at 6 o'clock, thus proving etiology of detachment. (From Hecht, S.: A method of estimating, the extent of planar Descemet's membrane detachment. In Emery, J. M., and Paton, D.: Current concepts in cataract surgery. Selected Proceedings of the Third Biennial Cataract Surgical Congress, St. Louis, 1974, The C. V. Mosby Co.)

tance of not more than half a millimeter and showed no tendency to curl up (Fig. 29-5, A). The detachment was seen to originate from a site near the limbus where a tiny hole could be seen in the membrane through which aqueous was obviously gaining access to the corneal stroma.

Since Descemet's membrane is not digested by the autolytic processes of the body, it remains undisturbed in ectopic locations or abnormal configurations indefinitely. Changes that occur in childhood are often observed during an examination many years later.

DIAGNOSIS

Usually the cataract surgery has been uneventful, but occasionally some difficulty has been encountered in the enlargement of the incision. The surgeon may observe the detachment of

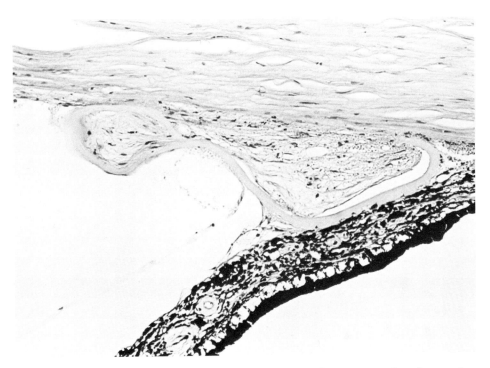

Fig. 29-3. Descemet's membrane curled back into place after apparent detachment during cataract extraction.

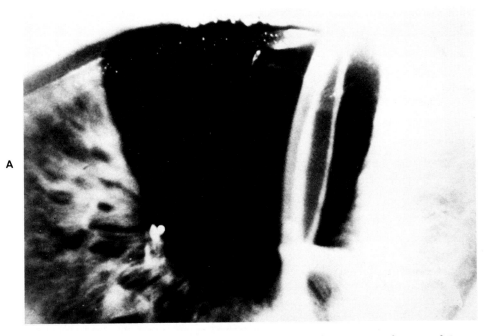

Fig. 29-4. A, Surgical detachment of Descemet's membrane. Detachment of Descemet's membrane following cataract extraction, with clear overlying cornea.

Continued.

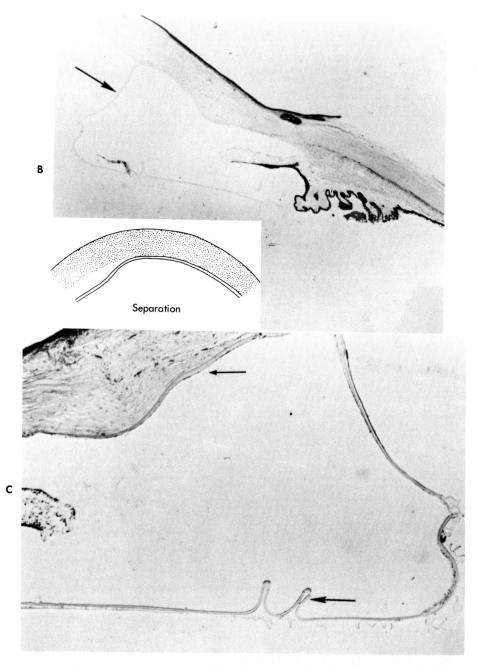

Fig. 29-4, cont'd. B, Detached Descemet's membrane *(arrow)* in eye of patient who had cataract extraction 14 years previously and maintained clear cornea because of formation of regenerated Descemet's membrane adjacent to wound. **C,** Detached Descemet's membrane shows folds and multilaminar pattern *(lower arrow).* Regenerated Descemet's membrane covers area of separation *(upper arrow).* (From Waring, G. O., Laibson, P. R., and Rodrigues, M.: Surv. Ophthalmol. **18:**325-368, 1974. Copyright © 1974, The Williams & Wilkins Co., Baltimore.)

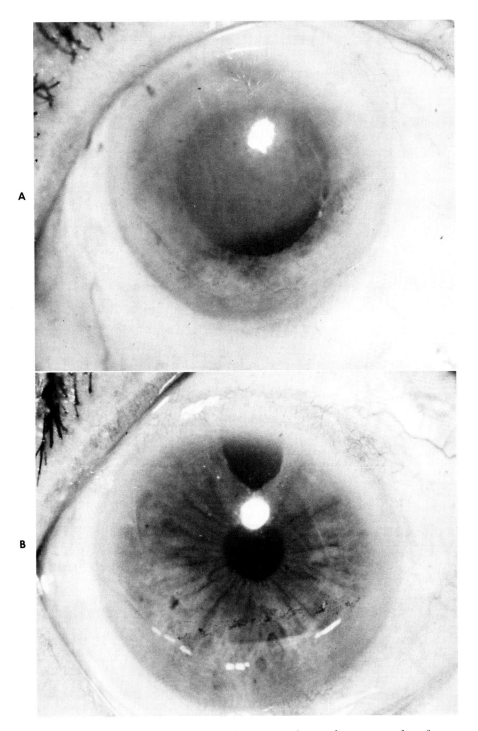

Fig. 29-5. A, Relatively flat detachment of Descemet's membrane extending from cataract incision to oblique line running from 3 to 7 o'clock. Bullous keratopathy and corneal opacification seen 11 weeks after surgery. Note clear cornea below. **B,** In same eye, perfectly clear cornea 6 weeks after second air injection into anterior chamber. Complete reattachment of Descemet's membrane. (From Sparks, G. M.: Arch. Ophthalmol. **78:**31-34, 1967.)

Descemet's membrane on making the incision. Corneal edema is present early and is usually mistaken for excessive Descemet's folds. If the cornea is cleared with glycerin or some other hyperosmotic agent, the diagnosis is usually made with the aid of the slit lamp. The presence of a sheet of Descemet's membrane curled inward or the detection of a separation of the membrane from the posterior stroma confined to the area of corneal edema is diagnostic.

If the condition remains undiagnosed for some time, a number of problems in differential diagnosis could appear. These problems would include the following postoperative conditions that cause a localized corneal edema restricted to the upper half of the cornea:

1. Epithelial downgrowth
2. Fibrous ingrowth
3. Vitreocorneal adherence
4. Malapproximation of the surgical wound
5. Shelved corneal incision

The first two are rarely present early, the third and fifth are diagnosed at the slit lamp examination, and the fourth tends to show progressive clearing as healing proceeds. Generally the diagnosis of detachment of Descemet's membrane is not difficult to make, and its differential diagnosis is rather simple.

PROGNOSIS

According to most reports, the prognosis for visual improvement is poor. Most minor detachments of Descemet's membrane cause no difficulty. The cornea overlying it may remain opaque or edematous, but this condition remains confined to the area of the detachment. When the detachment occurs over a wide area, the prognosis may be unfavorable, as emphasized by Scheie.[7] The condition may rapidly deteriorate from corneal edema to painful bullous keratopathy. In all three of his cases and in the two reported by Weve,[5] persistent corneal edema and bullous keratopathy resulted. Although this is the usual outcome, the final result may be more favorable. Sugar[8] reported three cases of extensive detachment, two of which cleared spontaneously; the third required surgical correction. Theodore[15] added another, and I can add one that had a favorable outcome without surgical intervention.

TREATMENT

Surgical correction of the detachment offers the only hope for a cure if the condition of the eye appears to be deteriorating. Descemet's membrane must be uncurled and kept in this position so that the corneal stroma is protected from aqueous. Sparks[9] utilized a simple technique that favorably influenced three cases. In cases where Descemet's membrane is curled inward a limbal stab wound is made, and the aqueous is removed. The anterior chamber is filled with air. The curled-up membrane is then manipulated back into place with a cyclodialysis spatula. In cases where Descemet's membrane is separated from the stroma but not curled inward, filling the anterior chamber with air may be sufficient to create reattachment (Fig. 29-5).

Since the patient may show an anatomic predisposition to detachment of Descemet's membrane, when the condition arises in one eye, it should be anticipated in the other eye. A deep scleral section in the second eye may prevent the complication. Since Descemet's membrane ends more peripherally than is usually anticipated at surgery, the incision should be made at least 2 mm posterior to the limbus. In addition, such an incision need not be made more than 150° in extent. If Descemet's membrane is seen to curl inward on making the incision, it is probably best to fill the anterior chamber with air and close the incision without proceeding with the cataract extraction. The latter may be performed at a subsequent date by employing a posterior incision.

Sugar[8] suggested reopening the central portion of the wound and unrolling the scroll of Descemet's membrane with an iris repositor. The edge of the membrane is then sutured to the cornea with a single suture. Air is placed in the anterior chamber, and the wound is resutured. This treatment was applied in a single case, and an excellent result was obtained.

In some cases it is possible to suture the detached edge of Descemet's membrane to the area of the surgical incision. The membrane is unfurled with air. A 10-0 nylon suture swaged onto a cutting edge needle is passed through the cornea about 1.5 mm inside the limbus, through the margin of Descemet's membrane, and out through the sclera 1.5 mm outside the limbus.

The suture is tied and left in situ. Additional suture bites may be taken.

If these simple methods fail, a penetrating keratoplasty should be performed. I have used a relatively large graft (8.5 mm donor, 8 mm recipient) in these cases. The results are usually good.

REFERENCES

1. Samuels, B.: Detachment of Descemet's membrane, Trans. Am. Ophthalmol. Soc. **26:**427-437, 1928.
2. Sallmann, L.: Ueber Verletzung der Membrana Deszemeti bei Glaukomoperationen, Verhandlung ophthalmologischen Gesellschaft in Wien, Dezember, 1924, Z. Augenheilk. **55:**200-202, 1925.
3. Böhm, F. M.: Cystenförmige Abhebung der Membrana Descemeti nach Cyclodialyse, Klin. Mbl. Augenheilk. **70:** 171-174, 1923.
4. Meller, J.: Ophthalmic surgery, ed. 6, New York, 1953, Blakiston Division of McGraw-Hill Book Co., p. 360.
5. Weve, H.: Ablsung der Membrana Descemeti nach Linsenextraktion, Nederl. T. Geneesk. **71**(2 Hälfte, Nr. 4): 398-400, 1927.
6. Wright, R. E.: Lectures on cataract. III. Anterior-segment and other complications in the postoperative period, Am. J. Ophthalmol. **20:**240-253, 1937.
7. Scheie, H. G.: Stripping of Descemet's membrane in cataract extraction, Trans. Am. Ophthalmol. Soc. **62:**140-152, 1964.
8. Sugar, H. S.: Prognosis in stripping of Descemet's membrane in cataract extraction, Am. J. Ophthalmol. **63:**140-143, 1967.
9. Sparks, G. M.: Descemetopexy. Surgical reattachment of stripped Descemet's membrane, Arch. Ophthalmol. **78:** 31-34, 1967.
10. Reese, A. B.: Discussion of Scheie, H. G.: Stripping of Descemet's membrane in cataract extraction, Trans. Am. Ophthalmol. Soc. **62:**151, 1964.
11. Monroe, W. D.: Gonioscopy after cataract extraction, South. Med. J. **64:**1122-1124, 1971.
12. Flaxel, J. T.: Histology of cataract extractions, Arch. Ophthalmol. **83:**436-444, 1970.
13. Bettman, J. W., Jr.: Pathology of complications of intraocular surgery, Am. J. Ophthalmol. **68:**1037-1050, 1969.
14. Hecht, S.: A method of estimating the extent of planar Descemet's membrane detachment. In Emery, J. M., and Paton, D., editors: Current concepts in cataract surgery. Selected Proceedings of the Third Biennial Cataract Surgical Congress, St. Louis, 1974, The C. V. Mosby Co., pp. 246-249.
15. Theodore, F. H.: Corneal complications after cataract surgery, Int. Ophthalmol. Clin. **4:**913-948, 1964.

CHAPTER 30

Retinal detachment in aphakia

The occurrence of a retinal detachment after cataract surgery is a serious complication. Not too long ago, such an event usually marked the termination of the visual life of the eye. Although the percentage of surgical reattachments of the retina has risen sharply during the past 20 years, a large percentage of these eyes are left with poorer vision than before the detachment occurred. Of those whose retinas are reattached, probably no more than 50% achieve better than 20/70 vision.

Because the inclusion of retinal detachment among the complications of cataract surgery implies acceptance of the cataract surgery as the direct cause of the detachment, I am stating at the outset that the relationship between the cataract surgery and the subsequent occurrence of the detachment is still largely unknown.

INCIDENCE OF RETINAL DETACHMENT IN APHAKIA

One has difficulty establishing the actual incidence of retinal detachment after cataract extraction (Table 30-1) because of the difficulty in obtaining long-term follow-up studies. Many aphakic patients die within a few years of their cataract surgery, and undoubtedly some of them would have developed a retinal detachment if they lived longer. In addition, some of these patients are lost to follow-up for other reasons. Nevertheless, it is probably reasonable to estimate that 1% to 3% of cataract extractions are followed by a retinal detachment. This percentage is compared to an incidence of retinal detachment of 0.005%[1] to 0.01%[2] among all patients.

In a study reported by Jaffe and co-workers,[12] the incidence of retinal detachment after a routine intracapsular cataract extraction was 1.74% in 2304 consecutive cases followed for at least 2 years, 6 months. This was compared to a rate of 0.62% after cataract extraction with intraocular lens implantation. The latter series included 650 consecutive cases, 86% intracapsular and 14% extracapsular cataract extractions. The lower rate in the implant series is directly related to case selection. For example, 18 of the 40 retinal detachments in the nonimplant series occurred in patients who were myopic (aphakic refractive error of +9.00 D or less) and young (less than 60 years of age).

The incidence of aphakia in any series of retinal detachments will vary from 7% to 40% (Table 30-2). This wide range occurs because of a tendency to refer aphakic retinal detachments to retinal centers, which therefore have more aphakic cases. In addition, more unfavorable cases are

Table 30-1. Incidence of retinal detachment in aphakia

Author	Year	Percent of retinal detachments after cataract extraction
Shapland[4]	1926-1929	2.2
Beach and McAdams[5]	1936	2
Knapp[6]	1936	1.2
Berens and Bogart[7]	1938	0.39
Schiff-Wertheimer[8]	1947	1.25
Sedan[8]	1947	1.35
Pasino and Santori[9]	1956-1966	2.76
Polychronakos[10]	1962	1.2
Scheie[11]	1973	2.2
Jaffe (personal series)	1975	1.8

Table 30-2. Incidence of aphakia among patients with retinal detachments

Author	Year	Percent of aphakia among retinal detachments
Shapland[4]	1933	7.6
Braley and Ostler[13]	1955	7
Schepens[14]	1951	22.7
Malbran and Dodds[15]	1964	15.2
Norton[16]	1963	32.8
Pasino and Santori[9]	1967	13.3
Knobloch and Cibis[17]	1965	33
Hawkins[18]	1974	33
Hagler[19]	1974	34
Norton[20]	1974	40

now referred for surgery, and a greater percentage of these occur in aphakic eyes.

A study[3] of the vitreous and peripheral retina in 200 nonmyopic aphakic eyes with a Goldman three-mirror lens revealed an incidence of retinal breaks in 9%. Retinal breaks were significantly more frequent in aphakic than in phakic eyes.

RELATIONSHIP OF CATARACT SURGERY TO THE SUBSEQUENT DEVELOPMENT OF A RETINAL DETACHMENT

There is probably some relationship between the cataract surgery and the retinal detachment in those cases where the detachment follows the cataract surgery by a relatively short interval and where the cataract surgery is marked by certain postoperative complications. However, many retinal detachment surgeons consider the predisposition to detachment to be a fundamental primary factor and the cataract surgery to be, perhaps, just a milestone along a degenerative trail. An intracapsular cataract extraction in the overwhelming majority of cases is probably a minimal trauma, but it may bear the same relationship to the subsequent development of a retinal detachment as a minor trauma to a phakic eye with myopia.

This view is strengthened by a consideration of patients with bilateral retinal detachments. In one eye the detachment may follow the cataract extraction, whereas in the other eye it may precede the cataract surgery. In some patients, cataract surgery is postponed in the second eye because of the development of a retinal detachment in the first eye after lens extraction. Despite this, a retinal detachment occurs in the phakic eye. In addition, some early or subclinical detachments (detachments too peripheral to cause a diminution of visual acuity and marked constriction of visual field) are present before the cataract surgery but are not recognized until the opaque lens is removed.

It is likely that except for very traumatic cataract extractions, the opposite eyes of patients who sustain a retinal detachment after cataract extraction show significant retinal degenerative changes that may predispose to a retinal detachment. As proposed by Schepens[14] about 25 years ago, there probably is a correlation between the disease process leading to cataract formation and that leading to peripheral retinal degeneration, thereby predisposing the patient to a retinal detachment when his cataract is removed. This accounts for the prevalent view that these are sick eyes and that probably both the lens and retina are diseased. Therefore it is probably not the trauma of the cataract extraction itself that causes the retinal detachment, but rather the aphakic state that exists after lens extraction that aggravates the preoperative retinal degeneration. One might then consider that these are abnormal eyes to begin with, and the condition is probably aggravated by the cataract extraction. As stated earlier, it is important to realize that the fellow eye will invariably show degenerative changes.

Most detachments occur within 6 months of cataract extraction. In the personal series of 1651 cataract extractions followed from 2 to 7 years there were 29 retinal detachments. The time of occurrence of these retinal detachments was as follows: 1 to 3 months, 17; 4 to 6 months, 2; 7 to 12 months, 3; 13 to 24 months, 4; 25 to 36 months, 2; 37 to 48 months, 1.

On a theoretical basis there are probably some valid reasons for the prevalence of retinal detachments in aphakic eyes.

The condition of aphakia

The extraction of the lens deprives the vitreous of its support at the level of the patellar fossa. An increase in the sagittal diameter of the vitreous cavity permits the vitreous to project partially into the anterior chamber and therefore to exert greater traction at the vitreous base or other foci of vitreoretinal attachments. The significance of this is clouded somewhat by the fact that the incidence of retinal detachment after extracapsular cataract extraction is no less than that after intracapsular extraction, in spite of providing the anterior vitreous with some support in the form of an intact posterior lens capsule. It is also possible that mechanical or chemical zonulysis alters somewhat the relationship between the vitreous and the ciliary body and retina at its base,[21] permitting greater traction in this region. Postoperative rupture of the anterior hyaloid membrane occurs in a relatively high percentage of cataract extractions.[22] The vitreous may become attached to the operative wound or the cornea. Subsequent fibroplastic changes may also contribute to increased traction on the retina in such cases.

Complications of the cataract surgery

Operative loss of formed vitreous is probably the most important complication of cataract surgery related to the pathogenesis of retinal detachment.[22] The multiple consequences of operative loss of vitreous have been considered on p. 255. The fibroplastic changes associated with this complication are well known. They cause marked distortion of the pupil, disruption of the wound with considerable postoperative astigmatism, intraocular inflammation, cystoid macular edema, and dense, fibroplastic bands of vitreous connecting the retina, on one hand, with the operative wound, on the other. These changes appear with greater virulence in younger patients. Many older patients have a partially liquefied vitreous, the disturbance of which is less serious. The loss of fluid vitreous is probably the least serious. Of course, any disruption of the vitreous is to be avoided, since those eyes with the most degenerated vitreous often show parallel changes in the retina.

Some support for operative loss of vitreous as a significant cause of subsequent retinal detachment is gathered by reviewing reports of several authors. Hughes and Owens[23] observed loss of vitreous in 13 of 30 cases (43%) with retinal detachment and aphakia. Of Bagley's[24] and Shapland's[25] cases, 20% had loss of vitreous. Schepens[14] reported eight cases of vitreous loss out of 72 cases (11%) of intracapsular cataract extraction followed by retinal detachments. In my personal series of 29 retinal detachments after cataract extraction referred to earlier, two patients had operative loss of vitreous, one had an aspiration of retrovitreal fluid because of a bulging vitreous, and one had a massive subchoroidal effusion. Although these series are admittedly small, the incidence of operative loss of vitreous among aphakic patients with detachment is considerably higher than what would be expected in any series of cataract extractions.

An intravitreal hemorrhage that follows a routine cataract extraction is a rare occurrence and may be associated with the subsequent development of a retinal detachment. It is difficult to determine cause and effect in such cases. The hemorrhage may cause the retinal detachment or it may be the result of a retinal tear. Malbran and Dodds[15] observed seven cases of early hemorrhage (3 to 15 days postoperatively) into the vitreous after uncomplicated cataract surgery that progressed to detachments. In four eyes the detachments occurred within a month of the cataract extraction. All seven eyes were myopic. In three eyes a careful examination of the fundus periphery was made preoperatively without finding any serious lesion that would contraindicate the lens extraction or justify prophylactic surgery.

We do not definitely know what role the intravitreal hemorrhage plays in the pathogenesis of a retinal detachment. Balazs[26] has postulated that the ferric ions from the blood latch on to the negatively charged hyaluronic acid to form insoluble hyaluronates. Hyaluronates favor vitreous retraction Schepens[27] has observed that when a sizable vitreous hemorrhage is present, the prognosis is less favorable and the danger of retinal detachment is increased because of a greater tendency to vitreous retraction. However, it is reemphasized that in some cases the hemorrhage may be the result of a retinal break and not the cause. Nonetheless, one must accept that when a routine cataract extraction is complicated by an intravitreal hemorrhage, and this in turn is followed by a retinal detachment, the cataract surgery is at least partly to blame for the detachment.

There has been a tendency to arbitrarily place a time limit on the interval after cataract surgery in determining whether the latter should be considered the cause of the retinal detachment. This probably makes little sense, except perhaps in those cases where an operative complication such as loss of vitreous or a postoperative complication such as an intravitreal hemorrhage leads to a retinal detachment within a short interval of time. However, the time span may not be as important as the degree of ocular aging at the time of cataract surgery. For example, it has been observed that retinal detachments are frequent after congenital cataract surgery, especially where multiple discissions have been performed. These detachments usually do not appear for many years after the lens surgery. The average elapsed time has been calculated by Cordes[28] at 22 years, Shapland[4] 24.6 years, and François[29] 27 years. There are as yet no long-term follow-up series of lens aspiration techniques.

PREDISPOSITION TO RETINAL DETACHMENT
Axial myopia

Axial myopia is frequently present in eyes with retinal detachments, whether aphakic or phakic. Schepens[13] found 37% myopic eyes in the aphakic detachments studied, whereas Malbran and Dodds[15] reported an incidence of 46%. Of the 29 retinal detachments in my recent series, nine patients had preexisting myopia (defined as an aphakic cataract spectacle prescription of 9.00 D spherical equivalent or less), and the strongest spectacle lens correction was 12.25 D. The incidence of myopia in this small series was 31%. That a myopic eye is predisposed to the development of a retinal detachment is well known. This can be proved by examining the opposite eye of myopic patients who have suffered a retinal detachment in the first eye after cataract surgery. In some, a retinal detachment will be found before cataract surgery; in others, the detachment occurs after the lens extraction; in still others, cataract surgery is not followed by detachment. Therefore it is risky to draw conclusions as to the role of the cataract surgery in causing the retinal detachments. However, a myopic eye is more predisposed to develop a retinal detachment after cataract extraction than an emmetropic or hypermetropic eye.

Retinal detachment present in the opposite eye

When a retinal detachment has occurred in one eye after cataract surgery, there is a much greater chance that it will occur in the second eye than if the cataract surgery in the first eye was not followed by a detachment. This is not surprising in view of the fact that the vitreoretinal degenerative changes associated with retinal detachments are often bilateral. It is likely that there is a greater risk of retinal detachment in an eye that suffered a retinal detachment while in the phakic state. This was found in four of the 29 retinal detachments in my recent series of 1651 cataract extractions.

Association of posterior cortical or subcapsular cataract, peripheral uveitis, open-angle glaucoma, and the age of the patient

That a certain type of cataract is found in those eyes that later go on to retinal detachment was emphasized by Schepens.[14] He observed a preponderance of posterior cortical cataracts sometimes associated with nuclear sclerosis in 71% of 62 eyes in his series of aphakic detachments. Nuclear sclerosis or senile wedge-shaped opacities were observed in only 21%. Eight percent showed some other type of lens opacity. He compared this with Kirby's[30] large series of 945 patients with cataracts but without retinal detachments in whom only 15% had posterior cortical cataracts, either alone or associated with other types of lenticular opacities. In Schepens' series the typical cataract showed a mixture of subcapsular opacities with scattered opacities in the posterior cortex. The subcapsular opacities began as apparent roughening of the affected area, which appeared irregular and iridescent. The changes spread from the posterior pole toward the equator of the lens. In some cases a mature cataract eventually developed.

The age of the patient may have some bearing on predisposition to development of retinal detachment. Many are in the presenile group. Malbran and Dodds[15] emphasized that a large number of detachments can be observed in patients under 50 years of age who have a posterior cortical or nuclear cataract. In their series, presenile cataracts were observed in 11 patients, all of whom suffered bilateral detachment with or without aphakia. It is unlikely that the detachment is the result of the greater traction required on the zonules in young patients, since many of them have fragile zonules. Moreover, the advent of enzymatic zonulysis does not seem to have lessened the tendency to detachment. As early as 1947, Schiff-Wertheimer and Sédan[8] stated that cataract surgical technique could not explain the frequency with which young aphakies subsequently developed retinal detachments. They pointed instead to a "pathological state of the peripheral choroid-retina or of the vitreous body." They quoted Sourdille as stressing the frequency with which equatorial or peripheral degenerations occur in eyes suffering from presenile cataracts.

Schepens[14] elaborated further on the factors that predispose to retinal detachment. Whereas only 8% of his aphakic detachment cases revealed a history of uveitis, 42% of those carefully examined with the slit lamp showed signs of inflammation. These signs included folds in Descemet's membrane, keratic precipitates, and flare and cells in the anterior chamber. Conceding that uveitis may result from a detachment, he was convinced after examining numerous aphakic and phakic eyes that in many instances the inflammatory process precedes the detachment and is probably an important etiologic factor in the disease. This seemed particularly likely when the inflammation is located near the ora serrata. In these cases the course is usually a protracted one, perhaps because of the poor vascularization in this area. What are the sequelae of such inflammation that ultimately lead to retinal detachment? Schepens included obliteration of the peripheral retinal vessels, thinning of the retina, formation of large retinal cysts, pigment proliferation in the choroid and retina, choroidal atrophy, dustlike opacities in the vitreous (more numerous in the extreme periphery), and vitreous retraction. He concluded that these changes create very favorable circumstances for the insidious development of a detachment, which may not become apparent for a long time after absorption of exudates in the ora region. They may also be the cause of other conditions often observed in these cases, such as posterior cortical cataracts and deep chamber glaucomas.

Some of these eyes exhibit a deep chamber glaucoma not unlike that seen in phakic patients with detachment, especially when there are lesions in the region of the ora serrata. This is not a very frequent occurrence, but when present, it should alert the ophthalmologist to the possible predisposition of such an eye to the development of a detachment after cataract surgery. Schepens[14] observed such an unexplained glaucoma in 9% of his aphakic detachment series and in 10% of another series of 49 cases with disseminated peripheral uveitis.

There are a variety of other situations where retinal detachment has been prone to follow cataract surgery. As mentioned previously, congenital cataract surgery has been followed by retinal detachment after a relatively long time interval with a strikingly high incidence. Doggart[31] established that an eye operated on for a congenital cataract has one chance in four of developing a detachment within 20 to 30 years. Whether this is attributable to the surgical techniques formerly employed or to an anatomic predisposition in these eyes is not yet known. Marfan's syndrome may be complicated by retinal detachment, with or without lens surgery. The association of atopic dermatitis and cataract has also shown a predisposition to the development of a detachment.

A special predisposing factor occurs in an eye that has already undergone a successful retinal detachment but in which a cataract requiring surgery has developed. In some eyes the cataract may in some unexplained way be related to the previous detachment or its surgery, since the lens opacity is unilateral. In other eyes the relationship is probably coincidental, since the cataracts are bilateral. In the great majority of cases the cataract surgery is not followed by a recurrent retinal detachment, although the surgery may be more complicated than a routine cataract extraction. These eyes may have uveitis associated with the retinal detachment. This may cause weakening of the lens capsule, posterior synechias, and adhesions between the posterior lens capsule and the anterior hyaloid membrane. Thus it is not surprising that Ackerman and co-workers[32] reported a high incidence of unplanned extracapsular cataract extractions (11 of 73 cases, or 15%) in such eyes. Nevertheless, of 73 cases, the retina was still attached in 70 eyes (96%) 6 months or longer after cataract surgery. Only three eyes (4%) suffered a redetachment, an incidence similar to that in eyes without a previous retinal detachment.

If one accepts that the predisposing factors to retinal detachments just described are valid, it becomes important to examine these eyes before the density of the cataract precludes it. If peripheral retinochoroidal lesions are associated with evidence of uveitis, deep-angle glaucoma, and myopia in a relatively young patient who has a posterior subcapsular or cortical cataract, there is strong reason to believe that such an eye will develop a retinal detachment some time after cataract surgery. These eyes should be examined at relatively short intervals after the cataract extraction, since treatment of suggestive lesions or the early recognition of subclinical retinal detachments may be possible. Binocular indirect ophthalmoscopy is indispensable in such examinations.

CLINICAL CHARACTERISTICS OF APHAKIC RETINAL DETACHMENTS
Retinal breaks

In spite of a frequent overlapping of morphologic characteristics in aphakic and phakic retinal detachments, there is sufficient clinical evidence to consider these as separate entities, particularly in regard to the location, shape, and number of retinal breaks.

The breaks in aphakic detachments are typically located near the ora, in contrast to the more typical equatorial predilection in phakic eyes. Schepens[14] compared 79 aphakic detachments and 143 phakic detachments as to the location of the breaks and reported the following:

	Aphakic	Phakic
Breaks at ora	66%	30%
Breaks at ora and equator	23%	23%
Breaks at equator	11%	47%

Malbran and Dodds[15] found retinal breaks in 75 of 81 surgically treated aphakic detachments. They found preequatorial breaks (ora serrata or its immediate vicinity) in 45% and equatorial breaks in 24%.

Norton[16] reached a similar conclusion, although he reported his results by noting the location of the most posterior retinal break in millimeters from the limbus. He found the following:

	10 mm or less	11 to 15 mm	16 mm or more
Aphakic (116 cases)	21%	60%	19%
Phakic (273 cases)	12%	52%	36%

His findings, although verifying that breaks in aphakic detachment frequently occur close to the ora, surprisingly reveal that 60% of the aphakic cases had their most posterior break at or near the equator.

Schepens and Bahn[33] studied the region of the ora serrata and found two characteristic types of retinal breaks. The first consisted of small dialyses or breaks parallel and closely related to the ora bays. Each dialysis occupied no more than one bay. The second consisted of breaks closely related to meridional folds of the ora. These folds were usually found over the teeth of the ora, seldom over its bays. They found meridional folds in 50%, a retinal break close to the posterior end of the fold in 26%, and one or several dialyses in 38%. Malbran and Dodds[15] likewise found dialyses of the ora serrata with greater frequency than breaks in the meridional folds. When retinal pathology predominated in the equatorial region, horseshoe-shaped breaks were those most frequently found.

Norton[16] found the following distribution of retinal breaks in his series of aphakic and phakic retinal detachments:

	Aphakic eyes (139)		Phakic eyes (285)	
	No.	%	No.	%
Superior temporal quadrant	78	56	184	65
Superior nasal quadrant	52	37	118	41
Inferior temporal quadrant	36	26	85	30
Inferior nasal quadrant	17	12	31	11
TOTAL	183		418	

These figures show a predilection for breaks to occur in the superior temporal quadrant in both groups and for a strikingly parallel distribution (1.5 to 1) between superior temporal and superior nasal breaks. Retinal breaks were found in the upper half of the retina about two and one half times more frequently than in the lower half. Hagler's[18] findings differed in that the most frequent site of retinal breaks in the aphakic eyes in his series was the upper nasal quadrant.

One of the more characteristic features of retinal breaks in aphakic eyes is their small size and the ease with which they may be overlooked during examination. This has been noted by many authors.[14,16,24,34] Norton[16] found small breaks in 92% of his aphakic cases where at least one break was discovered, in contrast to 67% of the phakic cases. He found no clear-cut break in 16% of his aphakic cases but in only 4% of his phakic cases. This is in conflict with Schepens'[14] figure of only 2.5% of aphakic detachments where no break was found. Norton explains this discrepancy by the differences in interpretation of the many suspicious areas one sees at the ora serrata in aphakic eyes. Such an area was classified as a break only if it was consistently identified and confirmed at surgery. In many aphakic eyes, he found breaks that were no larger than the caliber of a retinal vessel as it passes between the equator and the ora. Malbran and Dodds'[15] experience

lies closer to that of Schepens'. They found at least one break in 93% of their aphakic cases. However, Pasino and Santori[9] observed a retinal break in only 60% of their 44 aphakic retinal detachments, and this figure increased to 82% if only aphakias resulting from senile cataract extractions without surgical complications were considered.

These figures are all considerably higher than those reported by earlier investigators, before the current techniques of binocular indirect ophthalmoscopy with scleral depression and biomicroscopy with the Goldman three-mirror contact lens were introduced. Thus Bagley[24] found breaks in 38% of his cases and Shapland[25] in 48%. This is more dramatically shown by Schepens,[14] who with direct ophthalmoscopy found retinal breaks in only 33 of 79 (44%) aphakic eyes with detachments but with binocular indirect ophthalmoscopy found breaks in 77 of 79 eyes (97%).

Aphakic eyes with detachments show more retinal breaks than phakic eyes. Schepens[14] found

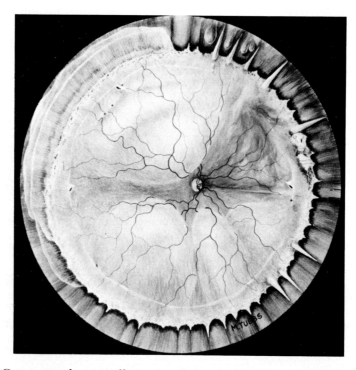

Fig. 30-1. Composite drawing illustrating features more commonly encountered in aphakic retinal detachment: (1) prominence of folds; (2) translucency (edema) of detached retina; (3) prominence of posterior vitreous base; (4) breaks, small along peripheral ridge; and (5) extension of detachment across ora serrata. (From Hawkins, W. R.: Aphakic retinal detachment: general considerations. In Emery, J. M., and Paton, D.: Current concepts in cataract surgery. Selected Proceedings of the Third Biennial Cataract Surgical Congress, St. Louis, 1974, The C. V. Mosby Co.)

an average of 4.45 breaks per eye in his aphakic cases. This, again, is somewhat refuted by Norton's[16] experiences. The latter found 183 breaks in 139 aphakic eyes and 418 breaks in 285 phakic eyes. However, Norton freely admits that because of the difficulty in absolutely identifying very small retinal breaks in aphakic eyes, he must have frequently missed some breaks.

There has been more written about the characteristics of retinal breaks in aphakic retinal detachments than about the detachment itself. Hawkins[18] has described the distinguishing appearance of aphakic retinal detachments (Figs. 30-1 and 30-2).

1. The detached retina shows high folds in aphakic eyes that he attributes to the marked collapse of the vitreous gel. When the retina detaches, there is no mechanical hindrance to prevent its forward movement.

2. The retinal detachment has a gray-colored, edematous appearance, and on occasion within the edematous areas there is a mosaic-like cobbling of the retinal surface. This latter phenomenon (retinal shagreen) has been found in animal studies[35] to be caused by extracellular fluid deposition within the inner nuclear layer. He found that the detached retina was more likely to become edematous when the vitreous is collapsed and liquefied.

3. A peripheral ridge may be noted approximately 2 to 3 mm posterior to the ora. Caused by traction of the posterior vitreous base, the ridge is often noted throughout the entire extent of the detached retina. Hawkins noted this ridge in 25 to 43 aphakic eyes with retinal detachments. The ridge tends to be more prominent in the superior fundus because of the gravity effect of the vitreous. These are less frequent in phakic eyes, since they do not tend to have prominent traction along the posterior vitreous base. He found this ridge in only five of 91 phakic eyes with retinal detachments.

4. There was extension of the retinal detachment into the pars plana, as described years ago

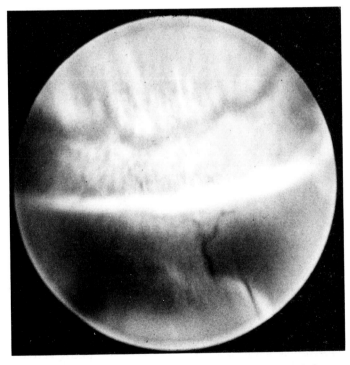

Fig. 30-2. Vitreous base traction ridge photographed with scleral depression. (From Hawkins, W. R.: Aphakic retinal detachment: general considerations. In Emery, J. M., and Paton, D.: Current concepts in cataract surgery. Selected Proceedings of the Third Biennial Cataract Surgical Congress, St. Louis, 1974, The C. V. Mosby Co.)

by Schepens,[36] in eight of the 43 aphakic eyes. This phenomenon occurs more frequently in aphakic eyes.[37]

Vitreous alterations

An important and ominous feature of detachment in aphakic eyes is a form of vitreous retraction that has been called massive vitreous retraction and massive preretinal organization.* In these eyes the retina never settles with bed rest. If the subretinal fluid is evacuated and fluid or air is injected into the vitreous, the retina flattens somewhat, but the folds retain their shape. Preretinal and intravitreal organization is usually present. In retinal detachments associated with massive vitreous retraction the identification of small peripheral breaks is often impossible because of the unevenness of the retina, the haziness of the media, and the loss of anatomic features.

It is difficult to compare the incidence of vitreous retraction in different series, since not all authors have broken this down according to the degree of involvement.

Schepens[14] found massive vitreous retraction in 24% of 88 aphakic eyes with detachments but in only 7.5% of 160 phakic eyes with detachments. Malbran and Dodds[15] found only 10% of their 81 aphakic patients with massive vitreous retraction and another 10% with the more developed types of fixed retinal folds. Norton[16] found 45% of his 139 aphakic eyes with evidence of vitreous traction and similar changes in 38% of 285 phakic eyes with detachments. He stated that the diagnosis of vitreous traction is extremely unsatisfactory and may be difficult for even the most skilled examiner. In his series, rolled edges of the breaks, stellate folds, meridional folds, equatorial folds, and rigid retinal folds were taken as evidence of vitreous traction.

It appears that aphakic patients under 50 years of age are more susceptible to massive vitreous

retraction than older aphakic patients. However, as shown by Schepens, younger phakic patients with detachments also show a greater tendency to massive vitreous retraction than those over 50 years of age. Therefore it is the age of the patient, perhaps the nature of his vitreous, and not the condition of aphakia, that predisposes to massive vitreous retraction.

Extent of detachment

Generally, when an aphakic retinal detachment is first recognized by the ophthalmologist, the detachment is more extensive than what is encountered when a phakic detachment is first examined. Norton[16] documented this by observing that 54% of his aphakic detachments at the time of initial examination had all four quadrants involved, whereas only 27% of the phakic detachments were this extensive. In addition, only 18% of the aphakic detachments presented without involvement of the macula, whereas 32% of the phakic detachments presented with the macula in place. Hagler[19] similarly found the macula in place in only 21% of eyes at the time of diagnosis of the retinal detachment. One would be tempted to explain this on the basis of what has been discussed previously, namely, that the fundus changes in aphakic detachments may be very subtle and may be missed at the time of the first examination. In addition, aphakic patients may be slower in recognizing the disturbance in vision and perhaps the detachment would be more extensive by the time it is first recognized. However, Norton[16] refutes this, since he found no difference in the estimated duration of the detachments in both groups, based on the history and findings at the time of the initial examination. This suggested to him that once the aphakic detachment becomes symptomatic, it is likely to spread much more rapidly than the phakic detachment.

Age of onset

Although, as has been noted earlier, patients with cataracts in the presenile group tend to develop a retinal detachment more frequently than older patients, aphakic eyes with detachments show the highest incidence in the 60-and-over age group, whereas in phakic eyes the highest incidence of detachment occurs in the 40- to 59-year age group.[16,24,34,38]

---

*Some controversy exists over the term "massive vitreous retraction," since an organization of vitreous occurs usually in association with an organization of preretinal tissue, which may arise from the retina but whose source of origin remains speculative. Although the terms "massive preretinal retraction" and "massive preretinal organization" have been employed more recently, understand that in this section "massive vitreous retraction" includes these other concepts.

TREATMENT OF APHAKIC RETINAL DETACHMENT

Cataract surgery or retinal detachment surgery—which one is operated on first when both coexist?

When a retinal detachment occurs in an eye with a cataract, there may be occasions when the surgeon must decide which should be operated on first—the detachment or the cataract. Since the decision is usually based on the degree of ophthalmoscopic visibility of the fundus, this question was a far greater problem before the introduction and popularization of the technique of binocular indirect ophthalmoscopy. A surgeon skilled in this method can visualize fundus details not seen by direct ophthalmoscopy, even in the presence of moderately advanced cataracts. Retinal detachment surgery is always given first priority over cataract surgery, except where visibility in unsatisfactory.

Norton's[16] impression is that uncomplicated iridectomy in phakic eyes creates little additional problem in the management of the detachment when better visualization of the retina is necessary. In contrast, lens extraction for better visualization of the detachment was frequently followed by massive vitreous retraction. Therefore if a retinal break cannot be found that adequately explains the detachment, detachment surgery is undertaken (even though lens opacities preclude proper visualization of the entire fundus), and all areas of detached retina are treated. Cryotherapy allows safe treatment of the entire circumference of the globe.

Prophylaxis

The predisposition of some eyes to bilateral retinal detachments justifies the application of prophylactic therapeutic measures, especially in the second eye. As discussed earlier, the incidence of retinal detachments after cataract extractions varies from 1% to 3%. If no operative complications or detachment occurred in the first eye, there is a greater risk of detachment in the second eye. The incidence is higher in those eyes showing a special predisposition to detachment (axial myopia, presenile cataracts, peripheral uveitis, congenital cataracts, Marfan's syndrome, and family history of retinal detachments with or without aphakia).

There is frequently an opportunity to satisfactorily examine the second eye, since the lens opacity is often not a serious obstacle. Because these eyes frequently show breaks without detachments or show subclinical retinal detachments, prophylactic therapy is possible.

The ophthalmologist occasionally encounters patients who will require a lens extraction in the future and have retinal breaks without detachment or with subclinical detachments. These patients lend themselves to prophylactic measures before cataract surgery in the first eye.

After a burst of initial enthusiasm regarding prophylactic treatment, a more conservative trend appears to be occurring in many areas. This is caused by the fact that many retinal breaks, such as small, round, peripheral holes, very often remain unchanged indefinitely. It is remarkable how often eye bank eyes show definite retinal breaks in eyes that produced no symptoms and do not have a retinal detachment. In addition, we now generally understand that prophylactic therapy may not be a benign procedure. Detachments at the site of the break may occur because of vitreous traction, as well as new breaks in other areas because of remote traction. Macular pucker is another unfortunate complication of prophylactic therapy.

Cryogenic applications may be safer for small, peripheral holes, since they are more amenable to this form of therapy, treatment is lighter, and fewer vitreous changes probably take place.

Most surgeons would treat the cataract patient prophylactically for the degenerated area, whereas they would not treat other patients with the same condition who have a clear lens. If the retina cannot be visualized preoperatively, a careful examination should be performed 2 months postoperatively and suspicious areas treated.

Advocates of the planned extracapsular cataract extraction often point to a lowered incidence of postoperative retinal detachment as a benefit of the procedure. However, the last study comparing the incidence of retinal detachment after an intracapsular extraction with that of an extracapsular extraction dates back more than 25 years. The incidence was equal at that time. Those who favor phacoemulsification also claim a lowered incidence of postoperative retinal detachment, but there have not been any age-matched series reported to support this view.

There is also some controversy over whether

the use of alpha-chymotrypsin during the lens extraction has any effect on the occurrence of retinal detachment. One very large series[11] reported no difference in incidence with or without this enzyme. Another study[39] claimed that the use of the enzyme in highly myopic eyes undergoing cataract extraction increased the likelihood of retinal detachment.

A prophylactic measure that has probably not received adequate attention is the use of routine finger counting visual fields by trained office personnel during routine examinations. This can probably reduce the frequency of macular involvement at the time of diagnosis of the detachment.

Surgical results in aphakic retinal detachments

No attempt will be made to discuss the surgical treatment of detachment of the retina, since it is beyond the scope of this book.

There has been a major improvement in the surgical results in aphakic retinal detachments during the last 20 years. The rate of surgical reattachment varied in earlier series from 7% to 35%. This prompted Woodruff,[40] to note in 1936 that retinal detachment after cataract extraction was for the most part incurable. When Schepens,[14] in 1951, in his series of 88 aphakic detachments reported a surgical cure rate of 56.5%, which improved to 72% when cases with fixed retinal folds and massive vitreous retraction were eliminated, the impact on ophthalmologists the world over was enormous. His surgical cure rate closely approximates his 80% rate in phakic retinal detachments.

Smith and Pierce,[41] in 1953, obtained 50% cures out of 84 aphakic eyes. If cases with fixed folds were excluded, the percentage rose to 66%. Malbran and Dodds,[15] in 1964, presented an impressive set of statistics. They obtained 51 cures in 81 cases (62%). In a group of aphakic retinal detachments where the cataract surgery was uneventful, they obtained a cure rate of 80% if cases of massive vitreous retraction, fixed folds, giant or very posterior breaks, and relapses from previous operations were eliminated from the series. In a group of 220 phakic eyes with detachment where the same types of cases were eliminated, their cure rate was 92%. Norton[16] presented an even more favorable set of statics in 1963 in

the largest series of aphakic detachments. In 139 aphakic eyes with detachments, including 30 cases that had undergone one or more previous detachment operations elsewhere, successful reattachment was achieved in 85%. In 285 phakic detachments, including 55 secondary cases, 89% were successfully reattached. Of the aphakic cases, 71% were reattached in one operation; 14% required a second operative procedure. Of the phakic cases, 81% were reattached in one operation; the remaining 8% required a second or third operation before they were reattached. When a difference of only 4% between aphakic detachments (considered almost incurable at one time) and phakic detachments can be obtained, it is a striking tribute to advances made in the methods of preoperative evaluation and surgical treatment.

An interesting point in this series is that Norton[16] achieved a reattachment rate of 87% in secondary cases (where one or more previous detachment operations were performed) and in 78% of secondary phakic detachments.

The markedly improved prognosis in aphakic retinal detachments is directly attributable to the following:

1. Improved methods of examination. Schepens deserves the major credit for the reintroduction in this country of the method of binocular indirect ophthalmoscopy with scleral depression; the technique of microscopy employing a multiple-mirrored lens such as that introduced by Goldman is an additional improvement in examination methods.

2. The Lindner technique of scleral resection, later modified by Shapland.[42] Scleral resection permits consistent diathermy to the choroid.

3. Scleral buckling procedures involving the use of synthetic materials, as introduced by Custodis[43] and modified by Schepens,[44] which effect apposition of the treated choroid and pigment epithelium to the retinal defects.

4. Photocoagulation as introduced by Meyer-Schwickerath.[45]

5. Cryogenic treatment, which apparently causes less scleral damage and a satisfactory chorioretinal adhesion.

Norton[16] provided the most comprehensive report of those factors that influenced the rate of reattachment and the final visual acuity.

The final visual acuity results were approximately the same in the aphakic and phakic groups: 50% with an acuity of 20/50 or better and 25% with visual acuity of 20/200 or less. Norton[20] recently revised this estimate in stating that no better than 50% of cured aphakic retinal detachment patients achieve better than 20/70 vision. The final visual acuity was related in both groups to vitreous traction, involvement of the macula, and the duration of the detachment. A higher rate of failure was noted in cases where the retina had shown fixed folds preoperatively, when the retina was totally detached, and when these were posteriorly located breaks or giant breaks.

Norton[16] found that a number of factors usually considered to influence the rate of reattachment had little or no effect on the final outcome. These included failure of previous detachment surgery in the fellow eye, vitreous hemorrhage, failure to find breaks in aphakic eyes, active uveitis, family history, multiple breaks, date of onset of the detachment after cataract surgery, the type of extraction (intracapsular or extracapsular), defects in the vitreous face, and the type of iridectomy (full sector or round pupil).

The surgical technique used in his series varied according to the preoperative appearance of the detachment, but usually scleral buckling operations were performed by using synthetic implants of polyethylene, silicone, or polyvinyl alcohol. The implants were made wide enough to cover the breaks and usually included an encircling component. The techniques, with some minor modifications, were similar to those previously reported by Schepens and co-workers.[44,46] Norton used an extensive resection combined with an encircling element to create a new ora to serve as a barrier against missed breaks. He attributed much of the success rate in the more difficult detachment cases to this method. Thus, although to close off all breaks is the object of the surgeon, "to wall off breaks is a useful compromise when the main objective cannot be achieved." The results of surgery using newer improved techniques have not been considered here.

The improvement in surgical techniques has been responsible for a permissive attitude in the postoperative care of the patient with a retinal detachment. Prolonged bed rest and hospitalization have given way to early ambulation and more rapid rehabilitation. Pulmonary, urologic, and cardiovascular complications are now rare during the immediate postoperative period.

This subject cannot be closed without paying a tribute to those tireless workers among the clinicians and research associates who have dedicated their lives to combating this problem. Ophthalmology owes a debt of gratitude to Custodis for innovations in treatment and to Schepens for methods of diagnosis and especially for teaching a vast group of retinal detachment surgeons who have assumed their responsibilities in various centers of the world.

Although the improvement in surgical results would naturally tend to create an air of optimism, the battle is far from ended. Problems such as massive vitreous retraction and giant breaks remain formidable obstacles. Intravitreal surgery will probably become more popularized and effective in the future in the surgical approach to these problems.

REFERENCES

1. Boehringer, H. R.: Statistisches zu Häufigkeit und Risiko der Netzhautablösung, Ophthalmologica **131**:331-334, 1956.
2. Rintelen, F.: Zur Frage der Häufigkeit der Netzhautablösung und zum Phänomen kompensatorisch-gerontologischer Processe, Ophthalmologica **143**:291-295, 1962.
3. Friedman, Z., Neumann, E., and Hyams, S.: Vitreous and peripheral retina in aphakia: a study of 200 nonmyopic aphakic eyes, Br. J. Ophthalmol. **57**:52-57, 1973.
4. Shapland, C. D.: Detachment of the retina in the aphakic eye, An. Inst. Barraquer **3**:420-448, 1962.
5. Beach, S. J., and McAdams, W. R.: Intracapsular extraction of cataract in the average practice. Report of one hundred cases in which Verhoeff's method was used, Arch. Ophthalmol. **15**:95-100, 1936.
6. Knapp, A.: Complications of the forceps intracapsular operation for cataract, based on an analysis of five hundred successful cases, Arch. Ophthalmol. **16**:770-775, 1936.
7. Berens, C., and Bogart, D.: Certain postoperative complications of cataract operations, with especial reference to a study of 1,004 operations, Am. J. Surg. **42**:39-61, 1938.
8. Schiff-Wertheimer, S., and Sédan, J.: Extraction totale du cristallin et décollement de la rétine, Ann. Oculist. **180**:513-520, 1947.
9. Pasino, L., and Santori, M.: Il distacco di retina dell'occhio afachico (analisi clinica di 44 casi), Ann. Ottal. **93**:497-518, 1967.

10. Polychronakos, D.: Clinical observations on 1,000 operations for cataract, Ophthalmologica **144**:375-384, 1962.
11. Scheie, H. G., Morse, P. H., and Aminlari, A.: Incidence of retinal detachment following cataract extraction, Arch. Ophthalmol. **89**:293-295, 1973.
12. Jaffe, N. S.: Results of intraocular lens implant surgery. The Third Binkhorst Medal Lecture, Am. J. Ophthalmol. **85**:13-23, 1978.
13. Braley, A. E., and Ostler, H. B.: Statistics on 100 cases of retinal detachment surgery, J. Iowa Med. Soc. **45**:473-476, 1955.
14. Schepens, C. L.: Retinal detachment and aphakia, Arch. Ophthalmol. **45**:1-17, 1951.
15. Malbran, E., and Dodds, R.: Retinal detachment and aphakia, Ophthalmologica **147**:343-384, 1964.
16. Norton, E. W. D.: Retinal detachment in aphakia, Trans. Am. Ophthalmol. Soc. **61**:770-789, 1963.
17. Knobloch, W. H., and Cibis, P. A.: Retinal detachment surgery with preserved human sclera, Am. J. Ophthalmol. **60**:191-204, 1965.
18. Hawkins, R. W.: Aphakic retinal detachment: General considerations. In Emery, J. M., and Paton, D., editors: Current concepts in cataract surgery. Selected Proceedings of the Third Biennial Cataract Surgical Congress, St. Louis, 1974, The C. V. Mosby Co., pp. 353-355.
19. Hagler, W. S.: Retinal detachment in the unilateral aphake. In Emery, J. M., and Paton, D., editors: Current concepts in cataract surgery. Selected Proceedings of the Third Biennial Cataract Surgical Congress, St. Louis, 1974, The C. V. Mosby Co., pp. 350-352.
20. Norton, E. W. D.: Discussion of retinal detachment. In Emery, J. M., and Paton, D., editors: Current concepts in cataract surgery. Selected Proceedings of the Third Biennial Cataract Surgical Congress, St. Louis, 1974, The C. V. Mosby Co., pp. 355-360.
21. Jaffe, N. S.: The vitreous in clinical ophthalmology, St. Louis, 1969, The C. V. Mosby Co., p. 111.
22. Jaffe, N. S., and Light, D. S.: Vitreous changes produced by cataract surgery: a study of 1,058 aphakic eyes, Arch. Ophthalmol. **76**:541-553, 1966.
23. Hughes, W. F., and Owens, W. C.: Extraction of senile cataract. A statistical comparison of various techniques and the importance of preoperative survey, Am. J. Ophthalmol. **28**:40-49, 1945.
24. Bagley, C. H.: Retinal detachment; survey of the etiology and results of treatment on phakics and aphakics, Am. J. Ophthalmol. **31**:285-298, 1948.
25. Shapland, C. D.: Retinal detachment in aphakia, Trans. Ophthalmol. Soc. U.K. **54**:176-196, 1934.
26. Balazs, E. A.: Physiology of the vitreous body. In Second Conference of the Retina Foundation, 1958; Schepens, C. L., editor: Importance of the vitreous body in retina surgery, St. Louis, 1960, The C. V. Mosby Co., pp. 29-48.
27. Schepens, C. L.: The preventive treatment of idiopathic and secondary retinal detachment. (Panel discussion) XVIII Concilium Ophthalmologicum Acta, Belgium, **1**: 1019-1027, 1958.
28. Cordes, F. C.: Failure in congenital cataract surgery: a study of 56 enucleated eyes, Ophthalmology (Rochester) **60**:345-367, 1956.
29. François, J.: Les cataractes congénitales, Paris, 1959, Masson & Cie., Editeurs, p. 780.
30. Kirby, D. B.: Pathogenesis of senile cataract, Arch. Ophthalmol. **8**:97-119, 1932.
31. Doggart, J. H.: The diagnosis and treatment of cataract in children, Med. Presse **224**:39-43, 1950.
32. Ackerman, A. L., Seelenfreund, M. H., Freeman, H. M., and Schepens, C. L.: Cataract extraction following retinal detachment surgery, Arch. Ophthalmol. **84**:41-44, 1970.
33. Schepens, C. L., and Bahn, G. C.: Examination of the ora serrata. Its importance in retinal detachment, Arch. Ophthalmol. **44**:677-690, 1950.
34. Hudson, J.: Late complications of aphakia, Trans. Ophthalmol. Soc. U.K. **81**:75-83, 1961.
35. Machemer, R.: Experimental retinal detachment in the owl monkey, Am. J. Ophthalmol. **66**:396-410, 1968.
36. Schepens, C. L.: Fundus changes caused by alterations of the vitreous body, Am. J. Ophthalmol. **39**:631-633, 1955.
37. Dobbie, F. G., and Phillips, C. I.: Detachment of ora serrata and pars ciliaris retinae, Arch. Ophthalmol. **68**:610-614, 1962.
38. Schepens, C. L., and Marden, D.: Data on the natural history of retinal detachment. I. Age and sex relationships, Arch. Ophthalmol. **66**:631-642, 1961.
39. Stein, R., Pinchas, A., and Treister, G.: Prevention of retinal detachment by a circumferential barrage prior to lens extraction in high myopic eyes, Ophthalmologica **165**:125-136, 1972.
40. Woodruff, H. W.: Management of complications in the operation for senile cataract, Am. J. Ophthalmol. **49**:146-150, 1936.
41. Smith, T. R., and Pierce, L. H.: Idiopathic detachment of the retina; analysis of results, Arch. Ophthalmol. **49**: 36-44, 1953.
42. Shapland, C. D.: Discussion on scleral resection and chemical coagulation operations for retinal detachment, Proc. R. Soc. Med. **44**:420-421, 1951.
43. Custodis, E.: Is the suturing of scleral implantations an advance in the surgery of retinal detachment? Ber. Deutsche Ophth. Ges. (Heidelberg) **58**:102-105, 1953.
44. Schepens, C. L.: Scleral buckling procedures, Ophthalmology (Rochester) **62**:206-218, 1958.
45. Meyer-Schwickerath, G.: Light coagulation. Translated by S. M. Drance, St. Louis, 1960, The C. V. Mosby Co.
46. Schepens, C. L., Okamura, I. D., Brockhurst, R. J., and Regan, C. D. J.: Scleral buckling procedures. V. Synthetic sutures and silicone implants, Arch. Ophthalmol. **64**:868-881, 1960.

CHAPTER 31

Behavioral disturbances

PREOPERATIVE PRIMING

The prevention of postoperative behavioral problems is mainly accomplished by the preoperative priming of the patient. Teamwork between surgeon and office personnel can place the patient in a favorable frame of mind so that he is able to face his impending surgery with a minimum of anxiety.

Surgeons should be forthright in making crystal clear why the surgery is necessary and what the goals are. They must inform patients that cataract surgery is not without risk but that because of progress made in recent years the overwhelming majority of patients achieve the anticipated result. Usually such directness will inspire confidence and set the stage for a meaningful patient-physician relationship.

Many patients dread the surgery because of a past surgical failure in a family member or a friend. The tales of prolonged bed rest, immobilization, wrist restraints, and binocular patches exaggerated by well-meaning acquaintances are enough to test even the hardiest of souls. Surgeons should be able to recite to patients in an organized manner the sequence of events that will confront them from the moment they enter the hospital admitting office. A medical report that includes the medications that are to be continued during the hospitalization of each patient should be obtained from the patient's personal physician. In most cases it is preferable, if only to relieve anxiety, to combine forces with the patient's internist during the hospital stay.

I inform the patient that although he is being admitted for an operation, he is not sick and will not require as much attention as others who are less fortunate. The implication is that demands made on an already overburdened nursing staff should be restricted to important matters. This will prevent some frustration for the patient if an unimportant request such as an extra napkin for meals is not responded to promptly. It is amazing how some patients will respond by disproportionate anxiety to the extent that they become totally incapable of cooperating. Introspective surgeons learn to beware of these individuals and alter their approach to meet the needs of the situation.

Because most cataract patients are old enough to recall tales of older methods of postoperative care of eye patients, surgeons can accomplish a great deal by informing patients that the better eye will remain open, that ambulation and bathroom privileges will be permited the day of surgery, that they may be permitted to watch television to pass the time, and that the hospital stay will be short. An outline of the routine after discharge from the hospital and the time for optical correction can only make the patient feel he is in capable hands. During all these discussions the surgeon must exhibit no tensions and anxieties, since the patient hangs on each word and manner of expression.

A capable, sympathetic, patient, and organized office assistant is invaluable in assuring that the patient's confidence in the surgeon is of the highest order. After my orientation of the patient is completed, I place him in the hands of one of my assistants who handles the details of admission and surgical scheduling. However, she does much more than that. She has become personally acquainted with the hospital personnel in the admitting office and in the operating room so that the patient, seated at the side of her desk, overhears a friendly, orderly conversation that inspires confidence and makes him feel that everything in his best interest is being done.

The office assistant discusses details such as the time to enter the hospital, the personal articles to take along, the surgical fee, insurance, and Medicare and, above all, creates an atmosphere of efficiency and the feeling that everyone in the office and hospital genuinely cares for the patient. The assistant is thoroughly versed in the routine of postoperative care and will not contradict statements made by the surgeon.

Hospital admission the afternoon before surgery is now routine in most areas of the country. Aside from the necessary routine physical examination and laboratory workup, it serves a valuable function. The patient becomes familar with his bed and its appurtenances. He meets the hospital personnel and feels pretty much at home by the day of surgery.

DURING THE SURGERY

A casual conversation with the patient as he is wheeled into the operating suite relaxes him. I prefer a lightly premedicated patient who has control of his sensorium. The soothing effect of music is beneficial. During the akinesia the patient is complimented profusely about his cooperation. If the preoperative priming has been successful, the patient will not be disturbed by the operating room and its apparatus. He has confidence in the surgeon and staff and will try to be a model patient. I insist on doing all the talking and making all requests of the nurses. The voice of the surgeon places the patient at ease.

Surgeons must alter routines according to personality and anticipated erratic patient behavior. They must learn to recognize unstable patients. Fortunately, the great majority of patients cooperate in a satisfactory manner. However, the rare "bad actor" severely tests the expertise of the surgeon. Such a patient starts complaining as soon as his stretcher reaches the operating suite. He cannot lie on his back, he cannot have anything on his face, he cannot breathe. His complaints increase and build to a resounding crescendo bordering on severe panic. He clenches his fists, grips the sides of the operating table, rolls his eyes, squeezes his eyelids, holds his breath, alternates between keeping himself rigid

and thrashing about on the table, and exhibits other signs of acute apprehension. In most instances if the procedure is delayed and the patient is encouraged by informing him that many people become frightened, he will calm down. I have found that meperidine (Demerol) given intravenously in amounts varying between 25 and 75 mg is very helpful in such a situation.

As the akinesia is begun, I immediately tell the patient that his behavior is superb and that I am grateful for his cooperation. After receiving such accolades, most patients do not dare complain. The patient is always relieved to hear after the retrobulbar injection that he has felt his last pain. During the surgery, all conversation directed at the patient is encouraging and optimistic.

POSTOPERATIVE PERIOD

At the conclusion of the surgery the patient is again complimented and told that he will be visited by his surgeon in a few hours. He is told that he may experience some postoperative pain for about 3 to 4 hours, which can be relieved by medication. If possible, the patient should be visited in his room before the surgeon leaves the hospital on the day of surgery. It greatly benefits him to hear again that the operation has gone well, and it is wise to state this aloud in front of any visitors. In this way, their anxiety is also relieved, and such relief will have a favorable effect on the patient.

The most serious psychiatric problems that complicate cataract surgery occur during the postoperative period. It has been almost traditional that patients undergoing cataract surgery suffer a high incidence of postoperative behavioral problems, including psychosis. However, these reactions have sharply declined in recent years. Evaluating reports on the incidence of behavior disturbances after cataract extraction in elderly patients is difficult. Most early reports (1900 to 1940) placed this figure at 3%. However, Linn and co-workers[1] found some degree of identifiably abnormal behavior during the period of hospitalization in 20 of 21 patients (95%). This wide discrepancy is based on the fact that if these patients are observed carefully over a 24-hour-period, disturbances in behavior will be observed that otherwise might have been missed. In addition, trained observers are able to detect minor alterations in mood. Unexpressed delusions or hallucinations can only be elicited by careful questioning.

There is no denying the fact that modern advances in the technique of cataract extraction—permitting early mobilization, uncovering one or even both eyes, and short hospital stay—have reduced the incidence of significant postoperative psychosis to a fraction of 1%.

Etiology of postoperative behavioral disturbances

Sensory deprivation. There is no simple explanation for the cause of postoperative behavioral disturbances. Stonecypher[2] has refuted the theory that psychoses after cataract extraction are caused by sensory deprivation. This theory supposedly received support from the discovery that a normal individual, suspended in a tank, alone, and in the dark, will have hallucinations. Therefore it was reasoned that an individual deprived of his sensory apparatus loses contact with the real world. He experiences difficulty telling reality from unconscious mental images. Thus, if both eyes of the recently operated cataract patient were covered, the night silence of the hospital would usher in the hallucinations of sensory deprivation. When one also considers that many elderly patients have small degenerative cerebral foci and therefore a declining sensorium, it was reasoned further that even minor sensory deprivations would be sufficient to decompensate their weakened apparatus.

When one examines closely the numerous factors responsible for postoperative behavioral disturbances and their often mutual interdependence, the theory of sensory deprivation seems to have little validity.

Senile psychosis. It appears far more likely that these postoperative disturbances represent an acute form of senile psychosis. The brains of such patients do not exhibit any characteristic changes when examined histologically. In addition, the response of these patients to psychotherapy points to the psychologic nature of the condition. The basic cause of this psychosis is psychologic stress. Stonecypher[2] has observed that the psychologic forces that cause senile psychoses parallel those which operate acutely in postoperative cataract patients.

If surgeons will acquaint themselves with the factors that comprise the etiology of most cases of senile psychosis, they cannot help but approach their elderly patients with greater understanding, sympathy, and gentleness, which will be amply rewarded by the sincere appreciation of these patients.

One cannot help but observe that the elderly, depressed patient has passed through an unending series of subtle frustrations. His retirement has made his life empty and lonely. He experiences a sense of purposelessness and uselessness. He notices a steady deterioration of his overall mental and physical acumen. He feels rejected by his children, who often live a great distance away; he is frequently saddened by the death of aquaintances; he is severely burdened by life on a retirement income. His retirement leaves him with excess time to dwell on his problems. He feels increasingly isolated. He reacts by developing defenses against threats that are largely imaginary. Whereas a stable individual can successfully combat these stresses, the individual whose personality is marked with defects will reaction with a pattern dictated by his basic personality. The surgeon will easily identify the hypochondriacal, the depressed, the suspicious, the paranoid, the flighty, and the rambling patient. When the stress becomes overwhelming, contact with reality ceases, and the senile psychosis becomes manifest.

In the comprehensive study made by Linn and his co-workers[1] on 21 consecutive patients undergoing cataract extraction, the following seven patterns of behavior disturbances were noted:

1. *Psychomotor disturbances (nine patients).* These included restlessness, attempts to climb over the side rails, tearing off the eye mask, and violence.
2. *Paranoid delusions (six patients).* Several interpreted their postoperative state as a form of punishment. Some thought they were in prison and insisted on being released.
3. *Somatic complaints (four patients).* One patient believed her eye had been enucleated, two had a severe hypochondriacal reaction, and one claimed he had not had a bowel movement for 3 months.
4. *Elation (four patients).* Elation was marked

by ravenous eating, high-spiritedness, talkativeness, and jocularity.

5. *Hallucinations (five patients).* Three had visual hallucinations, and two experienced auditory illusions.
6. *Disorientation (eight patients).* Because of spatial disorientation, the patients believed that they were somewhere else.
7. *Anxiety (two patients).* One feared his wife would no longer take care of him if the operation failed, and the other requested that the mask be removed so that she could see her husband.

Organic brain disease. Organic brain disease as an important factor in postoperative behavioral disturbances appears to be demonstrated in the work of Linn and co-workers.[1] This is supported by the puzzling finding that patients with senile cataract demonstrate abnormal electroencephalograms more frequently than other subjects of the same age group without cataracts. Strauss and co-workers,[3] after a carefully controlled study, have even concluded that cataract patients are subject to a specific degenerative process that concurrently strikes the cerebral cortex and the crystalline lens. They related this to the fact that these tissues have a common embryonal origin, the surface ectoderm. Others[4-7] have also emphasized the expression of a degenerative process affecting tissues of a common origin by relating the concurrence of cataracts and alopecia totalis.

Drugs. Weinstein and co-workers[8] established a diagnostic test based on the finding that patients with organic brain disease are prone to react to sedative medications with the development of disorientation and confusion, whereas patients without organic brain disease do not show these changes. The test is performed by injecting amobarbital sodium (Sodium Amytal) intravenously at a rate of 50 mg per minute until the patient shows marked nystagmus, dysarthria, drowsiness, and errors in counting backwards. He is then asked a series of questions to test orientation for place, time, person, and awareness of illness. In the patients studied by Linn and co-workers,[1] approximately 70% gave a positive response to the amobarbital test preoperatively. They found further that the most severe psychiatric disturbances occurred in patients who displayed both electroencephalographic abnormalities and a positive drug test prior to surgery.

Physical and psychologic stress of the surgery. Studies made in patients undergoing cataract surgery and in those of a similar age group not contemplating surgery are difficult to compare, since the anticipation of the surgery itself elicits a violent chain of stress reactions in many patients. The effect of the stress of the operation is emphasized when one compares the responses of patients to preoperative bandaging of both eyes as opposed to postoperative bandaging. Linn and co-workers[1] found that although preoperative bandaging aroused considerable anxiety in several of their patients, in no case did it result in psychotic phenomena like those observed postoperatively. The longer the eyes were covered, the greater the incidence and severity of behavior disturbance. Prior studies[9-13] have shown that the most frequent time of onset of postoperative delirium occurred on the second day in patients with both eyes bandaged.

Aside from bandaging both eyes, a rarely performed procedure today, other factors are also important. There are many psychologic and physical stresses associated with the operation and postoperative care. Uncertainty about the outcome is not as important a factor today as it was 20 years ago, but a history of surgical failure in the family or a neighbor is a real cause of anxiety. In some patients with a low pain threshold, small discomforts are grossly magnified. Limitation of mobility, side rails, constant admonishments about lying still, and numerous other restrictions provoke in many aged patients a desire to bolt from their restrictive prisons.

Although, as stated earlier, most of these traditional shackles have been lifted, stress anxiety is still a real problem. The surgeon must not lose sight of the fact that the patient has been bravely preparing for the surgery for weeks or months and that once it is over, his emotional reserve may be completely spent. Note how often then patients tremble, weep at the slightest provocation, move about feebly, and postoperatively appear to age before your eyes. This is the time for sympathetic understanding on the part of the surgeon.

From the preceding discussion one should understand the impossibility of pointing to a single etiologic factor in causing postoperative behavioral disturbances. The emotional aspect of aging is very complex. The degenerative processes in the cerebral cortex are difficult to evaluate. The impact of drugs on these patients is highly unpredictable. The effect of stress depends on the patient's emotional reserve, a parameter that defies careful estimation. Despite this reserve, one may safely say that all these factors are important, in varying degrees in different patients, and the surgeon would be well served by continued alertness to the impact of all of them.

Symptoms of postoperative behavioral disturbances

The two main psychiatric symptoms seen after cataract surgery in the aged are the depressive and the excited reactions. Depression may be extremely serious because it is difficult to treat in this group. These patients generally are more refractory to depth psychiatry. The excited reactions, although not as common as depression, include hallucinations of all sorts, hostility based on paranoid delusions, and elation with delusions of grandeur.

When one examines the behavior disturbances of these patients, one is struck by the impression that they appear to represent an attempt to deny illness, an observation made by Linn.[14] Male patients are often found looking for their clothes so that they can go to work or perform some other home routine. They may show a spatial disorientation when both eyes are covered. For example, when asked to describe his surroundings, a patient may describe his own bedroom. When asked why is he getting out of bed, he may answer that he is getting up to take his usual evening walk. Visual hallucinations are common, and through them the patient seems to deny that vision is absent. Weinstein and Kahn[15] have explained the paranoid and hypochondriacal reactions as expressions of an attempt to deny blindness and helplessness.

Prediction of postoperative behavioral disturbance

Ophthalmic surgeons do not require any special training in psychiatry to predict which patients are apt to become behavior problems during the postoperative period. With some experience in surgery they can readily perceive those behavior traits during the preoperative management that alert them to this problem.

Stonecypher[2] has summarized those factors in the makeup of an individual over 60 years of age that are likely to cause disturbing postoperative behavioral reactions.

The individual with a history of marginal social adjustment who drinks excessively, leaves home sporadically, and gets into fights frequently has been just barely managing to survive the stress of daily life. The sudden, additional burden of surgery may be more than he can bear.

Some patients appear excessively frail and helpless. If the patient has this attitude toward himself, he may succumb when faced with the ordeal of surgery.

If a patient has a long-standing history of disabling disease resulting in serious handicaps such as a colostomy, a prosthetic leg, or parkinsonism, he is acutely aware of his limited resources in combating additional burdens. The fear that his ability to cope with the problem of eye surgery will be inadequate makes him a prime candidate for disturbing postoperative behavior.

A patient who is a recent immigrant and who has a language barrier is less likely to feel safe in the hospital where he is unacquainted with the social customs of the strangers around him.

The patient who is already senile or who has a history of a prior psychotic episode while in a hospital is not likely to weather the postoperative period smoothly.

The effect of retirement on some patients has been discussed earlier. When it has produced numerous stresses such as lowered self-esteem, concern about declining health, financial worries, or loss of mental sharpness, the patient approaches cataract surgery with a depleted emotional reserve.

Prophylaxis

One should not adopt the attitude that nothing can be done about the patient who is a prime candidate for postoperative behavioral disturbances. If surgeons will take the time, they can often assess what is troubling the patient and adjust their standard postoperative routine according to the needs of the patient.

I have learned that a good deal can be accomplished by insisting that the patient verbalize his feelings about his attitude toward the impending surgery. It helps the patient to express his anxiety, especially when he is told that feeling tense and insecure about the operation is natural. At least he knows his surgeon is genuinely interested in him as a human being. I find it useful to drown the patient with compliments on his cooperation and his forthrightness in admitting his anxieties. He therefore seeks to win approval at every turn. It is important for surgeons to remember that this approach must not be abandoned once the surgery is over.

If the surgeon is convinced that trouble lurks, it seems reasonable to adopt measures that will reduce patient anxiety as much as possible. The patient may be hospitalized 2 days instead of 1 day before the surgery so that he will have more time to adjust to his surroundings. Having a member of the family or a close friend stay with the patient during the night is extremely useful. Nurses often frown on this, but I have made it clear that this will make their job easier. I make a special effort to admit the patient to the same room as another patient who is more stable and who is being prepared for surgery on the same day. Of course, doing so is not always possible.

Tranquilizers are of value during the hospitalization, and the preparation that has proved useful in the past may be prescribed. The use of a night light is also recommended. I often speak to the patient by telephone the evening before the surgery. This almost always eases the stress. If the patient habitually takes an alcoholic beverage in the evening, I see no reason to discontinue this practice while in the hospital. I avoid barbiturates. If used, a test dose should be prescribed the night before the surgery. Chloral hydrate is useful at bedtime along with whiskey.

Treatment

If, despite the prophylactic measures just outlined, the patient exhibits postoperative disturbed behavior, the surgeon should attempt to communicate with him and carefully evaluate his conversation. Side rails may be removed, but constant attendance is mandatory. If private duty nurses are in attendance, it is imperative that they understand the value of kindness, encouragement, and optimistic words. They must not be rigid in their restrictions. They must work in harmony with the family representative or friend who also is in the patient's room. Since many nurses are set in their ways, the surgeon should privately question the family or friend as to whether the relationship is amicable. A well-

meaning but dictatorial nurse can do more harm than good in this situation. The surgeon should not tolerate a tense interpersonal situation to persist, even if it means changing the nurse. The patient should be permitted to sit in a chair a good part of the day. The availability of a television set and a radio is important. A surplus of conversation is better than silence.

If the hospitalization routine appears to be affecting the patient adversely, early discharge may be helpful, provided that there is a trustworthy individual at home.

The drug treatment of the postoperative anxiety state is very helpful. Antianxiety agents produce mild sedation in doses unlikely to cause soporific effects or to adversely affect the clarity of consciousness and the quality of psychomotor performance. Particularly useful in this group are the following agents:

1. Chlordiazepoxide hydrochloride (Librium), 5 to 10 mg three or four times daily
2. Meprobamate (Equanil, Miltown), 400 mg three or four times daily
3. Diazepam (Valium), 4 to 40 mg daily in divided doses

The phenothiazines are also useful, since they are well tolerated by old patients and cause much less confusion than the usual sedatives. They are as follows:

1. Promazine hydrochloride (Sparine), 50 mg
2. Prochlorperazine dimaleate (Compazine), 5 mg
3. Thioridazine hydrochloride (Mellaril), 50 mg

They may be given orally or intramuscularly. If the patient appears very disturbed, it is best to start with the intramuscular route and change to oral administration every 3 to 4 hours when behavior improves. When using these drugs, one must be prepared for hypotensive and parkinsonian reactions. If the latter occurs, medication may be continued along with trihexyphenidyl hydrochloride (Artane Hydrochloride) or benztropine mesylate (Cogentin Methanesulfonate) in 2 mg doses with each dose of phenothiazine.

If depression becomes severe, several antidepressant drugs are available. Since hypotensive reactions are common side effects of this medication, they are best prescribed by the family physician or psychiatric consultant. If they are not available, amitriptyline hydrochloride (Elavil Hydrochloride) or imipramine hydrochloride (Tofranil) may be prescribed in divided doses totaling 100 to 150 mg per day. They may cause drowsiness and dryness of the mouth, but if the depression is overcome, these are minor side effects, which need not cause discontinuance of the drug. Continuing the medication for several weeks may be necessary.

Despite the availability of effective medications, the surgeon would be wise to consider their careful use in the senile or presenile patient. Overdosage or prolonged use is often counterproductive. It may take weeks or months for these patients to recover from this excess.

Surgeons should take pride in their ability to prevent postoperative behavioral disturbances and to treat them when they occur. Success in this area is truly the stamp of the well-rounded surgeon.

REFERENCES

1. Linn, L., Kahn, R. L., Coles, R., Cohen, J., Marshall, D., and Weinstein, E. A.: Patterns of behavior following cataract extraction, Am. J. Psychiatry **110**:281-289, 1953.
2. Stonecypher, D. D., Jr.: The cause and prevention of postoperative psychoses in the elderly, Am. J. Ophthalmol. **55**:605-610, 1963.
3. Strauss, H., Linn, L., and Ostrow, M.: Electroencephalographic and neuropsychiatric observations in patients with senile cataract, Mschr. Psychiatr. Neurol. **130**:321-327, 1955.
4. Brunsting, L. A., Reed, W. B., and Bair, H. L.: Occurrence of cataracts and keratoconus with atopic dermatitis, Arch. Dermatol. **72**:237-241, 1955.
5. Muller, S. A., and Brunsting, L. A.: Cataracts in alopecia areata: report of five cases, Arch. Dermatol. **88**:202-206, 1963.
6. Muller, S. A., and Winkelmann, R. K.: Alopecia areata: evaluation of 736 patients, Arch. Dermatol. **88**:290-297, 1963.
7. Winkelmann, R. K., Perry, H. O., Achor, R. W., and Kirby, T. J.: Cutaneous syndromes produced as side effects of triparanol therapy, Arch. Dermatol. **87**:372-377, 1963.
8. Weinstein, E. A., Kahn, R. L., Sugarman, L. A., and Linn, L.: The diagnostic use of amobarbital sodium ("Amytal Sodium") in organic brain disease, Am. J. Psychiatry **109**:889-894, 1953.
9. Boyd, D. A., Jr., and Norris, M. A.: Delirium associated with cataract extraction, J. Ind. Med. Assoc. **34**:130-135, 1941.
10. Brownell, M. E.: Cataract deliriums: a complete report of the cases of cataract delirium occurring in the ophthalmologic clinic of the University of Michigan between the years 1904 and 1917, J. Mich. Med. Soc. **16**:283-286, 1917.
11. Gat, L., and Orban, L.: Nach Staroperation auftretende Delirien, Ophthalmologica **112**:335-343, 1946.
12. Posey, W. C.: Mental disturbances after operations upon the eye, Ophthalmol. Rev. **19**:235-236, 1900.
13. Thomas, F. C.: Delirium following cataract operations, Ky. Med J. **24**:134-143, 1926.
14. Linn, L.: Psychiatric reactions complicating cataract surgery, Int. Ophthalmol. Clin. **5**:143-154, 1965.
15. Weinstein, E. A., and Kahn, R. L.: Denial of illness: symbolic and physiological aspects, Springfield, Ill., 1955, Charles C Thomas, Publisher (Am. Lecture Series. No. 249).

Index

Italicized page numbers indicate illustrations.

This book is to be returned on or before
the last date stamped below.